Science of Flexibility

Third Edition

Michael J. Alter, MS

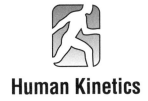

Human Kinetics

Library of Congress Cataloging-in-Publication Data

Alter, Michael J., 1952-
  Science of flexibility / Michael J. Alter.-- 3rd ed.
    p. cm.
Includes bibliographical references and index.
  ISBN 0-7360-4898-7
  1. Stretch (Physiology) 2. Joints--Range of motion. I. Title.
  QP310.S77A45 2004
  612.7'6--dc22

                              2003026043

ISBN-10: 0-7360-4898-7
ISBN-13: 978-0-7360-4898-9

Acquisitions Editor: Michael S. Bahrke, PhD; **Developmental Editor:** Anne Rogers; **Assistant Editor:** Sandra Merz Bott; **Copyeditor:** Ozzievelt Owens; **Proofreader:** Red Inc.; **Permission Manager:** Dalene Reeder; **Graphic Designer:** Fred Starbird; **Graphic Artist:** Dawn Sills; **Photo Manager:** Kareema McLendon; **Cover Designer:** Keith Blomberg; **Photographer (cover):** Al Bello/Getty Images; **Art Manager:** Kelly Hendren; **Illustrators:** Argosy, Mic Greenberg, Beth Young, Jennifer Delmotte, Michael Richardson, and Keith Blomberg; **Printer:** Sheridan Books

Printed in the United States of America   10   9   8   7   6

The paper in this book is certified under a sustainable forestry program.

Human Kinetics
Web site: www.HumanKinetics.com

United States: Human Kinetics
P.O. Box 5076
Champaign, IL 61825-5076
800-747-4457
e-mail: humank@hkusa.com

Canada: Human Kinetics
475 Devonshire Road, Unit 100
Windsor, ON N8Y 2L5
800-465-7301 (in Canada only)
e-mail: info@hkcanada.com

Europe: Human Kinetics
107 Bradford Road
Stanningley
Leeds LS28 6AT, United Kingdom
+44 (0)113 255 5665
e-mail: hk@hkeurope.com

Australia: Human Kinetics
57A Price Avenue
Lower Mitcham, South Australia 5062
08 8372 0999
e-mail: info@hkaustralia.com

New Zealand: Human Kinetics
P.O. Box 80
Torrens Park, South Australia 5062
0800 222 062
e-mail: info@hknewzealand.com

Blessed are You, L-rd our G-d, King of the universe,
who has formed man in wisdom and created
within him holes and holes[1] and spaces and spaces.[2]
It is revealed and known before your glorious throne
that if but one of them were to be closed
when it should be opened, or one of them should be opened
when it should be closed, it would be impossible to exist
even for a short while. Blessed are You L-rd,
who heals all flesh and performs wonders.

—A loose translation of the
traditional Jewish morning blessings

[1]Openings or orifices.
[2]Cavities, ducts, or tubes.

To Rainer Martens

Author,

Educator,

Visionary

Contents

Preface   viii

Acknowledgments   ix

Credits   x

Unit 1   Overview: Basic Sciences Related to Flexibility   1

Chapter 1   Modern Overview of Flexibility and Stretching   3

Defining Flexibility 3

Differences Among Flexibility, Hypermobility, Joint Laxity, and Joint Instability 3

Nature of Flexibility 4

Flexibility-Training Program 5

Benefits of a Flexibility-Training Program 6

Summary 14

Chapter 2   Topics in Osteology and Arthrology   15

Classifications of Study 15

Classification of Joints and Their Influence on Motion 15

Types of Motion 16

Relationship Between Bone Growth and Flexibility 17

Wolff's Law 18

Close-Packed Position and Its Relation to Flexibility 18

Loose-Packed Position and Its Relation to Flexibility 18

Summary 18

Chapter 3   Contractile Components of Muscle: Limiting Factors of Flexibility   19

General Overview of Skeletal Muscles 19

Composition of Myofibrils and Their Constituents 19

Regions of the Sarcomere 20

Ultrastructure of the Connecting, or Gap Filament: Titin 20

Sarcomere Structural Bridges 24

Theory of Contraction 25

Theory of Muscular Relaxation 25

Theoretical Limit of Muscular Elongation 27

Modifying the "Classic" Sliding Filament Model . 27

Additional Limitations to Range of Motion . . . 27

Effects of Immobilization 31

Mechanism of Passive Stretch on Myofibrillogenesis 33

Proposed Methods of Modulating Gene Expression via Stretching 33

Summary 35

Chapter 4   Connective Tissue: A Limiting Factor of Flexibility   36

Collagen 36

Ultrastructure of Collagen 36

Elastic Tissue 41

Relationship Between Collagenous and Elastic Fibers 44

Structures Composed of Connective Tissue . . . 44

Effects of Immobilization on Connective Tissue . 50

Metabolic and Nutritional Influences on Connective Tissue 51

Summary 52

Chapter 5   Mechanical and Dynamic Properties of Soft Tissues   53

Terminology 53

Soft Tissues 58

Muscle 62

Vascular Tissue 65

Peripheral Nerves 67

Factors Affecting the Mechanical Properties of Connective Tissues, Muscles, and Nerves . . 71

Need for Additional Research 71

Summary 71

Unit 2   Clinical Considerations   73

Chapter 6   Neuroscience of Flexibility   75

Sensory Receptors Related to Stretching 75

Reflexes and Other Spinal Neural Circuits 81

Coactivation/Cocontraction 82

Plasticity of the Spinal Cord Neural Circuits . . . 83

Neurological and Other Factors of
Flexibility Training 86
Summary 87

Chapter 7   Hypermobility of the Joint   88

Terminology 88
Assessment of Joint Hypermobility 88
Determining Factors of Hypermobility 89
Consequences of Hypermobility 90
General Management of Hypermobility 91
Inherited Syndromes 92
Research Perspectives in Heritable Disorders of
Connective Tissue 92
Additional Issues 93
Contortionism 93
Summary 96

Chapter 8   Relaxation   97

Defining Relaxation 97
Measuring Relaxation 97
Methodologies of Facilitating Muscular Relaxation 98
Summary 107

**Chapter 9   Muscular Injury and Soreness:
Etiology and Consequences   108**

Damaged or Torn Muscle Hypothesis 108
Damaged Connective Tissue Hypothesis 110
Hypothesis of Metabolic Accumulation or
Osmotic Pressure and Swelling 110
Lactic Acid Accumulation Hypothesis 110
Hypothesis of Localized Spasm of Motor Units . . 110
Predisposing Factors of Delayed-Onset Muscle
Soreness 111
Trauma and Overload Injury to the Musculature
and Connective Tissues 114
Medical Management of Acute Soft-Tissue
Injuries 115
Effects of Mechanical Stress on Elasticity and
Strength of Collagen in Scar Tissue 116
Summary 117

Chapter 10   Special Factors in Flexibility   118

Children and Flexibility Development 118
Gender Differences in Flexibility 120
Body Build and Flexibility 121
Racial Differences in Flexibility 124
Genetics and Flexibility 124

Dominant Laterality and Flexibility 125
Warming Up and Cooling Down 126
Strength Training and Flexibility 128
Circadian Variations and Flexibility 130
Summary 133

**Chapter 11   Social Facilitation and
Psychology in Developing Flexibility   134**

Effects of an Audience on Developing Flexibility
Through Stretching 134
Theoretical Aspects of Mental Training 135
Cybernetic Stretch 135
Ideokinetic Imagery 136
Psychosomatic Factors 137
Psychology of Compliance in Flexibility Training,
Injury Prevention, and Rehabilitation
Programs 138
Summary 142

Unit 3   Principles of Stretching   143

Chapter 12   Stretching Concepts   145

Homeostasis 145
Overstretching Principle 145
Flexibility-Training Methods 145
Retention of Flexibility 145
Requisite Knowledge for Stretching 147
Potential Factors Influencing Flexibility (ROM) . 147
Additional Principles of Stretching 148
Summary 156

Chapter 13   Types and Varieties of Stretching   157

Traditional Classifications of Stretching 157
Additional Classifications 161
Proprioceptive Neuromuscular Facilitation . . . 165
Additional Stretching Techniques 173
Mobilization 174
Manipulation and Chiropractic Adjustment . . . 174
Traction 177
Nontraditional Stretching Devices 179
Summary 181

**Chapter 14   Controversy Over Stretching
and Controversial Stretches   182**

Flexibility Continuum 182
X-Rated Exercises 187

No Absolute "No-Nos" 203

Summary 203

Chapter 15   Stretching and Special Populations   204

Flexibility and the Geriatric Population 204

Flexibility and Pregnancy 209

Flexibility and People With Physical Disabilities . . 210

Summary 211

Unit 4   Anatomical (or Regional) Aspects of Flexibility   213

Chapter 16   Anatomy and Flexibility of the Lower Extremity and Pelvic Girdle   215

The Foot and Toes 215

The Ankle Joint 216

The Lower Leg 218

The Knee Joint 220

The Upper Leg 221

The Pelvic Region 226

The Hip Joint 227

Summary 231

Chapter 17   Anatomy and Flexibility of the Vertebral Column   232

Gross Anatomy of the Vertebral Column 232

Function of the Vertebral Column 233

The Vertebrae 233

The Intervertebral Disks 234

The Vertebral Ligaments 236

Limits on Range of Motion of the Thoracic-Lumbar Region 238

Interrelationship of Stretching the Lower Back, Pelvis, and Hamstrings 239

The Cervical Vertebrae 243

Movements of the Cervical Region 243

Summary 245

Chapter 18   Anatomy and Flexibility of the Upper Extremity   246

The Shoulder Girdle and Arm 246

The Elbow Joint and Forearm Region 251

The Wrist Joint 252

Summary 253

Unit 5   Specific Disciplines   255

Chapter 19   Functional Aspects of Stretching and Flexibility   257

Aesthetic Aspect of Skills 257

Biomechanical Aspect of Skills: ROM 257

Additional Impediments 260

Jogging, Running, and Sprinting 260

Swimming and Water Polo 263

Throwing and Projecting 266

Wrestling 269

Weight Lifting, Power Lifting, and Bodybuilding 269

Rib Cage Flexibility, Performance, and Respiration 272

Springboard and Platform Diving 273

Golf 274

Ballet and Other Forms of Dance 277

Musicians 279

Summary 282

Appendix   283

References   299

Author Index   342

Subject Index   348

Preface

Historically, in the "Big Three" of exercise—cardiovascular fitness, muscular strength, and flexibility training—flexibility training has always assumed the role of Cinderella. For many years public attention to aerobic fitness as it relates to wellness and quality of life has been growing. Increasing information on the relationship between cardiovascular fitness, longevity, and quality of life has facilitated the boom in this area. The allure of muscular strength and power has existed since antiquity. Allusions to muscular strength are found in the Bible (Samson), ancient mythology (Hercules), and contemporary popular journals and movies (Arnold Schwarzenegger).

Knowledge regarding flexibility and stretching is conspicuously lacking compared with what is known about the advantageous functioning and optimal enhancement of the cardiovascular and muscular systems. Nonetheless, although the topics of flexibility and stretching has yet to receive the exposure, publicity, research time, and research dollars of other disciplines, an explosion in knowledge of flexibility and stretching has, in fact, occurred. Furthermore, as the present population ages, more people are beginning to appreciate the rewards of stretching. Flexibility and stretching are promoted as a possible means to offset age-related stiffness, reduce the risk of injury to the lower back, improve body posture and symmetry, enhance relaxation, relieve pain, augment physical fitness, and optimize functional movement in daily life. In sports, the beneficial claims of stretching include improved flexibility, improved muscle and athletic performance, improved running economy, prevention of injuries, reduction of the severity of injuries, possibly decreased delayed-onset muscle soreness, and promotion of healing during rehabilitation. These claims and other topics are examined throughout this text.

Many professionals are concerned about the limitations of flexibility and techniques for the optimal development of it. This book is written primarily for those professionals, to provide them with an up-to-date, comprehensive survey and critical view of knowledge on flexibility, including the factors that affect the quality and extent of it and range of motion. In the 15 years since the first edition, researchers have vastly expanded our understanding of the human body with novel approaches, concepts, and techniques. Quantum leaps in technology, such as the Human Genome Project and various imaging devices, have also contributed to our growing body of knowledge. Because science is tentative, research in basic and clinical sciences has disproved, substantiated, and explained many theories and exercise procedures from a variety of disciplines.

This third edition of *Science of Flexibility* expands the scope of its predecessors. The content has been enhanced and updated. Many of the figures from the second edition have been redrawn or replaced with photographs, older or poorer quality illustrations and tables were deleted, and a number of new figures have been added.

I have also reorganized and revised many of the chapters, substantially increasing the total textual content. In particular, chapter 19 includes golf, diving, dance, and physical movement required in producing music. In addition, the third edition includes an appendix, several new tables, and a number of special elements. The number of references has been expanded from about 1400 in the previous to about 2100 even though several hundred older references were deleted.

This book is an overview and therefore has its limitations. Entire books and journals are devoted to some of the individual concepts you will find in this survey. Furthermore, (repeating that science is tentative), scientists are continually expanding the knowledge of the body's workings. Therefore, all professionals must keep abreast of new information from various sources.

I hope the third edition of *Science of Flexibility* contributes to your appreciation of the capabilities of the human body and understanding of the subject of flexibility and its relationship to the body's optimal development.

Acknowledgments

This third edition of *Science of Flexibility* was made possible through the efforts of Michael S. Bahrke, PhD, (Acquisitions Editor for Human Kinetics, Scientific, Technical, and Medical Division), who proposed the writing of this third edition. As his predecessor, he facilitated the production of a more up-to-date text with additional educational material enhancing the previous editions.

I also wish to recognize the contribution of Anne Rogers, who is the edition's developmental editor. Her responsibility included coordination, direction and management of the production schedule. From our first correspondence in April 2003, Anne was encouraging and extremely helpful.

Many thanks to my "external reviewers." In particular, I wish to extend my gratitude to Marjorie Moore, PhD.

Many of her recommendations were incorporated into this new edition, resulting in an improved, "better read" text.

I also wish to thank the copy editor, Ozzievelt Owens, who enhanced the readability and clarity of the text.

Last, I wish to acknowledge the efforts of Sandra Merz Bott, assistance editor; production manager, Casey Rhodes; graphic artist, Dawn Sills; cover designer, Keith Blomberg; illustrators, Argosy, Mic Greenberg, Beth Young, Jennifer Delmotte, Michael Richardson, and Keith Blomberg; and all the other members of the Human Kinetics staff for their helpfulness throughout the production of this text.

Credits

Table 2.1 Reprinted by permission, from M.J. Alter, 1996, *Science of flexibility*, 2nd ed. (Champaign, IL: Human Kinetics), 15.

Figure 2.1 Reprinted by permission, from J.E. Donnelly, 1990, *Living anatomy*, 2nd ed. (Champaign, IL: Human Kinetics), 7-8.

Figure 3.1, 3.2a-c, and 3.4 Reprinted, by permission, from G.H. Pollack, 1990, *Muscles & molecules* (Seattle, Washington: Ebner & Sons), 81, 70, 71, 72, 152.

Figure 3.3 Reprinted, by permission, from L. Tskhovrebova and J. Trinick, 2000, *Elastic filaments of the cell*, edited by H.L. Granzier and G.H. Pollack (New York: Plenum), 171.

Figure 3.5 Reprinted, by permission, from A.M. Gordon, A.F. Huxley, and F.J. Julian, 1966, "The variation in isometric tension with sarcomere length in vertebrate muscle fibres," *Journal of Physiology (London)* 184(1), 185-186. Copyright Cambridge University Press.

Figure 3.6 Reprinted, by permission, from K. Wang, R. McCarter, J. Wright, J. Beverly, and R. Ramirez-Mitchell, 1993, "Viscoelasticity of the sarcomere matrix of skeletal muscles. The titin-myosin composite filament is a dual-stage molecular spring," *Biophysical Journal* 64(4), 1174.

Figure 3.7 Courtesy of Thomas K. Borg, PhD.

Figure 3.8 Reprinted, by permission, from A.J. McComas, 1996, *Skeletal muscle: Form and function* (Champaign, IL: Human Kinetics), 312.

Table 3.1 Adapted, by permission, from G.A. Jull and V. Janda, 1987, Muscles and motor control in low back pain: Assessment and management. In *Physical therapy of the low back*, edited by L.T. Twomey and J.R. Taylor (Edinburgh: Churchill Livingstone), 253.

Figure 4.1 Reprinted, by permission, from J. Kastelic, A. Galeski, and E. Baer, 1978, "The multicomposite structure of tendon," *Connective Tissue Research* 6(1), 21.

Figure 4.2 Reprinted, by permission, from S. Inoué and C.P. Leblond, 1986, "The microfibrils of connective tissue: I. Ultrastructure," *American Journal of Anatomy* 176(2), 136.

Figure 4.3 Reprinted, by permission, from E.R. Myers, C.G. Armstrong, and V.C. Mow, 1984, Swelling, pressure and collagen tension. In *Connective tissue matrix*, edited by D.W.L. Hukins (Deerfield Beach, FL: Verlag Chemie), 171.

Figure 4.4 Reprinted, by permission, from S. Mohan and E. Radha, 1981, "Age related changes in muscle connective tissue: Acid mucopolysaccharides and structural glycoprotein," *Experimental Gerontology* 16(5), 391.

Figure 4.5 Reprinted, by permission, from D.C. Taylor, J.D. Dalton, A.V. Seaber and W.E. Garrett, 1990, "Viscoelastic properties of muscle-tendon units: The biomechanical effects of stretching," *American Journal of Sports Medicine* 18(3), 300-309.

Figure 4.6 Reprinted, by permission, from National Strength and Conditioning Association, 2000, *Essentials of strength training and conditioning*, 2nd ed. edited by T.R. Baechle and R.W. Earle (Champaign, IL: Human Kinetics), 4.

Figure 4.7 Reprinted by permission, from W.H. Akeson, D. Amiel, and S. Woo, 1980. "Immobility effects on synovial joints: The pathomechanics of joint contracture," *Biorheology*, 17(1/2), 104.

Table 4.1 Reprinted, by permission, from M.J. Alter, 1988, *Science of stretching* (Champaign, IL: Human Kinetics), 24.

Table 4.2 Reprinted, by permission, from R.J. Johns and V. Wright, 1962, "Relative importance of various tissues in joint stiffness," *Journal of Applied Physiology* 17(5), 824-828.

Table 4.3 Reprinted, by permission, from D. Tinker and R.B. Rucker, 1985, "Role of selected nutrients in synthesis, accumulation, and chemical modification of connective tissue proteins," *Physiological Reviews* 65(3), 624.

Figures 5.1, 5.2, 5.3, and 5.4 Reprinted, by permission, from V. Wright and R.J. Johns, 1960, "Physical factors concerned with the stiffness of normal and diseased joints," *Bulletin of the Johns Hopkins Hospital* 106(4), 217.

Figure 5.5 Reprinted, by permission, from M.J. Alter, 1996, *Science of Flexibility, Second Edition* (Champaign, IL: Human Kinetics), 67.

Figure 5.6 Reprinted, by permission, from R.M. Alexander, 1988, *Elastic mechanisms in animal movement* (Cambridge: Cambridge University Press), 13.

Figures 5.7 and 5.8 Reprinted, by permission, from G.H. Pollack, 1990, *Muscles & molecules* (Seattle, Washington: Ebner & Sons), 68, 69.

Figure 5.9 Reprinted, by permission, from S. Sunderland, 1978, "Traumatized nerves, roots, and ganglia: Musculoskeletal factors and neuropathological consequences." In *The neurobiologic mechanism in manipulative therapy*, edited by T.M. Korr (New York: Plenum), 139.

Figure 5.10 Reprinted, by permission, from S. Sunderland, 1991, *Nerve injuries and their repair: A critical reappraisal*, 3rd ed. (Edinburgh: Churchill Livingstone), 66.

Figure 6.1 Reprinted, by permission, from J.H. Wilmore and D.L. Costill, 1999, *Physiology of sport and exercise*, 2nd ed. (Champaign, IL: Human Kinetics), 74.

Figures 6.2 and 6.3 Reprinted, by permission, from E.R. Kandel, J.H. Schwartz and T.M. Jessell, 1995, *Essentials of neural science and behavior* (Norwalk, CT: Appleton & Lange), 508, 511.

Figure 6.4 Reprinted, by permission, from J.R. Wolpaw, 1983, "Adaptive plasticity in the primate spinal stretch reflex: Reversal and redevelopment," *Brain Research* 278(1/2), 301.

Figure 6.5 Reprinted, by permission, from J.R. Wolpaw and J.S. Carp, 1990, "Memory traces in spinal cord," *Trends in Neuroscience* 13(4), 141.

Table 6.1 Reprinted, by permission, from B.D. Wyke, 1985, Articular neurology and manipulative therapy. In *Aspects of manipulative therapy*, edited by E.F. Glasgow, L.T. Twomey, E.R. Scull and A.M. Kleynhaw (London: Churchill Livingstone), 73.

Figure 7.1 Michel Louis. Reprinted with permission.

Figure 7.2 Reprinted with permission. Circus World Museum Library.

Figure 7.3 Reprinted by permission, M. Louis.

Figure 7.4 Reprinted by permission, M. Louis.

Figure 8.1 Reprinted by permission, from J.H. Wilmore and D.L. Costill, 2004, *Physiology of sport and exercise*, 3rd ed. (Champaign, IL: Human Kinetics), 246.

Figure 9.1 Reprinted, by permission, from J.H. Wilmore and D.L. Costill, 2004, *Physiology of sport and exercise*, 3rd ed. (Champaign, IL: Human Kinetics), 101.

Figure 9.2 Based on ideas presented in: D.L. Morgan, 1990, "New insights into the behavior of muscle during active lengthening," *Biophysical Journal* 57, 209-221. Reprinted, by permission, from R.L. Lieber, 2002, *Skeletal muscle structure, function, & plasticity*, 2nd ed. (Philadelphia: Lippincott Williams & Wilkins), 327.

Figure 9.3 Reprinted, by permission, from A.L. Vujnovich, 1995, "Neural plasticity, muscle spasm and tissue manipulation: A review of the literature," *Journal of Manual & Manipulative Therapy* 3(4), 153.

Figure 10.1 Reprinted, by permission, from W.W.K. Hoeger and D.R. Hopkins, 1992, "A comparison of the sit and reach and the modified sit and reach in the measurement of flexibility in women," *Research Quarterly for Exercise and Sport* 63(2), 191-195.

Figures 10.2 and 10.3; Table 10.1 Reprinted, by permission, from M.A. Adams, P. Dolan, and W.C. Hutton, 1987, "Diurnal variations in the stresses on the lumbar spine," *Spine* 12(2), 136.

Figure 11.1 Reprinted, by permission, from G. Batson, 1994, "Stretching technique: A somatic learning model. Part II: Training purposivity through Sweigard Ideokinesis," *Impulse* 2(1), 52, 53, 54, and 56.

Table 11.1 Reprinted, by permission, from P. Ley, 1988, *Communicating with patients: Improving communication, satisfaction, and compliance* (London: Croom Helm), 180.

Table 11.2 Modified from "Dimensions of compliance-gaining behavior: An empirical analysis" by G. Maxwell and D. Schmitt, 1967, *Socimetry* 30(4), 357-358.

Figure 12.1 Photo courtesy of J.V. Ciullo, MD.

Table 12.2 Reprinted, by permission, from S.J. Hartley-O'Brien, 1980, "Six mobilization exercises for active range of hip flexion," *Research Quarterly for Exercise and Sport* 51(4), 627.

Figure 13.1 Reprinted, by permission, from J.E. Zachazewski, 1990, Flexibility for sports. In *Sports physical therapy*, edited by B. Sanders (Norwalk, CT: Appleton & Lange), 234.

Figure 13.2 Reprinted, by permission, from M.J. Alter, 1988, *Science of stretching* (Champaign, IL: Human Kinetics), 88.

Figure 13.3 Reprinted, by permission, from R.E. McAtee and J. Charland, 1999, *Facilitated stretching*, 2nd ed. (Champaign, IL: Human Kinetics), 26.

Figure 13.4 Reprinted, by permission, from P.A. Houghlum, 2001, *Therapeutic exercise for athletic injuries* (Champaign, IL: Human Kinetics), 255.

Figure 13.5 Adapted, by permission, from M.J. Alter, 1988, *Science of stretching* (Champaign, IL: Human Kinetics), 92.

Figures 13.6 and 13.7 from "Some physical mechanisms and effects of spinal adjustments," by R.W. Sandoz, 1976, *Annals of the Swiss Chiropractors' Association*, 6, p. 92. Copyright 1976 by the Swiss Chiropractors' Association. Reprinted by permission.

Figure 13.8 Photo courtesy of Carson Hurley.

Figures 14.1, 14.2, and 14.3 Reprinted, by permission, from R. Cailliet and L. Gross, 1987, *The rejuvenation strategy* (Garden City, NJ: Doubleday), 34, 37, 35.

Figure 14.4 Reprinted, by permission, from M.J. Alter, 1990, *Sports stretch* (Champaign, IL: Human Kinetics), 118-119.

Figure 14.5 Reprinted, by permission, from S. Gracovetsky, M. Kary, I. Pitchen, S. Levy, and R.B. Said, 1989, "The importance of pelvic tilt in reducing compressive stress in the spine during flexion-extension exercises," *Spine* 14(4), 415.

Figures 14.6 and 14.7 Reprinted by permission, from M.J. Alter, 1990, *Sports stretch* (Champaign, IL: Human Kinetics), 108-110, 117-118, 128-130.

Table 15.1 Adapted from U.S. Census Bureau, National Population Projections—Summary Tables, January 13, 2000. www.census.gov/population/www/projections/natsum-T3.html.

Figure 16.1 Reprinted, by permission, from G.W. Warren, 1989, *Classical ballet technique* (Tampa, FL: University of South Florida Press), 11. Photo by Juri Barikin.

Figure 16.2 from *Living Anatomy* (p. 139) by J.E. Donnelly, 1982, Champaign, IL: Human Kinetics. Copyright 1982 by J.E. Donnelly. Reprinted by permission.

Figure 16.3 Reprinted, by permission, from P.I. Sallay, R.L. Friedman, P.G. Coogan, and W.E. Garrett, 1996, "Hamstring muscle injuries among water skiers: Functional outcome and prevention," *American Journal of Sports Medicine* 24(2), 131.

Figure 16.4 Reprinted, by permission, from P.A. Houglum, 2001, *Therapeutic exercise for athletic injuries* (Champaign, IL: Human Kinetics), 349.

Figure 16.5 Reprinted, by permission, from B. Calais-Germain, 1993, *Anatomy of movement* (Seattle, WA: Eastland Press), 185.

Figures 17.1 and 17.2 Reprinted, by permission, from I.A. Kapandji, 1978, *The physiology of the joints: Vol. 3. The trunk and the vertebral column* (Edinburgh: Churchill Livingstone), 29.

Figure 17.3 Reprinted, by permission, from J.W. Fisk and B.S. Rose, 1977, *A practical guide to management of the painful neck and back* (Springfield, IL: Charles C Thomas), 37.

Figure 17.4 Reprinted, by permission, from M.J. Alter, 1988, *Science of stretching* (Champaign, IL: Human Kinetics), 130.

Figure 17.5 Reprinted, by permission, from J.W. Fisk and B.S. Rose, 1977, *A practical guide to management of the painful neck and back* (Springfield, IL: Charles C Thomas), 37.

Figure 17.6 Adapted, by permission, from A.A. White and M.M. Panjabi, 1990, *Clinical biomechanics of the spine*, 2nd ed. (Philadelphia: Lippincott), 59.

Figures 17.7, 17.8, 17.9, 17.10, 17.11, and 17.12 Reprinted, by permission, from R. Cailliet, 1981, *Low back pain syndrome*, 3rd ed. (Philadelphia: F.A. Davis), 40, 44, 64, 65, 132, 133.

Table 17.1 Reprinted, by permission, from M.J. Alter, 1988, *Science of stretching* (Champaign, IL: Human Kinetics), 130.

Table 17.2 Reprinted by permission, from M.J. Alter, 1996, *Science of flexibility*, 2nd ed. (Champaign, IL: Human Kinetics), 276-277.

Figures 18.1, 18.2, and 18.3 Reprinted, by permission, from R. Cailliet, 1966, *Shoulder pain* (Philadelphia: F.A. Davis), 65.

Figure 19.1 from *Lower Extremity Injuries in Runners Induced by Upper Body Torque (UBT)* by B. Prichard, 1984, presented at the Biomechanics and Kinesiology in Sports U.S. Olympic Committee Sports Medicine Conference January 8-14, 1984, in Colorado Springs, CO. Copyright 1984 by Bob Prichard/SOMAX Posture & Sport. Marin Medical Center, 711 D Street #208, San Rafael, CA 94901. Reprinted by permission.

Figure 19.2 Reprinted, by permission, from D. Martin and P. Coe, 1997, *Better training for distance runners*, 2nd ed. (Champaign, IL: Human Kinetics), 27.

Figure 19.3 Reprinted, by permission, from D. Martin and P. Coe, 1997, *Better training for distance runners*, 2nd ed. (Champaign, IL: Human Kinetics), 14.

Figure 19.4 Reprinted, by permission, from G.S. Fleisig, J.R. Andrews, C.J. Dillman, and R.F. Escamilla, 1995, "Kinetics of baseball pitching with implications about injury mechanisms," *American Journal of Sports Medicine* 23(2), 238.

Figure 19.5 Reprinted, by permission, from M. Mysnyk, B. Davis, and B. Simpson, 1994, *Winning wrestling moves* (Champaign, IL: Human Kinetics), 151.

Figure 19.8 Reprinted by permission, from G. Carr, 1997, *Mechanics of sport* (Champaign, IL: Human Kinetics), 136-137.

Figure 19.9 Reprinted, by permission, from W.T. Hardaker, L. Erickson, and M. Myers, 1984, The pathogenesis of dance injury. In *The dancer as athlete*, edited by C.G. Shell (Champaign, IL: Human Kinetics), 12-13.

Table 19.1 Reprinted, by permission, from G. Dintiman, R. Ward, and T. Tellez, 1988, *Sport speed* (Champaign, IL: Human Kinetics), p. 149.

1

OVERVIEW: BASIC SCIENCES RELATED TO FLEXIBILITY

1

Modern Overview of Flexibility and Stretching

The outcome of any flexibility program can be made more predictable and less haphazard if certain biological and biomechanical principles are applied. In evaluating one's flexibility and formulating a flexibility-training program, one must consider not only the benefits but also the potential for injury and impairment of function and performance if rehabilitation or training occurs under suboptimal conditions. The development and maintenance of optimal flexibility often involves multiple stakeholders, including coaches, instructors, trainers, therapists, physicians, dancers, professional and recreational athletes, and laypersons, who should all take advantage of every opportunity to develop optimal flexibility. The development of optimum flexibility is often a bidirectional process.

DEFINING FLEXIBILITY

The word *flexibility* can be defined in several different ways depending on the discipline or the nature of the research. For example, the term may be applied to both animate and inanimate objects. The word is derived from the Latin *flectere* or *flexibilis*, "to bend," and is defined as the "ability to be bent, pliable."

Little agreement can be found on the definition of so-called normal flexibility. In physical education, sports medicine, and allied health sciences, perhaps the simplest definition of flexibility is the range of motion (ROM) available in a joint or group of joints (de Vries 1986; Hebbelinck 1988; Hubley-Kozey 1991; Liemohn 1988; Stone and Kroll 1991). For others, flexibility also implies freedom to move (Goldthwait 1941; Metheny 1952), the ability to engage a part or parts of the body in a wide range of purposeful movements at the required speed (Galley and Forster 1987), the total achievable excursion (within limits of pain) of a body part through its potential ROM (Saal 1998), normal joint and soft-tissue ROM in response to active or passive stretch (Halvorson 1989), the ability to move a joint smoothly through its complete ROM (Kent 1998); the ability to move a single joint or series of joints

smoothly and easily through an unrestricted, pain-free ROM (Kisner and Colby 2002), and the ability to move a joint through a normal ROM without undue stress to the musculotendinous unit (Chandler et al. 1990). Another alternate definition of flexibility has been offered by Halbertsma et al. (1996): it should refer to extensibility rather than ROM.

Many researchers have used ROM or maximal ROM of a limb as an index of the musculoskeletal flexibility (Halbertsma et al. 1996; Magnusson et al. 1996b; McHugh et al. 1998). However, this usage raises a pertinent question: Is maximal ROM an appropriate index? In addition, Gajdosik (2001) and Halbertsma et al. (1996) have raised concern about the use of confusing terminology (i.e., using different terms to describe similar phenomena). Several alternative terms have been suggested along with their rationales. Halbertsma et al. (1996) suggest that flexibility should refer to extensibility rather than to the ROM. Several investigators (Gajdosik 1995, 2001; Gajdosik and Bohannon 1987; Gajdosik et al. 1999) recommend that flexibility be defined as a ratio of change in muscle length or change in joint angle to change in force or torque. These ratios are actually measures of compliance. However, Krivickas (1999) cautions that in this concept, the "definition does not encompass the concept of dynamic vs. static flexibility, since [this] requires that the muscle be lengthened without muscle activation" (p. 84). The confounding definitions reiterate the necessity of carefully reading and completely understanding how the term flexibility is used in a specific research paper or text.

DIFFERENCES AMONG FLEXIBILITY, HYPERMOBILITY, JOINT LAXITY, AND JOINT INSTABILITY

The terms *flexibility*, *hypermobility*, *joint laxity*, and *joint instability* are not synonymous. As previously stated, *flexibility* commonly refers to ROM of a joint. In contrast, *laxity* refers to the stability of a joint (Brody 1999; Saal 1998). Excessive joint laxity can be a result of a chronic injury or a congenital or hereditary condition, such as Ehlers-Danlos syndrome (EDS). Joint derangement and dysfunction resulting from a loss of joint stability is referred to as *joint instability*. Often, the terms *joint hypermobility* and joint instability are used interchangeably, and there is no standard definition of these terms. Peterson and Bergmann (2002) have made a simplified attempt to distinguish clinical joint instability from hypermobility. Hypermobility is associated with an increased ROM, normal ratio of translational movements, and normal coupled movements, whereas joint instability is characterized by increased or normal ROM, increased proportion or aberrant translational movements, and aberrant coupled movements. Throughout this text, *flexibility* will refer to the degree of normal motion unless otherwise stated; *laxity* will refer to the degree of abnormal motion of a given joint; and in general, *hypermobility* will refer to the ROM in excess of the accepted normal motion in most of the joints or excessive length of a tissue.

NATURE OF FLEXIBILITY

Goniometry is the measurement of joint ROM. ROM may be measured in either *linear units* (e.g., inches or centimeters) or *angular units* (degrees of an arc). Regardless of the method, the data should be clear, simple, and understandable. Clinical investigations of flexibility in humans have used maximal joint ROM as the dependent variable. As previously mentioned, this practice has been criticized (Magnusson et al. 1996b; Siff 1993a). Specifically, Siff (1993a) points out that (1) joint ROM, a single measurement in time in a static system provides limited information about the behavior of the muscle-tendon unit, (2) mechanical characteristics of tissues change dynamically during exercise, and (3) other biomechanical variables, such as maximal load, damping ratio, energy absorbed, and stiffness, are important.

Physical fitness is an important part of total development that includes flexibility, cardiorespiratory endurance, strength, and muscular endurance. Over time, numerous batteries of tests have been developed to assess physical fitness. Although flexibility is commonly thought of as being more or less uniform throughout the body (i.e., people are generally very flexible or inflexible in all the body joints), research studies do not substantiate this point (American College of Sports Medicine 2000; Holland 1968). In fact, flexibility does not exist as a general characteristic but is *specific* to a particular joint and joint action (Bryant 1984; Corbin and Noble 1980; Harris 1969a, 1969b; Holland 1968; Merni et al. 1981; Munroe and Romance 1975). Adequate ROM in the hip does not ensure adequate ROM in the shoulder. Similarly, sufficient ROM in one hip may not mean sufficient ROM in the other hip. In short, "no single flexibility test

can be used to evaluate total body flexibility" (American College of Sports Medicine 2000, p. 86). The differences in ROM reflect genetic variation, personal activity patterns, and specialized mechanical strains imposed on connective tissue.

Static flexibility relates to ROM about a joint with no emphasis on speed. Two examples of static flexibility are slowly bending to touch the floor or performing a "split." Knudson, Magnusson, and McHugh. (2000) caution that several complications are associated with static flexibility measures. Significantly, the limits of static flexibility tests are subjectively defined by either the subject or the tester. Therefore, such tests cannot be truly objective.

Ballistic flexibility is usually associated with bobbing, bouncing, rebounding, and rhythmic motion. Another term somewhat related to rhythmic motion is *dynamic flexibility*, which refers to the ability to use a range of joint movement in the performance of a physical activity at either normal or rapid speed (Corbin and Noble 1980; Fleischman 1964). Hence, dynamic flexibility does not necessarily denote ballistic or fast types of movement. However, a rigorous definition of dynamic flexibility has not been universally accepted (Hubley-Kozey 1991). A review of the literature (Knudson, Magnusson, and McHugh 2000) showed dynamic flexibility accounts for about 44% to 66% of the variance of static flexibility. However, the reviewers acknowledge that "there is insufficient research to determine whether static and dynamic flexibility are two distinct properties or two aspects of the same flexibility component" (p. 3). An alternative term is *functional flexibility* (Clippinger-Robertson 1988). An example of "slow" dynamic, or functional, flexibility is the ability of a ballet dancer to slowly raise and hold her leg at a 60° angle, whereas a split leap is an example of "fast" dynamic flexibility. Obviously, most athletic events involve dynamic flexibility. Here too, the type of flexibility is specific to the type of movement (speed and angle) of a given discipline and thus is not necessarily related to just ROM. Siff and Verkhoshansky (1999) break down functional stretching conditioning into three components: (1) flexibility-speed, the ability to produce efficient full ROM at speed; (2) flexibility-strength, the ability to produce efficient, powerful static and dynamic movements over a full ROM; and (3) flexibility-endurance, the ability to repetitively produce efficient full ROM under static and dynamic conditions.

Passive flexibility is a measure of the ROM in the absence of active contraction (i.e., voluntary muscular effort). Instead, a partner or special equipment often maintains the ROM. Passive flexibility can also be applied to oneself by having one part of the body exert a stretching force on another part, such as pulling the thumb back with the opposing hand or using the weight of upper torso when stretching forward to touch the toes while seated on the floor. Toft et al. (1989) have suggested "passive tension measurements seem to be more objective range of motion measurements, since psychologic factors do not interfere with the results" (p. 493). However, Gajdosik (2001) points out that measuring passive extensibility ultimately depends on accurately defining the end point of maximal muscle length, which is based on psychophysiological phenomena such as a subject's perception of discomfort or pain (stretch tolerance).

Passive ROM is more difficult to measure reliably than active ROM (Gajdosik and Bohannon 1987). As elaborated by Amis and Miller (1982), "Passive movements are extremely difficult to reproduce, because the stretching of soft tissues at the limits of motion depends on the force applied to the limb, which must, therefore, be carefully controlled" (p. 576). Accordingly, Gajdosik and Bohannon (1987) suggested the use of "force dynamometers to standardize the amount of passive force applied and thereby decrease the potential for error" (p. 1869).

Flexibility is specific to a given group of sports as well as to a given joint, a given side, and a given speed. Furthermore, even within sports groups, particular patterns of flexibility are related to frequent or unique joint movements. Those joints demanding flexibility are characteristic of a given sport and of each subgroup within a sport. For example, a number of sports and arts disciplines require the development of specific flexibility patterns. These disciplines include ballet (DiTullio et al. 1989; Hamilton et al. 1992), baseball (Fleisig et al. 1995; Gurry et al. 1985; Magnusson et al. 1994; Tippett 1986), ice hockey (Agre, Casal et al. 1988; Song 1979), power lifting (Chang et al. 1988), swimming (Bloomfield et al. 1985; Oppliger et al. 1986), and tennis (Chandler et al.

Compensatory Relative Flexibility

"Compensatory relative flexibility" is a concept emphasized by Sahrmann (2002), based on the assumption that to achieve a particular range of motion, the body will move through the point of least resistance. This point is the area of greatest relative flexibility. A practical example is a rower at the bottom of the catch position (Mallac 2003). In this position, the rower's hands (and the oar) must reach past the feet in order to generate the drive required to transfer force from the body to the oar. If the rower has extremely tight hips and cannot bend forward (flex at the hips), the body must move somewhere else to compensate for the lack of hip flexibility. Most often, the rower will flex the lumbar and thoracic regions of the spine. The back has more "relative flexibility," and consequently contributes to the overall range of motion. However, the back movement is detrimental and may possibly result in lumbar and thoracic dysfunction and pain.

1990). Therefore, flexibility training should be prescribed accordingly (Zernicke and Salem 1996).

FLEXIBILITY-TRAINING PROGRAM

In athletics, training in general is defined as "a multi-sided process of the expedient use of aggregate factors (means, methods and conditions) so as to influence the development of an athlete and ensure the necessary level of preparedness" (Matveyev 1981, p. 22). Training programs often concentrate on strength training, power training, aerobic (endurance) training, and anaerobic training. However, an essential component of any training program is flexibility training. To obtain maximum benefits from a training program to enhance ROM, participants must know and understand the capabilities and limitations of the program and know how to differentiate between various types of programs.

A flexibility-training program is defined as a planned, deliberate, and regular program of exercises that can permanently and progressively increase the usable ROM of a joint or set of joints over a period of time (Aten and Knight 1978). Often, the term *flexibility exercise* is used synonymously with stretching exercise (Pezzullo and Irrgang 2001). However, Kisner and Colby (2002) emphasize

> Remember, stretching and ROM exercises are not synonymous terms. Stretching takes soft tissue structures *beyond* their available length to *increase* ROM. ROM exercises stay within the limits of tissue extensibility to *maintain* the available length of tissues. (p. 187)

Evjenth and Hamberg (1993) divide stretching into two categories: self-stretching and therapeutic muscle stretching (TMS). Frequently, the self-stretching is utilized in fitness exercises, athletic training, and dance. Related, but more specific in design, TMS is specific muscle stretching performed, instructed, or supervised by a therapist for patients with dysfunctions of the musculoskeletal system (Mühlemann and Cimino 1990). Such patients may or may not be athletes. TMS and self-stretching may supplement each other (Evjenth and Hamberg 1993).

A common and distinct entity that should be employed in most exercise regimens is a flexibility warm-up/cool-down program, which is a planned, deliberate, and regular program of exercises that is done immediately before and after an activity to improve performance or to reduce the risk of injury. (The term *cool-down* is synonymous with *warm-down*.) A flexibility warm-up/cool-down program alone will not improve flexibility during the weeks after the program (Aten and Knight 1978; Corbin and Noble 1980). In contrast to cool-down, self-stretching and TMS retain improved flexibility during the weeks after activity (Zebas and Rivera 1985).

BENEFITS OF A FLEXIBILITY-TRAINING PROGRAM

The potential benefits of a flexibility-training program are virtually unlimited. The quality and quantity of these benefits are ultimately determined by two factors: the ends, that is, the participant's goals or objectives, the context of which may be biological, psychological, sociological, or philosophical, and the means, the methods and techniques used to attain the ends. If the ends are purely emotional or psychological, as opposed to biological or physiological, then certain stretching techniques would be employed and others would not. What benefits, then, can one expect from a flexibility-training program? In light of the recent proliferation of material on the subject, this unit will examine the question.

Union of the Body, Mind, and Spirit

From a purely esoteric point of view, a flexibility-training program can serve to unify one's body, mind, and spirit. Yoga is probably the most widely known of such programs. The word *yoga* is derived from the Sanskrit root *yuj*, meaning "to bind, attach, and yoke" (Iyengar 1979). An equivalent idea is conveyed by the English phrase "getting into harness" or "yoking up." The yogi undoubtedly "gets into harness" in his or her work of controlling the body and mind by the will (Ramacharaka 1960). Similarly, Iyengar (1979) points out that the term *yuj* implies "to direct and concentrate one's attention; to use and apply" (p. 19). It also means union or communion.

According to the *Yoga Sutras*, an ancient writing, yoga comprises several categories of physiological practices and spiritual exercises, called *angas*, or "limbs." Classical yoga comprises eight limbs whose end is final liberation, *enstasis*:

1. Yama: abstentions
2. Niyama: observances
3. Asanas: postures
4. Pranayama: control of breath
5. Pratyahara: withdrawal of the senses
6. Dharana: concentration
7. Dhyana: meditation
8. Samadhi: a state of superconsciousness; a state of oneness or unifying concentration

Unfortunately, asanas are commonly thought of as merely physical exercises or postures that display flexibility and suppleness. Lists and descriptions of asanas are found in many ancient Indian texts, manuals, and manuscripts. According to one ancient text, the *Gheranda Samhita*, "There are eighty-four hundreds of thousands of Asanas described by Siva, [however] only thirty-two have been found useful for mankind in this world" (Vasu 1933, p. 25).

In brief, numerous sources on yoga emphasize the following basic principles that are mystical and transcendental, yet highly logical and rational:

- The body is the temple that houses the Divine Spark.
- The body is an instrument of attainment.
- The yogi masters the body by the practice of asanas.
- The yogi performs asanas to develop complete equilibrium of the body, mind, and spirit.
- The body, mind, and spirit are inseparable.

As an analogy, Iyengar (1979) explained yoga as follows:

> To the yogi, his body is the prime instrument of attainment. If his vehicle breaks down, the traveler cannot go far. If the body is broken by ill-health, the aspirant can achieve little. Physical health is important for mental development, as normally the mind functions through the nervous system. When the body is sick or the nervous system is affected, the mind becomes restless or dull and inert and concentration or meditation becomes impossible. (pp. 24-25)

Thus, whether one practices the asanas to improve the mind or attain Samadhi, an additional side benefit can be flexibility.

Relaxation of Stress and Tension

Stress is an inescapable part of life that generally can be described as "wear and tear." It is the body's generalized reaction to stimuli. The buildup of stress without release of tension leads to problems. For example, induced psychological stress causes an increase in EMG amp in the upper trapezius both during standardized static contractions and in the absence of physical loads (Larrson et al. 1995; Lundberg et al. 1994). The literature contains abundant evidence that therapeutic exercise alleviates stress (de Vries et al. 1981). Empirical evidence indicates that individualized flexibility-training programs may be similarly beneficial.

Muscular Relaxation

One of the most important benefits of a flexibility program is the potential promotion of relaxation. Physiologically, relaxation is the cessation of muscular tension. Undesirably high levels of muscular tension have several negative side effects, such as decreasing sensory awareness and raising blood pressure. It also wastes energy; a contracting muscle requires more energy than a relaxed muscle. Furthermore, habitually tense muscles tend to cut off their own circulation. Reduced blood supply results in a lack of oxygen and essential nutrients and causes toxic waste products to accumulate in the cells. This process predisposes one to fatigue, aches, and even pain. Moulton and Spence (1992) proposed that muscular hypertension might eventually lead to ischemia of the affected muscles, generating a pain-tension-pain cycle. Larsson et al. (1999) studied 76 workers (with long-standing unilateral neck pain and diagnosed chronic trapezius myalgia) using laser Doppler flowmetry to measure blood flow and surface EMG of both upper trapezius muscles during a fatiguing series of stepwise increased static loads. They concluded that the increased muscle tension on the painful side ($p < .05$) might be secondary to impaired microcirculation of the muscle ($p < .05$) and the consequent release of nociceptive substances, thereby maintaining the pain-tension-pain cycle. Common sense and everyday experience show that a relaxed muscle is less susceptible to these ailments and many others.

When a muscle stays partially contracted, a *contracture*, an abnormal state of prolonged shortening develops. Contracture and chronic muscle tension not only shorten the muscle but also make the muscle less supple, less strong, and unable to absorb the shock and stress of various types of movement. Consequently, excess muscular tension can produce excessive muscular tightness.

Simons et al. (1999) have written extensively on the subject of trigger points. They define a trigger point as a "highly irritable localized spot of exquisite tenderness in a nodule in a palpable taught band of muscle tissue." The "nodule" is the trigger point itself, a mass of contracted sarcomeres in individual muscle fibers forming a lump that can range in size from a pinhead to a pea. In the large muscles of the thigh, a trigger point can feel like a knot the size of a thumb. The "palpable taut band of muscle tissue" that contains the trigger point nodule often feels like a cord or cable and is easily mistaken for a tendon. Taut bands of muscle fiber tend to restrict ROM by limiting a muscle's ability to lengthen, keeping it both tight and weak.

The most appropriate remedy for such a disorder is to facilitate muscular relaxation and immediately follow with some type of stretching. de Vries and Adams (1972) found exercise to be more effective than medication in decreasing muscular tension.

Self-Discipline and Self-Knowledge

Most of us live undisciplined lives; that is, our responses are often conditioned by mindless habit. Therefore self-discipline must be cultivated. Because the body is controlled by the mind, if the body is mastered, then the mind must be mastered. Herein lies the fundamental importance of the asanas in yoga. The yogi masters the body by the practice and self-discipline of asanas and thus makes the body a fit vehicle for the spirit. The concept that disciplining the mind disciplines the body also holds true for the athlete, artistic performer, and layperson. If one aspect of life can be mastered, then other aspects can

be mastered. A flexibility-training program offers an ideal opportunity to seek mastery over oneself. Stretching can give one something to struggle for and against, just as a marathon race does for a runner.

Stretching also offers a unique opportunity for spiritual growth by providing quiet intervals for thought, meditation, or self-evaluation. During such moments, one can also listen to and monitor one's own body, something most of us today seldom do. Moreover, the beauty of stretching is that it can be done anywhere at any time.

In artistic performances and sports, successes and failures are visible for all to see, and the measures of success are objectively accurate. One can do little to hide a poor arabesque or a failed split jump. A stretching program (or any exercise program) can enable us to understand our own development and abilities. Each of us has different abilities and talents, some of which go unrecognized. Stretching can teach us lessons about our abilities and provide opportunities to test ourselves physiologically.

Body Fitness, Posture, and Symmetry

The desire to be healthy and attractive is almost universal. The best way to improve bodily measurements and proportions is through a combination of appropriate diet and exercise. *Posture* is the position of body parts in relation to each other. According to Magee (2002), "Correct posture is the position in which minimum stress is applied to each joint" (p. 873). To develop body symmetry and good posture, one should engage in gross motor activities rather than specialize in an activity that develops only one area of the body. Presumably, by incorporating an individualized flexibility program into an overall fitness program, one can improve not only health and fitness but also bodily appearance.

Advocates of good posture claim it can potentially eliminate the causes of many dysfunctions (e.g., low back) and decrease fatigue and pain. Some claim that posture is a window to a person. Consequently, good posture can improve interpersonal power because it inspires greater confidence in other people and results in greater respect. The most common cause of poor posture is poor postural habit (Magee 2002). Structural deformities, which are the result of congenital anomalies, developmental problems, trauma, disease, may also cause a modification of posture. Additional causes of poor posture include weak muscles, pain, obesity, pregnancy, poor-quality beds, stress, and involuntary muscle tension. Strategies and techniques to improve posture include exercise, stretching, massage, and other soft-tissue techniques; modalities such as diathermy and ultrasound; and re-education in movement patterns and positions during activities.

The relationship of flexibility to posture is both theoretical and clinical. Crawford and Jull (1993) found that increased kyphosis (flexion in the thoracic region) in older subjects is related to reduced range of arm elevation. Corbin and Noble (1980) suggested that an imbalance in muscular development and inflexibility in certain muscle groups contributes to poor posture. Rounded shoulders, for example, may be associated with poor flexibility in the pectoral muscles and less endurance in the scapular girdle adductors (i.e., rhomboids and middle trapezius). This condition may be alleviated by stretching the shortened connective tissue and muscles and by strengthening the weakened muscles.

Another popular clinical notion is that short hamstrings cause posterior pelvic tilting posture and a decreased lumbar angle (flatter curve) in standing. However, clinical studies by Toppenberg and Bullock (1986) and Gajdosik et al. (1994) determined that hamstring muscle length was not significantly related to pelvic angle. Klee et al. (2002) investigated the relationship of muscular balance and posture to pelvic inclination of 53 subjects, 40 volunteered to participate in a 10-week training experiment. This study, and another by Wiemann et al. (1998), concluded, "muscular balance should 'not' be treated with stretching but with resistance exercises" (Klee et al. 2002, p. 95). Additional research is needed to determine the optimal protocols to produce optimal posture and symmetry in those with muscular imbalance.

Relief of Low-Back Pain

Low-back pain (LBP) is one of the most prevalent complaints in modern society. Thousands of people seek relief from LBP by various treatments every year. In fact, most people will probably be affected by LBP at some point in their lives. The question is "What is the relationship between flexibility, or lack of it, and low-back pain?" A review of the literature will unequivocally demonstrate a vast array of contradictory findings. Numerous researchers (Biering-Sørensen 1984; Burton et al. 1989; Chiarello and Savidge 1993; Elnagger et al. 1991; Marras and Wongsam 1986; Mayer et al. 1994; Mayer et al. 1984; Mellin 1987; Waddell et al. 1992) reported a general decrease or deficit in spinal mobility associated with a history of back problems. In contrast, Howes and Isdale (1971) reported increased spinal mobility associated with back problems. However, Nadler et al. (1998) demonstrated no association between tight hip flexors and the development of LBP in 257 college athletes. A study of 15 subjects by Li et al. (1996) also showed that a history of back pain had no effect on spinal flexion ROM. Similarly, a study of subjects with and without a history of significant LBP found no differences between the two groups in the amount of lumbar or hip motion during forward bending (Esola et al. 1996). Yet, another investigation of 2,747 adults with a mean age of 44.6 years indicated no relationship between the sit-and-reach performance and reported LBP (Jackson et al. 1998). An investigation by Lundberg and Gerdle (2000)

of 607 women working as homecare personnel reported that peripheral joint mobility, spinal sagittal posture, and thoracic sagittal mobility showed low correlations with disability. However, their study also found lumbar sagittal hypomobility was associated with higher disability.

Decreased lumbar flexion in those with chronic LBP is based on a theoretical model. Tight hip extensors decrease the lordotic curve that naturally exists in the lumbar spine, which can also exaggerate the posterior tilt of the pelvis. This condition diminishes the shock-absorbing capacity of the lumbar segments and increases compressive forces on the lumbar spine. Furthermore, decreased lumbar flexion increases tension on the surrounding ligaments and musculature. Ballistic movements performed during athletics are thought to greatly magnify these forces (Ashmen et al. 1996).

The lack of lateral flexibility of the torso may also be a factor in LBP. Ashmen et al. (1996) write

> The oblique musculature, which helps control lateral flexion, is believed to be a key trunk stabilizer. The primary role of the oblique complex is to reinforce the erector spinae fascia by pulling it laterally. This widened, reinforced fascia is a more efficient support and decreases strain on the lumbar vertebra. A unilateral reduction in oblique flexibility could result in asymmetrical forces on the lumbar fascia and pelvic girdle. (p. 283)

Mellin (1987) substantiated that lateral flexibility of the torso has a direct correlation to LBP. Similarly, Ashmen et al. (1996) found deficits in right lateral flexibility in subjects experiencing LBP. However, Ashmen et al. (1996) caution that "these differences may also be explained by hand dominance or side-dominated sports. [Furthermore], to what degree the oblique muscles support the lumbar spine and chronic low back pain has yet to be determined" (p. 283).

Although the etiology of LBP remains controversial, strong evidence supports the need for adequate mobility of the trunk. Farfan (1978) reported that flexibility of the lumbar spine provides a mechanical advantage for function and efficiency. Dolan and Adams (1993) concluded: "Poor mobility in the lumbar spine and hips increases the bending moments acting on the spine during forward bending and lifting activities. This may lead to an increased risk of injury to the intervertebral discs and ligaments" (p. 191). Furthermore, numerous authorities and studies suggest that adequate flexibility or stretching may help reduce the risk or severity of LBP (American College of Sports Medicine 2000; Cailliet 1988; Deyo et al. 1990; Khalil et al. 1992; Locke 1983; Rasch and Burke 1989; Russell and Highland 1990). However, doubts regarding the relationship between flexibility and LBP have been raised in various quarters.

Battié et al. (1990) point out the common public perception "that greater spinal flexibility is associated with improved back health and lesser risk of injury" (p. 768). They state that improved ROM may be associated with symptomatic relief in patients with subacute and chronic back problems (Mayer et al. 1985; Mayer et al. 1987; Mellin 1985). Another example of the supposed relationship between ROM and LBP is discussed by McGill (1997):

> Most often, judgement regarding a back injured person's fitness to return to work is based on their trunk range of motion. Perhaps, it was rationalized that back injured people have a reduced range of motion and therefore to regain that range of motion is a desirable objective. However, investigation of spine mechanics demonstrates a variety of ills associated with moving the spine to the end range of motion (including increased risk of damage to the disc, ligaments and vertebral components), not to mention moving an already injured spine to the end range of motion. (p. 473)

However, there is little evidence to support the use of exercises to maintain or increase spinal ROM as a protective measure against back problems (Battié et al. 1987; Battié et al. 1990; Elnagger et al. 1991; McGill 1999). Nonetheless, Battié et al. (1990) emphasize that

> Lack of such an association does not prove that a program that induces changes will have no effect . . . However, these data suggest that it is unlikely that increasing flexibility alone in the sagittal and frontal planes will reduce back pain reports. (p. 771)

McGill (1998) writes

> Despite the notion held by some people, there are few data to support a major emphasis on trunk flexibility to improve back health and to lessen the risk of injury. Some exercise programs that have included loading of the torso throughout the ranges of motion (in flexion and extension, lateral bending, or axial twisting) have had poorer outcomes (Biering-Sorensen 1984; Battié et al. 1990), and greater mobility in some cases has been associated with low back trouble (Biering-Sorensen 1984; Burton, Tillotson and Troup 1989). Furthermore, spinal flexibility has been shown to have little predictive value for future low back trouble (Biering-Sorensen 1984; Battié et al. 1990). (p. 759)

Therefore, McGill (1998, 1999) recommends that

- end of ROM for specific injuries should be contraindicated;

- torso flexibility exercises should be limited to unloaded flexion and extension for individuals who are concerned with safety;
- sufficient hip and knee flexibility is imperative to spare the spine excessive motion during the tasks of daily living;
- hip and knee flexibility can be achieved through several movements that emphasize the trunk stabilization through exercise with a neutral spine; and
- spine flexibility should not be emphasized until the spine has stabilized and has undergone strength and endurance conditioning (some may never reach this stage).

Other factors may be associated with the cause or prevention of injury, including length discrepancy, poor endurance, strength deficits in the abdominals, erector spinae, gluteals and hip extensors, and hip muscle imbalance (Ashmen et al. 1996; McGill 1998; Nadler et al. 2001). Comparisons between spinal mobility and the prevalence of current or previous back pain may also be ambiguous because a painful back may be more mobile because of ligamentous instability (Dolan and Adams 1993; Howes and Isdale 1971; Lankhorst et al. 1985; Stokes et al. 1981). Additional factors associated with a program may also influence the eventual outcomes. Thus, "[f]lexibility measurements may be influenced by a number of factors such as pain, fear, and motivation, in addition to anatomic or physiologic limitations" (Battié et al. 1990, p. 772). This notion of a nonanatomic or nonphysiologic limitation of ROM has been raised by a number of researchers (Dolan and Adams 1993; Marras and Wongsam 1986; Pearcy et al. 1985; Seno 1968; Stokes et al. 1981). Consequently, changes in flexibility resulting from injury may be a form of protective behavior to reduce pain or irritation (fear avoidance) or to reduce moment (force times the perpendicular distance from a fulcrum) and thus the force about the spine (Burton et al. 1989; Dolan and Adams 1993; Mayer et al. 1984; Pearcy et al. 1985). However, Zuberbier et al. (2001) found "correlations between lumbar range of motion scores and spinal disability and function were inconclusive" (p. E-472). Their conclusion was "absolute lumbar range of motion scores may not be suitable as the sole determinants of low back pathology diagnosis" (p. E-472). Yet, the findings of an investigation (Kuukkanen and Mälkiä 2000) of 86 chronic LBP subjects who participated in a 3-month therapeutic exercises program to enhance flexibility suggested that "flexibility does not play an important role in coping with chronic low back pain for subjects whose functional limitations are not severe" (p. 46).

Parks et al. (2003) point out that traditionally, lumbar range of motion (LROM) is the standard used to determine disability for the purposes of compensation and work readiness. However, "a discrete physical impairment associated with LBP and diminished ROM often is never found" (p. 380). Furthermore, their study concluded, "The relationship between LROM measures and functional ability is weak or nonexistent" (p. 380).

Another important factor related to LBP is trunk (i.e., lumbar spine) velocity. Marras and Wongsam (1986) found significant differences for both angle and velocity measures between patients with LBP and a normal control group. Their investigation suggested "trunk velocity be used as a quantitative measure of low back disorder and that it be used as a means to monitor the rehabilitative progress of patients with LBP" (p. 213).

In conclusion, two important issues must be recognized. First, longitudinal studies assessing premorbid spinal flexibility are needed to clearly define the relationship between spinal flexibility and back problems (Battié et al. 1987). Second, as Jackson and Brown (1983) pointed out over 20 years ago, clinical assessment of sufficient mobility remains undefined. Consequently, until adequate flexibility can be scientifically defined and the clinical means are developed to measure the achievement of goals (i.e., of ROM), the use of mobility and flexibility exercises to reduce the risk of LBP will remain theoretical. Hunt et al. (2001) echoed and expanded the concerns raised by Jackson and Brown (1983). Their thoughtful words deem consideration:

> The current system for impairment determination recommended by the AMA *Guides* is based on a medical model and consists of either ROM or diagnosis-related estimates. In the current article and two companion articles, we describe serious limitations to the ROM approach. Beyond this, we question the appropriateness of an exclusively medical approach for the measurement of physical disability. A vast literature is currently accumulating with an emerging consensus that a multifactorial, biopsychosocial approach to disability may be far more fruitful than a purely medical model. We recommend movement toward this new approach to disability. Moving away from an exclusively medical model will eliminate the need to use biometrically limited physical impairment determinations to prove functional disability. Although models, such as ROM, are appealingly simple and apparently objective, future work should focus on a more thorough concept of disability. The field now sits in an ideal position to evaluate many years of empirical research and, in so doing, to enhance the accuracy and sophistication of its approach to disability quantification. (p. 2717)

Relief of Muscular Cramps

Painful, involuntary skeletal muscle contractions are generally called *cramps* (McGee 1990), of which several types

are known. Ordinary cramps are neural, not muscular, in origin, and they begin when muscles already in the most shortened position involuntarily contract (Norris et al. 1957; Weiner and Weiner 1980). This process may explain the susceptibility of swimmers to calf cramps. Good kicking form, with the toes pointed, involves contraction of the shortened gastrocnemius (calf) muscle (Weiner and Weiner 1980). Ordinary cramps cease when the involved muscle is passively stretched (Bertolasi et al. 1993; Davison 1984; Graham 1965; Weiner and Weiner 1980) or with active contraction of its antagonist (Fowler 1973). Both of these maneuvers have been found to decrease a muscle's electrical activity (de Vries 1966; Helin 1985; Norris et al. 1957). The mechanisms proposed to explain the ability of these techniques to relieve cramps are conjectural (McGee 1990). Because stretching relieves acute cramps, some individuals propose that stretching exercises will prevent cramps (Daniell 1979; Matvienko and Kartasheva 1990; Sontag and Wanner 1988). One study found that a group of 44 patients was cured of nocturnal cramps after 1 week of brief calf-stretch exercises performed three times a day (Daniell 1979).

A cause of cramping in some women is *dysmenorrhea*, or excessively painful menstruation. A number of theories have been propounded to explain its cause, ranging from an imbalance in the normal estrogen-progesterone equilibrium to poor posture. Theoretically, the postural deviation involves shortening of fascial and ligamentous connective tissue around the uterus that restricts the posterior tilt of the pelvis, resulting in the subsequent pain (Billig 1943, 1951; Golub 1987; Rasch and Burke 1989). The poor-posture theory has led to a number of studies on the effect of exercise on dysmenorrhea.

The findings of several investigators (Billig and Lowendahl 1949; Golub 1987; Golub and Christaldi 1957; Golub et al. 1958; Golub et al. 1968) indicate that dysmenorrhea can be prevented or at least reduced through regular stretching of the pelvic area. Presumably, stretching the fascial bands and ligamentous tissue relieves the compression irritation of the involved nerves and prevents recurrence of the symptoms (Billig 1943, 1951).

Relief of Muscular Soreness

Slow stretching exercises may reduce and sometimes eliminate muscular soreness. Two types of pain are associated with muscular exercise: (1) pain during and immediately after exercise, which may persist for several hours, and (2) delayed, localized soreness, which usually does not appear until 24 to 48 hours after exercise (i.e., delayed-onset muscle soreness, or DOMS). Currently, disagreement regarding the physiological cause or causes of muscular soreness and how stretching supposedly reduces or eliminates it continues. Two questions will be explored here: Is stretching effective in relieving or preventing DOMS? If so, how does stretching produce these desired effects?

Through a series of experiments, de Vries (1961a, 1961b, 1966) found that electromyography (EMG) demonstrated no reduced soreness after stretching. Rather, EMG demonstrated reduced muscle activity level after stretching, which correlated with reduced complaint of soreness by test subjects. The explanation of this reduction is based on the notion that muscle soreness and spasms are associated with elevated muscle action potentials (MAPs). Thus, reducing excess muscular tension will reduce soreness (de Vries 1966). Muscle soreness should therefore be prevented if stretching reduced MAPs. The studies show that static stretching can significantly decrease electrical activity in the muscle to bring symptomatic relief of muscle soreness. In a study by Thigpen et al. (1985), static stretching brought about a statistically significant reduction of the H/M ratio (this term relates to the level of α–motor neuron excitability). The M and H waves are two discrete muscle action potentials. However, not all research supports these findings.

The effects of static stretching on muscle pain were also investigated by McGlynn et al. (1979b) and McGlynn and Laughlin (1980). They observed perceived pain of the static-stretching group was not significantly lower than that of the control group. Buroker and Schwane (1989) found that exercise-induced DOMS in eccentrically contracting muscles was not reduced either over the prolonged postexercise period by a regimen of intermittent stretching or immediately after the exercise by a bout of short-term stretching. Similarly, High et al. (1989) found no significant differences in soreness between volunteers who performed a preexercise stretching protocol, with or without warm-up, and subjects who performed the DOMS-inducing exercise without any preexercise activity. Wessel and Wan (1994) concluded that "a stretching protocol, performed before or after eccentric exercise, does not reduce delayed-onset muscle soreness" (p. 83). However, Rodenburg et al. (1994) found that the combination of a warm-up, stretching, and massage reduced some negative effects of eccentric exercise, but the results were inconsistent. Lund et al. (1998) studied the effect of passive stretching on DOMS after eccentric exercise. They concluded that "passive stretching did not have any significant influence on increased plasma CK, muscle pain, muscle strength, and the PCr/P_i ratio, indicating that passive stretching after eccentric exercise cannot prevent secondary pathological alterations" (p. 216). Johansson et al. (1999) suggested that "preexercise static stretching has no preventative effect on the muscular soreness, tenderness and force loss that follows heavy eccentric exercise" (p. 219). Ernest (1998) has criticized this study because the protocol did not allow a decision on whether the preexercise preparation or the postexercise massage brought about the decrease in DOMS. Ernest also criticized several

other studies because of their "serious methodological flaws" (p. 212). In conclusion, he writes: "Even though massage has some potential in reducing the symptoms of DOMS, its effectiveness has not been demonstrated convincingly. A definitive study seems to be warranted" (p. 214). Gulick et al. (1996) compared six different treatment groups (a nonsteroidal anti-inflammatory drug, high-velocity concentric muscle contractions, ice massage, 10-minute static stretching, topical ointment, and sublingual *Arnica montana* pellets) and one control group. There were no significant differences between the groups and "none were effective in abating the signs and symptoms of DOMS" (p. 145). Herbert and Gabriel (2002) conducted a systematic review of the current literature. Their finding was that stretching before or after exercise does not confer protection from muscle soreness and had no effect on DOMS.

There have been many theories on the mechanism by which stretching alleviates pain associated with exercise. Bobbert et al. (1986) postulated that stretching after exercise disperses the excess fluid that accumulates as a result of muscle damage and thus alleviates pain. However, Clarkson et al. (1992) demonstrated that peak swelling occurred 5 days after exercise. Consequently, peak swelling does not correspond with peak soreness (2 to 3 days). Armstrong (1984) proposed that stretching provides enough of a mechanical stimulus to alter the response of the group IV fibers that perhaps transmit sensations of DOMS. Additional research is required to determine how various stretching protocols may alleviate pain in some individuals.

Injury Prevention

The use of stretching exercises to increase flexibility is based on the idea that stretching decreases the incidence, intensity, or duration of musculotendinous and joint injury (Aten and Knight 1978; Brown 2002; Bryant 1984; Corbin and Noble 1980; Davis et al. 1965; Fredette 2001; Garrett et al. 1989; Hilyer et al. 1990; Smith 1994; Wiktorssohn-Möller et al. 1983). In theory, the risk of injury to the muscle-tendon unit is based on the notion that "tight" muscles are more likely to be strained. The assumption is that a more compliant muscle can be stretched further and to a higher ultimate strain and is therefore less susceptible to injury (Garrett 1993; Hunter and Spriggs 2000; Safran et al. 1998). Furthermore, increased flexibility is thought to increase a muscle's ability to absorb energy and control joint motion (Garrett 1993). This assumption has led to the long-held belief that stretching is important to reducing the risk of muscle-tendon unit injury (Fredette 2001; Garrett 1993; Hubley-Kozey and Stanish 1990). Currently there is "no" conclusive or substantive support for this claim (Comeau 2002; Garrett 1993; Gleim and McHugh 1997, 1999; Herbert and Gabriel 2002; Hunter and Spriggs 2000;

Knudson 1999; Pope et al. 1998; Pope et al. 2000; Shrier 1999, 2000, 2002; Shrier and Gossal 2000; Watson 2001). A review of the literature by Watson (2001) found only one prospective study (Ekstrand and Gillquist 1983) that indicated poor flexibility is a factor predisposing to injury in field games.

A four-year study of 136 physical education students by Twellaar et al. (1997) included 16 flexibility indices and four anthropometric characteristics. "No influence of flexibility or anthropometric variables on the total number of injuries or the number of several specific injuries (ankle sprain, muscle rupture, dislocation, shin splints, backache) could be established" (p. 66). In contrast, an investigation by Witvrouw et al. (2003) examined 146 male professional soccer players before the 1999–2000 Belgium soccer competition. The results indicated that "soccer players with an increased tightness [decreased ROM] of the hamstrings or quadriceps muscles have a statistically higher risk for a subsequent musculoskeletal lesion" (p. 41).

In two other studies (Jones et al. 1993; Knapik et al. 1992), the research suggested that the relationship between flexibility and injury may be bimodal or U-shaped: athletes with either very low or very high levels of flexibility in the hip/low back region have a higher incidence of various lower extremity injuries. However, other studies fail to support these findings (Hennessy and Watson 1993; Shambaugh et al. 1991; van Mechelen et al. 1993). Elaborating, Gleim and McHugh (1999) write

> The notion that decreased flexibility is associated with increased risk of sports injury has persisted despite the lack of any conclusive supporting evidence. Sports injury risk is multifactorial, and flexibility is a single intrinsic factor that tends to be studied in isolation. At best it could be concluded that the extremes of flexibility (both 'tight' and 'loose') may represent increased injury risk. However, flexibility patterns are specific to particular sports, and risk may be different for different sports. (p. 63)

The American College of Sports Medicine Position Stand (1998) has also acknowledged that "there is a lack of randomized, controlled clinical trials defining the benefit of flexibility exercise in the prevention and treatment of musculoskeletal injuries" (p. 984). Furthermore, Saal (1998) states, "The inability to clearly define injuries by a 'gold standard' diagnostic test has made it difficult to draw definitive conclusions regarding the relevance of any of the interventions used in daily practice on all levels of sports medicine" (p. 86). This controversial issue is further elaborated in chapter 14.

The claim that enhanced flexibility can reduce the risk of injury has been criticized because muscle-tendon unit injuries have multiple causes (Gleim and McHugh 1997; Hunter and Spriggs 2000). Furthermore, the claim is erroneous and misleading because several types of flexibility and stretching exercises (static, ballistic, active, and passive) are performed. Instead, Hunter and Spriggs (2000), Krivickas (1999) and Wilson et al. (1991) suggest that the measurement of muscle stiffness may be a more valid measurement than flexibility. Wilson, Wood, and Elliott (1991) write

> The musculo-tendinous unit represents the link between the skeletal system and muscular structures. As an external force is imposed on the musculature, a compliant system will extend to a greater extent allowing the applied force to be absorbed over a larger distance and greater time as compared to a stiff system. As such, the cushioning effect of a compliant system reduces the trauma on the muscle fibers decreasing the incidence of muscular injury as compared to a stiff musculo-tendinous system. (p. 407)

McHugh et al. (1999) found that stiffer subjects demonstrated symptoms of greater muscle damage in the hamstrings as compared with compliant subjects after eccentric exercise. McHugh et al. (1999) also proposed that the strain imposed by the active lengthening of stiff muscles is transferred from a rigid tendon-aponeurosis complex to the muscle fibers, resulting in myofibrillar strain. In compliant muscles, the tendon-aponeurosis complex is thought to absorb lengthening, thereby limiting myofibrillar strain. These researchers further suggested, "a theoretical explanation of the present results assumes that passive muscle stiffness reflects tendon-aponeurosis extensibility" (p. 598). Therefore, they also claim their study provides experimental evidence that "more-flexible people are less susceptible to exercise-induced muscle damage" (p. 598).

Research by McHugh et al. (1996) demonstrated that stiffness during the central portion of the ROM is related to terminal ROM measurements in individuals of varying flexibility ($r = -.91$). Furthermore, investigations (Halbertsma and Göeken 1994; Halbertsma et al. 1996; Magnusson et al. 1996a, 1996c) have demonstrated that an increase in ROM does not necessarily equate with a decrease in passive stiffness. Rather, improvements of ROM can be attributed to improved "stretch tolerance." However, this hypothesis was recently challenged by a novel investigation by Krabak et al. (2001).

Fifteen volunteers (mean age, 31.7 years) scheduled for arthroscopic surgery for unilateral knee injuries received either (1) spinal anesthesia with bupivacaine, (2) epidural anesthesia with lidocaine, (3) general anesthesia, or (4) femoral nerve block of injured leg only. The investigators hypothesized that potential neurologic contributions to ROM restriction could be neutralized by the anesthesia used during knee surgery. The intervention resulted in an increase in ROM, which reflected a neurologic contribution to hamstring length independent of pain. This finding contradicts earlier studies that related increase ROM to patient stretch tolerance, viscoelastic effects, or both (Magnusson, Simsonsen et al. 1995; Magnusson et al. 1996b, 1996d; Magnusson et al. 1997). Consequently, Krabak et al. (2001) point out

> The relative contribution of the neurologic system and the mechanical properties of the muscle-tendon unit to muscle flexibility continue to be investigated. Previous studies have attempted to divide these influences into either neural or predominantly viscoelastic muscle effects. Such a division, however, may represent an oversimplification of the various process involved." (p. 244)

Another aspect of the effectiveness of stretching to reduce injury is the concept of kinetic chain. A pertinent question is "[Do] studies of the ineffectiveness of stretching look at stretching one link in the kinetic chain to reduce injury elsewhere or were they concerned with merely local effects?" (Schur 2001a, p. 138). Clearly, the kinetic chain must be precisely delineated. "[I]t is important to be precise about what is being done to what, when, and for how long for comparisons to be made or for valid debate to proceed" (Schur 2001b, p. 364).

The validity of extrapolating research studies is also a significant factor in the supposed prophylaxis effect of stretching. Shrier (1999, 2000, 2001) points out that a review of the literature finds very little clinical evidence that stretching "immediately before" exercise and not stretching in general reduces injury. Furthermore, most studies have confounding results because they test the effects on injury of a pregame warm-up routine that includes both light cardiovascular exercise and a stretching routine. Consequently, which aspect of the warm-up routine exerts the protective effect is not known. Additional research is required before definitive conclusions can be reached.

More than minimal joint extensibility appears to be advantageous in some sports and vocations. However, several studies have contradicted the belief that increased flexibility correlates with improved performance. The jury is still out on whether enhanced flexibility can prevent muscle strain or joint sprain. Perhaps, an ideal or optimal range of flexibility exists that can prevent injury when muscles and joints are accidentally overstretched. However, this statement should not be interpreted to mean that maximum joint flexibility prevents injury. The question of whether any benefit is gained from stretching a muscle to an "extreme" ROM must be asked. In addressing this question, Hubley-Kozey and Stanish (1990) point out that some athletes, such as gymnasts, must be able to reach an extreme ROM without damaging the surrounding tissues. Not all athletes, however, need extreme ROM. Distance runners, for example, require a smaller ROM. Nevertheless, their ROM should be adequate to allow them to run without excessive soft-tissue resistance.

Insufficient data are available to assess the average ROMs required for different athletic activities. Normal ROMs have been determined only for healthy, nonathletic subjects. Physicians, therapists, and trainers must rely on their empirical experience and knowledge when suggesting how far athletes should stretch. Thus, in determining whether stretching a muscle to an extreme ROM provides any benefit, Hubley-Kozey and Stanish (1990) conclude, "most athletes do not need, and therefore should not attempt to reach, maximum or extreme ranges of motion" (p. 22). Furthermore, available data do not document the minimal amount of flexibility necessary to prevent injury or whether a lack of flexibility predisposes one to injury.

Almost 25 years ago, Corbin and Noble (1980) stated that conventional wisdom suggested that shortness of muscle and connective tissue limits joint mobility and may predispose a tight muscle or connective tissue to injury. Thus, they concluded that despite a wealth of empirical data on the subject, "common sense suggested that adherence to lengthening (stretching) and strengthening programs for athletes, vocational or avocational, would be wise" (p. 59). More recently, the American College of Sports Medicine Position Stand (1998) has also recommended the inclusion of flexibility exercises into an overall fitness plan. Its rationale was "based on the growing evidence of its [flexibility exercises] multiple benefits" (p. 984).

Enhanced Sleep

Another postulated side benefit of stretching is improved quality of sleep. One rationale is that stretching is relaxing and, hence, has a direct influence on the quality of sleep (Laughlin 2002b). This explanation is appealing but has numerous deficiencies. First, no clinical research supports this claim. Second, the claim is too broad. Third, specifics about the time or type of stretching are lacking. Presumably, slow, gentle, gradual stretching has the greatest likelihood of promoting sleep.

A second rationale for stretching is to prevent leg cramps during sleep. The argument is rejected because this condition probably has little to do with muscle extensibility. The Cooper Fitness Center (2002) is of the opinion that muscle cramping is most often caused by muscle dehydration and electrolyte imbalance. Therefore, stretching may relieve the symptoms, but a better remedy is increasing one's water intake and making dietary changes to include high sources of potassium.

A third rationale for stretching is that sleep positions and position shift during sleep impacts the quality of sleep (de Koninck et al. 1992; Gordon et al. 2002; Jamieson et al. 1995). Good sleep is associated with little nocturnal movement. de Koninck et al. (1992) found a progressive disappearance of prone sleep position and a progressive preference, very marked in the elderly, for right-side sleep position. They attribute the abandonment of prone positions "most likely attributable to the lack of flexibility of the spinal cord and/or the extra effort required for breathing from the respiratory cage" (p. 148). Gordon et al. (2002) suggest, "Decreasing range of cervical spine motion may protect against nocturnal postural stress or perhaps as subjects age they are simply adjusting their sleep posture accordingly" (p. 13). Jamieson et al. (1995) analyzed 22 subjects, 11 with ankylosing spondolylitis and 11 control subjects, and found, "A better sleep integrity with little nocturnal movement was related to a decrease in lumbar flexibility" (p. 73). Additional clinical evidence is required to substantiate whether stretching improves sleep hygiene. If so, dosages must be determined for specific populations: time to stretch, type of stretch, duration of stretch, and intensity of stretch.

Sex

A number of books, popular magazines, and Web sites discuss how stretching and improved flexibility can enhance one's sex life. The rationale is very direct.

- Greater flexibility allows partners a greater variety of unusual and athletic love positions. For example, the *Kama Sutra*, an ancient text, details 529 sexual positions.
- Stiffness can lead to fatigue, tiredness, or exhaustion and diminish sexual feelings. Therefore, optimum flexibility can enhance the sex act by improving muscular strength and endurance.
- Stretching and improved flexibility enhances kinesthetic pleasure because of better sexual movements.

- Stretching and an increased ROM enhance the quality of the orgasms.

In addition, proponents of stretching claim stretching helps fine-tune one's instrument to get the most out of his or her sex life.

Enjoyment and Pleasure

A flexibility-training program can provide many physical and mental advantages, not the least of which are enjoyment and pleasure. Stretching is refreshing and often results in a tingling and warm sensation. It is a simple way to both relax and reenergize. Yet, for some, a flexibility-training program may provide personal gratification and pleasure from just doing something good for themselves and from the pride in accomplishing set goals.

SUMMARY

Simply stated, flexibility is the range of motion available in a joint or group of joints. Flexibility is usually classified as ballistic, dynamic/functional, or static. Research indicates that flexibility is specific to particular joints or directions of movement. In addition, research has substantiated that patterns of flexibility are specific to groups of sports and even within groups of sports. Proponents contend that a flexibility-training program can have qualitative or quantitative benefits such as relaxation of stress and tension; muscular relaxation; self-discipline; improvement in body fitness, posture, and symmetry; relief of muscular cramps; relief of muscular soreness; reduced risk of low-back injury or pain; enhanced sleep; and improved sex life. In particular, optimal flexibility increases efficiency of movement.

2

Topics in Osteology and Arthrology

Osteology is the study of bones, and *arthrology* is the classification of the major joints and the movement potential of each joint. A basic understanding of both subjects is prudent because these topics relate to a major focus of this text: flexibility. (Note that conventional stretching procedures are not effective in cases where loss of motion is caused by abnormal joint structure.)

CLASSIFICATIONS OF STUDY

Virtually every bone moves at some joint (except the hyoid bone, which is situated at the base of the tongue and does not articulate with any other bone). Furthermore, the range of movement at most joints is restricted by both bone and joint structure. Thus, some knowledge of arthrokinesiology and osteokinematics is prudent. *Arthrokinesiology* is the study of the structure, function, and movement of skeletal joints (Neumann 2000). This term is derived from the combination of *kinesiology*, the science of movement, with the Greek prefix *arthro*, or joint. *Osteokinematics* describes the motion of a rotating bone about an axis of rotation oriented perpendicular to the path of the moving bone. In contrast, *arthrokinetics*, or intraarticular kinetics, describes the relative rotary and translatory movements of one articular surface on another (Williams et al. 1995).

CLASSIFICATION OF JOINTS AND THEIR INFLUENCE ON MOTION

The junction of two or more bones is an *articulation*, commonly known as a *joint*. Joints are classified according to the amount of movement they allow and according to their structural composition. The simpler classification is the one based on the amount of gross movement. According to this classification, *synarthroses* are immovable joints, *amphiarthroses* are slightly movable joints, and *diarthroses* are freely movable joints.

Articulating bones of diathroses have a variety of shapes. The classification based on structural composition has six different types of joints.

- *Ball-and-socket joints.* These joints provide the greatest amount and ROM, allowing movement in three directions. In this type of joint, a bone with a more or less rounded head (ball) lies in a cuplike or bowl-shaped cavity (socket). The hip is a ball-and-socket joint.

- *Condyloid or ellipsoid joints.* This type of joint permits movement in two directions: flexion-extension and abduction-adduction. The surface of the articulation is oval shaped, with an elliptical cavity on one bone receiving the other bone. The wrist joint between the radius and carpal bones is such a joint.

- *Hinge joints.* This type of joint allows angular movement in only one plane. Therefore, motion is limited to flexion and extension. This movement is similar to a door on a hinge, hence the name. The ankle, elbow, and knee are hinge joints.

- *Pivot joints.* These joints permit only a rotary movement in one axis. A ring rotates around a pivot, or a pivotlike process rotates within a ring that is formed of bone and connective tissue. This kind of joint occurs between the first and second cervical vertebrae (atlas and axis, respectively), where head rotation occurs on the neck, and between the radius and ulna, where forearm pronation and supination take place.

- *Plane or gliding joints.* This type of joint permits gliding movements only. The facet joints of the vertebrae in the spine and the intercarpal joints of the hand are such joints. In this type of joint, the articular surfaces are nearly flat, or one surface may be slightly convex and the other slightly concave.

- *Saddle joints.* This joint resembles a saddle on a horse's back. The surface of each bone is concave in one direction but convex in the perpendicular direction. This joint allows movement in two directions: flexion-extension and abduction-adduction. The best example of a saddle joint is the carpometacarpal joint at the base of the thumb.

TYPES OF MOTION

Six primary types of osteokinetic (voluntary or active) movement that a body segment can pass through and several special types of movements are described below.

- *Flexion* is a movement that generally decreases an angle (see figure 2.1a)

- *Extension* is lengthening or stretching. When extension continues beyond the anatomical position, it is called *hyperextension* (see figure 2.1b).

- *Abduction* is the movement of a body segment away from the midline of the body or of the body part to which it is attached (i.e., away from the median plane of the body) (see figure 2.1c).

- *Adduction* is the opposite of abduction. It is the movement of a body segment toward the midline of the body or of the body part to which it is attached (see figure 2.1d).

- *Rotation* is the pivoting or moving of a body segment around its own axis (see figure 2.1e).

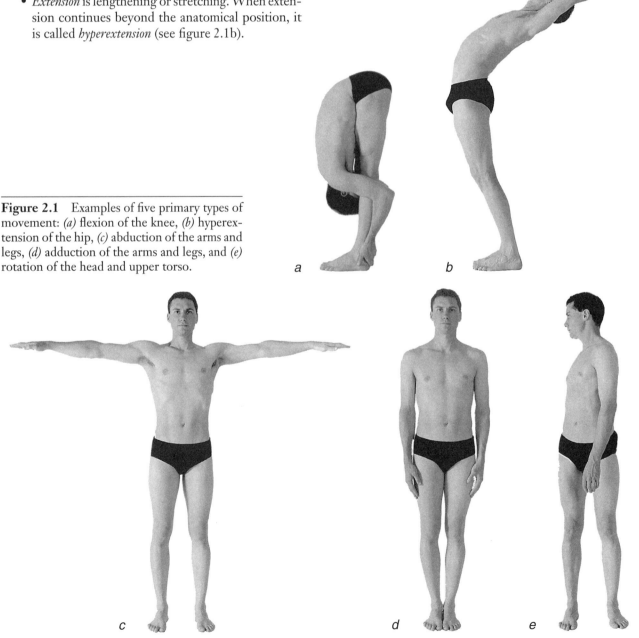

Figure 2.1   Examples of five primary types of movement: *(a)* flexion of the knee, *(b)* hyperextension of the hip, *(c)* abduction of the arms and legs, *(d)* adduction of the arms and legs, and *(e)* rotation of the head and upper torso.

a   b

c   d   e

- *Circumduction* is movement that allows the end of the segment to describe or trace a circle. Circumduction is often a combination of flexion, abduction, extension, and adduction.
- *Supination* is the outward rotation of the forearm.
- *Pronation* is the inward rotation of the forearm.
- *Inversion* is the turning of the sole of the foot inward.
- *Eversion* is the outward rotation of the sole of the foot.
- *Dorsiflexion* is bending the ankle so that the dorsum (top) of the foot comes closer to the anterior (front) surface of the shin.
- *Plantar flexion* is straightening the ankle, or pointing the foot, so that the foot's dorsum moves away from the shin.
- *Protraction* is a pushing, or forward, motion of the shoulder, scapula, and clavicle.
- *Retraction* is a pulling, or backward, motion of the shoulder, scapula, and clavicle.

RELATIONSHIP BETWEEN BONE GROWTH AND FLEXIBILITY

Sutro (1947) proposed a growth hypermobility hypothesis suggesting that hypermobility was probably a disproportion in the relative rate of growth of the bones and their attached ligaments. In other words, an excess of ligament may lead to hypermobility. In a footnote, Sutro (1947) stated

> In certain stages of development of the skeleton the rate of bone growth may not be parallel to that of the ligamentous and capsular tissues. This may lead to a relative excess of insufficiency of ligaments with either laxity or rigidity of the bones comprising the joint. (p. 74)

In the subsequent years, this secondary hypothesis that growth rate may result in rigidity of bones composing a joint was expanded and clarified by others to explain the observed phenomenon of reduced flexibility and increased "tightness." It has been postulated that an increase in muscle-tendon tightness about the joints and a loss of flexibility can occur during periods of rapid skeletal growth. The increase is possibly caused by the bones growing much faster than the muscles grow and stretch (Bachrach 1987; Howse 1987; Kendall and Kendall 1948; Leard 1984; Micheli 1983). Today, longitudinal growth is known to occur in bones along with the soft tissues, such as the muscles and tendons. However, there is a time variable between the growth of bones and the soft tissues. Since the muscles and their respective connective tissues lag behind in growth, greater tension, tightness, and growing pain results. Therefore, this disproportion in

relative growth of the bones and their connective tissues has been suggested as a partial explanation for increased tightness of children growing into adolescence.

A specific area of concern is increased tension and tightness in the lower back. The lumbar fascia may possibly be unable to keep up with bony growth during the adolescent growth spurt, leading to a tethering effect and subsequent hyperlordosis (Bachrach 1987; Micheli 1983b; Poggini et al. 1999). This issue is a potential concern for ballet dancers.

Eventually, this increased passive tension stimulates the production of additional sarcomeres (the functional unit of a muscle), resulting in a subsequent decrease in tightness. Consequently, Micheli (1983b) recommends that children consistently perform stretching exercises to maintain flexibility and prevent injuries. Baxter and Dulberg (1988) reported that stretching decreased the duration of growing pains in children 5 to 14 years of age. Howse (1987) states, "It is extremely important that the child be actively discouraged from any excessive stretching during these periods [i.e., when the growth spurt ceases and the soft tissues catch up in growth and the previous mobility is restored], as stretching muscles that have weakened during the growth can cause damage" (p. 110). The question remains: Is there a transient loss of flexibility associated with peak height velocity during adolescence?

Pratt (1989) found no evidence of such deficits in a cross-sectional sample of 84 male students. Pratt employed the Tanner staging (TS) assessment, which determines sexual maturity using a rating of I (immature) to V (mature), based on pubic hair growth and pattern. His hypothesis was that the TS had greater predictive value than chronological age for strength and flexibility. He found boys at TS II and TS III to be markedly less flexible than boys at TS IV and TS V.

Naish and Apley (1951) challenged the hypothesis that growth is the cause of growing pains. They pointed out that most growing pains occur between the ages of 8 and 12 years, or slightly earlier than the adolescent growth spurt, which normally occurs between 10 and 14 years of age. Consequently, they recommended that "The term 'growing pains' should be discarded since the pains have no demonstrable connexion with growth" (p. 138). In addition, most sites of pain did not correspond to sites of maximal growth. Another shortfall of the hypotheses is that toe-touch flexibility appears to decrease from young childhood to young adolescence (Gurewitsch and O'Neill 1944; Kendall and Kendall 1948; Kraus and Hirschland 1954), even though the growth rate is slowing during this period (Feldman et al. 1999).

Feldman et al. (1999) attempted to determine whether adolescent growth is associated with decreases in flexibility. Over 600 students, 13 to 14 years of age, were measured at 0 months, 6 months, and 12 months. The investigators concluded that, "growth could not cause a decrease in flexibility, but rather is only associated with it" (p. 28). However, Micheli (2000) raised several points of concern about the conclusions of the Feldman et al. (1999) study. First, a time interval of every 3 months was necessary to capture the growth spurt phase. Second, "the prepubescent growth spurt in girls and boys occurred with 95% confidence between the ages of 11 and 13 years and 12 and 14 years, respectively, whereas Feldman's girls and boys were somewhat older, and thus may have had their peak growth spurt before the study" (p. 76). Third, neither chronological nor skeletal age was an accurate predictor of peak growth, and a wide deviation from "normality" in growth occurred.

WOLFF'S LAW

Wolff's law states that bone growth and remodeling is directly dependent on the mechanical load placed on it. The law is based on three principles: (1) reduced biomechanical stress leads to reduced tissue formation; (2) the more stress placed on bones, the stronger they become; and (3) increased biomechanical stress increases bone density and potentially size. Bone can be modified by excessive stress. For example, excess stress applied to the ankle decreases range of motion because of the formation of spurs on the anterior and posterior lips of the talus and osteophytes on the tibia impinging on the front of the ankle. Conversely, architectural modifications in the tarsal bones promoting increased ROM occur in dancers who begin training before 12 years of age.

CLOSE-PACKED POSITION AND ITS RELATION TO FLEXIBILITY

The *close-packed position* is the final position in which "the joint surfaces become fully congruent, their area of contact is maximal, and they are tightly compressed having in a sense been 'screwed-home,' while the fibrous capsule and ligaments are maximally spiralized and tense, and no movement is possible" (Williams et al. 1995, p. 483). Close-packed joint surfaces can be described as having their articulating bones temporarily locked together, as if no joint existed between them. Thus, it is the position of maximum joint stability (Magee 2002). See table 2.1.

LOOSE-PACKED POSITION AND ITS RELATION TO FLEXIBILITY

The *loose-packed position* is the position in which the articulating surfaces are not congruent, and some parts of the articular capsule are lax. In this position, the joint capsule has its greatest capacity. This position is important because an examiner will utilize it to test joint play movement. In addition, it is the most common position for treatment using joint play mobilizations (Magee 2002). See table 2.1.

SUMMARY

Arthrokinesiology is the study of the structure, function, and movement of skeletal joints. Basic knowledge of the terminology and methods of classifying joints and their motions is essential for describing joint movements with accuracy and precision. Ultimately, range of motion at a joint is restricted by both bone and joint structure. Research has yet to determine whether, during periods of rapid skeletal growth, an increase in muscle-tendon tightness about the joints and a loss of flexibility results from the bones growing much faster than the muscles grow and stretch.

Table 2.1   Close-Packed Versus Loose-Packed Position

Joint	Close-packed position	Loose-packed position
Ankle	Dorsiflexion	Neutral
Knee	Full extension	Semiflexion
Hip	Extension + medial rotation	Semiflexion
Vertebrae	Hyperextension	Neutral
Shoulder	Abduction + lateral rotation	Semiabduction
Wrist	Hyperextension	Semiflexion

Reprinted, by permission, from M.J. Alter, 1996, *Science of flexibility,* 2nd ed. (Champaign, IL: Human Kinetics), 15.

Contractile Components of Muscle: Limiting Factors of Flexibility

The three categories of muscle tissue are skeletal (striated), smooth (nonstriated), and cardiac. Skeletal muscle most directly relates to flexibility and will be the major focus. This chapter will review the major lines of research regarding the ultrastructure of skeletal muscle as it relates to stretching and flexibility. In later chapters, this information will provide a foundation for the theoretical mechanisms of muscle injury and soreness. Knowledge of the primary structure of skeletal muscle is necessary for understanding the critical role of skeletal muscle's components and their respective functions.

GENERAL OVERVIEW OF SKELETAL MUSCLES

Skeletal muscles vary in shape and size. The central portion of a whole muscle is called the *belly*. The belly comprises smaller compartments called *fasciculi*. Each fasciculus consists in turn of approximately 100 to 150 individual muscle *fibers* that range from 1 to 40 μm (micrometers) in length and 10 to 100 μm in diameter (1 mm = 0.03937 in.; 1 in. = approximately 25.4 mm; 1 μm = 0.000039 in.). Each muscle fiber constitutes a single muscle cell. When viewed under a microscope, individual muscle fibers have a banded or striated structure. This banding pattern reflects the ultrastructural organization of each myofibril. Thus, to understand how muscles contract, relax, and elongate, one must understand the structure of the myofibril.

COMPOSITION OF MYOFIBRILS AND THEIR CONSTITUENTS

Each muscle fiber is actually composed of many smaller units called *myofibrils*. Myofibrils range in diameter from 1 to 2 μm. They are grouped in clusters and run the length of the muscle fiber. In turn, each myofibril comprises long, thin strands of serially linked sarcomeres (*sarco* = flesh; *mere* = unit). *Sarcomeres* are the functional unit of a muscle. Sarcomeres measure approximately 2.3 μm in length and repeat themselves in a specific pattern in each myofibril. At the end of each sarcomere is a dense boundary, termed the Z-line (also known as the Z-band or Z-disk). The term Z-line is derived from the German word *zwischen*, meaning *between*. Thus, the segment between two successive Z-lines represents the functional unit of a myofibril.

Myofibrils comprise even smaller structures called *myofilaments*, or *filaments* for short. (The term *filament* will be used throughout the text.) Originally, two types of filaments, one thin (*actin*) and one thick (*myosin*), were thought to reside within the sarcomere. Based upon early research, a typical myofibril was determined to contain about 450 thick filaments in the center of the sarcomere and about 900 thin filaments at each end of the sarcomere. From this data, a single muscle fiber 10 nm in diameter and 1 cm long was then calculated to contain about 8,000 myofibrils and each myofibril to consist of 4,500 sarcomeres. Consequently, a single fiber contains 16 billion thick and 64 billion thin filaments (Vander et al. 1975)!

At the molecular level, the chemical composition of the filaments can be determined. The filaments are made of protein formed by a sequence of amino acids and manufactured within the muscle cell. The synthesis of amino acids is controlled by the chromosomes in the muscle cell nucleus. These chromosomes are a spiraled form of deoxyribonucleic acid (DNA), which contains the sequence of genes necessary to tell the muscle how to order the amino acids correctly. Stretching theoretically modifies gene expression (see Effects of Immobilization, page 31).

REGIONS OF THE SARCOMERE

Myofibrils are characterized by alternating light and dark areas when observed with an optical microscope. Altogether, there are five well-defined bands or zones within a sarcomere. The Z-line, or Z-disk, forms the dense line at either end of the sarcomere (i.e., the terminal point of the sarcomere). Under high-resolution microscopy, the Z-line has a zigzag appearance, partially because the thin filaments on either side of the Z-line are not collinear. They are offset by half the filaments' lateral separation. This two-line configuration has the capacity to accommodate substantial variation in the myofibrillar diameter by either increasing or decreasing the lateral separation between the filaments. This structural malleability can possibly contribute to muscle's pliability.

Adjacent to the Z-line is the *I-band*, an optically less dense band of the muscle striations. When passed through the muscle's I-band, the velocity of the emerging light is *isotropic* (the same in all directions). The I-band contains actin filaments, titin filaments, and I-bridges (see figure 3.1). The I-band measures approximately 1.5 µm in length. The dark areas of the sarcomere are called *A-bands*, so-called because a light wave passing through them is *anisotropic* (its velocity is not equal in all directions). The A-bands measure approximately 1.0 µm and correspond to the length of the thick filaments. A relatively less dense and lighter area, the H-zone, occupies the center of each A-band, between the tips of the thin filaments. Its size depends on the muscle length or the extent of overlap of the filaments. Last, there is the *M-line*, a dense, transverse structure located at the center of the sarcomere, corresponding to several closely spaced, parallel M-bridges.

ULTRASTRUCTURE OF THE CONNECTING, OR GAP FILAMENT: TITIN

Originally, sarcomeres were thought to consist of just two filaments: actin and myosin. However, after years of research a third filament, *titin*, was discovered (see figure 3.2). The significance of this discovery will be elaborated below.

Titin's Structure

Titin is a giant protein (approximately 3,000 to 4,000 kd; approximately 1 µm long) that spans half of the striated muscle sarcomere, from the Z-discs to the M-lines (Furst et al. 1988; Itoh et al. 1988; Wang et al. 1985; Whiting et al. 1989). Titin constitutes about 10% of myofibril mass (Trinick et al. 1984; Wang et al. 1984). It is primarily composed of approximately 300 modules in two motif types: immunoglobulin (Ig) and fibronectin type III (FnIII) domains. Proteins of the titin family are the longest single polypeptide chains currently known (Kurzban and Wang 1988; Maruyama et al. 1984). Furthermore, human titin has 234 exons, the largest number in a single human gene (Wang, Forbes, and Jin 2001). In the I-band region of a sarcomere, four amino acids P (proline), E (glutamate), V (valine), and K (lysine) constitute 70% of this element. Therefore, Labeit and Kolmerer (1995) coined the term, the PEVK, to describe this region of titin. The PEVK region is mainly responsible for passive tension (i.e., elasticity) generation and acts as extensible springs under stretch.

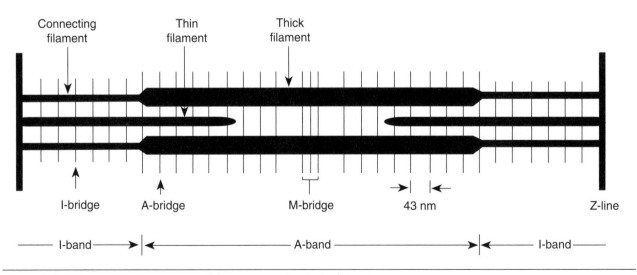

Figure 3.1 Diagrammatic summary of the sarcomere's principal structures.
Reprinted from Pollack 1990.

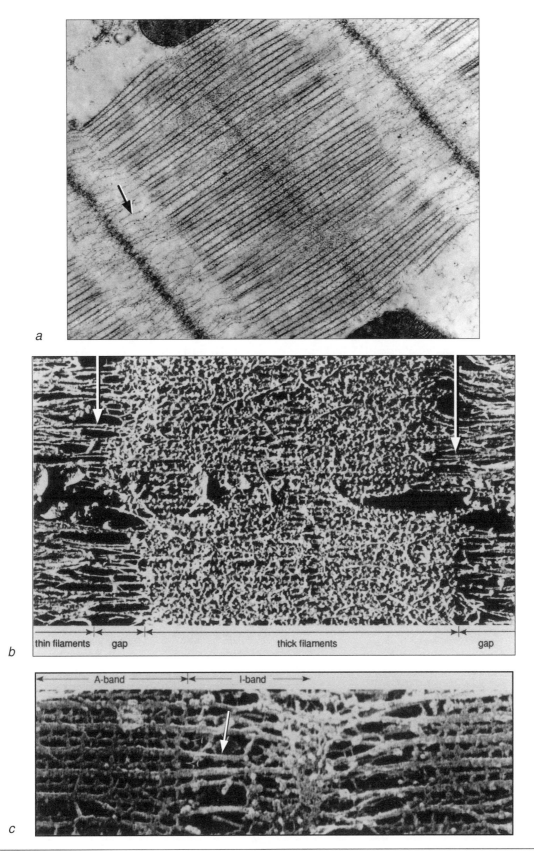

a

b

c

Figure 3.2 *(a)* Direct evidence for connecting filaments in flight muscle of honeybee. During fixation, thin filaments were depolymerized and washed away. Connecting filaments remain intact and visible (arrow). Photo by Trombitás and Tigyi-Sebes. *(b)* Examples of connecting filaments (titin). Overstretched frog muscle, prepared by freeze-fracture, deep-etch method. Thick filaments (center) do not terminate; they give way to thinner "connecting" filaments (arrows), which run out of the field toward the Z-line. Thin-filament tips, seen at edges of figure, do not overlap the thick filaments. Photo by M.E. Cantino and G.H. Pollack. *(c)* Freeze-fracture image of honeybee flight muscle in rigor. Thin filaments dislodged from Z-line (arrowheads). Connecting filaments are visible in the I-band (arrow).

Reprinted from Pollack 1990.

Tskhovrebova and Trinick (2001) suggest a three-zone scheme with a different organization of titin present in the I-band: (1) Outside the tip of the thick filament, 0.1 μm long segments of titin molecules are associated side-by-side in bundles consisting of several molecules; (2) between approximately 0.1 μm from the end of the thick filament and 0.1 μm from the center of the Z-line, the molecules appear separate; and (3) at approximately 0.1 μm from the Z-line center, titin binds to thin filaments (see figure 3.3).

What Makes the Titin Filament So Extensible?

The extensibility of titin appears to be over fourfold, while remaining elastic (Kellermayer and Granzier 1996). Several factors theoretically contribute to titin's tremendous extensibility. Titin is rich in the amino acid *proline*, which breaks the α-helical chains that ordinarily confer rigidity on polypeptides (Pollack 1990). A single titin molecule does not contain any α-helical structure. Instead, it consists of *random coils* (Trinick et al. 1984). A single peptide of 3 million daltons could have a length up to 7.0 μm. However, at rest, a sarcomere's length is about 2.4 μm, and at extreme stretch, it is 7.0 μm. Tskhovrebova and Trinick (2000) suggest two types of mechanisms to explain the extensibility associated with the I-band of titin: *entropic*, involving straightening the molecular from an originally coiled state, and *enthalpic*, involving mechanical unfolding of the titin's internal structure. In either case, the result is the high capacity for extensibility.

What Is Responsible for Titin's Elasticity?

Elasticity refers to the property of a tissue to return to its original shape after a force is removed. Politou et al. (1996) suggest elasticity may be caused in part by the exposure of the hydrophobic residues during elongation of the titin molecule, thus resulting in a strong tendency to return to its original folded state. Another possible explanation is the unfolding sequence of the various titin domains (Politou et al. 1995), with each domain influenced by the adjacent domains.

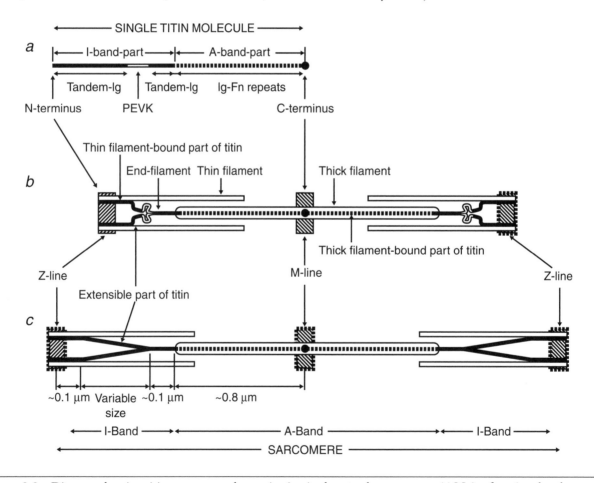

Figure 3.3 Diagram showing titin structure and organization in the muscle sarcomere. *(a)* Major functional and structural regions of the titin molecule. *(b)* Probable titin arrangement in muscle at slack sarcomere length and *(c)* during sarcomere extension and developing passive tension.

Reprinted from Tskhovrebova and Trinick 2000.

Elasticity

In the literature about titin, "elasticity" is sometimes confused with "extensibility." Elasticity is a thermodynamically reversible material property. Any elastic specimen is necessarily also extensible, but extensibility is a much more loosely defined term. It means simply the ability to extend with no implication of reversibility. This distinction is of particular relevance to titin, which is extensible but is known to suffer irreversible damage if stretched too far (Politou et al. 1995, pp. 2607-2608).

Regulation of Muscle Extensibility

Two critical questions need to be raised: (1) What regulates muscle extensibility? (2) Can the factor(s) regulating this muscle extensibility be modified to enhance one's flexibility? Wang et al. (1991) investigated the first issue. They found that the length and size of titin appears to be an important factor in determining when sarcomeres will develop resting tension and where the sarcomere will yield under stress. For example, muscles that express larger titin *isoforms* (structural variants) initiate tension at longer sarcomere lengths and reach their elastic limit at higher sarcomere lengths. In addition, muscles that express the longest titin develop the lowest tension. Wang et al. (1991) also concluded that different muscle groups express various types of titin isoforms and thus exhibit various stress-strain curves.

Thus, the data suggested "skeletal muscle cells may control and modulate stiffness and elastic limit coordinately by selective expression of specific titin isoforms" (Wang et al. 1991, p. 7101). Observed anatomical variations in titin isoforms have been reported in muscles from various regions of the body (Akster et al. 1989; Hill and Weber 1986; Horowits 1992; Hu et al. 1986; Wang and Wright 1988). Mutungi and Ranatunga (1996) have also raised the intriguing possibility that viscoelastic differences between fast-slow twitch muscle fibers (discussed below in Muscle Fiber Type and Fiber Architecture, p. 27) may reflect differences in titin isoforms. Existence of these isoforms raises the question: Can differences in titin isoforms in slow or fast muscle fiber be deliberately modified by rehabilitation and training? Avela et al. (1999) postulated that sustained passive stretching could modify titin and result in some irregularities of filament overlapping. Consequently, this overlapping could lead to increased compliance of the sarcomere and to a decrease in the number of attached cross-bridges, which, in turn, would lead to "a reduced external force response to stretch and, therefore, a decrease in the mechanical effect on the muscle spindles" (p. 1290). Thus, the modified titin could result in an altered reflex sensitivity.

Why differential titin isoform expression occurs in healthy, mature skeletal muscle or what influence this expression may have on performance is not clear (Fry et al. 1997). McBride et al. (2003) have speculated, "If in fact titin plays such a significant role in contributing to human movement via elastic energy storage and re-utilization then it would stand to reason that a more elastic muscle via altered titin isoforms would be related to a more powerful performance" (p. 554). Assuming differential titin isoforms can influence performance, a pertinent question is once again raised: Can training be tailored to deliberately influence specific titin isoforms? To date, no research has been carried out in this arena. Nevertheless, a study could be conducted to compare and contrast the titin isoforms in identical muscle groups among performers involved in various disciplines known for their outstanding flexibility (e.g., ballet, rhythmic gymnastics, and long-term adherents of hatha yoga) and compare the results to those of practitioners of other disciplines (e.g., marathon runners or shot putters). Any differences found might help determine what type of stretching program could most efficiently and safely be implemented to enhance the optimal titin isoform production. Another crucial question arises: Does the body experience critical periods during which titin is being manufactured and its structure can be modified? One may speculate that the earlier one starts on a stretching program, the greater the titin isoform modification.

The relationship between titin degradation and various neuromuscular diseases such as Schwartz-Jampel syndrome (Soussi-Yanicostas et al. 1991) and Duchenne muscular dystrophy (DMD) has been investigated. Defects in titin have now been linked to several types of muscular dystrophy (Haravuori et al. 2001; Sorimachi, Ono, and Suzuki 2000; van der Ven et al. 2000). Matsumura and colleagues (1989) state that the degradation of titin "even though secondary, is presumed to play an important role in the pathogenesis of myofibrillar degeneration in DMD" (p. 147). The role of titin in cardiac tissue is also receiving increasing attention (Granzier et al. 2002; Linke et al. 2002). An important issue that needs to be investigated is the influence of various medications upon titin isoforms.

For those involved in athletic training and rehabilitation, the following questions are significant: Does titin isoform modification occur as a result of trauma? If so, how does the body react in the case of a macrotrauma (e.g., a car accident)? Similarly, can isoform modifications be caused by microtraumatic insults (e.g., long-term poor posture)? What are the effects of immobilization or reduced movement on titin isoforms? What is the influence of stretching on titin as a consequence of a traditional flexibility-training program or rehabilitation regimen?

Function of Titin

Titin is speculated to serve a variety of functions. (1) It plays a major role in muscle's elasticity. Because the elastic elements link each end of the thick filament to the Z-line, the titin filaments can produce resting tension, which is present when the muscle fiber is at its normal physiological length and increases as a relaxed fiber is elongated. (2) Titin contributes to stability because it also provides a force that tends to center the thick filaments within the sarcomere (Horowits and Podolsky 1987a; Horowits 1992; Liversage et al. 2001). (3) Titin may facilitate the transition of intermolecular interactions between the arrays of thick and thin filaments (Tskhovrebova and Trinick 2000). (4) Goulding et al. (1997) suggest that a major function of titin is to ensure uniform sarcomere length over the entire muscle and thus prevent localized myofibril overstretch during isometric contraction. (5) Klee et al. (2002) believe that restoring sarcomere length after stretching is the most important function of titin. (6) Titin is responsible for the sarcomere's extraordinary extensibility. (7) Titin may play a role in the morphogenesis of the myofibril (Fulton and Isaacs 1991; Liversage et al. 2001; Pollack 1990). (8) An elastic portion of titin has an affinity for calcium ions and has binding sites. This property could impact the contraction-relaxation cycle of skeletal muscle (Tatsumi et al. 2001) and affect cardiac contractile properties (Linke et al. 2002).

Desmin

Desmin (also known as skeletin), another protein found in the sarcomere, is a 53-kd protein composed of some 300 amino acids. It is the major subunit of the intermediate protein filaments forming the Z-discs (Wang and Ramirez-Mitchell 1983). Desmin connects Z-discs transversely and to organelles (Goebel 2002). It also extends longitudinally from Z-disc to Z-disc (Wang et al. 1993; Wang and Ramirez-Mitchell 1983). Desmin contributes to the exosarcomeric cytoskeleton and lengthens as the sarcomere is stretched. Consequently, desmin may contribute to the passive resistance of a stretched muscle (Gajdosik 2001). "Desmin-related disorders are myopathies that develop sporadically or in families following autosomal-dominant or recessive modes of inheritance" (Goebel 2002, p. 265).

SARCOMERE STRUCTURAL BRIDGES

The myofibrillar sarcomere not only is held together in the axial direction but must also be supported in the transverse direction. Something must protect a muscle when it is squeezed or sat upon (as are the gluteals), and the source of the transverse resistance that maintains the sarcomere's integrity are three bridgelike structures: the M-bridges, A-bridges, and I-bridges (see figures 3.1 and 3.4).

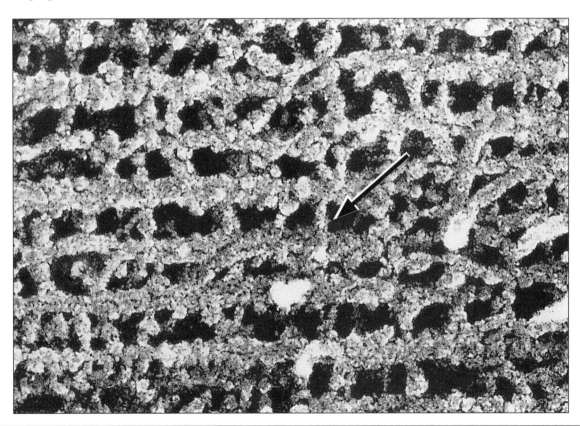

Figure 3.4 Runglike interconnections between thick filaments. Photo by K. Trombitás.
Reprinted from Pollack 1990.

M-Bridges, A-Bridges, and I-Bridges

In some muscles, the organizing center of the sarcomere contains transverse, runglike interconnections between the thick filaments called M-bridges. Their function is to help organize and stabilize the filament lattice (Pollack 1990). Because some muscles lack M-bridges, additional structures called A-bridges and I-bridges must help to stabilize the filament lattice. (Pollack 1990). A-bridges are runglike interconnections between adjacent, parallel thick filaments (Baatsen et al. 1988; Magid et al. 1984; Pollack 1983, 1990; Suzuki and Pollack 1986). A-bridges organize and stabilize the myosin filaments. I-bridges are runglike interconnections that span the gap between the titin and actin filaments. First noted by Franzini-Armstrong (1970) and then Reedy (1971), I-bridges are believed to be built of troponin. Pollack (1990) has suggested that the function of these struts is to confer lateral stability and maintain separation of the filaments.

THEORY OF CONTRACTION

The function of muscle is to develop or generate tension in a process called *contraction*, which, in turn, produces movement. Contraction also maintains posture and produces body heat. Once a muscular contraction is initiated, a reversible chain of physical and chemical events is set into motion.

Ultrastructural (Physical) Basis of Contraction

The exact mechanism that regulates muscle contraction, relaxation, and elongation is not yet completely understood. The best-known theory, the sliding filament theory (see figure 3.5, a-c), asserts that the changes in sarcomere length are mediated exclusively by relative sliding of thick and thin filaments. A maximally contracted sarcomere may shorten from 20% to 50% of its resting length. When passively stretched, it may extend to about 120% of its normal length. Measurements of the A-bands and I-bands from intact muscle in the contracted, relaxed, and elongated states have conclusively proved that the A-bands, and thus the thick filaments, always remain constant in length. Similarly, the distance between the Z-line and the edge of the H-zone also remains constant during normal contraction, indicating that the thin actin filaments likewise undergo no change in length. Based on these observations, researchers have concluded that change in muscle length must result from the sliding of the thick and thin filaments along each other.

For contraction to occur, the Z-line of the sarcomere must be drawn in toward the A-band, resulting in the gradual narrowing and eventual elimination of the I-bands and H-zone. Thus, muscles pull but do not push.

Molecular (Chemical) Basis of Contraction

The immediate source of energy for muscular contraction is the breakdown of adenosine triphosphate (ATP), which is triggered by nerve impulses. When nerve impulses reach a skeletal muscle fiber, they spread over its sarcolemma and move inward via its T-tubules. This process increases the permeability and triggers the release of calcium ions (Ca^{2+}) from the sacs of the sarcoplasmic reticulum. In the resting state, tropomyosin molecules are believed to lie on top of active sites on the actin filaments, preventing binding of the myosin cross-bridges and actin filament. Ca^{2+} binds with the troponin molecules on the actin filament, thereby "turning on" the active sites on the actin filament. Simultaneously, the ATP cross-bridge complex is charged, permitting the actin and myosin to form an actomyosin complex. This process activates myosin ATPase, an enzyme component of the myosin filament. Myosin ATPase breaks down ATP into ADP (adenosine diphosphate) and P_i (inorganic phosphate), releasing energy. This energy release allows the cross-bridges to swivel to and slide over the myosin filament toward the center of the sarcomere. Consequently, the muscle shortens and develops tension. Thus, muscles depend on nerve impulses for activation and subsequent generation of muscular tension.

THEORY OF MUSCULAR RELAXATION

Muscular relaxation is essential for optimal movement and health. Hence, the process of muscular relaxation has been studied intensively. Like contraction, the exact mechanism of relaxation is not fully understood. The physical and chemical basis of relaxation will be analyzed in the following sections.

Ultrastructural (Physical) Basis of Relaxation

Muscular relaxation is completely passive. Muscle fibers relax when they no longer receive nerve impulses, that is, at cessation of muscular tension. As the cross-bridges detach and separate, the internal elastic force that accumulated during contraction is released. Thus, the recoil of the elastic components restores the myofibrils to their uncontracted lengths. A second possible restoring force could arise when overlapping thin filaments repel one another because of their similar net charge. Pollack (1990, p. 142) suggests "such restoring forces may be more than mere luxuries; they reduce the energetic cost of relaxation." In addition, the elasticity of the connective tissues that attach muscle to the bone restores the muscle to its original length.

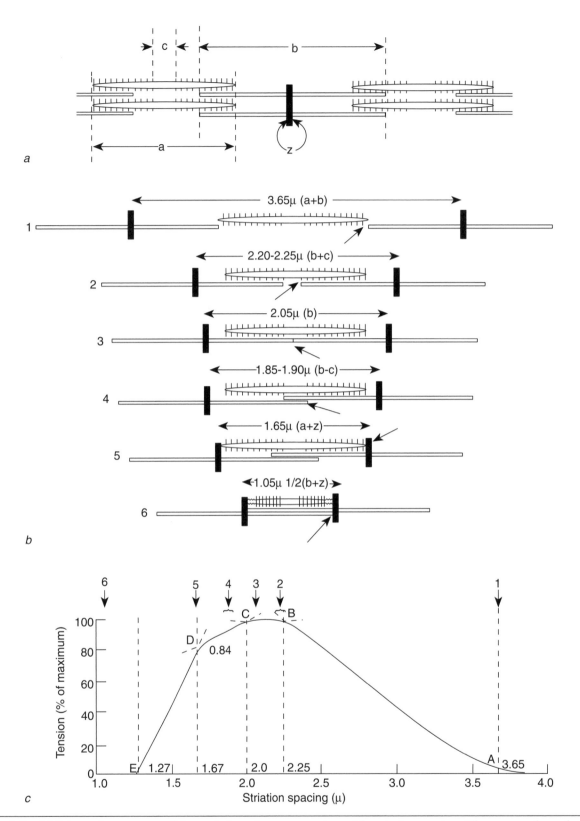

Figure 3.5 (*a*) Schematic summary of the variation of tetanus tension with striation spacing. The arrows along the top are placed opposite the striation spacing at which the critical stages of overlap of filaments occur, numbered as in (*c*). (*b*) Schematic diagram of filaments, indicating nomenclature for the relevant dimensions. (*c*) Critical stages in the increase of overlap between thick and thin filaments as a sarcomere shortens.

Reprinted from Gordon, Huxley, and Julian 1966b.

Molecular (Chemical) Basis of Relaxation

Most scientists believe that muscle relaxation is brought about by a reversal of the contraction process. In relaxation, calcium-troponin combinations separate, and Ca^{2+} reenters the sarcoplasmic reticulum. Because the troponin is no longer bound to the calcium, it prevents actin from interacting with myosin. This inhibition allows dissociation of actin and myosin and "resliding" of the filaments back to their resting positions. In short, contraction is "turned on" by the release of calcium and "turned off" by its withdrawal.

THEORETICAL LIMIT OF MUSCULAR ELONGATION

Muscular fibers are incapable of lengthening or stretching themselves. A force must be received from outside the muscle, such as gravity, momentum (motion), the force of antagonistic muscles, or the force provided by another person or by some part of one's own body.

The theoretical limitation of a muscle cell's contractile component, based on the sliding filament theory, can be determined by microscopic measurements of the length of the sarcomere (2.30 μm), the myosin filaments (1.50 μm), the actin filaments (2.00 μm), and the H-zone (0.30 μm). When a sarcomere is stretched to the point of rupture, it can reach a length of approximately 3.60 μm. The length at which the filaments slightly overlap, without rupture of the sarcomere and with at least one cross-bridge maintained between the actin and myosin filaments, is approximately 3.50 μm. Thus, with the sarcomere's resting length 2.30 μm, the contractile component of the sarcomere is capable of increasing by 1.20 μm. This increase is more than 50% of the resting length. If the sarcomere's resting length is 2.10 μm and all other factors remain constant, the contractile component of the muscle can then increase by 67%. This extensibility enables our muscles to move through a wide ROM. Chapters 4 through 6 examine how connective tissues and the nervous system (e.g., muscle spindles) interact with muscle to limit ROM. The theoretical limitation of sarcomere elongation is significant in terms of the "popping hypothesis" as it relates to muscle soreness and force deficit (Morgan 1990, 1994b). This topic is examined in chapter 9.

MODIFYING THE "CLASSIC" SLIDING FILAMENT MODEL

According to the classic sliding filament model, the sarcomere is primarily composed of two filaments: actin and myosin. During contraction, these filaments slide over each other so that each fiber shortens. In contrast, when a sarcomere is stretched, the thick and thin filaments merely slide further apart. Neither the thick nor thin filaments change length, but simply have less overlap between them (see figure 3.5). The mechanism by which the sarcomere elongates is now known to be more complex than originally hypothesized.

The modified sliding filament model includes a third filament, titin. In this model, the tandem Ig and PEVK segments of slack sarcomeres (approximately 2.0 μm) are folded. Under external force, each domain "yields" and unfolds at threshold values of force and loading rates (Wang, Forbes, and Jin 2001). From approximately 2.0 to 2.7 μm, the "contracted" tandem Ig segments straightened while their individual Ig domains remained folded. This initial extension at low forces is caused by their high bending rigidity (Trombitás et al. 1998). Subsequent extension of the PEVK segment occurs only upon reaching sufficiently high external forces resulting from its low bending rigidity (Trombitás et al. 1998). With increasing elongation, the extensible segment becomes longer by recruiting previously inextensible titin when its anchorage to thick filaments starts to slip or when the distal ends of the thick filaments become distorted (see figure 3.6). Eventually, further elongation will break the titin strand.

This section has dealt almost exclusively with the relationship of stretch and the sarcomere's filaments. However, the most important component of muscle related to ROM is the connective tissues that envelop and surround the muscle at its various levels of organization (i.e., muscle fiber, bundle, and whole muscle). These tissues, the endomysium, perimysium, and epimysium, are discussed in chapter 4.

ADDITIONAL LIMITATIONS TO RANGE OF MOTION

Additional factors that may limit a joint's ROM include muscle fiber type, muscle fiber architecture, contracture, spasticity, improper muscle balance, inadequate muscle control, and whether the muscle is immobilized.

Muscle Fiber Type and Fiber Architecture

Human skeletal muscles contain two types of fibers. They can be categorized as lying on a continuum between slow contracting, slow fatiguing fibers and fast contracting, fast fatiguing fibers. Slow-twitch (ST) fibers are classified as type I. ST fibers have a reddish coloration because of their higher content of myoglobin. In general, ST fibers are associated with muscles that maintain posture and sustain prolonged, low-intensity activity such as distance running. Consequently, ST fibers have a high level of

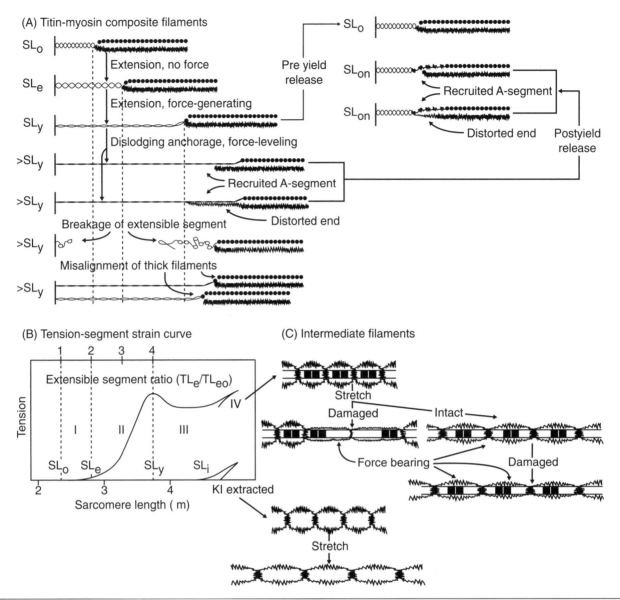

Figure 3.6 Proposed structural correlates of tension-segment strain curves of sarcomere-associated cytoskeletal lattices. The resting tension-sarcomere length curve (*b*) is characterized by four zones (I to IV) and interpreted by structural behaviors of the sarcomere matrix (*a*) and the intermediate filament lattice (*c*). *Zone I.* From SL_o to SL_e. The stretching of the sarcomere in this range generates no significant tension, perhaps reflecting a straightening of a flaccid network of titin filaments without a change in contour length. *Zone II.* From SL_e to SL_y. The stretching of sarcomere generates exponential rise in tension and causes a net change in the contour length of the extensible segment of titin filaments. Release of the preyield fibers returns the sarcomeres to prestretch slack length (SL_o). *Zone III.* Yield point and beyond (> SL_y). Yield point tension causes distortion of distal ends of thick filaments and the dislodging of titin-myosin anchorage. The recruitment from the anchored segment causes a net distortion of distal ends of thick filaments and the dislodging of titin-myosin anchorage. The recruitment from the anchored segment causes a net increase in the length of the extensible segment and a reduction of stiffness. Misalignment and breakage of titin may also contribute to the broad transition near the yield point. Release of postyield fibers at the (*n* – 1)th cycle returns it to a new slack sarcomere length SL_{on} that is longer than the SL_o of preyield sarcomeres. The increase in slack length reflects the net length of the newly recruited titin filaments. The net length of the extensible segment increases further when sarcomeres are stretched beyond the yield point, resulting in a leveling of tension. *Zone IV.* Intermediate filaments. The intermediate filament lattice that links adjacent sarcomeres at the Z-line (shown) and M-line (not shown) is normally slack and begins to elongate and bears tension around 4.5 μm. Below 4.5 μm, the intermediate filaments may also elongate locally if sarcomeres lose the ability to generate and transmit active force. In such cases, intermediate filaments may serve as a bypass mechanism to transmit tension to prevent a total breakdown of force transmission between the adjacent sarcomeres in the myofibril. The generalized tension-segment strain curve is plotted against the extensible segment ratio (TL_e/TL_{eo}), which is approximated by the ratio of I-band width at various sarcomere lengths. The resting tension-sarcomere length curves of many types of muscles can be normalized to this tension-segment strain curve.

Reprinted from Wang, McCarter, Wright, Beverly, and Ramirez-Mitchell 1993.

aerobic endurance. The soleus muscle is representative of predominantly ST fibers. Gosselin et al. (1994) and Kovanen et al. (1984a, 1984b) have shown that ST muscles contain a greater collagen concentration and more extensive cross-linkings of collagen than do fast-twitch (FT), or type II, muscles and therefore are less compliant, or stiffer. These biochemical properties of ST muscle correlate with a higher ultimate tensile strength (i.e., the point at which a muscle tears when stretched) than that of FT fibers (Gosselin et al. 1998). Kovanen et al. 1984a speculates, "the different functional demands of different skeletal muscles are also reflected in the structure of intramuscular connective tissue, even at the level of endomysial collagen" (p. 235). However, another possible explanation for ST muscle fibers having greater passive stiffness than FT muscle fibers is that each fiber type contains different isoforms of titin (Mutungi and Ranatunga 1996).

The second type of muscle, FT fibers, are low oxidative but possess a high glycolytic capacity. FT fibers are capable of greater strain (i.e., change in length before mechanical failure) than ST fibers (Kovanen et al. 1984b). Three types of FT fibers have been identified: type a (IIA or FT_a), type b (IIB or FT_b), and type c (IIC or FT_c). "In humans, fast twitch fibers predominant in muscles that span more than one joint, such as the hamstrings, rectus femoris and the tricep surae, are the most commonly strained muscles in athletes" (Garrett et al. 1987, p. 451). The differences between the three types of FT fibers are not fully understood.

Every muscle group contains a different ratio between FT and ST fibers, depending on their function and training history. For example, world champions in the marathon are reported to possess 94% to 99% ST fibers in their gastrocnemius. In contrast, world-class sprinters have only about 25% ST fibers in this muscle (Wilmore and Costill 1999). In addition, Fridén et al. (1983) demonstrated that myofibrillar damage after eccentric exercise predominantly occurred in the FT fibers.

Knowledge of muscle fiber types is important for several reasons. (1) It may explain why some muscles are stiffer than others. (2) It may explain why muscle damage is associated with muscle groups composed predominantly of FT fibers. (3) It may elucidate why muscle groups of predominantly FT fibers may be more susceptible to muscle strain.

Architecture is another factor that has significant influence on muscle function. Muscle architecture is the angle of pennation of the muscle fibers in relation to the muscle-tendon axis and the line of force generation (i.e., the direction of the fibers) (Garrett et al. 1988). The four architectural arrangements are fusiform, unipennate, bipennate, and multipennate. The arrangement of fibers varies in different muscles. Differences in passive tension per gram of muscle may be related to the degree of fiber pennation. For example, in the rat soleus muscle, where

muscle fibers have a more parallel arrangement, a more direct pull of the longitudinally arranged fibers should produce a greater passive tension than a muscle with a greater angle of fiber pennation, such as the gastrocnemius (Gillette and Fell 1996; Sacks and Roy 1982). Muscle adaptation has been induced by training changes in fiber type distribution in rat (Almeida-Silveira et al. 1996) and humans (Komi 1984).

Garrett et al. (1988) found that architecture had no effect on the ultimate site of rupture of the musculotendinous unit. However, architecture had a pronounced effect on elongation to failure. "Muscles with more pinnate structure tended to elongate further to their resting fiber length" (p. 11). Perhaps, these differences in muscle architecture and arrangement of connective tissue help explain the differences in response to stretching before and after warm-up in various muscles (Mohr et al. 1998). Top-caliber ballerinas, rhythmic gymnasts, or practitioners of yoga may have modified the architecture of their muscles because of years of intensive stretching.

Contracture

A contracture is a shortening of a muscle or other tissues that results in loss of motion. A contracture develops when normally elastic connective tissues are replaced with inelastic fibrous tissues. Contractures are either neurally or nonneurally mediated. Neurally mediated contractures are caused by spasticity (i.e., involuntary relax contractions of muscles). They are often common sequelae of upper motor neuron lesions. "While some believe that stretching also induces functionally important and lasting reductions in spasticity, this is yet to be verified with good quality studies (Harvey and Herbert 2002, p. 1). Nonneurally mediated contractures are caused by structural adaptations of soft tissues, usually a result of soft tissues habitually held in a shortened position after orthopedic procedures or immobilization.

Contractures can be treated by a variety of strategies and techniques, either singly or in combination, including manual mobilization or stretching, mechanical traction, and use of modalities such as deep heat. Harvey and Herbert (2002) recommend that therapists move away from the labor-intensive tradition of manually applying stretches with their hands and instead use "positioning programs" incorporated into patients' rehabilitation routines and daily lives. This change can be achieved by using relatively simple equipment and devices such as splints.

Spasticity

Spasticity is another factor that can result in increased muscle stiffness and reduced ROM. Spasticity may be defined as a velocity-dependent hypertonia, that is, a rate-dependent, increased resistive (tone) to passive stretch of the muscles (de Lateur 1994). The definition of spasticity implies that an increase in motor neuron response to muscle lengthening may be the primary mechanism for increased resistance to passive joint movement, decreased joint ROM, and some exaggerated reflexes (Bressel and NcNair 2002). Numerous relaxation strategies are used to treat patients with spasticity (see chapter 8). Bressel and McNair (2002) explained, "although evidence for increased motor neuron excitability is strongly supported, some researchers have argued that changes in passive mechanical properties of muscle may be the additional mechanisms responsible for symptoms observed in people with spasticity" (p. 881). Those who have experienced a stroke often experience spasticity. Bressel and McNair (2002) continued with the suggestion "that interventions for stroke may need to focus on passive mechanical properties of muscle and not just motor neuron excitability" (p. 881). Additional research is necessary to determine the mechanism(s) responsible for the symptoms observed in people with spasticity and the optimal means to treat them.

Improper Muscle Balance

Healthy muscles maintain a structural homeostasis, a key to which is an equal pull by antagonistic, or opposing, muscles located on the opposite sides of the joint. An imbalance in these forces can affect ROM. Muscle imbalance can be caused by several factors, including the presence of *hypertonic* muscles (i.e., muscles in a state of contracture or spasm) or weak muscles. Postural antigravity ST muscles tend to tighten, whereas the phasic FT muscles tend to weaken (see table 3.1). Treatment in such cases is to strengthen the weak muscle (Klee et al. 2002) and stretch the shortened muscle.

However, according to Hammer (1999), "it is imperative to evaluate and treat short tightened muscles before prescribing exercises for weak muscles" (p. 416). His rationale is that an often-inhibited muscle will regain strength spontaneously after its tight antagonist is normalized. Therefore, an examiner can determine whether a muscle is inhibited by facilitating it. Additional clinical research is necessary to determine the optimal means of restoring muscle imbalance.

Table 3.1   Functional Division of Muscle Groups

Prone to tightness	Prone to weakness
(Postural)	(Phasic)
Gastrocnemius	Peronei
Tibialis posterior	Tibialis anterior
Short hip adductors	Vastus medialis and lateralis
Hamstrings	Gluteus maximus, medius, and minimus
Rectus femoris	Rectus abdominis
Iliopsoas	Serratus anterior
Tensor fascia latae	Rhomboids
Piriformis	Lower trapezius
Paravertebral back extensors	Short cervical flexors
Quadratus lumborum	Extensors of upper limb
Pectoralis major	Scalenes
Upper trapezius	
Levator scapulae	
Sternocleidomastoid	
Flexors of upper limb	

Adapted, by permission, from G.A. Jull and V. Janda, 1987, "Muscles and motor control in low back pain: Assessment and management." In *Physical therapy of the low back,* edited by L.T. Twomey and J.R. Taylor (Edinburgh: Churchill Livingstone), 253.

Inadequate Muscle Control

Even a person endowed with natural flexibility and suppleness may lack local muscular control necessary to execute specific flexibility skills because many flexibility skills have additional components. For our purposes, *muscular control* is adequate balance, coordination, or control of one's body part(s) or sufficient muscular strength to perform a given skill. For example, to perform a skill as delicate and elegant as an arabesque (scale) in ballet, one must have the necessary balance. One must also have enough strength to achieve, support, and maintain the desired position. Sufficient coordination, rhythm, or timing are also necessary. Complex motor skills can be performed only with the proper combination of all these components.

Monoarticular and Biarticular Muscles

Muscles that cross more than one joint can potentially impact flexibility, stretching strategy, and present a potential risk for injury. These muscles are known as biarticular, or two-joint, muscles because they can affect more than one joint. The hamstrings for instance, can extend the hip, flex the knee, or rotate the hip or knee. In contrast, monoarticular muscles cross only one joint and can have only one action on a joint. Biarticular muscles are at risk for injury during activities that simultaneously place high demands on the muscles. Biomechanically, the synchronization between two joints is a complicated proprioceptive and mechanical problem (see chapter 16). Physiologically, full stretch occurs in the hamstrings group only if the knee is fully extended with the hip fully flexed. Even well-conditioned and highly trained athletes may fail when required to pass through their full amplitude under rapid and stressful situations. A classic example is the hamstrings during hurdling or kicking with the leg kept straight. To improve ROM in two-joint muscles they must be stretched by putting both involved joints in positions opposite to the functions of the muscle.

Effects of Aging on Muscle

The normal aging process brings about an almost imperceptible diminution in normal muscle functions, including strength, endurance, agility, and flexibility. When complicated by the deconditioning of inactivity, disease, or injury, these functions decline rapidly. Physiologically, one of the most conspicuous degenerative changes associated with aging is the progressive *atrophy*, or wasting away, of muscle mass. This loss results from the reduction in both size and number of muscle fibers (Hooper 1981). According to Wilmore (1991), "This decrease in sarcomere number may contribute to the reduced mobility commonly associated with old age" (p. 236). The age at which these changes begin is highly variable. These changes also vary in degree, depending on the muscles

involved and their degree of use as one grows older. The number of nerve cells in the musculoskeletal system also decreases with age (Gutmann 1977). A decrease in muscle length is also associated with aging (Gajdosik 1997).

As muscle fibers atrophy, replacement by fatty and fibrous (collagen) tissue occurs. (Overend et al. 1992; Rice et al. 1989; Vandervoort et al. 1986; Vandervoort and McComas 1986). Collagen, the chief component in connective tissue, has an extremely low compliance, which implies that small increases in the quantity of collagen in a muscle considerably increases the stiffness of the tissue. This phenomenon was investigated by Alnaqeeb et al. (1984), using the soleus and extensor digitorum longus muscles of rats. Their research confirmed that total collagen content increased continuously with age. Furthermore, the investigation revealed a lower rate of passive tension development for every unit increase in length in young muscle than in adult muscle.

> The data for the stiffness of the muscles and those for connective tissue are in accord [with one another] at the ages studied, with the exception of the soleus in the senile animal. With this exception, the passive mechanical behaviour of the muscle appears to be related directly to collagen concentrations. (p. 677)

However, research by Gajdosik (1997) did not support the finding that the muscle of older men had increased amounts of connective tissue. Further research is required to ascertain the content of adipose tissue, collagenous tissue, and elastic connective tissue of aged muscles and their effects.

EFFECTS OF IMMOBILIZATION

Research has shown that muscle will adapt to its optimal mechanical efficiency when immobilized. This characteristic was demonstrated by the experiments of Marvey (1887). Since the late 1960s, the mechanisms of length adaptation have been studied at the cellular and ultrastructural levels. Goldspink (1968, 1976) and Williams and Goldspink (1971) have shown that the increase in muscle fiber length during normal growth is associated with a large increase in the number of sarcomeres along the length of the fibers. Because the length of the actin and myosin filaments is constant, the adaptation of adult muscles to a different functional length presumably must involve the production or removal of a certain number of sarcomeres in series to maintain the correct sarcomere length in relation to the whole muscle (Goldspink 1976; Tabary et al. 1972).

Adult cat soleus muscle immobilized in a lengthened position by plaster casts adapts to its new length. Tabary et al. (1972) found that this lengthening is accomplished by a production of approximately 20% more sarcomeres in series. Williams and Goldspink (1973) found that the new sarcomeres are added on the end of the existing myofibrils. In the case of denervation (loss of nerve supply to the muscle) and immobilization in a lengthened state, 25% more sarcomeres in series were produced (Goldspink et al. 1974). Upon removal of the plaster cast, both the normal and the denervated muscle rapidly readjusted to their original lengths (Goldspink et al. 1974; Tabary et al. 1972; Williams and Goldspink 1976). A study by Scott (1994) to determine whether the extraocular muscle system of three monkeys adapted in the same way as cats' limb muscles found that the eye muscles lengthened 18%, 25%, and 33% because of suturing. The data substantiated previous findings that an addition of sarcomeres was responsible for the increase in muscle length. Bohannon (1984) passively loaded the hamstrings of 10 young, healthy volunteers to toleration during a passive straight-leg raising (SLR) test for 8 minutes on 3 consecutive days. Twenty-four hours after 3 days of loading, the experimental group increased its angle of straight-leg raising 4.4 degrees suggesting that muscle lengthened. Bohannon's findings tended to support the "clinical reports and the findings of experiments that suggest that loading for more than 20 minutes should be practiced if adequate soft-tissue lengthening is to occur" (p. 496).

On the other hand, when a limb was immobilized with the muscle in its shortened position, the muscle fibers lost 40% of the sarcomeres in series (Tabary et al. 1972). Denervation and immobilization in the shortened position caused a 35% reduction of sarcomeres in series (Goldspink et al. 1974). The sarcomere number of these muscles also readjusted rapidly on return to their original length (Goldspink et al. 1974; Tabary et al. 1972).

Thus, the results indicated that the adjustment of sarcomere number to the functional length of the muscles does not appear to be directly under neuronal control. Rather, it appears to be a myogenic response to the amount of passive muscle tension (Goldspink 1976; Goldspink et al. 1974; Williams and Goldspink 1976). The mechanism appears to reside within the muscle tissue directly, independent of neurological activity (Gajdosik 2001).

Another possible factor for increased muscle stiffness because of injury is the modification of its titin isoform. Lieber (2002) writes: "It is possible that altered muscle stiffness that is observed secondary to chronic length changes, immobilization, stroke, head injury, spinal cord injury, or cerebral palsy may be strongly affected by the amount and isoform of titin expressed in various muscles" (p. 59). Fridén and Lieber (2003) raised the question of whether observed changes in spastic muscle cells could be attributed to variation in titin isoforms, titin concentrations, or other structural components.

Reduced extensibility (increase in passive resistance) of the muscles immobilized in the shortened position is associated with reduction in fiber length and in the number and length of the sarcomeres (Goldspink 1976;

Goldspink and Williams 1979; Tabary et al. 1972). This loss of flexibility occurred whether or not the muscle was denervated (Goldspink 1976). Goldspink and Williams (1979) found that connective tissue was lost at a slower rate than muscle contractile tissue. Hence, the relative amount of connective tissue increased (Goldspink 1976; Goldspink and Williams 1979; Tabary et al. 1972). Williams and Goldspink (1984) documented that collagen fibers in immobilized muscle were arranged at an angle more acute to the axis of the muscle fibers than was the axis in normal muscle. This change would be expected to affect the compliance of muscle. Ahtikoski et al. (2001) also found that stretch seems to partially counter the effects of immobilization in rat fibrillar collagens in skeletal muscles. Specifically, stretch appeared "to counteract the negative effects of immobilization on the mRNAs for their fibrillar collagens" (p. 137).

A modified immobilization study by Gillette and Fell (1996) employed whole-body suspension of rats for 14 days to investigate passive tension in posterior hindleg. The animals were suspended in a horizontal position with their hindlegs unable to contact any supportive surface and therefore non–weight bearing. In suspended animals, increased passive tension was caused by musculotendinous units (75%) rather than by the joint (25%). The investigators suggested that the "increased passive tension in the hindleg muscle be due to changes in muscle architecture, viscoelastic properties of the muscle, connective tissue elements, or cytoskeletal protein alterations" (p. 729).

The decrease in extensibility appears to be a safety mechanism that prevents the muscle from being suddenly overstretched (Goldspink 1976; Goldspink and Williams 1979; Tabary et al. 1972). This mechanism is particularly important in shortened muscle (i.e., muscle that has lost sarcomeres) because stretching even through the normal ROM would cause the sarcomeres to be pulled out to the point where the myosin and actin filaments do not interdigitate or overlap, thus causing permanent damage (Goldspink 1976; Tabary et al. 1972). In contrast, changes do not occur in the elastic properties of the muscle immobilized in the lengthened position, because the adaptation is in the reverse direction and the chance of the muscle being overstretched is no greater than for a normal muscle (Tabary et al. 1972).

However, the decrease in extensibility is not just a protective function. The main effect is a shift in the muscle's length-tension curve to the left (for shortened immobilized muscle) or to the right (for lengthened immobilized muscle). These length changes adapt the muscle to generate optimal tension levels at its new position and length.

Williams et al. (1988) investigated whether lack of stretch or lack of contractile activity is responsible for the loss of serial sarcomeres, for the increase in the proportion of collagen, and for the increased muscle stiffness that occurs when muscles are immobilized in a shortened position. They determined that the connective tissue accumulation in inactive muscles can be prevented by either passive stretch or active (i.e., electrical) stimulation.

A logical question arises: Are short periods of stretch effective in preventing the changes in muscle connective tissue, in fiber length, and in sarcomere number and thus in maintaining joint ROM? To answer this question, Williams (1988) had the soleus muscle of mouse immobilized in a shortened position for 10 days by means of a plaster cast. Every 2 days, the cast was removed and the muscle passively stretched for 15 minutes. The study demonstrated that only 15 minutes of passive stretch every other day was necessary to maintain normal connective tissue proportions. However, it did not prevent the reduction in muscle fiber length, which in itself resulted in considerable loss of ROM. If extrapolated for human subjects, the practical significance of this study for therapists is that "connective tissue changes which occur in immobilized muscle and which affect joint movement can be prevented by a simple, short regimen of passive stretching exercise" (p. 1016).

MECHANISM OF PASSIVE STRETCH ON MYOFIBRILLOGENESIS

Immobilization in the lengthened position results in an increase in muscle fiber length. This increase in length is associated with an increase in the number of sarcomeres in series along the myofibrils and hence along the length of the fibers. The newly synthesized sarcomeres form near the muscle-tendon junction. The cellular control mechanism behind muscle fiber elongation and hypertrophy (i.e., myofibrillogenesis) continues to be investigated.

Dix and Eisenberg (1990, 1991a, 1991b) found that the accumulation of slow oxidative myosin mRNA at the end of the muscle in stretched fibers was greater than in control fibers. "These local accumulations of mRNA provide for regional synthesis of contractile proteins, rapid sarcomere assembly, and extension of the myofibrils" (Dix and Eisenberg 1990, p. 1893). In particular, "a large cytoplasmic space containing polysomes opened up between the myofibrils and the sarcolemmae of the myotendon junction of lengthening fibers and many developing myofibrils were found" (Russell et al. 1992, p. 192). In addition, stretched muscles also lengthen by the addition of proliferating myotubes, which may later fuse with existing fibers (Moss and LeBlond 1971; Williams and Goldspink 1973).

How does stretch increase mRNA production? A review of several proposed "master regulators" is presented by Russell et al. (1992). However, an additional area that needs to be explored is the potential relationship of *streaming potentials* on myofibrillogenesis (see chapter 4). Sutcliffe and Davidson (1990) investigated the transduction of mechanical force (i.e., stretching) into gene expression by smooth muscle cells. Additional research is needed in this area.

PROPOSED METHODS OF MODULATING GENE EXPRESSION VIA STRETCHING

Muscle cells consist of several structural compartments that are all interrelated and involved in the perception of mechanical signals during contraction and stretching. These interfacing units are three-dimensional, tissue-specific networks that reflect the unique functions of each tissue. In striated muscle cells, these compartments are extracellular, cytoplasmic, and nuclear. Each compartment transmits information across at least one membrane interface along the boundary of the compartment (Simpson et al. 1994). This integration of mechanical stimulation within and between these three arbitrary compartments has been described as a system of dynamic reciprocity (Bissell et al. 1982). Mechanical stimulation affects gene expression, but how muscle converts mechanical stimuli into growth signals is a longstanding question.

Sadoshima and Izumo (1993) proposed three possible mechanisms through which cell stretch can lead to the activation of multiple intracellular second messengers. The first possibility is that mechanical stress can directly activate signal-transducing molecules. Watson (1991) postulated that mechanical forces applied to the cell surface might generate direct conformation changes in the molecules associated with the plasma membrane, which may activate the downstream second messenger systems. However, Sadoshima and Izumo state, "there is little direct evidence for this hypothesis" (p. 1690).

The second possibility is that mechanical stretch activates putative cellular mechanotransducers. The proposed pathway begins with mechanical stimulation transmitted to the extracellular matrix (ECM). The ECM consists primarily of collagen, noncollagenous glycoproteins, and proteoglycans. Then signals from the ECM are transmitted across the sarcolemma (i.e., the membrane surrounding the muscle cell) at specific sites near Z-bands. This interaction appears to be mediated in part by specific receptors identified and termed *integrins* (Tamkun et al. 1986). These receptors link the externally located ECM components with the elements of the cytoskeleton (CKS) and are important in the transmission of mechanical information (Ingber 1997; Ingber et al. 1990; Tamkun et al. 1986; Terracio et al. 1989; Vandenburgh 1992; N. Wang et al. 2001). Researchers have proposed several tensegrity models to explain how mechanical forces regulate cell function by linking mechanics to microstructure and molecular biochemistry. These models "predict that living cells and nuclei may be hard-wired to respond immediately to mechanical stresses transmitted over cell surface receptors that physically couple CKS to ECM or to other cells" (Ingber 1997, pp. 576-577) (see figure 3.7).

The precise mechanisms of the transmission of mechanical stimulation are not understood (Goldspink et al. 1992; Simpson et al. 1994). Several cytoskeletal components include vinculin, talin, nonsarcomeric actin, titin, and desmin. These cytoskeletal components play an important role in the generation of force and transmission of mechanical tension (Price 1991; Wang and Ramirez-Mitchell 1983) and provide positional information to the contractile fibers. In turn, the cytoskeleton attaches to the contractile apparatus and to the nuclear compartment. This interconnection is important in positioning the nucleus within the cell. Little is known about nuclear positioning in striated muscle, although it is thought to be very important in other systems (Simpson et al. 1994).

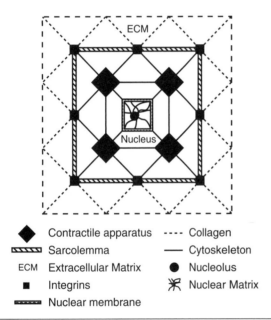

Contractile apparatus · · · · Collagen
Sarcolemma ——— Cytoskeleton
ECM Extracellular Matrix ● Nucleolus
■ Integrins ✳ Nuclear Matrix
▬▬ Nuclear membrane

Figure 3.7 A schematic diagram of the three major compartments that play a role in the transmission of mechanical forces. The extracellular matrix transmits forces from adjacent cells and tissues to the sarcolemma, where it is attached to the cell by integral membrane protein receptors known as integrins. Integrins appear to be pivotal molecules for transmitting force since they span the sarcolemma and are attached to the cytoskeleton. The cytoskeleton in turn attaches to the contractile apparatus and to the nucleus, thus serving to organize the complex cytoplasm and to transmit force to the nucleus. The nucleus in turn is composed of a system of filaments known as the nuclear matrix, which organizes the chromatin and nucleolus into specific functional domains. Thus, the same basic organizational pattern exists to integrate forces from outside the cell, move them across the cell membrane, through the cytoplasm to the nucleus, and affect gene expression.

Courtesy of Thomas K. Borg, PhD.

Nuclear positioning may be important in establishing the regional domains of protein synthesis that may be essential for myofibrillogenesis and the turnover of myofibrillar components (Blau 1989; Russell and Dix 1992). Next, these mechanical stimulation forces are transmitted to the nuclear membrane complex and, in turn, to the nuclear matrix that contains the genetic material necessary for cellular functions. Research on the spatial and positional organization of DNA has caused speculation that mechanical alteration of the nuclear membrane would in turn cause an alteration of the DNA; these forces thereby may alter gene expression (Simpson et al. 1994). Potentially, altered gene expression may be responsible for enhanced flexibility.

The third and most favored possibility offered by Sadoshima and Izumo (1993, p. 1690) is "that mechanical stress causes the release of some growth factor(s) and that this factor activates its receptor and subsequent second messenger cascades." Vandenburgh et al. (1991) suggest that some of these factors are prostaglandins. Goldspink (2002) and Goldspink et al. (2002) have discussed the possibility that a "MGF" (mechano–growth factor) is the end product of mechanotransduction signaling pathway in muscle and other cell types. McComas (1996) has developed a simplified sequence of intracellular events that results in muscle fiber hypertrophy after stretch (figure 3.8).

What are the underlying mechanism(s) by which muscle and connective tissues modulate their isoforms (i.e., structural variants) in response to mechanical stimulation? The possibilities, which might operate singly or in combination, include neurological stimulation, transmission of biochemical signals (Ingber 1997; Kornberg and Juliano 1992), stretch-activated ion channels, or streaming potentials (see chapter 4).

Investigators have used several animal models, including cats, rabbits, rodents, and chickens, to study length-associated changes in muscles and suggested applicability to humans. However, Goldspink (2002) cautions that "extrapolation of data derived from this species to others, particularly large animals, is sometimes misleading" (p. 287). Several problems must be addressed when relating the animal studies to humans. First, there has been no documented proof of an increase of sarcomeres in humans via a "traditional" stretching program (i.e., stretching in a recreational or athletic program). Second, the applicability of investigations of immobilization in a lengthened position is dubious at best. The lengths of time muscles were under stretch varied from 4 days to 4 weeks. How can this stimulus relate to a typical stretching regime consisting of one set of 6 repetitions, each held for approximately 10 seconds? Third, most of the studies employed traction (passive and static force). Therefore, what is their practical relationship to the development of active (functional) or even ballistic flexibility? Fourth,

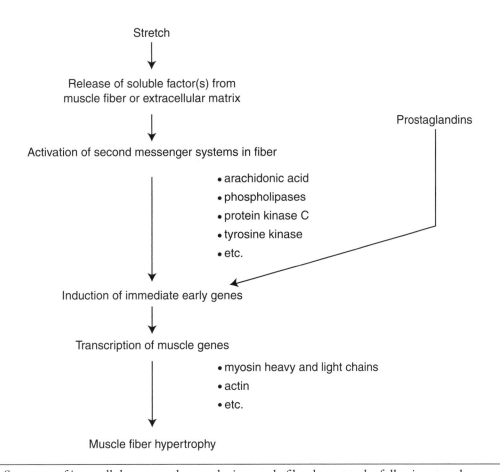

Figure 3.8 Sequence of intracellular events that results in muscle fiber hypertrophy following stretch.
Reprinted, by permission, from A.J. McComas, 1996, *Skeletal muscle: Form and function* (Champaign, IL: Human Kinetics), 312.

training in animal models does not exactly mimic training in humans.

SUMMARY

Muscle is a complex structure comprising progressively smaller units that in part determine one's flexibility. The discovery of a third filament, titin, has shown that the sliding filament theory of the 1950s was incomplete. This filament has proved primarily responsible for the sarcomere's resting tension. Furthermore, muscle tissue is very adaptable. The theoretical limit of a sarcomere's elongation while still maintaining at least one cross-bridge between the actin and myosin filaments exceeds 50% of its resting length. Thus, the contractile elements of a muscle are capable of increasing over 50% from resting length, thereby allowing muscles to move through a wide ROM.

Sarcomere number, sarcomere length, and fiber length adjust to the functional length of the whole muscle. Currently, stretching is speculated to modulate gene expression and influence muscle extensibility. Additional research is needed to identify the rehabilitation and stretching regimens that produce the optimal amount of flexibility. Modern molecular biology, the availability of new technologies, and knowledge about the human genome, and advances in sports medicine will continue to contribute to our understanding of flexibility.

Connective Tissue:
A Limiting Factor of Flexibility

This chapter reviews the present state of knowledge about the mechanical properties, mechanical ultrastructure, and biochemical constituents of connective tissues and the effects of aging and immobilization on connective tissues. The goal is to understand how these variables affect and determine the function of connective tissues. This information will allow a better understanding of the behavior of connective tissue, which, to a major extent, determines one's degree of flexibility.

Connective tissue contains a wide variety of specialized cells that perform the functions of defense, protection, storage, transportation, binding, connection, and general support and repair. This chapter concentrates on cells that provide binding and support functions, specifically the tendons, ligaments, and fascia, which play a significant role in determining flexibility and stiffness. Before exploring those tissues, one must analyze their primary constituents: collagen and elastin.

COLLAGEN

Collagen, the most abundant protein in the mammalian body, is generally regarded as a primary structural component of living tissue. In higher vertebrates, collagen constitutes one-third or more of the total body proteins. Collagen contains three chains of amino acids wound in a triple helix. The two major physical properties of collagen fibers are their great tensile *strength* and relative *inextensibility*.

Collagenous fibers appear virtually colorless or off-white. They are arranged in bundles and, except under tension, are characteristically wavy. Collagen fibers are capable of only a slight degree of extensibility but are very resistant to tensile stress. Therefore, they are the main constituents of structures such as ligaments and tendons that are subjected to a pulling force.

At least five classes of collagen have been identified, each of which has subclasses (Jungueira et al. 1989). Types of collagen are identified by roman numerals that indicate the order in which the types were discovered. Type I collagen is the most common form and is important to ROM. Type I collagen is located in skin, bone, ligament, and tendon. Genetic mutations that affect the structure or processing of the chains of type I collagen are often expressed as generalized connective tissue disorders.

ULTRASTRUCTURE OF COLLAGEN

The structural organization of collagen is analogous to that of muscle (see figure 4.1; table 4.1). However, the classification system is not widely agreed upon because of a lack of consistent terminology (Benjamin and Ralphs 2000; Kastelic et al. 1978; Strocchi et al. 1985). Under a microscope, individual collagen fibers display a banded or striated structure. The characteristic pattern of cross-striations of collagen reflects its ultrastructural organization, the knowledge of which is fundamental to understanding the mechanism of collagen's great tensile strength and relative inextensibility.

The collagen of a tendon is arranged in wavy bundles called *fascicles* (see figure 4.1). Fascicles vary from 50 to 300 mm in diameter and are composed of bundles of 50 to 500 nm *fibrils*. Fibrils, in turn, are composed of bundles of 10 to 20 nm *subfibrils*. Each subfibril is composed of bundles of approximately 3.5 nm *microfibrils* or *filaments*. The sizes of the filaments in a given tissue vary with age and other factors.

According to Inoué and Leblond (1986), collagen microfibril is the least known fibrous component of connective tissue. The microfibril was given its present name by Low (1961a, 1961b, 1962). Various and conflicting descriptions have been made of this structure. To clarify these uncertainties, Inoué and Leblond (1986) examined microfibrils of the connective tissue of a mouse at high resolution under an electron microscope. Their study revealed that microfibrils are composed of a *tubule* and a *surface band*.

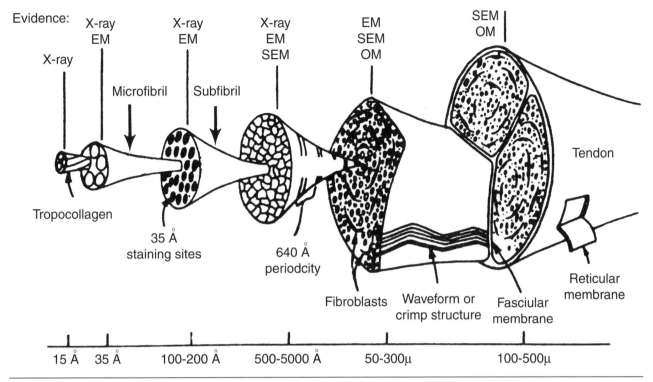

Figure 4.1 Collagen hierarchy.
Reprinted from Kastelic, Galeski, and Baer 1978.

Table 4.1 A Comparison of Muscle and Collagen Structures

Muscle	Collagen
Muscle	Tendon
Muscle bundle (fasciculus)	Fascicle
Muscle fiber	Fibril
Myofibril	Subfibril
Filament (myofilament)	Microfibril
Sarcomere (functional unit)	Collagen molecule (functional unit)
Actin	Alpha$_1$ chains (2)
Myosin	Alpha$_2$ chains (1)
Titin	
Cross-bridges	Cross-links

Adapted, by permission, from M.J. Alter, 1988, *Science of stretching* (Champaign, IL: Human Kinetics), 24.

The tubule is characterized by an approximately pentagonal wall and an electron-lucent lumen containing a bead called a *spherule*. The surface band is a ribbonlike structure wrapped around the tubule. The band has dense borders called *tracks* with *spikes* attached at intervals (see figure 4.2). Additional research is recommended to confirm whether this structure is also present in human microfibrils and to determine its relationship to ROM.

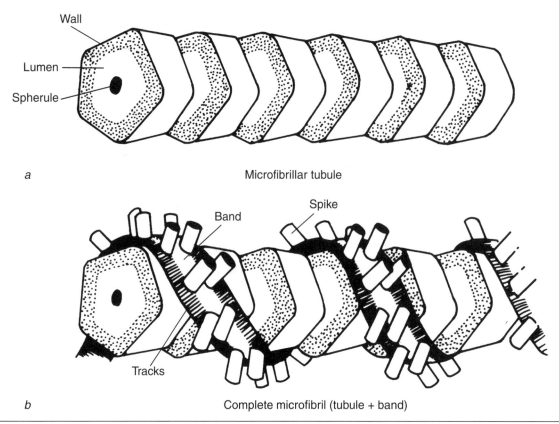

Wall

Lumen

Spherule

a   Microfibrillar tubule

Band   Spike

Tracks

b   Complete microfibril (tubule + band)

Figure 4.2 Model of the tubular portion of a typical microfibril. It is composed of pentagonal segments associated in a column *(a)*. Segments are all the same size, but larger and smaller spaces alternate between them. *(b)* Model of a typical microfibril. At the surface of the tubular portion, represented as in *(a)*, the surface band is associated with protruding spikes. The band is depicted as a helix but may be differently organized. In any case, it is in close association with the surface of the segments. Approximate magnification × 2,700,000.

Reprinted from Inoué and Leblond 1986.

The collagen microfibril is composed of regularly spaced, overlapping collagen molecules that are analogous to the sarcomeres of muscle cells. The collagen molecules are, in turn, made of coiled helices of amino acids. The collagen molecules measure about 300 nm in length and 1.5 nm in diameter. They lie in parallel alignment with a staggered overlap of almost one-fourth their length. This overlap creates the prominent cross-bands, or striations. Collagen fibrils have a cross-band periodicity of 60 to 70 nm, depending on their source and degree of hydration. Actual measurements indicate that a gap or hole of about 41 nm occurs between the end of one collagen molecule and the beginning of the next in the same line.

Extreme magnification reveals the collagen molecule as three polypeptide chains coiled in a unique type of rigid helical structure. Two of the three intertwining amino acid chains in human collagen are identical (the α_1 chains), and one is distinct (the α_2 chain). The three chains are thought to be held together by hydrogen bonds that form cross-links.

In addition to a cross-banding periodicity or striation pattern, connective tissues possess wavelike undulations of the collagen fibers. This undulating phenomenon, known as *crimp*, is one of the major factors behind the viscoelastic response of connective tissue. Collagen is composed of crimped fibrils that are aggregated into fibers. Each collagen fibril can be considered a mechanical spring and each fiber can be considered an assemblage of springs. Consequently, the crimp "acts as a buffer allowing small longitudinal elongation of the fiber without damage to the tissue, and thus, acting as a shock absorber along the length of the tissue" (Järvinen et al. 2002, p. 252).

Straightening the crimp in collagen fibers is estimated to result in a 1% to 2% stretching of the collagenous tissue (Kannus 2000). Therefore, whenever a fiber is pulled, its crimp straightens, and its length increases. Like the energy in a mechanical spring, the energy supplied to stretch the fiber is stored in the fiber, and release of this energy returns the fiber to its normal configuration when the applied load is removed (Özkaya and Nordin 1999). Fibril crimp has been attributed to collagen ground substance interactions, properties of the molecular structure, and cross-linking effects, but the exact cause is not known.

Collagenous Tissue Cross-Links

The presence of both *intramolecular* cross-links between the α_1 and α_2 chains of the collagen molecule and *intermolecular* cross-links between collagen subfibrils, filaments, and other fibers adds tensile strength to collagenous structures. In a sense, cross-links weld the building blocks (i.e., the molecules) into a strong, ropelike unit. Generally, the shorter the length between cross-links or the larger the number of cross-links in a given distance, the higher the elasticity (Alexander 1975, 1988).

The number of cross-links may be related to collagen turnover; that is, collagen is continuously and simultaneously being produced and broken down. If production exceeds breakdown, more cross-links are established and the structure is more resistant to stretching, as in the case of scar tissue (Delforge 2002; Tillman and Cummings 1992). Conversely, if the breakdown exceeds production, the opposite holds true. For those developing a scar, collagen breakdown exceeding collagen production could lead to a more flexible and less bulky scar mass (Delforge 2002; McCune and Sprague 1990). Gosselin et al. (1998) demonstrated in rats that exercise decreases the number of cross-links by increasing the collagen turnover rate and thereby reduces muscle stiffness. The duration, frequency, and intensity of exercise required to achieve a reduction in muscle stiffness and hydroxylysylpyridinoline (HP) cross-links in aged rats is unclear. Findings (Cummings and Tillman 1992; Spielholz 1990) have also suggested that exercise or mobilization may play a determining factor in preventing cross-linking. Additional research is needed to quantify the exercise variables as they pertain to specific human populations (e.g., senior citizens or athletes).

Biochemical Composition of Collagen

The collagen molecule is a complex helical structure whose mechanical properties result both from its biochemical composition and from the physical arrangement of its individual molecules. Although collagen is composed of many amino acids, three are most prominent: *glycine*, which constitutes one-third of the total, *proline*, and *hydroxyproline*. Each of the latter constitutes one-fourth or more. Proline and hydroxyproline keep the ropelike packing arrangement of collagen stable and resistant to stretching. Thus, the higher the concentration of these amino acids, the higher the stretch resistance of the molecules. Because the nitrogen of proline is fixed in a ring structure, proline prevents easy rotation of the regions in which it is located (Grant et al. 1972). To help visualize this idea, think of these additional amino acids as being comparable to eggs added to a meat loaf or tin combined with copper to make bronze. In all these cases, the result is increased rigidity and stability of the end product.

Influence of Ground Substances on Collagen

A major factor affecting the mechanical behavior of collagen is the presence of *ground substances*, which are widely distributed throughout connective tissue and supporting tissues. They are also known as *cement substances*, and they form the viscous, gellike matrix in which cells and other components are embedded. They are composed of glycosaminoglycans (GAGs), plasma proteins, a variety of small proteins, and water.

Water makes up 60% to 70% of the total connective tissue content. The enormous water-binding capacity of GAG is considered partially responsible for this high water content. According to Viidik et al. (1982), the importance of the hyaluronate molecule cannot be overestimated, because it takes up a hydrodynamic volume 1,000 times the space occupied by the chain itself in an unhydrated state.

Hyaluronic acid and its attached or entrapped water is the principal fibrous connective tissue lubricant. It is believed to serve as a lubricant between the collagen fibers and fibrils, maintaining a critical distance between them and permitting them to glide freely past each other. The lubricant may also prevent excessive cross-linking (see figure 4.3).

Ground substances impart a viscous fluid factor into tissue. Viscous material such as putty responds slowly to maintained stretch with gradual creep and elongation. The lengthening of viscous substances is inversely related to the velocity of stretch. Therefore, the slower the stretch, the greater the elongation. After a release of tension, recovery is incomplete—the tissue does not return to its original length. The permanent deformation or lengthening is believed to be caused by bond disruption and fiber slippage, with resultant structural change in the tissue (Laban 1962; Sapega et al. 1981).

Electromechanical and Physiological Properties

Solid crystalline materials demonstrate electromechanical properties when deformed. This phenomenon is the *piezoelectric effect* (Athenstaedt 1970; Shamos and Lavine 1967). A similar effect is present in biological tissues. The knitted tropocollagen molecules that make up the native collagen fibril are electrically dipolar rods that have a permanent electric moment in the direction of the longitudinal tropocollagen axis (Athenstaedt 1970). Hulliger (2003) has suggested that "a Markov-chain mechanism takes place during collagen fibril self-assembly in extracytoplasmic channels . . . by a stochastic process of fibril elongation" (p. 3501).

In biologic tissues, the piezoelectric effect is called *electrokinetics* or *streaming potentials*. When a connective tissue such as cartilage is compressed, a mechanical-to-electrical transduction occurs, resulting in measurable electrical

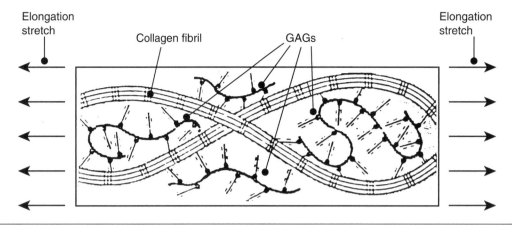

Figure 4.3   The action of GAGs. Stretch is applied to collagen fibrils, but the GAGs keep the fibrils separated and aligned.

Reprinted from Myers, Armstrong, and Mow 1984.

Glycosaminoglycan

A glycosaminoglycan (GAG) is a polysaccharide composed of repeating disaccharide (two-sugar) units. The four major GAGs found in connective tissue are hyaluronic acid, chondroitin-4-sulfate, chondroitin-6-sulfate, and dermatan sulfate. Generally, GAGs are bound to a protein and collectively referred to as *proteoglycans.* Connective tissue proteoglycans combine with water to form proteoglycan aggregates. By definition, a proteoglycan consists of a protein or a polypeptide to which one or more GAG chains are covalently attached. Each disaccharide group in the GAG chain often has two negatively charged groups. Their high fixed negative charge attracts counterions, and the osmotic imbalance caused by a local high concentration of ions draws water from the surrounding areas. Lederman (1997) has likened this action to dipping a bud of cottonwool into water: the cotton bud swells and expands as the water separates the cotton fibers. Proteoglycans thus keep the matrix hydrated by creating a water-filled compartment. Proteoglycans are not rigid because the GAG chains are freely mobile and can be forced together. This proximity produces a rise in internal charge density that counterbalances compressive forces.

potentials (Grodzinsky 1983). Deformation of biologic tissues can also produce hydrostatic pressure gradients, fluid flow, and cell deformation in the matrix. The mechanisms of these responses are unknown, although several theories have been proposed. However, an electrokinetic or a streaming-potential mechanism is the primary source of this transduction response (Grodzinsky 1987). (For overview of the relationship between electromechanical and physiochemical properties of connective tissue, see Grodzinsky [1983].) At present, two important questions are being investigated: (1) What is the mechanism that makes it operate? (2) What is the transduction phenomenon at the cellular level?

Mechanical Properties

The streaming potentials possibly represent the mechanism by which the mechanical forces of stretching are transduced into various types of gene expression and therefore into protein synthesis (e.g., developing specific isoforms of titin and other tissues). Sutcliffe and Davidson (1990) demonstrated that transduction of mechanical force into elastin gene expression by smooth muscle cells during stretching may contribute to their specific adaptations.

Currently, most research concentrates on articular cartilage under compression. Nonetheless, important information can be extrapolated from such studies on two grounds. First, articular cartilage is in the family of connective tissue. Second, elongation occurs simultaneously as a result of compression. Electrostatic forces are among the intermolecular interactions that can significantly affect rheological behavior of biological tissues (Grodzinsky et al. 1978). In particular, the extracellular matrix has the important function of resisting tensile, compressive, and shear mechanical stresses. Electrostatic repulsion forces between GAG fixed-charge groups tend to stiffen the matrix, thereby increasing its ability to withstand deformation and loading (Grodzinsky 1983, 1987; Muir 1983). Thus, proteoglycans act like "molecular springs" (Muir 1983).

The swelling pressure of certain tissues (e.g., intervertebral disks or cartilage) is crucial to the tissue's ability to withstand compressive loads. Urban et al. (1979) investigated the swelling pressure of proteoglycan solutions and found that swelling was independent of molecular size and aggregation state. The final hydration of intact tissues is determined not only by fixed-charge density but also by various other factors, including the arrangement of collagen fibrils, intramolecular and intermolecular cross-linkages, and proteoglycan-collagen interactions. Additional research is needed to investigate the effect of tensile forces applied under varying conditions (e.g., ballistic and static) on muscle fascia, ligaments, and tendons.

Effect of Static Versus Dynamic Loading

Studies of articular cartilage in vivo has demonstrated that static immobilization, reduced loading, or static compression of a joint results in regions of increased fixed-charge density, an increased concentration of positive counterions, and an increased osmotic pressure. Such factors inhibit proteoglycan synthesis and processing (Gray et al. 1988; Schneiderman et al. 1986; Urban and Bayliss 1989) and impair cartilage nutrition. In contrast, dynamic or oscillatory compression increases hydrostatic pressure, fluid flow, and streaming potentials and alters cell shape, possibly stimulating biosynthesis (Hall et al. 1991; Kim et al. 1994; Sah et al. 1992). Therefore, cyclic loading and unloading is good for maintaining cartilage health. However, during impacts or excessive loading, fluid flow, strain, and strain rate increase. High levels of strain or strain rate may cause matrix disruption, tissue swelling, and accentuate diffusion within cartilage (Sah et al. 1991), resulting in permanent cartilage damage.

Based on the preceding information, certain types of stretching techniques (e.g., ballistic) or specific stretches (e.g., hurdler's stretch, inverted hurdler's stretch, or bridges) may seem potentially harmful. However, those studies utilized high-amplitude, 24-hour cyclic compression in 2-hours-on/2-hours-off intervals. Does this information, then, have practical implications and relevance for those people who incorporate into an exercise program "traditional" stretches that maintain a stretch for 5 to 10 seconds, up to 1 minute? Additional research is needed to determine any advantageous or detrimental effects of loading for such brief periods of time.

Effects of Aging on Collagen

As collagen ages, specific physical and biochemical changes take place that reduce minimal extensibility and increase rigidity. For instance, aging increases the diameter of the collagen fibers in various tissues. Fibrils also become more crystalline, which strengthens the intermolecular bonds and increases resistance to further deformation. Furthermore, aging is believed to be associated with an increased number of intramolecular and intermolecular cross-links that apparently restrict the ability of collagen molecules to slip past each other. Dehydration also occurs with the aging process. Although the degree of reported dehydration varies from source to source, tendon water content declines from approximately 80% to 85% in babies to 70% in adults (Elliott 1965) (see figure 4.4). Another impact of age is a gradual decrease in collagen crimp. Martin et al. (1998) suggest that the reduced crimping may be two sides of the same

coin. That is, the reduced crimping may just be a "manifestation of the altered conformation of the collagen molecules caused by their additional cross-linking and the straightening of the collagen may promote additional cross-linking" (p. 323).

Studies using animal and human cadavers have shown that the mechanical properties of tendons change with aging. However, imaging techniques such as magnetic resonance imaging (MRI) and brightness-mode (B-mode) ultrasonography have revealed the architecture of the muscle-tendon complex and elastic properties of human tendon structures in vivo. The first such investigation by Kubo, Kanehisa, Kawakami, and Fukunaga (2001a) substantiated "that elastic properties of tendon structures are more compliant in younger boys than in adults" (p. 138). Their research also suggested that, "the observed properties of tendon structures in the younger boys may play a role in protecting younger boys from athletic injuries associated with immature muscle-tendon complex" (p. 138).

Ultrastructural Basis and the Physiological Limit of Collagen Elongation

Unlike a sarcomere, a collagen fiber is comparatively inextensible. A weight 10,000 times greater than its own will not stretch it (Verzar 1963). Under a microscope, elongated collagen displays progressive alteration in intrafibril periodicity and lateral dimensions.

Such an extension is believed to occur initially through a straightening of the fibers followed by a gradual slip of one fiber relative to the next. This movement results in an increase in crystallinity or orientation that strengthens the intermolecular bond and increases resistance to further elongation. With an increase in crystallinity, the intermeshing of the adjacent molecules increases. Consequently, increased regularity in packing and enhanced interchain forces permits increased resistance to deformation. Thus, simply stated, collagenous fibers allow elongation until the slack of their wavy bundles is taken up. However, if stretch continues, a point will be reached where all intermolecular forces are exceeded and the tissue parts (Goldberg and Rubinovich 1988; Laban 1962).

ELASTIC TISSUE

Elastic tissue is a primary structural component of living tissue and is found in various quantities throughout the body. Electron photomicrographs show a large amount of elastic tissue in the sarcolemma of a muscle fiber (the connective tissue that surrounds the sarcomere). Thus, elastic tissue plays a major role in determining the possible range of extensibility of muscle cells. In certain locations, large amounts of almost pure elastic fibers can

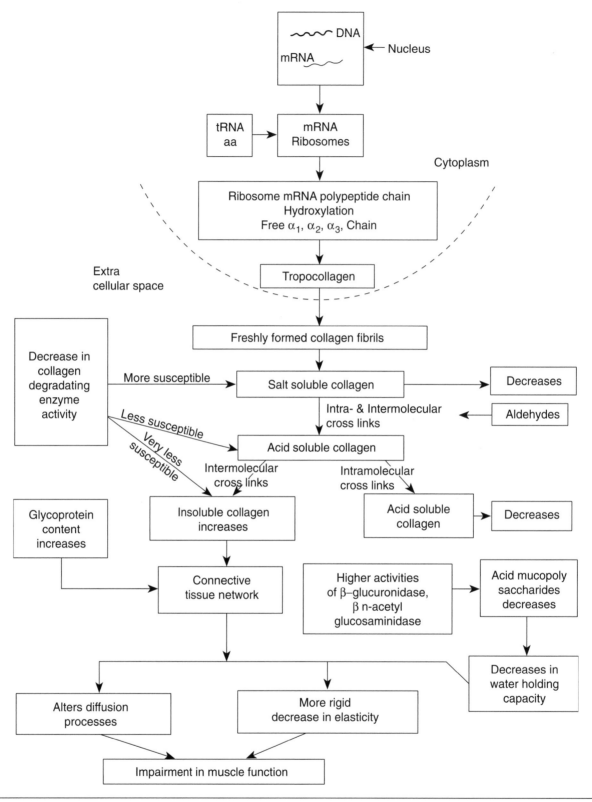

Figure 4.4 Schematic representation of age changes in connective tissue leading to impairment in muscle function. Reprinted from Mohan and Radha 1981.

be found, particularly in the ligaments of the vertebral column. Consequently, to a major extent, elastic tissue determines ROM.

Elastic fibers perform a variety of functions, including disseminating stresses that originate at isolated points, enhancing coordination of the rhythmic motions of the body parts, conserving energy by maintaining tone during relaxation of muscular elements, providing a defense against excessive forces, and assisting stretched organs in returning to their natural configuration (Jenkins and Little 1974).

Composition of Elastic Fibers

Unfortunately, elastic fibers have not been studied as extensively as collagen fibers and therefore are less understood. This situation is primarily the result of technical difficulties encountered in solubilizing elastic fibers (Modis 1991). Another reason is that elastic and collagen fibers are usually very closely associated anatomically, morphologically, biochemically, and physiologically. In fact, elastic fibers may have collagen fibers interwoven with their principal components and are usually dominated by them.

Elastic fibers are optically homogeneous. Hence, they are highly refractile and almost isotropic. Under an electron microscope, each fiber appears to consist of a fused mass of fibrils twisted in ropelike fashion. Unlike collagenous fibers, elastic fibers display a complete lack of banding or striation.

Elastic Tissue Cross-Links

Elastic fibers are thought to be composed of randomly coiled chains, probably joined by covalent (shared electrons) cross-links. However, the noncovalent interchain forces are considered weak, and the cross-links themselves are believed to be widely spaced (Goldberg and Rubinovich 1988). Consequently, elastic cross-links do not weld the molecules into a strong, ropelike unit similar to collagen. The significance of this difference will be discussed later.

Elastin

The term *elastic tissue* or *elastic fiber* has a structural connotation. In contrast, *elastin* refers to the biochemical character of elastic fibers. Elastin is a complex structure with a mechanical property of elasticity resulting both from its biochemical composition and from the physical arrangement of its individual molecules. Like collagen, elastin is also composed of amino acids, but elastin is composed mostly of nonpolar, hydrophobic amino acids, and it has little hydroxyproline and no hydroxylysine. Also, elastin contains *desmosine* and *isodesmosine*, which function as covalent cross-links in and between the polypeptide chains. The cross-link arrangement is not random. Rather, cross-linking domains must be specifi-

cally aligned during the polymerization process (Akagawa and Suyama 2000). Similar to collagen, about one-third of the residues of elastin are *glycine* and about 11% are *proline*.

Effects of Aging on Elastic Fibers

As a result of aging, elastic fibers lose their resiliency and undergo various other alterations, including fragmentation, fraying, calcification and other mineralizations, and an increase in cross-linkages. Biochemically, amino acids containing polar groups (e.g., desmosine, isodesmosine, and lysinonorleucine) increase as well. Other changes are an increase in the proportion of chondroitin sulfate B and keratosulfate. Altogether, these alterations appear to be responsible for age-related loss of resiliency and increased rigidity (Bick 1961; Gosline 1976).

Ultrastructural Basis and the Physiological Limit of Elastin Elongation

Elastic fibers yield easily to stretching but return to virtually their former length when released. Only when elastic fibers are stretched to about 150% of their original length do they reach their breaking point; a force of only 20 to 30 kg/cm^2 is required (Bloom et al. 1994).

Several models have been developed to explain the elastic force associated with elastin. One theory is the two-phase model proposed by Partridge (1966) and later adopted by Weis-Fogh and Anderson (1970a, 1970b). According to this model, elastin exists as distinct particles attached to one another by cross-linkages, with water in spaces between the particles. The globules are initially spherical, but during stretching, they are drawn out and form an ellipsoid shape. This change of shape is opposed by the surface tension. When the stretch is released, surface tension makes the globules become spherical again and so drives the elastic recoil. This model has been challenged by Hoeve and Flory (1974), based on thermodynamic considerations.

A second theory is that the elastin is composed of a network of randomly coiled chains joined by covalent cross-links. These cross-links impose a restriction on the relative movement of the elastic fibers, so that when the tissue is stretched, the individual chains are constrained and cannot slip past one another (Franzblau and Faru 1981). However, the covalent interchain forces are weak, and the cross-links widely spaced. As a result, minimal unidirectional force can produce extensive elongation of chains before the cross-links begin to restrict movement. Thus, like the collagenous fibers, elastic fibers allow extensibility until the slack and spacing between the chains are taken up.

A third theory, proposed by Urry (1984), also relies on an entropy-driven mechanism to provide the elastomeric force. However, this theory relies on a different molecular conformation, which has been summarized by Rosenbloom et al. (1993):

> The entropic elasticity derives from the b-spiral structure, with essentially fixed end-to-end chain lengths. The peptide segments suspended between the b-turns are free to undergo large-amplitude, low-frequency rocking motions called librations. Upon stretching, there is a decrease in amplitude of the librations that results in a large decrease in the entropy of the segment, and this provides the driving elastomeric force for return to the relaxed state. (p. 1217)

Recently, Li and Daggett (2002) reconfirmed that "Water plays a critical role in determining elastin's conformational behavior, making elastin extremely dynamic in its relaxed state and providing an important source of elasticity" (p. 561). Further studies are required to determine the molecular basis for the extensibility of elastin. A final working model must account for elastic proteins ability to withstand low force, stretch and not break at high force, and recover upon release of the force.

RELATIONSHIP BETWEEN COLLAGENOUS AND ELASTIC FIBERS

Elastic fibers are almost always found in close association with collagenous tissues. Furthermore, the performance of the combined tissue is a result of blending and integrating the distinctly different mechanical properties of the two tissues. The elastic fibers themselves are typically responsible for what may be called reverse elasticity (the ability of a stretched material to return to its resting state). The collagen meshwork provides the rigid constraints that limit the deformations of the elastic elements and that are largely responsible for the ultimate properties (tensile strength and relative inextensibility) of those composite structures. Logically, where collagenous fibers dominate, rigidity, stability, tensile strength, and a restricted ROM will prevail (Eldren 1968; Gosline 1976).

The difference in male and female subjects' responses to various stretching treatments may be caused by the unique properties of connective tissue in each sex (Starring et al. 1988). Males have more connective tissue than females, especially collagen. Consequently, the extensibility of a male's muscle tissue is less. This fact may also explain why a male will not gain as much ROM as a female after stretching treatment. Furthermore, the different connective tissue network of males provides even greater mechanical strength than that of females. Consequently, a male's "connective tissue composition is more resistant to passive stretching, resulting in lower ROM gains" (Starring et al. 1988, p. 319).

STRUCTURES COMPOSED OF CONNECTIVE TISSUE

The human body contains numerous structures composed of connective tissue. Classification systems of connective tissue vary but can be broken down into five main categories: (1) loose connective tissue, which is further divided into areolar (ordinary tissue located between other tissues and organs) and adipose (fat); (2) dense connective tissue located in tendons, ligaments, aponeuroses, deep fascia, the dermis, and scars, which can also be subcategorized as regular and irregular; (3) cartilage; (4) bone; and (5) blood. In terms of flexibility and stretching, the three structures that are of greatest concern are tendons, ligaments, and fascia.

Tendons

Tendons are tough and fibrous cords that attach muscles to bones. The primary function of tendons is to transmit tension from muscles to bones, thereby producing motion. Additional functions of tendons include joint stabilization, serves as mechanical pulleys, and motor control (Nordin and Frankel 2001). Tendons are extremely important in determining one's quality of movement. Verzar (1964) vividly described this concept:

> The importance of inextensibility, from a physiological point of view, is that the smallest muscular contraction can be transmitted without loss to the articulations. If tendons, i.e., collagen fibers, were only slightly extensible, the finest movements, such as those of the fingers of a violinist or pianist, or the exact movements of the eye, would be impossible. (p. 255)

Tendons are also believed to prevent or reduce injury to a muscle during high-velocity action or the sudden application of external force (Moore 1992). One important role of tendons is proprioception. Mechanoreceptors called Golgi tendon organs sense tension and provide feedback control to muscles (see chapter 7). Another function of tendon is energy storage (see chapter 19).

The chief constituents of tendons are closely packed, parallel, collagenous bundles that vary in length and thickness. They show a distinct longitudinal striation and in many places fuse with one another. The fibrils making up the tendon are virtually all oriented toward the long axis, which is also the direction of normal physiological stress. The tendon is thus especially adapted to resist movement in one direction. However, "during various phases of movements, the tendons are exposed not only to longitudinal but also to transversal and rotational forces. In addition, they must be prepared to withstand direct contusions and pressures" (Kannus 2000, p. 310). Tendons have the highest tensile strength of any soft tissue. Elastic fibers within tendons may contribute to the shock-absorbing capacity of tendons and maintenance of the collagen crimp pattern (Hyman and Rodeo 2000). The greater the proportion of collagen to elastic fibers, the greater the density of stable (pyridinoline) cross-links, the greater the number of fibers that are oriented in the direction of stress, and the greater the cross-sectional area or width of the tendon, the stronger the tendon.

Because muscle fibers are organized in a staggered fashion, the macroscopic transition from muscle to tendon is gradual rather than abrupt (Moore 1992). The myotendinous junction (MTJ) is the region where tension generated by muscle fibers is transmitted from intracellular contractile proteins to extracellular connective tissue proteins (collagen fibrils) (Józsa and Kannius 1997). At the MTJ, the collagen fibrils insert into deep recesses that are formed between fingerlike processes (endings) of the muscle cells. This type of folding increases the contact area between the muscle fibers and tendon collagen fibers, by 10 to 20 times. Consequently, this folding arrangement can significantly reduce the force applied per surface unit of the MTJ during muscle contraction (Józsa and Kannius 1997; Whiting and Zernicke 1998). Experimental evidence (Garrett et al. 1987), clinical evidence (Safran et al. 1988), computed tomography (CT) scanning (Garrett et al. 1989), and MRI (De Smet and Best 2000; Fleckenstein et al. 1989) have shown that most muscle strain injuries occur at the musculotendon junction or tendon-bone junction (Garrett 1990). Whiting and Zernicke (1998) speculate several factors contribute to the MTJ's susceptibility to injury:

- The structural folding configuration aligns the junctional membrane so that it experiences primarily shear forces rather than tensile forces.
- The folding may increase the adhesive strength of the muscle cell to the tendon.
- The sarcomeres near the junction are stiffer than those farther from the junction and thus have limited extensibility.

Additional research is needed to identify the optimal means to prevent injury at this weak link.

An important character of tendons is that the stress-strain relationship is nonlinear (Kuo et al. 2001). When stretch tension is applied to tendon, the amount of deformation follows a load-deformation curve. A tendon displays a typical stress-strain curve with three characteristic regions (Abrahams 1967; Lucas et al. 1999; Rigby et al. 1959): a toe region, an elastic region, and a plastic region.

At the lowest levels of tension, the tendon's crimped fibrils merely straighten. Abrahams (1967) has termed this portion of the curve the primary region, while others refer to it as the "toe region" (Lucas et al. 1999). This region corresponds to approximately 0% to 1.5% strain (Abrahams 1967). The crimping arrangement of the

collagen fibrils permits tendons to have an initial low stiffness. Two possible explanation for this viscoelastic behavior include:

> (1) internal friction caused by sliding of one microstructural element past another (for example, collagen fibrils rubbing against collagen fibrils). Viscous drags of interstitial fluid as it flows through the porous-permeable solid matrix (analogous to the resistance encountered when water is forced through coffee grounds in an espresso machine) . . . For ligaments and tendons under tensile loads, the major cause of internal friction arises from the "uncrimping" of the collagen fiber bundles as they slide through the thick viscous proteoglycan gel. (Mow et al. 2000, p. 159)

Abrahams (1967) demonstrated that repeated loading within this region is associated with complete recovery without residual strain or permanent deformation. For tendons, the stress needed to flatten the "toe region" was found to be equal to maximal contraction of the muscle (Viidik 1980). "This implies that during passive muscle stretching most of the elongation will take place in the muscle belly rather than its tendon" (Lederman 1997, p. 26).

The second region of the curve is the elastic, or linear, region. As applied tensile load increases, the crimping straightens out and the collagen fibrils become more fully oriented. This secondary region of the curve corresponds to a strain of approximately 1.5% to 3.0%. However, some sources report strains as high as 5% (Abrahams 1967; Crisp 1972; Lederman 1997; Zachazewski 1990). The elastic region is characterized by deformations that rise in a linear manner related to the amount of tension. This region represents the elastic modulus of the tendon. Within this range of loads, the tendon will return to its original length when unloaded.

The plastic region, or Zone III, is the region of primary failure (Zachazewski 1990). At loads greater than the elastic range, permanent length changes will occur, accompanied by microtrauma to the tendon's structural integrity (the "yield" point of the curve). Abrahams (1967) reported physical rupture of fibers commenced at the 5% to 6% strain level. Because fewer fibrils remain to absorb the tensile force, the tendon has a reduced effective cross-sectional area (Moore 1992). If strain continues, the tendon will ultimately reach a point of total failure. Estimates of strain at the point of ultimate failure range from 5% to 30% (Abrahams 1967; Woo 1982; Zachazewski 1990).

Taylor et al. (1990) investigated the viscoelastic properties of rabbit extensor digitorum longus and tibialis anterior muscle-tendon unit. Their experiments attempted to simulate cyclic stretching and static stretching. Figure 4.5a depicts the data from 10 controlled stretches to 10%

beyond resting length. Each stretch resulted in a progressive decrease in the peak tension. The first four stretches show significant difference from the other nine peak tensions. Figure 4.5b shows the relaxation curves that followed each stretch. Only the first three stretches show a statistical difference. Figure 4.5c depicts the lengthening associated with each stretch. The study demonstrated that

80% of the total change in length was accomplished in the first four stretches when 10 repeated stretches were applied at the same level of tension. Figure 4.5d shows representative waveforms from a single muscle during the first series of stretches. Figure 4.5e shows the energy absorbed (hysteresis) during cyclical stretching to 10% beyond the resting length at different rates.

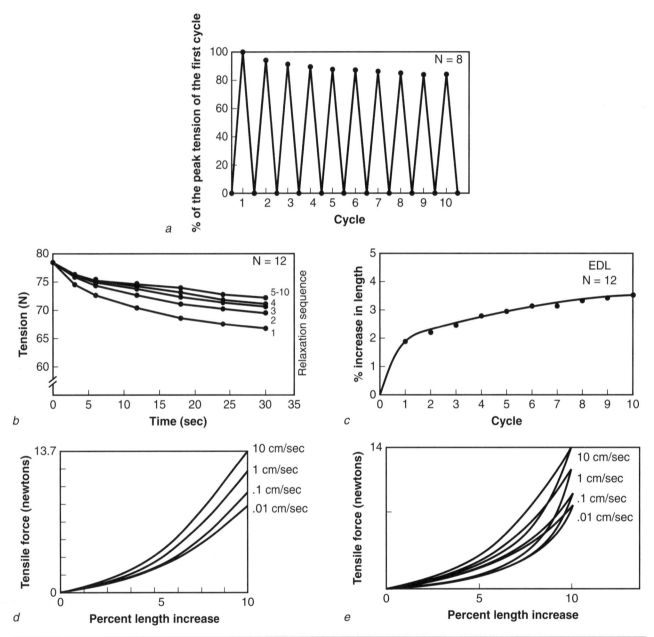

Figure 4.5 (*a*) Tension curves of EDL muscle-tendon units repeatedly stretched to 10% beyond resting length. Each of the peak tensions for the first four stretches showed a statistically significant ($p < .05$) difference from the other peak tensions. The overall tension decrease was 16.6%. (*b*) Relaxation curves for EDL muscle-tendon units stretched repeatedly to 78.4 N. The relaxation curves of the first two stretches demonstrated statistically significant differences from the other curves. There were no significant differences in curves 4 through 10. (*c*) Graphic representation of EDL lengthening with repeated stretching to the same tension. Eighty percent of the length increase occurred during the first four stretches. (*d*) Representative force-length relationships demonstrating the effect of stretch rate on a single TA muscle-tendon unit. (*e*) Hysteresis loops observed in TA muscle during loading at constant rates of 0.01, 0.1, 1 and 10 cm/s.

Reprinted from Taylor et al. 1990.

Based on the research of Taylor et al. (1990), little benefit might be expected after four stretches. However, readers are cautioned about extrapolating this data to humans. Significantly, the study does not factor in various neurological processes that also impact the muscle-tendon unit while it is under tensile force.

What is the effect of repetitive loading on a tendon? Kubo, Kanehisa, and Fukunaga (2002b) has demonstrated that repeated static stretching and isometric contractions made the human tendon structures decrease stiffness, indicating an increase in elongation of the tendon structures. Thus, the tendon was more compliant *in vivo*. One possible explanation was that contractions were responsible for an actual increase in temperature. In turn, this temperature increase would alter the viscoelastic properties of the intramuscular connective tissue. With 5 minutes of static stretching, stiffness decreased by 8% and hysteresis decreased by 29%. In another study, stiffness and hysteresis decreased significantly 9% and 34% after stretching for 10 minutes (Kubo, Kanehisa, Kawakami, and Fukunaga 2001b). These studies substantiate that stretching makes tendon structure more compliant. Considering these findings Kubo, Kanehisa, and Fukunaga (2002a) speculate that stretch training increases flexibility but not the elasticity of tendon structures. Rather, it affects the viscosity of tendon structure and significantly decreases the hysteresis. An investigation by Fukashiro et al. (2002) found no significant difference in tendon elasticity among African American and Caucasian athletes.

Ligaments

Ligaments bind bone to bone. Consequently, unlike tendons, they attach (insert) to bones at both ends and stabilize and support a joint (the place where two or more bones meet) by holding the bones in place. Abundant research information exists about the types of neural sensory receptors located in ligaments (Brand 1986; Rowinski 1997) that function as sensors for the nervous system. Thus, "they may have played a larger role in normal joint function than has been realized and may make a correspondingly large contribution to the pathological consequences of injuries" (Armstrong et al. 1992, p. 276). Additional functions of ligaments are guiding movement, maintaining body posture, and motor control (Nordin and Frankel 2001).

Ligaments are similar to tendons, except they have a lower percentage of collagen and a higher percentage of ground substance, and the elements are more randomly arranged (Lucas et al. 1999). Like tendons, ligaments are composed mainly of bundles of collagenous fibers parallel to, or closely interlaced with, one another. Ligaments occur in different shapes, such as cords, bands, and sheets. However, they lack the glistening whiteness of tendons because they have a greater mixture of elastic and fine collagenous fibers woven among the parallel bundles.

Consequently, they are pliant and flexible enough to allow freedom of movement but strong, tough, and inextensible enough to be resistant to applied forces.

Ligaments contain mostly collagenous tissue. The exceptions are the ligamentum flavum and ligamentum nuchae, which connect the laminae of adjacent vertebrae in the lower spine and neck, respectively. These ligaments are made up almost entirely of elastic fibers and are quite elastic. Another reason for differences in viscoelastic properties among some ligaments and tendons is the percentage of GAGs. Woo et al. (1985) found that only 1% to 1.5% of tendons are made up of GAGs. Similarly, collateral ligament also consists of 1% to 1.5% GAGs. In contrast, the cruciate ligaments total 2.5% to 3.0% GAG concentration. Part of ligament's viscoelastic nature results from the interaction of the collagen and ground substance (Lucas et al. 1999). A study to find out whether quantitative differences exist between the GAG content of ligaments of gymnasts, dancers, or contortionists and those of the "normal" population would be interesting. Does a higher percentage of GAGs increase the extensibility of ligaments?

Johns and Wright (1962) determined that tendons provide only about 10% of the total resistance to movement. In contrast, the ligaments and joint capsule contribute about 47% (see table 4.2). Consequently, the latter tissues are extremely significant in determining the ultimate ROM of a joint. As a general rule, laypeople should not direct their stretching exercises toward elongating the joint capsule and normal-length ligaments, because stretching these structures may destabilize the joint and increase the likelihood of injury. However, the application of a chiropractic adjustment or general manipulation under the care of a trained and certified practitioner (e.g., chiropractor, osteopath, or physical therapist) has been demonstrated in many cases to be effective in correcting subluxations, increasing ROM, reducing pain, and improving performance in many patients. In fact, stretching a joint capsule is absolutely essential if it has

Table 4.2 Comparison of the Relative Contribution of Soft Tissue Structures to Joint Resistance

Structure	Resistance
Joint capsule	47%
Muscle (fascia)	41%
Tendon	10%
Skin	2%

Reprinted, by permission, from R.J. Johns and V. Wright, 1962, "Relative importance of various tissues in joint stiffness," *Journal of Applied Physiology* 17(5), 824-828.

become shortened and is limiting ROM (as in adhesive capsulitis at the shoulder).

Fascia

The word *fascia*, taken from Latin, means a band or bandage. The term is used in gross anatomy to designate all fibrous connective structures not otherwise specifically named. Like previously mentioned tissues, fascia varies in thickness and density according to functional demands, and it usually forms membranous sheets.

The fascia can be broken down into three general types. (1) The *superficial fascia* lies directly below the dermis (i.e., skin). It is composed of two layers. The outer layer, called the *panniculus adiposus*, contains an accumulation of fat that varies in amount among individuals and regions of the body. The *inner layer*, by contrast, is a thin membrane that ordinarily has no fat. In many parts of the body, the superficial fascia glides freely over the deep fascia, producing the characteristic movability of skin (Clemente 1985). (2) The *deep fascia* is directly beneath the superficial fascia and is usually tougher, tighter, and more compact than the superficial fascia. Deep fascia covers and is fused with the muscles, bones, nerves, blood vessels, and organs of the body. It compartmentalizes the body by separating such things as muscles and the internal visceral organs. (3) The *subserous fascia* is innermost around body cavities. It forms the fibrous layer of the serous membranes that cover and support the viscera. Examples include the pleura around the lungs,

the pericardium around the heart, and the peritoneum around the abdominal cavity and organs.

The deep fascia that envelops and binds down skeletal muscle into separate groups is named according to where it is found (see figure 4.6). The deep fascia that encases the entire muscle is called the *epimysium*. The *perimysium* surrounds the bundles of muscle fibers known as *fasciculi* and interconnects them to the epimysium. Within the perimysium, as many as 150 individual fibers may be found. The perimysium also binds each muscle fiber within a bundle to its immediate neighbor (Rowe 1981). Surrounding each muscle fiber is the *endomysium*, which also interconnects to the perimysium (Borg and Caulfield 1980). Beyond the individual muscle fiber is the sarcomere, the functional unit of the muscle. This level of muscle is surrounded by a connective tissue called the *sarcolemma*.

In a comparison of six bovine muscles, Light et al. (1985) found that the ratio of dry mass of perimysium to dry mass of endomysium was between 2.8 to 1 and 64 to 1. Thus, generally speaking, muscle contain far more perimysial connective tissue than endomysial connective tissue (Purslow 1989). Furthermore, although several components of connective tissue that package the muscle belly contribute to resistance when a muscle is passively stretched, the relatively large amount of perimysium has been considered the major contributor to extracellular passive resistance to stretch (Purslow 1989). According to Gajdosik (1997), the perimysium is important because its influence is associated with aging:

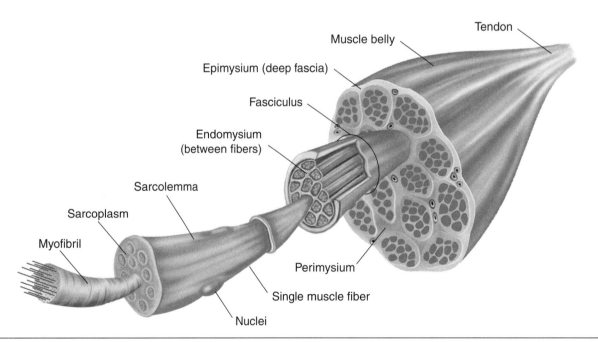

Figure 4.6 Schematic drawing of a muscle illustrating three types of connective tissue: epimysium (the outer layer), perimysium (surrounding each fasciculus, or group of fibers), and endomysium (surrounding individual fibers).

Reprinted from National Strength and Conditioning Association 2000.

Increased amounts of the perimysium [associated with aging] would potentially contribute to increased passive stiffness because lengthening the relatively inextensible collagen fibers would mechanically realign the criss-cross array of the collagen fibers. This realignment should cause increased stiffness because of greater tension per unit of length change, particularly near the end of muscle lengthening. (p. 164)

Function of Fascia

According to Rowe (1981), intramuscular connective tissue has at least three probable functions. First, it provides a framework that binds the muscle together and ensures the proper alignment of muscle fibers, blood vessels, nerves, and so on. Second, it enables forces, either actively developed by the muscle or passively imposed on the muscle, to be transmitted by the whole tissue safely and effectively. Third, it provides the necessary lubricated surfaces between muscle fibers and muscle fiber bundles that enable the muscle to change its shape.

As much as 30% of muscle mass is connective tissue. This tissue allows muscle to change length. During passive motion, the sum of the muscle's fascia accounts for 41% of the total resistance to movement. In comparison, the resistance of the joint capsule, tendon, and skin are 47%, 10% and 2%, respectively (Johns and Wright 1962). Hence, the fascia represents the second most important factor limiting the ROM. Consequently, a stretching program should be directed primarily toward elongating the fascia but not the ligaments, because stretching these structures may result in destabilization of the joint.

The functional relationships between fascia and the forces and pressures generated by underlying muscular contractions are still poorly understood. Few research projects have studied the biomechanical effects of fascia on muscle or explored the effect that removal of the fascia has on the underlying muscle and osseofascial compartment (Manheim 2001). One early research study clearly demonstrated the importance of the fascial tissues. Garfin et al. (1981) found that using a surgical fascial release to create a small slit in the epimysium of a dog's hindlimbs resulted in an approximately 15% reduction in force produced and a 50% decrease in the intracompartmental pressure developed during muscle contraction. Huijing (1999), Huijing and Baan (2001) and Huijing et al. (1998) proposed and supported the proposition that intramuscular connective tissue is indeed a major path for force transmission. They termed this mechanism "myofascial force transmission."

As discussed in chapter 3, views on adaptation of muscle are shifting to a possibility of direct mechanical deformation of the cell nuclei (Ingber 1997; N. Wang et al. 1993). Furthermore, even autocrine muscular activity (Goldspink 1999) may be related to processes of myofascial force transmission. "These pathways could conceivably be active as a path in exerting direct effects from a whole compartment onto nuclei within muscle fibres and fibrocytes of muscle" (Huijing and Baan 2001, p. 309).

Myofascial Restrictions and the Anatomy of Fascia

Often, medical practitioners and allied health professionals view the body from a myopic point of view determined by their practice, philosophy, mastered techniques, or time limitations. Traditionally (and of course stereotypically), physical therapists are concerned with movement dysfunction as the basic problem addressed by their intervention, chiropractors are concerned with a subluxation of the vertebrae, osteopaths are concerned with an osteopathic lesion, medical doctors are concerned with pain or symptom relief, acupuncturists are concerned with treating a trigger point, and so on. However, what happens if the problem is in the fascia and not the joints, muscles, or nerves? As described by Kegerreis (2001), "Soft tissue injury is the injury that 'falls between the cracks' of medical specialists" (p. 5). Fascia has the capacity to adapt to various conditions. Furthermore, fasciae must be recognized as continuous (fasciae can be traced from one area of the body to another) and contiguous (they all touch). To better understand myofascial interaction, imagine that the body is like a giant balloon filled with smaller balloons that are attached to it inside. These smaller balloons represent the body's various organs and muscles. If just one part of the balloon is distorted by tightness or restriction, then all parts of the balloon must be distorted to compensate. A variety of models can be employed to represent this concept (Kegerreis 2001; Kuchera and Kuchera 1992).

Diagnosis of Myofascial Restrictions

Diagnosing myofascial restrictions requires a similar approach as that used in an auto body shop: evaluating areas of the rest of the patient's body for symmetry/asymmetry and looseness/tightness. For example, if your car is hit in the rear bumper by another car at a moderate speed, damage may occur to the rear bumper and fenders, but body damage may also occur throughout the vehicle. Thus, the body shop would not only need to replace the damaged fender but also repair the damage throughout the car. Patients in a health practitioner's office may not be treated as well as a car in a body shop—the "rear fender" is fixed, but the subtle damage to the rest of the body is ignored. With a car, this oversight may reduce its efficiency and decrease its life expectancy. With a human being, uneven stress transmitted through the fascia to other parts of the body may result in short and tight connective tissue and muscle causing stiffness, decreased ROM, pain, and decrease in quality of life. The evaluating process of myofascial restrictions can be easily demonstrated.

Fascial interconnections can be demonstrated visually and tactilely. First, visualize a skeleton with a tight plastic overlay representing the muscles and fascia. As the overlays are stretched, they change to white along the lines of stress. Similarly, trained therapists can often visually detect uneven stress transmitted to the skin. Second, fascial connections can be sensed by palpation. Specifically, the therapist monitors tissue tightness by developing a kinesthetic link with the patient through touch. For example, have a partner lie on a table. Place your fingers gently on his or her scalp, close your eyes, and concentrate on any movement transferred to the scalp. Have the partner move his or her head, and feel the subsequent movement transmitted to the scalp. Next, have the partner shrug his or her shoulders, and once again feel the movement transmitted to the scalp. Gradually, work down the body, having the hips, knees, ankles, and even toes flex and extend. Even the most subtle movements of the most distal parts of the extremities will be detected. Readers interested in learning how to evaluate areas of the body of symmetry-asymmetry and looseness-tightness are referred to the references below.

Treatment Strategies for Compromised Fascia

When the body is subjected to insult, fascial restrictions may occur in all directions: parallel, perpendicular, and oblique to the muscle fibers. To relieve such restrictions, biomechanical forces of tension, compression, shearing, bending, stress, and strain can be applied to the tissue (Spoerl et al. 1994). Dennis Morgan (1994) has identified at least nine soft-tissue treatment variables:

1. Location: (the placement of the hand or hands in relation to the lesion)
2. Area (the surface area contacted)
3. Direction (the direction the force is applied)
4. Depth (the distance tissue is depressed)
5. Force (the force applied to the area)
6. Time (the length of time the force is applied to the area)
7. Amplitude (the range the tissue is moved)
8. Rhythm (the rhythm the force is applied)
9. Rate (the speed the force is applied)

Based upon these nine variables a variety of techniques can be performed (e.g., general massage, rolfing, mobilization, manipulation, and stretching). One technique that has received much notoriety is the *myofascial release technique* (MRT). MRT can target connective tissues or muscles. Several books and chapters of books have been written on MRT, from which this discussion was culled (Barnes 1999; Cantu and Grodin 2001; Keirns 2000; Manheim 2001; Souza 1994; Ward 1993, 2001). "Unfortunately, very few articles concerning Myofascial Release have been published in peer reviewed journals" (Manheim 2001, p. xv).

Manheim (2001) has identified five basic steps of myofascial release: feedback, stretch, hold, release, and end-feel. A grossly overgeneralized version of this technique follows. The patient is evaluated by "reading the tissues" for areas of symmetry-asymmetry and looseness-tightness. A body region or limb is moved in multiplanar directions of relative ease until a distinct motion barrier is encountered. Then, a force is applied in the appropriate direction and held until the soft tissues are relax and the barrier is released. This "softening" or "letting go" is called a *release*. This release also includes the somewhat esoteric concept of "unwinding" (Bilkey 1992). The process is then repeated until the targeted tissues are fully elongated. A variety of force application techniques can be employed using MRT. In the method termed *transverse muscle play*, a shearing force is applied by both palms of the therapist. The hands do not slide over the skin. Rather, the fascial layers slide on one another. Another method is *stripping*. Here, the therapist uses a broad contact over the area of tightness and applies firm pressure as the patient actively moves through a full range. In a variation of this technique, the therapist performs a stripping massage while the muscle is under stretch with no active movement by the patient. *Strumming* is a deep-release technique that is usually performed with the therapist's fingers held in rigid extension or hand cupped in a clawlike position. Deep pressure is then applied to the restricted site across and perpendicular to the muscle fibers. For a more detailed discussion, the reader is referred to the works of Cantu and Grodin (2001), Keirns (2000), and Manheim and Lavett (2001).

EFFECTS OF IMMOBILIZATION ON CONNECTIVE TISSUE

As a result of abnormal physical and chemical states, fascia may thicken, shorten, calcify, or erode, often causing pain. In particular, when joints are immobilized for any length of time, the connective tissue elements of the capsules, ligaments, tendons, muscles, and fascia lose their extensibility. Of significance, "immobilization results in the rapid down-regulation of total muscular collagen synthesis" and "decrease in mRNA levels of type I and III collagens" (Ahtikosli et al. 2001, p. 131). In addition, immobilization is associated with a concomitant change in chemical structure: 40% decrease in hyaluronic acid, 30% decrease in chondroitin-4-sulfate and chondroitin-6-sulfate, and 4.4% loss of water (Akeson et al. 1967; Akeson et al. 1977; Akeson et al. 1980; Woo et al. 1975). If distances between fibers are assumed to be reduced when GAG and water volumes decreases, the loss of GAG and water will result in a reduction of the critical fiber distance between collagen fibers. Consequently, the connective tissue fibers will come into contact with each other and eventually stick, thereby encouraging the formation of abnormal cross-linking. The result is the loss of extensibility and an increase in tissue stiffness (see figure 4.7) (Akeson et al. 1980; McDonough 1981).

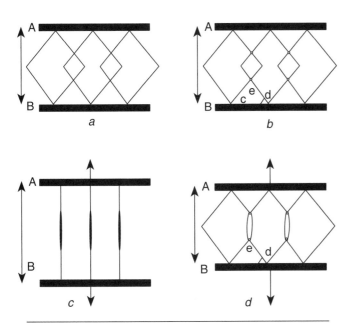

Figure 4.7 The idealized weave pattern of collagen fibers. It can be demonstrated that fixed contact at strategic sites (e.g., points d and e) can severely restrict the extension of this collagen weave. (*a*) Collagen fiber arrangement; (*b*) collagen fiber cross-links; (*c*) normal stretch; and (*d*) restricted stretch due to cross-link.

Reprinted from Akeson, Amiel, and Woo 1980.

In addressing the significance of immobilization and mobilization, Donatelli and Owens-Burkhart (1981) succinctly point out:

> If movement is the major stimulus for biological activity, then the amount, the duration, the frequency, the rate, and the time of initiation of the movement are all important in producing the desired therapeutic effects on connective tissue structures. These factors must be determined before we can comprehend the optimal benefits of mobilization. (p. 72)

METABOLIC AND NUTRITIONAL INFLUENCES ON CONNECTIVE TISSUE

Normal tissue growth and wound healing are a highly dynamic, integrated series of cellular, physiologic, and biochemical events that occur exclusively in whole organisms. Two factors that have significant implications for optimal function, growth, and wound healing are metabolic and nutritional influences (e.g., vitamins A, E, and C and the minerals calcium, copper, iron, magnesium, and manganese). A number of dietary deficiencies, excesses, and imbalances influence the metabolism and maturation of connective tissue proteins (see table 4.3). Furthermore, inherited genetic disorders influence enzyme activity and, in turn, influence the metabolic pathways involved in the synthesis of connective tissue. Because several enzymes participate in tissue formation, defects in any of the several steps of modification could become manifest. In turn,

Table 4.3 Roles of Selected Nutrients in Maintenance of Connective Tissue

Nutrient	Functions important for connective tissue maintenance
Copper	Collagen and elastic cross-linking, perhaps in sulfation or glycosylation of proteoglycans
Manganese	Cofactor for glycosyl transferases
Zinc	Cell differentiation and histone assembly and structure
Ascorbic acid	Cofactor in prolyl and lysyl hydroxylation, perhaps a cofactor in certain glycosylation reactions
Pyridoxine	Elastin and collagen cross-linking (?)
Thiamine	Collagen synthesis (?)
Vitamin A	Differentiation of epithelium and putative role in proteoglycan synthesis
Vitamin E	Collagen cross-linking (?)
Vitamin D	Bone collagen synthesis and osteoblast differentiation
Vitamin K	Cofactor in carboxylations of glutamyl residues in osteocalcin

Reprinted, by permission, from D. Tinker and R.B. Rucker, 1985, "Role of selected nutrients in synthesis, accumulation, and chemical modification of connective tissue proteins," *Physiological Reviews* 65(3), 624.

these connective tissue defects may ultimately influence tissue elasticity, stiffness, ROM, and wound healing.

Tinker and Rucker (1985) offers the most detailed analysis on the subject of the proposed mechanisms by which diet changes can modify connective tissue metabolism. Mead (1994) provides an interesting examination of how research suggests that diet may improve one's suppleness. Unfortunately, the article does not provide any references.

A factor discussed widely in the popular media and on the Internet is the importance of drinking plenty of water. Dehydration is another postulated factor in muscle stiffness. "Thirsty muscles" are believed to be less flexible and more prone to injury. Supposedly, it is also easier to stretch when your body is well hydrated. Therefore, water proponents claim muscle tissue beginning to

"dry" for lack of water will be more difficult to stretch adequately. Clinical research is required to substantiate these claims.

SUMMARY

Connective tissue plays a significant role in determining one's ROM. This tissue is influenced by a variety of factors, such as aging, immobilization, insults to the body, metabolic disorders, and nutritional deficiencies or excesses. Total resistance to movement has been determined to be 10% from tendon, 47% from joint capsule and ligament, and 41% from fascia. Because connective tissues are one of the most influential components in limiting ROM, they must be optimally stretched.

Mechanical and Dynamic Properties of Soft Tissues

Biophysics is the study of biological structures and processes by applying the principles of physics. Understanding the biophysics of muscle and connective tissue under various types of stress is essential for determining the optimal means of increasing ROM. Unfortunately, the principles of physics do not always readily lend themselves to the study of biological tissues, which often behave in nonlinear ways. When dealing with such tissues, one must simultaneous take into consideration their mechanical, electrical, and biochemical responses, particularly at the micro level (Lee 1980). In addition, when dealing with living human beings, one must take into consideration nonbiophysical factors such as feelings (e.g., pain and pleasure) and emotions (e.g., fear and joy).

TERMINOLOGY

Authors of review articles and researchers have expressed criticism regarding the confusing nomenclature and terminology in the literature (Gajdosik 2001; Gajdosik et al. 1999; Kotoulas 2002). This lack of consistency creates difficulty in making comparisons between studies and interpreting results across studies. Standardized terminology is essential for accurate intradisciplinary and interdisciplinary communication. A lack of standardized terminology creates a high risk of misinterpreting published results. For example, some studies use the term *elasticity* to describe the extensibility of tissue, whereas others use the term to refer to the property of tissue to return to its original shape. Occasionally the terms flexibility (ROM) and compliance are used interchangeably within a paper. However, these terms can have completely different meanings. For knowledge to optimally progress, standardized nomenclature must be established and implemented. The most precise and accurate terminology possible has been adopted for use in this text.

Types of Force and Deformations

Whenever a material is subjected to a *force* (i.e., a pull or a push), a change in the shape or size of the material can occur. This response is, of course, dependent upon such variables as the type of material, the amount of force, the duration of the force, and the temperature of the material, to name a few. An obvious goal in flexibility training or rehabilitation is to use optimal force to produce an intended change.

These changes are called *deformations*, and the types of force and the resulting deformations experienced by biological tissues and other materials fall into three major categories. A material subjected to a *compressive* force, for instance, decreases in length and increases in width. This type of deformation is called *compression*. An example of compression is weight bearing on the cartilage of a joint surface. In rehabilitation, compression can be a valuable tool because of its influence on fluid flow. It can be used in a pump-like technique to facilitate the flow of fluids. However, compression is ineffective as a stretching technique. As with a wet mop, squeezing or compression produces an outflow of liquid without elongation of the mop's fibers (Lederman 1997).

In contrast, when a *tensile*, or *horizontal*, force is applied to a material, its length is increased. The increase in length is an *axial*, or *tension*, deformation. In layperson's terms, *stretching* is the process of elongation and *stretch* is the elongation itself. Hence, the application of a tensile force is the cornerstone and foundation of any flexibility training or rehabilitation program to enhance ROM. *Shear* deformation results from shear forces that, when applied to a material, cause one layer to slide over another. Shear produces complex patterns of compression and elongation. This force is also a formidable tool in the arsenal to enhance optimal ROM.

Elasticity

Elasticity is the property that enables a tissue to return to its original shape or size when a force is removed. Elasticity is the amount of counterforce within the material itself. Because elastic stretch represents springlike behavior, it is often symbolized pictorially by a zigzag line representing a spring. It is sometimes called the *Hookean element* (see figure 5.1). In the literature, the term *stiffness* is often used interchangeably with elasticity. However, stiffness has other, nonrelated meanings (discussed later). A term often mistakenly interchanged for elasticity is *extensibility*.

Elasticity, or stiffness, is important for several reasons. First, musculotendinous stiffness is significantly related to static flexibility (Wilson et al. 1991). Second, it is a vital component in human performance (e.g., running, hopping, or jumping) (Arampatzis et al. 2001; Farley and Gonzalez 1996; Nigg and Liu 1999). Third, elasticity (i.e., stiffness) is at least implicated in muscular injury (Walshe and Wilson 1997; Walshe et al. 1996). Fourth, tissue elasticity can be modified by training (Kubo, Kanehisa, Kawakami, and Fukunaga 2001a, 2001b). This concept is referred to as "muscle tuning" (Nigg and Liu 1999, p. 849).

Stress

When an external force acts on a body or material, internal resistance forces called *stresses* within the body react. Stress is measured by the force applied per unit area that produces or tends to produce deformation in a body, that is, the applied force divided by the cross-sectional area of the material that resists the force. Examples of stress units are lb/ft^2, N/m^2, and $dynes/cm^2$. Thus,

Stress = Force/Area of surface on which it acts
= F/A

The three principal kinds of stresses are compressive, tensile, and shear. A *compressive* stress is the force in the material that resists its being pushed together. Compressive stress results from two forces that are directed towards each other along the same straight line. *Tensile* stress is the force in a material that resists the pulling apart or separating of the material. Tensile stress is produced when two forces are directed away from each other along the same straight line. *Shear* stress is the force in a material that opposes or resists two forces directed parallel to each other but not along the same line. Stress is a vital component in both injury and rehabilitation and training.

Strain

Strain is the change in length or amount of deformation caused by the applied force. Strain is defined as the ratio of length after stress is applied to original length. Because it is a ratio, it has no dimensions or units. It is a pure number or a percentage of original length. Thus,

Longitudinal strain = Change in length/Initial length
= L/1

The amount of strain produced by a stress is determined basically by the electrochemical forces between the material's atoms. The stronger these forces are, the greater the stress needed to produce a given amount of strain. Mathews et al. (1964) have clearly described this concept. The molecules of a material are held together by attractive forces. When no external force is applied, the length of a material is determined by a balance between attractive and repulsive forces. When a material is lengthened, the molecules spread farther apart; the attractive forces then grow stronger while the repulsive forces grow weaker. "Therefore, there is a force generated within the

Factors in Joint Stiffness

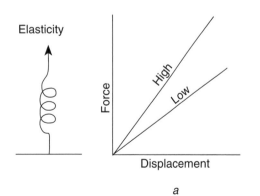 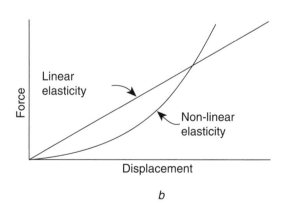

a   b

Figure 5.1 Elastic stiffness as exemplified by an ideal spring showing a linear relationship between force and displacement. (*a*) A stiffer spring exhibits a higher degree of stiffness (steeper slope). (*b*) Linear and nonlinear elasticity of the common type in which stiffness (slope) increases with displacement.

Reprinted from Wright and Johns 1960.

molecules of the material itself which tends to pull the ends of the sample back toward the unstressed condition. This is the elastic force" (p. 69).

The use of the term *strain* should not be confused with the strain that refers to a specific type of injury. When muscles are subject to a tensile force beyond their capacity to sustain, injury can result. A common example of a term synonymous with a muscle strain is a *pulled muscle*. Obviously, the appropriate meaning of the term strain is determined by its context.

Stiffness

Stiffness is another term that means different things to different people or in different disciplines. Common words that are synonymous with stiffness are resistance, soreness, tension, and tightness. Pezzullo and Irrgang (2001) define tightness as "a nonspecific term used to describe mild shortness of the musculotendinous unit that does not result in loss of joint motion" (p. 113). According to Gajdosik (1991), what is meant by "tight" hamstring muscles is unclear, but the term probably refers to muscles with decreased length, decreased extensibility, and decreased compliance. In everyday usage, stiffness can imply anything from a difficulty in moving a joint to a low level of discomfort at the end of the ROM (Gifford 1987). To the manipulative therapist, stiffness is generally taken to mean a painless abnormal restriction of movement or concern with a concept referred to as end-field or end-play (Maitland 2001). To the rheumatologist, it is a diagnostic criterion of morning stiffness and rheumatoid arthritis (Helliwell 1993). To the exercise physiologist, stiffness can describe postexercise soreness in muscles that is exacerbated when the affected tissues are stretched or contracted. (The topic of delayed-onset muscle soreness will be discussed in chapter 9.) To the psychiatrist and psychologist, stiffness may reflect a psychosomatic disorder.

Numerous problems face manual testers of stiffness. In the opinion of Maher (1995), two possible approaches enhance the objectivity and accuracy of stiffness assessment. The first approach is to rely upon instrumentation to measure stiffness. The second approach encompasses continuing manual assessment, but refines the current methods. Additional research is needed to resolve the problems associated with manual assessment of stiffness.

In biophysics, stiffness is the ratio of stress to strain, or of force to deformation. In other words, stiffness is the ratio of the change in force to the change in length. The reciprocal of stiffness is *compliance*. As force increases, deformation also increases, but the amount of deformation from any given force depends on the material being stretched. In the case of muscle, resistance to stretch is determined by neural factors as well as mechanical factors.

Stiffness can be plotted on a stress-strain, or load-deformation, curve and is indicated by the slope of the stress-strain relationship. A tissue with a steep load-deformation plot (such as bone) has a high stiffness. It will exhibit relatively less deformation for a given amount of force. In contrast, a tissue with a more gradual slope for a given amount of force (such as cartilage) has less stiffness. It will exhibit relatively more deformation. Similarly, a more compliant muscle will lengthen with less resistance. Research suggests that inflexible ("stiff") individuals have a greater resistance to stretch throughout the ROM (McHugh et al. 1992). Wilson et al. (1991) determined that static flexibility tests were significantly correlated with the maximal stiffness values ($r = -.544$, $p > .05$) of the glenohumeral joint in 14 experienced male weight lifters. Additional research is necessary to substantiate that these findings are consistent with other parts of the body and in different populations.

Hooke's Law and the Modulus of Elasticity

The numerical relationship between stress and strain was first discovered by Robert Hooke. *Hooke's law* states that a constant or proportional arithmetical relationship exists between force and elongation. One unit of force will produce one unit of elongation, two units of force will produce two units of elongation, and so forth. Within the context of Hooke's law, body tissues may be *perfectly elastic*. Two requirements must be fulfilled for a material to be perfectly elastic. First, the elastic element must have full recovery and regain its exact original dimensions from the deformation. Second, an instantaneous application or removal of force must be accompanied by an instantaneous change in dimension.

The equation constant in Hooke's law is the material's *modulus of elasticity*. This modulus value varies for different tissues. With materials of a higher modulus, stiffness is greater. Therefore, a stiffer material will require a greater stress for a certain strain or a greater load for a given deformation than will a more flexible tissue. The modulus of elasticity is the ratio of the unit stress to the unit of deformation or strain, where Y is the proportional constant. Thus, the modulus of elasticity equals the stress required to produce one unit of strain.

$$Y = \frac{\text{Longitudinal stress}}{\text{Longitudinal strain}} = \frac{F/A}{L/l} = \frac{FL}{AL}$$

Because the strain is a dimensionless ratio, the units of Y are identical with those of stress, namely, force/length^2. Thus, Y may be expressed in lb/in.^{2}, N/m^2, or dynes/cm^2. The value of Y differs for different material and does not depend on the material's dimensions. The value for a cross-linked polymer (i.e., a material that has molecules built up from large numbers of more or less similar units) depends on the spacing of the cross-links. The shorter the length of molecules between one cross-link and the next, the higher the modulus of elasticity and thus the harder the material is to stretch (Alexander 1975, 1988).

Elastic Limit

In materials that are not perfectly elastic, the arithmetical relationship between force and elongation reaches the *elastic limit*. The elastic limit is the smallest value of stress required to produce permanent strain in the body. Below the elastic limit, materials return to their original length when the deforming force is removed. However, when a force beyond the elastic limit is applied, the stressed material will not return to its original length when the force is removed. The difference between the original length and the new length is the *permanent set*, or *sprain*; it is also called *plastic stretch*. When stress is applied beyond the elastic limit, deformation and force are no longer linearly proportional. The material elongates much further for each unit of force above the elastic limit than below it.

When stress slightly beyond the elastic limit is applied, a deformation occurs without additional stress. This transition is the *yield point*. As force increases beyond this point, the curve tends to flatten. As further stress or force is applied, gradual tissue failure occurs. Eventually, the maximal force that can be tolerated by the tissue is reached. The maximum stress recorded—that is, the unit stress that occurs just at or below rupture—is the *ultimate strength* of the tissue.

These concepts are extremely significant for athletes and laypeople alike. If one wishes to reduce the probability or degree of tissue damage from overstretching, one must strengthen those parts of the body most likely to receive insults. This practice is commonly seen in athletes who engage in resistance training (e.g., free weights or machines) to strengthen the musculature and appropriate tissues (e.g., ligaments and tendons). The tissues adapt to a higher level of stress as a result of the overload, and their ultimate strengths are increased. Strengthening may have a protective effect by increasing the ability of muscle to absorb injury (Garrett 1993).

Thixotropy

Thixotropy is associated with time-dependent effects (Campbell and Lakie 1998; Enoka 2002; Lakie and Robson 1988; Mewis 1979; Proske et al. 1998). "The term thixotropy was originally coined to describe an isothermal, reversible, gel-solid (solid-liquid) transition due to mechanical agitation . . . At present, there exists a rather general agreement to call thixotropy the continuous decrease of apparent viscosity with time under shear and the subsequent recovery when the flow is discontinued" (Mewis 1979, p. 2). Muscle, like tomato ketchup, exhibits thixotropic properties: both become stiff and semisolid with disuse and are temporarily made more mobile by agitation (Lakie and Robson 1988). Lakie and Robson (1988) revealed a linear relationship between the time a muscle remains still and the stiffness of that muscle in response to a stretch. In contrast, movement, whether active or passive, always produces a decrease in stiffness.

Wiegner (1987) suggested that thixotropic effects serve "to increase the stiffness of relaxed joints and muscles, rendering them less susceptible to displacement as a result of random torques arising within and without the body" (p. 1621).

Several investigators (Campbell and Lakie 1998; Hagbarth et al. 1985; Hill 1968; Lakie and Robson 1988; Proske and Morgan 1999) suggest the molecular arrangement in muscle involves the development or maintenance of stable bonds between the actin and myosin filaments. With inactivity, additional bonds are formed, making the muscle stiffer. The initial steep tension rise during stretch has been speculated to result from strain and detachment of these bridges (Hill 1968). In contrast, with stretching or activity, many of the bonds are broken and consequently, muscle stiffness decreases (Hagbarth et al. 1985; Lakie and Robson 1988; Lakie et al. 1984). Lakie and Robson (1988) suggest, "thixotropy may explain the beneficial effects of limbering up before exercise and the efficacy of certain forms of physiotherapy in the treatment of muscle stiffness" (Lakie and Robson 1988, p. 499). A possible relationship between proprioceptive neuromuscular facilitation (PNF) stretching techniques and thixotropy is discussed in chapter 13.

Plasticity

Plasticity is the property of a material to permanently deform when it is loaded beyond its elastic range. Past the yield point, a tissue's plastic response involves considerable amount of deformation with very small increases in force. Probably no perfectly plastic materials exist (see figure 5.2). However, modeling clay is an example of a material that exhibits extremely plastic behavior.

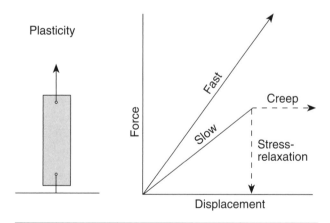

Figure 5.2 Plastic or viscoelastic stiffness. The elastic stiffness of a plastic substance is typically greater with faster stretch (steeper slope). Maintenance of a constant force results in continued elongation (creep). If stretched and maintained at constant length, the force required wanes (stress-relaxation).

Reprinted from Wright and Johns 1960.

Plasticity is crucial to both the cause and the treatment of various injuries. Long-term, repetitive microtrauma can result in deformed (i.e., plastic) tissues that exhibit reduced stability, leading to reduced efficiency and quality of life. A classic example is long-term improper sitting posture. Over time, the body adapts to the stresses by deformation of the back tissues and shortening of anterior trunk tissues, leading to reduced ROM and discomfort and pain.

Conversely, stretching exercises, traction, and other remodeling procedures play an important part in improving performance or in rehabilitation. Most athletes are aware that proper stretching (i.e., plasticity training) increases flexibility. That is, the tissues adapt to the stretching forces with increased flexibility. For many disciplines, this adaptation is essential to success. In rehabilitation, the achievement of plasticity is essential. Therapeutic stretching procedures are used to create a beneficial deformation back to a more efficient position (Garde 1988).

Viscosity

Viscosity is the property of materials to resist loads that produce shear and flow. Unlike elasticity and plasticity, it is truly time dependent. A plunger immersed in a fluid (e.g., a syringe) classically illustrates viscosity. The faster one tries to move the plunger, the higher the pressure within the fluid (see figure 5.3). A practical implication is the advantage of slow versus rapid flexion and extension of the spine. The former results in less viscosity and stiffness in the spine (McGill 1998; Yingling 1997) and reduces the passive stresses that otherwise would develop.

Viscosity is especially important in sports. Athletes are commonly told to warm up. One reason is to reduce their tissue viscosity. During warm up, the bodily tissues and fluids become warmed, reducing viscosity and consequently enhancing extensibility. As an analogy, think of a syringe filled with warm honey and another filled with cold honey. The warm honey will flow faster.

Viscoelasticity

Biological tissues are neither perfectly elastic nor perfectly plastic. They exhibit a combination of properties, referred to as *viscoelasticity*. At low loads, tissues exhibit elastic behavior; at higher loads, they exhibit plastic behavior. In addition, when loads are applied over time, tissues exhibit viscous deformation.

Hysteresis

During stretching, a discrepancy exists between the mechanical energy used to stretch tissues and the energy required to return the tissues to their original length. *Hysteresis* is a phenomenon associated with energy loss by viscoelastic materials subjected to loading and unloading (see figure 5.4). The stress-strain curve of an elastic tissue is identical during loading and unloading. In contrast, for viscoelastic material, the curves are not identical. If the loading ceases before tissue failure, the descending curve for the decreasing stress will not precisely coincide with the ascending curve, despite the absence of permanent

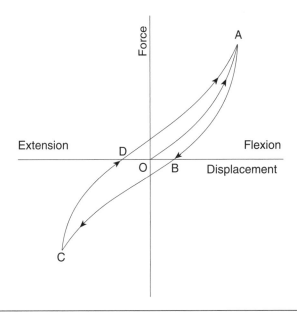

Figure 5.4 Diagram of the stiffness of joints, with extension to the left, flexion to the right, and force (torque) vertically. Joint rotation begins at the midposition (O) and proceeds to full flexion (A). It is then extended (A, B, C) and flexed (C, D, A). It is apparent that the elastic stiffness (slope) is nonlinear and that there is hysteresis.

Reprinted from Wright and Johns 1960.

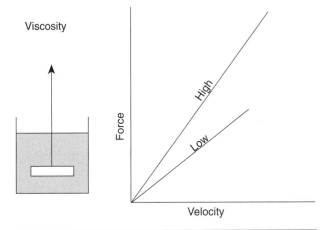

Figure 5.3 Viscous stiffness as exemplified by a plate moved through an ideal viscous fluid showing a linear relationship between force and velocity. Increased viscosity results in higher viscous stiffness (steeper slope).

Reprinted from Wright and Johns 1960.

deformation at the end. The area between the loading and unloading curves (i.e., within the loop) represents energy lost (converted into heat). In contrast, the area under the unloaded curve represents the energy recovered in the elastic recoil. In athletics (and in all people), the significance of hysteresis is that not all energy is conserved as elastic strain energy. Consequently, less mechanical energy is available for the recoil associated with the relaxation phrase. These discrepancies are in part caused by the rate of fluid flow in the tissues (Lederman 1997). The strain energy stored in tendon structures is necessary for the optimum performance of athletes involved in sprinting and jumping activities (Kubo et al. 1999; Kubo et al. 2000).

Passive stretching and repeated contraction decreases tendon stiffness and hysteresis. For example, stiffness and hysteresis decreased 9% and 34%, respectively, after subjects stretched for 10 minutes (Kubo et al. 2002). An earlier investigation by the same team (Kubo, Kanehisa, Ito, and Fukunaga 2001a), also employing a 10-minute stretching protocol, found that stretching for 10 minutes significantly decreased stiffness and hysteresis from 22.9% ± 5.8% to 20.6% and from 20.6 ± 8.8% to ± 13.5%. In another study, just 5 minutes of static stretching decreased hysteresis by 29% (Kubo, Kanehisa, Ito, and Fukunaga 2001b). The mechanisms that result in these decreases after stretching are unknown. In contrast, Kubo, Kanehisa, and Fukunaga (2002a) found the effects of an isotonic resistance-training program of the plantar flexor muscles in 8 subjects decreased the hysteresis by approximately 17% and significantly increased stiffness of the tendon structures by 19%. The mechanism that resulted in the increased stiffness remains unknown. However, the researchers suggested the increased stiffness might have resulted from induced changes in the internal structures of the tendon, aponeurosis, or both. The significance of these studies is the suggestion that training programs can enhance performance.

As with plasticity, hysteresis is important in therapeutic remodeling procedures such as traction. Hence, two points made by Garde (1988) deserve mention. First, hysteresis is the desired effect of those procedures that produce a beneficial deformation back to a more efficient position. If the tissues remained resilient after their initial and negative deformation, no change in condition occurs. Consequently, a beneficial deformation back to a more efficient position could not take place. Second, hysteresis is also part of the pathological deforming cycle caused by macrotrauma or repetitive microtrauma.

SOFT TISSUES

Tissues may be divided into two categories: hard and soft. Hard tissues include bone, teeth, nails, and hair. Soft tissues include tendons, ligaments, muscles, skin, and most of the other tissues. Soft tissues are divided into two groups: contractile and noncontractile.

Properties of Soft Tissues

Soft tissues vary in physical and mechanical characteristics. Both contractile and noncontractile tissues are extensible and elastic, but contractile tissues are also contractible. *Contractility* is the ability of a muscle to shorten and develop tension along its length. *Distensibility* (commonly known as *extensibility* or *stretchability*) is the ability of a muscle to stretch in response to an externally applied force. The weaker the forces generated within the muscle, the greater the amount of stretch.

Relationship of the Mechanical Properties of Soft Tissues to Stretching

The greater the stiffness of a soft tissue, the greater the force needed to produce an elongation. A tissue of low stiffness cannot resist a stretching force as well as a tissue of high stiffness, and the former will need a lesser force than the latter to produce the same degree of deformation. Therefore, soft tissues with greater stiffness are less susceptible to injuries such as sprains (which involve tears of ligamentous and capsular tissues) and strains (which involve tears of muscle and tendon tissue).

Soft tissues are not perfectly elastic. Beyond their elastic limit, they cannot return to their original length once the stretching force is removed. The difference between the original length and the new length is the *permanent set* (plastic stretch or deformation), and it correlates to minor tissue damage. Thus, when one suffers a sprain or strain, the soft tissues do not return to their original length after the excessive stress is removed. In some cases, ligament sprains can lead to permanent laxity and joint instability.

Questions then arise: To develop flexibility, should one stretch to the elastic limit or slightly beyond it? Most authorities recommend stretching to the point of "discomfort" or "tension" but not pain. What, then, is the difference between discomfort and pain? The meanings of these terms in medicine (and other disciplines) can be interpreted in various ways (de Jong 1980; Merskey and Bogduk 1994). In 1979, the International Association for the Study of Pain (IASP) was organized to develop an internationally acceptable definition of pain and a classification system of pain syndromes. Eventually, pain and 18 other common terms were defined. A revised list was developed by Merskey and Bogduk (1994). Three terms are most relevant to this discussion: *Pain* is "an unpleasant sensory and emotional experience associated with actual or potential tissue damage, or described in terms of such damage." *Pain threshold* is "the least experience of pain which a subject can recognize." *Pain tolerance level* is "the greatest level of pain which a subject is prepared to tolerate."

Most authorities state that the stretch should be at least to the pain threshold point. "The meaning of pain is given primarily by each individual's subjective reactions, sensory perceptions, experiences, emotions, memories and ideas" (Borg 1998, p. 10). Therefore, coaches or trainers cannot determine the pain threshold for anyone under their charge, because each person is unique in his or her own sensory and emotional experience, and this experience continually changes.

Another point deserves special consideration and caution. For individuals who are undergoing rehabilitation and have healing tissues, the point before pain is reached may be sufficient to rupture already weakened tissues. After injury, the tissue architecture is less capable of withstanding the stress of tensile loading (Hunter 1998). Hence, extreme caution must be employed when applying tension to previously damaged tissues.

Another question arises: Is the point of discomfort below, at, or beyond the elastic limit? Although the literature is not conclusive on this subject, research (Laban 1962; Lehmann et al. 1970; Warren et al. 1971, 1976) indicates that the type of force, the duration of the force, and the temperature of the tissue during and after stretching determine whether the elongation is recoverable or permanent.

Length-Tension and Stress-Strain Relationship

The length of a soft tissue depends on the relation of the internal force developed by the tissue to the external force exerted by the resistance or load. If the internal force exceeds the external force, the tissue shortens; if the external force exceeds the internal force, the tissue lengthens.

Stress-Relaxation and Creep During Passive Tension

Living tissues are characterized by the presence of time-dependent mechanical properties, including creep and stress-relaxation. When a resting muscle is suddenly stretched and held at a constant length for a period of time, a slow loss of tension occurs. This behavior is called *stress-relaxation* (see figure 5.5a). In contrast, the lengthening that occurs when a constant force or load is applied is called *creep* (see figure 5.5b).

We are most interested in how these time-dependent mechanical properties operate on muscle cells and connective tissues. Among the pertinent questions that should be addressed in future research are the following:

- How is tensile force transmitted through the sarcomere and the structures of the various connective tissues?
- What is the effect of tensile force on the sarcolemma, sarcoplasm, and cytoskeleton (i.e., the supporting framework of minute filaments and tubules within every cell)?

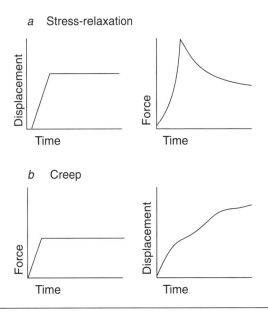

Figure 5.5 Responses of tissues to applied force. (*a*) Stress-relaxation results when there is a reduction in force that occurs when a tissue is held at a constant length. (*b*) Creep is the lengthening that occurs over a period of time when a constant force is applied.

Reprinted, by permission, from M. Alter, 1996, *Science of Flexibility, Second Edition* (Champaign, IL: Human Kinetics), 67.

- Where and through what mechanisms in the sarcomere do the creep and stress-relaxation phenomena operate?
- What is the relationship (if any) of creep and stress-relaxation in sarcomeres to pressure gradients, fluid flow, and streaming potentials of the structures of the various connective tissues?

Molecular Mechanism of Connective Tissue's Elasticity Response

Connective tissues are composite materials linked to form long, flexible chains. Two essential variables that influence the stiffness (or elasticity) of connective tissues are the spacing of their cross-links and the temperature. For example, assume a long, flexible molecule composed of *n* number of segments. Each segment has a length *a*. Each segment in itself is stiff, but the joints between the segments are flexible. Also assume that the molecules of the segments are free to move.

All molecules move in a random fashion. However, as temperature decreases, molecules become less active. At the temperature of absolute zero (–273° C), all movement ceases. Because of random molecular movement, at a particular instant, the distance from one end of a segment to another may have any value from 0 (if the ends are in contact) to *na* (if the molecule is stretched out straight). However, the maximum-length position is unlikely. The most probable length for the molecule is its midlength, $n^{1/2}a$. (This value is a root mean square, not a simple mean.)

In a "normal" state, molecular chains in a network will continue to move, and the junctions at which they end will move together and move apart. The distance between the ends of a particular chain will vary, but the average distance among many chains will always be $n^{1/2}a$.

Assume an external tensile force is applied to the connective tissue shown in figure 5.6a. The network will be deformed as in figure 5.6b, and the chains will align in the direction of stretch. Consequently, the chains aligned in the direction of the tensile force (for example, A-B) now have average lengths greater than $n^{1/2}a$. In contrast, those chains aligned across the direction of stretching (B-C) have average lengths less than $n^{1/2}a$. The arrangement is no longer random, but when the distorting force is removed, the chains move back into random configurations. The connective tissue returns to its original shape; that is, it recoils elastically.

As described by Alexander (1988),

a theory developed from these ideas predicts the force required for equilibrium of the deformed network, and hence the modulus of elasticity. The shear modulus G and Young's modulus E are given by the equation:

$$G = NkT = E/3$$

where N is the number of chains per unit volume of material, k is a physical constant (Boltzmann's constant), and T is the absolute temperature. *Notice the importance of the number of chains. If more cross-links are inserted, dividing the molecules into a larger number of shorter chains, the material becomes stiffer. Also, the modulus is proportional to the absolute temperature because the energy associated with the writhing of the molecules increases with tem-*

perature. Similarly, the pressure exerted at constant volume by a gas increases with temperature, because the kinetic energy of the molecules increases with temperature. (p. 14, emphasis added)

Research Findings Regarding Stretching of Connective Tissue

With a basic knowledge of the biophysics of connective tissues and muscles, we can examine the research findings. When a tensile force is applied to connective tissue or muscle, the original length increases and the cross section (i.e., width) decreases. Can different types of forces, or different conditions under which a force is applied, create an optimal change in connective tissue?

When tensile forces are continuously applied to connective tissue or muscle, the time required to elongate the tissue a specific amount varies inversely with the forces used (Warren et al. 1971, 1976). Warren et al. (1971, 1976) and Laban (1962) demonstrated that a low-force stretching method requires more time to produce the same amount of elongation as a high-force method. However, the proportion of tissue lengthening that remains after tensile stress is removed is greater for the low-force, long-duration method. Therefore, "by permitting time for more yielding at the higher force, a slower-stretch cycle results in greater plastic deformation" (Sun et al. 1995, p. 261). Consequently, these studies appear to support proponents of static stretching. Others (Becker 1979; Glazer 1980; Jackman 1963; Kottke et al. 1966; Light et al. 1984) have also demonstrated that stretching at low to moderate tension levels is effective. In addition, research (Sapega et al. 1981) has demonstrated that the application of high-force, short-duration stretching favors recoverable, elastic tissue deformation. In contrast, the application of a low-force, long-duration tensile force enhances permanent, plastic deformation (Warren et al. 1971, 1976; Laban 1962).

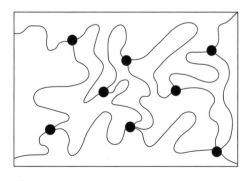

a

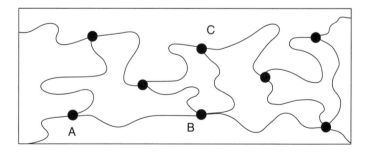

b

Figure 5.6 A diagram of a rubbery polymer (*a*) unstrained and (*b*) stretched horizontally. The sinuous lines represent polymer molecules and the dots represent cross-links.

Reprinted from Alexander 1988.

Furthermore, laboratory studies (Rigby et al. 1959; Warren et al. 1971, 1976) have demonstrated that some degree of mechanical weakening takes place in permanently elongated connective tissue structures,. However, mechanical weakening is not necessarily associated with an outright rupture (Rigby et al. 1959; Warren et al. 1971, 1976). Rydevik et al. (1990) demonstrated that multiple ruptures do occur in what appear to be grossly intact nerves placed under tensile force.

The amount of structural weakening depends on the velocity at which the tissue is stretched as well as how much it is elongated. Significantly, for the same amount of tissue elongation, a fast, high-force stretching method produces more structural weakening than a slow, low-force method (Warren et al. 1971, 1976). Faster stretch rates result in greater tensions and more absorbed energy within the tissue for a given length of stretch (Taylor et al. 1990). Also, the velocity of the high-force stretch does not provide an opportunity for time-dependent stress-relaxation or creep to reduce the tension or increase the length (Taylor et al. 1990). Thus, ballistic stretching presents a greater risk of injury than static stretching.

Temperature also has a significant influence on the mechanical behavior of connective tissue and muscle under tensile stress. As tissue temperature rises, stiffness decreases and extensibility increases (Laban 1962; Noonan et al. 1993; Rigby 1964). Raising the temperature of tendon tissues above 103° F increases the amount of permanent elongation that results from a given amount of initial stretching (Laban 1962; Lehmann et al. 1970). At about 104° F, a thermal transition in the microstructure of collagen occurs, significantly enhancing the viscous stress-relaxation of collagenous tissue and allowing greater plastic deformation during stretch (Mason and Rigby 1963; Rigby 1964; Rigby et al. 1959). The mechanism behind this thermal transition may be the destabilization of the intermolecular bonding or enhanced viscous flow properties of the collagenous tissue (Rigby 1964; Rigby et al. 1959). The important point is that heat and stretch have a cumulative effect on collagen structural changes (Hardy and Woodall 1998).

Sapega et al. (1981) have postulated that when connective tissue is stretched at an elevated temperature, the conditions under which the tissue cools can significantly affect the amount of elongation that remains after the tensile stress is removed. Their hypothesis is based on the earlier research of Lehmann et al. (1970), which found that after heated tissue is stretched, maintaining tensile force during tissue cooling significantly increases the relative proportion of plastic deformation compared with unloading the tissue while its temperature is still elevated. Lehmann et al. (1970) speculated that cooling the tissue before releasing the tension apparently allows the collagenous microstructure to restabilize more toward its new stretch length.

However, the benefit of cooling a tissue while it remains on stretch is now questioned (Hardy and Woodall 1998). Lentell et al. (1992), in a study of normal shoulders stretched under various conditions, found heat with stretch to be the superior method for lengthening tissues. The application of cold in all study groups diminished the gains made in flexibility. These findings suggest that the application of ice after stretching is unnecessary. Additional clinical studies that combine tissue temperature manipulation and therapeutic stretching are necessary to resolve this controversy

When connective tissue is stretched at temperatures within the usual therapeutic range (102° to 110° F), the amount of structural weakening produced by a given amount of tissue elongation varies inversely with the temperature (Warren et al. 1971, 1976). This condition is apparently related to the progressive increase in the viscous flow properties of the collagen as it is heated. As pointed out above, thermal destabilization of intermolecular bonding possibly allows elongation to occur with less structural damage. However, "despite evidence supporting the heat and stretching theory, research has not been conclusive" (Peres et al. 2002, p. 47).

Summarizing the research, Sapega et al. (1981) state the following:

> The factors influencing the viscoelastic behavior of connective tissue can be summarized by stating that elastic or recoverable deformation is most favored by high-force, short-duration stretching at normal or colder tissue temperature, whereas plastic or permanent lengthening is most favored by lower-force, longer-duration stretching at elevated temperatures, but allowing the tissue to cool before releasing the tension. In addition, the structural weakening produced by permanent tissue deformation is minimized when prolonged, low-force application is combined with high therapeutic temperatures, and it is maximal when higher forces and lower temperatures are used. (p. 61)

Scientific Rationale for Stretching to Prevent Injuries

Stretch can at least temporarily increase ROM for a given period of time. Such increase in ROM may in fact improve performance in a number of disciplines (athletics and dance). However, a fundamental reason for incorporating a stretching regimen (not to be confused with a warm-up regimen) is to prevent injuries. The causes of injuries are multifactorial. Nonetheless, the premise is that stretching can reduce the risk or severity of injury. The most common proposed mechanisms are based on either a mechanical or a neurophysiological model.

The mechanical model is predicated on the premise that a decrease in muscle stiffness (i.e., elasticity) reduces the risk of injury. As explained by McNair and Stanley (1996), "Intuitively, a less stiff muscle would be beneficial as it can be extended to a greater extent, allowing the applied forces to be absorbed over a greater range and longer time. In so doing, this 'cushioning effect' may reduce the stress on the musculotendinous structures" (pp. 316-317). In support of this premise, proponents of stretching cite several classic studies. Taylor et al. (1990) applied stretch to rabbit extensor digitorum longus muscles. An initial force of 1.96 N to 78.4 N was held for 30 seconds before returning to the initial length. Ten trials were performed on each muscle. A 3.45% increase in muscle length occurred to withstand the predetermined stretch force. Similarly, 10 trials were performed stretching the muscles to 10% of their resting length and immediately returning them to their initial positions. A 16.6% decrease in peak tension occurred at the assumed stretched position. Thus, the study substantiates a decrease in muscle stiffness, force per unit length, as a significant effect of stretching. Elaborating, Cross and Worrell (1999) write

> The previous study concerning muscle stiffness suggests that, at a given muscle length, cyclic stretching will reduce the force that is placed upon the muscle and associated connective tissue. Theoretically, less tension will be applied within the musculotendinous tissue when it is subject to the changes in joint motion that accompany sport or recreational activity. Thus, the potential for musculotendinous strain throughout the normal range of motion will be reduced by elongation of the musculotendinous unit. (pp. 11-12)

Garrett (1996) administered 10 cycles of stretching to 50% of the previously determined failure length of a rabbit muscle-tendon unit (MTU). The MTU achieved greater length before injury. At failure, no difference existed in force or energy absorption between the stretch groups and control groups. However, when the MTUs were stretched to 70% of the previously determined failure length, macroscopic disruptions in the muscle's integrity appeared before the 10 stretching cycles were completed. These findings indicated the maximum amount of force and energy that can be accommodated before MTU failure in individual muscles. After a moderate stretching program, the MTU will not experience these maximum values until it reaches a greater length (Garrett 1996). Thus, during a specific sport activity, less force will be placed on the MTUs throughout the required arcs of motion, and, consequently, less energy will need to be attenuated.

The neurophysiological model is based on the hypothesis that stretching will result in an indirect decrease in stiffness because of reflex inhibition and consequent viscoelastic changes from decreased actin-myosin cross-bridging. Decreased muscle stiffness would then permit an increased joint ROM (Shrier 2002; Shrier and Gossal 2000).

Scientific Rationale That Stretching Does Not Prevent Injuries

Recently, a number of articles were published that challenged the long-held belief that stretching prevents injuries (Black and Stevens 2001; Shrier 1999, 2000, 2001, 2002; Shrier and Gossal 2000). These investigators presented five arguments.

1. *Compliance:* Compliance refers to the length change that occurs when a force is applied but is not necessarily related to a tissue's resistance to injury. Increased compliance is associated with an inability to absorb as much energy as generated by the applied force. Consequently, increased compliance may actually increase the risk of injury.

2. *Sarcomere heterogeneity:* Not all sarcomeres within a muscle fiber are homogeneous. Some sarcomeres lengthen during a contraction, while others may be shortening. Thus, the issue of an increase in total-muscle compliance is irrelevant (see popping hypothesis in chapter 9).

3. *Eccentric contractions:* Active muscle has a much lower compliance than resting muscle but absorbs significantly more energy.

4. *Overstretching:* Strains as little as 20% beyond the resting fiber length can produce muscle damage. Thus, "correct" stretching techniques may be more difficult to define and elaborate than previously thought.

5. *Analgesic effect:* Stretching may provide short-term relief for muscle aches and discomfort. However, this relief does not mean that the risk of injury is decreased.

MUSCLE

Muscle is composed of three independent mechanical components or elements, which may be classified as either *elastic* or *viscous*. These mechanical components resist deformation and therefore play a major role in determining flexibility. Elastic components exert a restoring force in response to a change in length. Viscous components exert a force in response to the rate (velocity) and duration of a change in length. The three mechanical components are (1) the *parallel elastic component* (PEC), (2) the *series elastic component* (SEC), and (3) the *contractile component* (CC).

Parallel Elastic Component

The parallel elastic component is responsible for passive or resting tension in muscle. The PEC is so named because it lies parallel to the contractile mechanism. A muscle removed from a body will naturally shorten by about 10% of its original, intact (in situ) length (Garamvölgyi 1971). This shortening is independent of contraction (passive). The length of the isolated, uncontracted muscle is called its *equilibrium length*; thus, shortening means that muscles are under tension at their intact length. The in situ length of an uncontracted or unstretched muscle is called its *resting length*, symbolized as Rl or L_o.

Resting muscle is elastic and resists lengthening. At less than equilibrium length ($0.90L_o$) no resting tension exists, and the PEC is slack. However, when an unstimulated muscle is stretched, it develops tension in a nonlinear fashion. That is, little tension is developed with initial stretch, but increasingly more tension is developed as stretch continues. The same effect is seen when a knitted stocking is stretched (Carlson and Wilkie 1974). What is the composition of PEC, and what structures are responsible for a muscle's resting tension?

Originally, the PEC was thought to consist primarily of the sarcolemma, sarcoplasm, and elastic fibers of the epimysium, perimysium, and endomysium. Later, Huxley and Hanson (1954) proposed the S-filament, which was thought to link the ends of the actin filaments on either side. However, 1 year later, S-filaments were dropped without explanation from the muscle model of Huxley (1957). Another explanation for the passive resting tension was an *electrostatic force*. For example, the volume of muscle fibers remains constant when muscle is stretched, but the cross-sectional area (i.e., width) must decrease, and so must the side spacing between the actin and myosin filaments as they move closer to each other. If a mutual electrostatic repulsive force exists between the filaments, work must be done to move the filaments closer together. That is, some force must maintain the filaments in a regular array. Consequently, the force necessary to move the filaments closer against the electrostatic repulsion would appear as the resting tension or the "parallel" resistance to stretch (Davson 1970; Huxley 1967). Although the electrostatic force may contribute to resting tension at high degrees of stretch, it cannot be a dominant source.

Unequivocal evidence has demonstrated that titin is the major source of muscle elasticity. This proof has been accomplished by destroying the titin filament while recording the muscle's degree of tension under stress. In the first study of this type, titin was preferentially destroyed by radiation (Horowits et al. 1986). The result was a reduction in resting tension. A year later, Horowits and Podolsky (1987b) published additional data from another study that supported the hypothesis that the elastic titin filaments produce most of the resting tension in muscle. In another study (Yoshioka et al. 1986), titin was preferentially destroyed via controlled proteolysis (i.e., the use of digestive enzymes). Once again, resting tension was reduced. Similarly, in a more recent study (Funatsu et al. 1990), resting tension decreased with the degradation of titin via its enzymatic digestion (by plasma gesolin).

What then happens as the sarcomere is stretched and released? During stretch, neither the thin filament (actin) nor the thick filament (myosin) changes length. Instead, the filaments merely slide past one another (the sliding filament theory). During stretch, the sarcomere resists the deforming force by its resting tension. At first, the resting tension is modest. After a considerable stretch, the resting tension rises steeply and resists any further extension (elastic stiffness). Titin causes this behavior. Upon release, the stretched titin filaments retract. Hence, titin can store potential energy.

If titin contributes to resting tension, what about nebulin? Wang and Wright (1988) have suggested that nebulin constitutes a set of inextensible filaments attached at one end to the Z-line and that nebulin filaments are in parallel, not in series, with titin filaments. However, nebulin is not a factor in the resting tension. When nebulin is degraded, resting tension does not decrease (Funatsu et al. 1990; Wang and Wright 1988). Therefore, nebulin does not produce the elasticity.

Another possible factor contributing to passive tension (stiffness) in muscle relates to the extensibility of the tendon and aponeurosis (McHugh et al. 1999). However, Kubo et al. (2001b) suggest that passive stiffness of muscle is unrelated to tendon-aponeurosis stiffness. In a study of the straight-leg raise, 79% of the variability in maximum straight-leg raise ROM could be explained by the passive response to stretch (McHugh et al. 1998).

Series Elastic Component

When a muscle is stretched, the CC (i.e., the actin and myosin filaments and their cross-bridges), PEC, and SEC all contribute to the development of tension. The SEC is so named because the elastic components occur directly in line with the contractile components. The SEC has the important function of smoothing out rapid changes in muscle tension. Wilson et al. (1991) demonstrated that 30% of the variation in the glenohumeral ROM could be explained by stiffness of the SEC.

The SEC consists of both passive and active elements (Walshe et al. 1996). A chief passive element is thought to be tendon. Active elements include the intracellular cross-bridges of actin and myosin (Walshe et al. 1996). However, Pollack (1990) postulated that the Z-line may also constitute a modest source of the sarcomere's series elasticity. This function is accomplished by the thin filaments pulling on the Z-line. For example, when a force on the thin filaments is transmitted to the Z-line, the lateral separation between the filaments is reduced (see figure 5.7). Yet, to accommodate a decrease in interfilament spacing, the fold angle in the Z-line structure simply becomes accentuated and more acute (see figure 5.8). Consequently, the Z-line effectively thickens, creating a kind of "elasticity." "Studies of isolated muscle preparations have shown that the relative contribution of these structures to overall musculotendinous stiffness

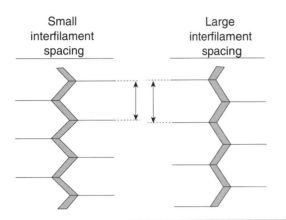

Figure 5.7 Effect of change of interfilament spacing on Z-line structure. The Z-line accommodates such changes through variation of the angle between contiguous elements.

Reprinted from Pollack 1990.

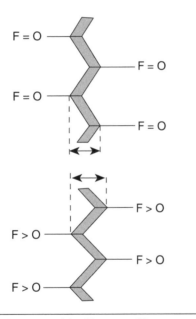

Figure 5.8 Force on thin filaments (F) accentuates the zigzag pattern of Z-line structure, resulting in changes of effective "width" of the Z-line. Such accordionlike changes may give rise to series elasticity.

Reprinted from Pollack 1990.

is dependent upon the proportions of these structures within the MTU, contraction type and load" (Walshe et al. 1996, p. 337).

Contractile Component

The contractile component is the muscle's ability to increase tension, and so may be regarded as a tension generator. The CC consists of the filaments and their cross-bridges. If tension is proportional to the number of chemical links between the two filaments, then the greater the overlap between the filaments, the more binding sites can interact and the greater the tension that can be developed. Maximal contractile tension is assumed to develop when sarcomere lengths are such that maximal single overlap of actin and myosin filaments exists. At greater muscle length, the number of cross-links diminishes as filament overlap decreases, resulting in reduced tension. As the stretch continues, the tension becomes less until, finally, it is no greater than the tension in a passive muscle. At such lengths, actin and myosin filaments no longer interdigitate. Thus, they can develop little or no tension.

Total Tension of Active Muscle During Stretch

In general, the maximum total active tension is found at about 1.2 to 1.3 times the muscle's original, or rest, length. At greater lengths, total active tension diminishes until the muscle is at about 1.5 times its rest length, at which point, active tension is zero. At lengths beyond $1.3L_o$, the number of cross-links diminishes as overlap decreases, resulting in reduced tension. Furthermore, although the PEC increases its passive tension output, this total does not match the corresponding decline in active tension of the CCs. Consequently, total tension decreases. At extreme muscle lengths, passive tension generated by the SEC increases substantially, compensating for the decline in active tension, resulting in an increase in total tension. Other explanations for the mechanism underlying the extra tension during slow lengthening to contraction include heterogeneity of sarcomere lengths, an elastic structure other than the cross-bridges recruited or formed during activation, and axial shifts of cross-bridges (Morgan 1990, 1994b; Yagi and Matsubara 1984).

Muscle Stretches Applied During Contraction at Long Muscle Lengths

When tissues are stretched, they develop tension known as the *stretch response*, which is independent of the central nervous system (CNS) and is a mechanical property of the tissues. On the other hand, the *stretch reflex* is a response mediated by the CNS that causes the stretched muscle to contract in response to stretch stimulus (Gowitzke, Milner, and O'Connell 1988).

One of the major arguments against the use of ballistic stretching (i.e., bobbing or bouncing) is that it initiates a stretch reflex. However, if stretching is begun beyond the length of $1.5L_o$, the stretch reflex should not result in any increase of tension in the CC, because, at such lengths, the filaments are no longer capable of interdigitating and developing tension. This reasoning would be valid if all sarcomeres in the muscle fiber were stretched to the same extent. However, when a muscle is stretched, sarcomeres near tendons stretch much less than sarcomeres in the middle of a muscle. Hence, filament in sarcomeres at the end of the muscle may still have considerable overlap, whereas filaments in the middle sarcomeres are stretched beyond the point of overlap (Davson 1970; Morgan 1990, 1994). Therefore, the sarcomeres near tendons can still develop reflex tension and influence the degree of extension. Furthermore, the resistance to continued stretching likely arises either from the reattachment of previously broken cross-bridges or from the attachment of additional cross-bridges to sites on the actin filament that are not available initially but become accessible as a result of the movement (Flintney and Hirst 1978; Morgan 1990, 1994). Thus, activation of the stretch reflex, even when the muscle fiber is beyond $1.5L_o$, will probably result in production of additional tension by the CC.

VASCULAR TISSUE

Numerous structures of the body are exposed to a wide range of forces during movement, particularly during stretch. Among the most obvious structures subjected to forces are the connective tissues (e.g., tendons, ligaments, and fascia) and the muscles. However, two other broad categories of structures must not be overlooked—the gross structures of the vascular system and nervous system.

Anatomy of the Vascular System

Upon leaving the heart, the blood enters the vascular system, which is composed of numerous types of blood vessels that transport the blood throughout the body. In addition, blood vessels permit the exchange of nutrients, metabolic end products, hormones, and other substances between the blood and the interstitial fluid. Eventually, the blood returns to the heart. The three major kinds of blood vessels are arteries, veins, and capillaries.

An *artery* carries blood away from the heart. All arteries (except the pulmonary artery and its branches) carry oxygenated blood. When an arterial vessel has a diameter of less than 0.5 mm, it is referred to as an *arteriole*. Arteries are classified as either *elastic* or *muscular*, according to the prevalent tissue component in their walls. Examples of elastic arteries are large vessels such as the aorta, common carotid, subclavian, and common iliac. The great majority of arteries are muscular. Blood flow is regulated through the constriction and dilation of arteries.

A *vein* carries blood toward the heart. All of the veins (except the pulmonary vein) contain deoxygenated blood. Small veins (less than 0.1 mm) are called *venules*. The main difference between the veins and the arteries is the comparative weakness of the vein wall's middle coat. Its much smaller content of muscle and elastic fibers is related to the much lower venous blood pressure. In addition, unlike arteries, veins have valves.

Capillaries are microscopic blood vessels that connect arterioles with venules. Their walls are composed of a single layer of endothelial cells. The average diameter of capillaries varies from 7 to 9 mm. Their length usually varies from 0.25 mm to 1 mm, the latter length being characteristic of muscle tissue. Capillaries serve a variety of functions, such as transporting the blood with all its necessary components and permitting them to be exchanged with the surrounding tissues, maintaining normal blood pressure and circulation, and serving as a blood reservoir.

Applications of Stretch to Blood Vessels

When blood vessels are loaded (stretched by blood flow or subjected to the effects of stretch on blood vessels), they display typical viscoelastic properties in response to the constantly changing stress of each cardiac cycle. The effect of skeletal muscle sarcomere length on total capillary length was investigated by Ellis et al. (1990) in the extensor digitorum longus of the rat. Normalized data from six capillaries "indicated that four [vessels] stretched to the same degree as the muscle, one stretched more and another less" (p. 63). The variations in capillary distensibility were suggested to be the result of variations in vessel diameter, wall thickness, and degree of tethering to adjacent muscle cells. Lee and Schmid-Schonbein (1995) demonstrated that removal of the overlying fascia from the spinotrapezius muscle enlarges the perivascular space, and the muscle fibers become more circular. Thus, removal of fascia alters the spatial orientation and interaction between the muscle fiber and the capillary by disrupting the structural integrity of the capillary-to-myocyte and myocte-to-myocyte collagenous struts. Ellis et al. (1990) essentially substantiated the hypothesis that capillaries are generally in a tortuous (winding) configuration, and muscle extension will merely cause them to straighten, with no change in vessel length. Once capillaries have been straightened, further muscle extension will result in capillary stretching and a linear increase of individual vessel length from L_o. Significantly, each individual capillary does not stretch in a direct 1:1 relationship to changes in sarcomere length. For example, one capillary actually stretched more than did its adjacent muscle fibers, whereas another stretched less. In addition, research (Mathieu-Costello 1987; Mathieu-Costello et al. 1991; Mathieu-Costello et al. 1989; Nako and Segal 1995; Poole et al. 1997) has shown that capillary and arteriole geometry changes with sarcomere length.

Artery length changes very little in vivo (i.e., in the living body). Dobrin (1983), citing Lawton (1957) and Patel and Fry (1964), reported a 1% increase in length of the thoracic aorta and a 1% decrease in length of the abdominal aorta during each cardiac cycle. The ascending aorta and pulmonary arteries change 5% to 11% in length, but this effect results from gross motion of the heart (Patel et al. 1963). Although artery length changes negligibly over a wide range of pressures, it may change with shifts in body position. Browse et al. (1979) radiographically determined the changes in arterial length and diameter, as well as the patterns of blood flow, in the femoral and brachial arteries of 10 males. Beginning with the leg straight (i.e., a knee joint angle of 180°), the knee was then fully flexed. The average amount of flexion was 100° (from a straight leg to one bent to 80°), and this movement caused a mean shortening of 4.5 cm in the femoral artery, 20% of the initial mean length, but the vessel's diameter was maintained. The only noticeable change in the vessel was crinkling of the internal surface when the artery was fully bent. Measurements on a human brachial artery showed that at the elbow, this vessel shortened by 2.3 cm to 16.3 cm at 180° (arm straight) to 14 cm at 105° (elbow flexed); that is, 3 mm per 10° of joint movement, with no measurable change in vessel diameter.

The mechanical characteristics of blood vessels are attributable, in part, to the properties of the connective tissues in the wall, specifically elastin and collagen. With maturation, the collagen-to-elastin ratio of arteries increases, and therefore their stiffness also increases. Vessel stiffness under distention may be plotted as a function of several parameters and depends on whether the vessels are constricted or relaxed. Dobrin (1983) deals with these complexities in greater detail.

Influence of Stretch on Muscle Oxygen Consumption and Regional Blood Flow

Exercise dramatically increases the amount of blood transported through the cardiovascular system. However, what is the effect when a stretched muscle is relaxed, contracting isometrically in an elongated state, contracting eccentrically, or under compression before, during, or after stretching? Improved technologies have allowed this question to be investigated.

Gaskell (1877) showed that dogs' muscular blood flow decreased during contraction of calf muscles, a finding confirmed in many later works. In general, blood flow is reduced in proportion to the force of contraction. However, what happens to the blood flow of a muscle and its oxygen consumption during and after stretch? This question was investigated by Stainsby et al. (1956), who found that when the gastrocnemius-plantaris muscle group of the dog was stretched, oxygen consumption fell on the average to half the resting rate and remained at this low level until tension was released. When the tension was released, the oxygen consumption returned to the previous resting rate with little payment of the oxygen debt created during stretch. Several hypotheses were proposed to explain this phenomenon.

Gray and Staub (1967) observed that less reduction of blood flow occurred during passive stretching than during the same degree of active tension. They suggested the decreased blood flow resulting from stretch was caused by local pinching of vessels. Hirche et al. (1970), working on muscles dilated with papaverine (a vasodilator drug), found the increased resistance to blood flow to be the same in both passive and active muscle tension. Wisnes and Kirkebø (1976) determined that active contraction or stretching of the calf muscles of rats mechanically impeded muscular blood flow, most pronouncedly in the central inner zone at high tensions. The blood flow in the inner, central zones of the muscle groups was reduced far more than flow in the outer, peripheral zones. As a result, Wisnes and Kirkebø (1976) suggest that "since blood flow may vary regionally within a single muscle, measurements of total organ flow should not be regarded uncritically to represent a similar flow in every locality of the organ" (p. 265). Kirkebø and Wisnes (1982) explained the disproportionate reduction of blood flow in the central zones as caused by differences in regional tissue pressure. In addition, they suggested "the heterogeneous pattern of muscle fiber directions and relative displacement of various elements during work, may induce shear forces causing focal vessel obstructions that are different during contraction and stretch" (p. 551).

Matchanov, Levtov, and Orlov (1983) reported that a longitudinal stretch of cat gastrocnemius muscles by 10% to 30% of initial length increased the passive strength and regularly decreased the blood flow. The decreased blood flow was dependent on the value of the passive tension and not on the degree of deformation. Postelongation hyperemia (increased blood flow) developed after stretching. Matchanov, Shustova et al. (1983) found that longitudinal stretch of cat gastrocnemius muscle to between 111% and 117% of its initial length was followed by increases in passive strength and in mechanical displays of the 15-s isometric tetani. In addition, blood flow in the muscle vessels decreased at rest during the longitudinal stretching, whereas oxygen (O_2) extraction from the blood increased, but oxygen consumption did not change. Shustova, Maltsev et al. (1985) once again applied stretch to the gastrocnemius of cats. Longitudinal stretch of the muscle by 1 to 2 cm decelerated the capillary blood flow up to its complete rest. After 1 minute of stretch, the blood flow velocity increased by 0.30 ± 0.06 mm per second in 148 capillaries, decreased by 0.22 ± 0.07 mm per second in 35 capillaries, and remained the same in five capillaries. Responses of individual capillaries seemed to be unrelated to the initial flow velocity at their location within the vessel network. Shustova, Matchanov et al. (1985) investigated the effect of the compression of cat gastrocnemius muscle vessels on the muscle blood supply during stretching. A 10% to 20% longitudinal stretch of the muscle reduced the blood flow from 5.0 to 3.0 ml per minute. However, the decrease of the blood flow in stretching and the postelongation hyperemia could not be reproduced by external compression of the muscle equal to the balancing pressure at a given extent of stretching. Furthermore, the effect of longitudinal muscle stretch on its vessels is not limited to their compression by the intramuscular pressure. Levtov et al. (1985) found that mean blood velocity increased in capillaries during postelongation hyperemia. However, the velocity was slower in distal capillaries. The blood flow velocity in the capillaries was determined to depend on the ratio of the total resistance of incoming and outgoing vessels to the resistance of the capillary.

Poole et al. (1997) examined whether muscle extension in vivo would impair capillary red blood cell hemodynamics. At increased sarcomere length, mean capillary red blood cell velocity is reduced, and a greater proportion of capillaries in which red blood cell flow is stopped or intermittent. Significantly, not only does muscles stretching reduce bulk blood (and oxygen) delivery but it also alters capillary red blood cell flow dynamics, which may further impair blood-tissue oxygen. Consequently, this condition could impair muscle performance and enhance fatigability. Kindig and Poole (1999) determined that the relationship between capillary diameter and mean arterial pressure is dependent on skeletal muscle sarcomere length.

Two explanations originally evolved to elucidate the reduced muscle blood flow caused by changes in length: (1) passive reductions in vessel diameter resulting from compression and axial stretch and (2) kinking and pinching of vessels by shear forces generated between muscle fibers and fiber bundles. Two alternative explanations have been offered by Welsh and Segal (1996). First, muscle lengthening elicits an active vasomotor response that results in vasoconstriction. Specifically, "muscle length activates stretch-sensitive ion channels in perivascular nerve fibers, causing depolarization and the generation of action potentials. Such an effect could be mediated by integrin binding to extracellular matrix" (p. 558). Second, "muscle extension may increase the release of a paracrine substance that gives rise to action potentials in perivascular nerves, perhaps via a local axon reflex" (p. 558). However, such a mechanotransduction mechanism has yet to be identified.

PERIPHERAL NERVES

Normally both active and passive joint movements can be freely carried out over a wide range. During such movements, nerves are subjected to various stresses and strains that usually are tolerated without pain or any functional impairment. However, under certain conditions, nerve injuries do occur. Traumatic and stretch injuries to peripheral nerves represent considerable clinical problems to allied health practitioners and to those involved with treating athletes and performing artists. Knowledge of those features that relate to nerve compression and stretch is important on several levels. The athlete, dancer, coach, and trainer must know the limiting factors that can influence performance or predispose to injury. Nerve compression and stretch represent practical treatment and rehabilitation problems to the medical community. For instance, peripheral nerves may be subjected to stretching during suturing of severed nerve trunks under tension. Similarly, physical therapists must be cognizant of nerve vulnerability during mechanical traction procedures. Health-care practitioners who employ adjustment and manipulative techniques must be vigilant to avoid causing, or compounding preexisting, nerve damage.

Nerve Structure and Sheaths

For over 100 years, researchers have investigated the structure of peripheral nerves (nerves lying outside of the CNS). With improved microscopic techniques and technologies, a greater understanding of the nature of peripheral nerves has become possible. In the peripheral nervous system, the nerve fibers are grouped in bundles to form the nerves.

Nerves have three separate connective tissue sheaths: the *epineurium*, the *perineurium*, and the *endoneurium*. The obvious functions of the connective tissue sheaths are to provide structural support to the peripheral nerves and to contribute to the elasticity that allows nerves to be stretched during body movement. In addition, some of the sheaths serve as a blood-nerve barrier that protects the nerve fibers from various noxious agents, limits the penetration of macromolecules, and possibly controls the passage of ions. The sheaths also separate and compartmentalize the nerve fibers.

Epineurium

The epineurium is a fibrous coat of dense connective tissue that encloses the entire nerve and lies between fiber bundles. It contains connective tissue fibers, blood vessels, and some small nerve fibers that innervate the vessels. The components of the epineurium, the most prominent of which are collagen fibrils, are mainly oriented longitudinally. Elastic fibers are also present.

Perineurium

The perineurium lies deep within the epineurium and separately encloses each bundle (fascicle) of nerve fibers. Therefore, each bundle is surrounded by the perineurium, which consists of three to 10 concentric layers of cells. The number of layers depends on the size of the enclosed nerve fascicle and its proximity to the CNS. The cells in these layers are joined at their edges by tight junctions, an arrangement that makes the perineurium a barrier to most macromolecules. The collagen fibrils are thinner than those of the epineurium and contain only a few scattered elastic fibers.

Endoneurium

The endoneurium is the deepest of the nerve sheaths and encloses each individual nerve fiber. The endoneurium consists of a thin layer of collagen fibrils that are mainly oriented longitudinally and are generally similar in diameter to perineurium fibrils.

Application of Stretch to Nerves

Studies on the behavior of peripheral nerves subjected to stretching (i.e., tensile load) date from the latter half of the nineteenth century. Still, little is known about the biomechanical properties of peripheral nerves or about the limits of stretching that the nerve may undergo before structural damage occurs. Chronically injured nerves may have altered mechanical properties, such as increased stiffness (Beel et al. 1984). However, the available data regarding tensile properties and the critical limits of stretching are limited and often conflicting (Beel et al. 1986; Denny-Brown and Doherty 1945; Haftek 1970; Highet and Sanders 1943; Hoen and Brackett 1970; Rydevik et al. 1989; Sunderland 1991; Sunderland and Bradley 1961). In the following sections, we will review the research regarding stretching forces as related to the biomechanics of nerves, the blood flow to the nerves, and the effect on neural transmission.

Comparison between the reported experiments is often impossible because of a lack of biomechanical standardization (Wall et al. 1992). Among some of the variables relating to the nerve to be tested are in situ versus in vitro experimentation, the type of animal, the specific nerve, the age of the nerve, the preparation of the nerve, and the test itself.

In general, when a nerve is subjected to a gradually increasing tensile load, a linear relationship exists between load and elongation until a certain point is reached. Beyond that point, the nerve ceases to behave as an elastic structure (Sunderland 1978, 1991). The principal component imparting elasticity to the nerve trunk and giving it tensile strength is the perineurium. The elastic range is between 6% and 20% of resting length. Beyond the elastic limit, deformation and force are no longer linearly proportional. As greater force is applied, the curve flattens until the maximum stress or ultimate strength level—the point at or before rupture—is reached. Existing data regarding the amount of stretching that leads to structural changes are limited, with values from 11% to 100% elongation. These structural changes are highly dependent on the magnitude and character of the deforming force, as well as on the length of time the force is applied. Grewal et al. (1996) graphically describe the significance of stretch damage to the perineurium.

> Damage to the perineurium changes its diffusion properties, which causes an increase in its permeability and results in leakage of proteins into the fascicles. This produces intrafascicular edema, leading to fibrosis within the nerve, which jeopardizes the recovery of normal function. (p. 201)

Stress-Strain Properties of the Peripheral Nerve Trunk

Sunderland and Bradley (1961) performed a series of experiments on the stress-strain properties of stretched human peripheral nerves that are subjected to progressively increasing loads up to the point of mechanical failure. Specimens of human median ($n = 24$), ulnar ($n = 24$), medial popliteal ($n = 13$), and lateral popliteal ($n = 15$) nerves were obtained from the autopsy room within 12 hours of death and tested immediately. All specimens were from adults 30 to 50 years of age. The tests provided the following data about the range of maximum load irrespective of size:

Median	7.3 to 22.3 kg
Ulnar	6.5 to 15.5 kg
Medial popliteal	20.6 to 33.6 kg
Lateral popliteal	11.8 to 21.4 kg

Maximum Tensile Strength of the Nerve Trunk

Nerves are not homogeneous structures and do not behave as perfect cylinders. The range of maximum tensile stress (kg/mm^2) on the cross-sectional area of the nerve trunk is as follows:

Median	1.0 to 3.1 kg/mm^2
Ulnar	1.0 to 2.2 kg/mm^2
Medial popliteal	0.5 to 1.8 kg/mm^2
Lateral popliteal	0.8 to 1.9 kg/mm^2

Maximal Elongation of the Nerve Trunk

If a nerve was not strained beyond its elastic limit, Sunderland and Bradley (1961) found that the specimen regained its original length. It also retained its elastic properties when the load was removed. However, once the elastic limit was exceeded, the specimen did not regain its original length but acquired a permanent set, or deformation. The linear (elastic) relationship between load and elongation over a range of elongation may be summarized as follows:

Median	6% to 20%
Ulnar	8% to 21%
Medial popliteal	7% to 21%
Lateral popliteal	9% to 22%

Percentage of Elongation at Mechanical Failure

Although substantial individual variations existed among the nerve samples tested by Sunderland and Bradley (1961), the greatest elongation at the elastic limit was about 20%. Complete mechanical failure occurred at maximal elongations of approximately 30%. The elongations at mechanical failure, as a percentage of resting length, were

Median	7% to 30%
Ulnar	9% to 26%
Medial popliteal	8% to 32%
Lateral popliteal	10% to 32%

Implications of Nerve Stretch for Health-Care Practitioners

Rydevik et al. (1990) made several important observations that have implications for health and medical practitioners. First, when the nerve failed mechanically, it appeared to be grossly intact, although multiple ruptures of the perineurial sheaths were seen. "It is thus not reliable to assess the structural integrity of a nerve trunk through visual examination" (p. 699). Furthermore, the perineurial sheath did not rupture at one given point, but over some distance. Hence, this observation "indicates that stretch injuries to a peripheral nerve may not be localized and may occur along the length of the nerve" (pp. 699-700) (see figure 5.9).

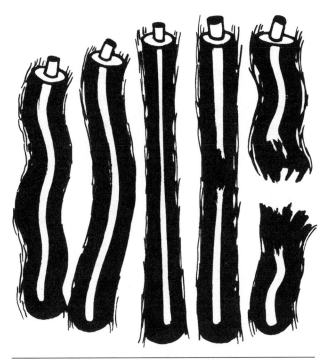

Figure 5.9 The behavior of the fascicle and contained nerve fibers of a nerve trunk stretched to the point of mechanical failure.

Reprinted, by permission, from S. Sunderland, 1978, "Traumatized nerves, roots, and ganglia: Musculoskeletal factors and neuropathological consequences." In *The neurobiologic mechanism in manipulative therapy*, edited by T.M. Korr (New York: Plenum), 139.

Intraneural Microvascular Flow

Stretching a nerve seriously affects the intraneural microvascular blood flow. Stretching a nerve causes elevated intrafascicular pressure and gradual reduction of the nerve's cross-sectional area. These changes cause compression that results in further deformation of the nerve fiber as well as impairment of its blood supply. Lundborg (1975), Lundborg and Rydevik (1973), and Ogata and Naito (1986) found that intraneural microvascular flow was impaired beyond an 8% elongation of the nerve. Complete intraneural ischemia (a decrease in blood supply) occurred at a 15% elongation. After stretches to these lengths, complete return of arteriolar and capillary circulation recovers after relaxation, but venous flow was restored incompletely. Prolonged stretch at 15% caused irreversible ischemic damage. Therefore, stretching that interferes with the intraneural microvascular flow can impair nerve function.

Effect of Stretch on Nerve Transmission

Another significant consequence of stretching nerves is the failure of electrical conduction. Failure to conduct is reported (Grewal et al. 1996; Wall et al. 1992) to begin at stretch extents ranging from 6% to 100%, depending on the animal tested. Wall et al. (1992) suggested that mechanical deformation, not ischemia, is responsible for early conduction loss.

Protective Structures of Nerve Trunks

Most peripheral nerves have four features that protect them from physical deformation: (1) slackness, (2) the course of the nerves in relation to the joints, (3) extensibility, and (4) elasticity.

Slackness of the Nerve Trunk and Nerve Fibers

A nerve trunk runs an undulating course in its bed. So, too, the fiber bundles (fasciculi) run an undulating course within the epineurium sheaths, and each nerve fiber runs an undulating course inside the fasciculi. With little or no tension, nerves shorten in an accordionlike arrangement (Smith 1966). As a result, the length of a nerve trunk and its nerve fibers traveling between any two fixed points on the limb is considerably greater than the linear distance between those points (see figure 5.10).

During initial stretching, the undulations are taken out of the nerve. With continued stretching, the undulations are eliminated in the fasciculi and finally in the individual nerve fibers. Only at this last point is all the slack taken up and the nerve fibers subjected to tension. If stretching continues, conduction in the nerve fibers is

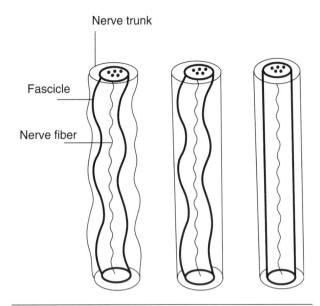

Figure 5.10 Diagram illustrating the undulations in nerves, fasciculi, and nerve fibers, which protect nerve fibers when nerves are stretched during a full range of limb movements.

Reprinted from Sunderland 1991.

progressively impaired and then fails completely. Finally, the nerve fibers fracture inside the fasciculi. The perineurium is the last component to fail structurally.

The importance of this slack system cannot be overstated. As explained by Sunderland (1991), "The slack provided in the system in this way absorbs and neutralizes traction forces generated during limb movements so that the contained nerve fibers are at all times protected from being overstretched" (p. 66).

Course of the Nerve in Relation to Joints

The course or path of the nerve in relation to the joints protects nerves and facilitates ROM. With two notable exceptions, nerves typically cross the flexor aspect of joints (the "inside" of the joint when flexed). Because the range of joint flexion is much greater than that of extension, a nerve crossing the flexor aspect of a joint remains relaxed during flexion and is only slightly stretched during extension. In contrast, a nerve crossing the extensor aspect of a joint is relaxed during extension but is put under considerable tension during flexion. In other words, there is a greater "safety margin" and more "nerve play" with flexion than extension. Nerves crossing the extensor aspect of a joint are at a disadvantage in regard to exposure to forces generated during limb movements.

The exceptions are the ulnar nerve, which crosses the extensor aspect of the elbow joint, and the sciatic nerve, where it crosses the extensor aspect of the hip joint. These two nerves are repeatedly subjected to undue tension during full flexion. Because movements involving forward trunk flexion with the knees extended are common to many sports and activities, this fact is particularly relevant to physically active individuals.

Where the sciatic nerve crosses the extensor aspect of the hip joint, the epineurial tissue represents as much as 88% of the cross-sectional area of the nerve (Sunderland 1991). This structure is probably a special protective feature, for much time is spent squatting or sitting on the sciatic nerves with the thighs flexed, putting stretch on that nerve.

Extensibility of the Nerve Trunks

Extensibility protects nerves from excessive elongation. Nerves can deform or elongate when subject to a tensile force. As in all tissues, this ability is subject to eventual failure.

Elasticity of the Nerve Trunks

Elasticity is a material's resistance to distortion—the property that enables it to return to its original shape or size. As previously stated, when a nerve is subjected to a gradually increasing tensile load, a linear relationship exists between load and elongation until the nerve ceases to behave as an elastic structure. The principal component responsible for elasticity in the nerve trunk and for giving it tensile strength is the perineurium. Various test data have been published regarding the stress-strain values for different peripheral nerves. Research (Sunderland and Bradley 1961) indicates that in peripheral nerves the elastic range is between 6% and 20%.

Factors Reducing the Elasticity, Extensibility, and Mobility of Nerves

Peripheral nerves display the attributes of strength, elasticity, extensibility, and mobility, but these characteristics can be modified. Factors that can alter the mechanical characteristics of nerve fibers include

- adhesions and scar tissue,
- changes in the ratio of collagenous tissue to elastic tissue of the nerve,
- deformities,
- trauma, and
- sutures.

Can Training Modify Peripheral Nerves?

To date, no known studies have attempted to determine how different types of traditional stretching regimens or protocols influence peripheral nerve characteristics. Thus, whether, or how, stretching (as employed in athletics, dance, yoga, and physical therapy) affects peripheral nerve elasticity, extensibility, and mobility is not known. Research is needed to explore these issues.

FACTORS AFFECTING THE MECHANICAL PROPERTIES OF CONNECTIVE TISSUES, MUSCLES, AND NERVES

The behavior of connective tissues (collagenous or elastic) and of muscle and nerves under stress are influenced by a number of related factors, including the following:

- The alignment or orientation of the fibers
- The influence of different interweaving patterns of fibers within specific tissues
- The influence of different interweaving patterns of collagen molecules within each fibril
- The presence of interfibrillar substances
- The number of fibers and fibrils
- The cross-sectional area of the fibers
- The proportion of collagen and elastin
- The chemical composition of the tissues
- The degree of hydration
- The degree of relaxation of the contractile components
- The tissue temperature before and during the application of force
- The tissue temperature before releasing the applied force
- The magnitude of applied force (load)
- The duration of the applied force (time)
- The type of applied force (ballistic versus static)
- The duration of the recovery interval between force applications
- The number of cycles of repeated loading

NEED FOR ADDITIONAL RESEARCH

Research is a never-ending process. In the area of soft-tissue mechanics, an array of issues must be addressed. Two issues pointed out almost 25 years ago by Lee (1980) remain relevant:

1. Soft tissue contains largely fluids. Movement of this fluid within the tissue greatly influences the tissue's response to deforming forces. The deformational responses of the tissue are also dependent on the mechanical, electrical, and biochemical characteristics of the tissue's cellular and molecular constituents. These factors are likely responsible for the loading path–dependent and rate-dependent nature of the biomechanical response of soft tissues. However, additional quantitative research is needed in this area.

2. Most soft-tissue responses are more or less controlled and coordinated by the nervous system. The passive mechanical properties of elastic fibers and biological membranes have been studied separately by many investigators. The interactive nature of the muscles with the passive soft-tissue components must be clearly established. (pp. 30-33)

SUMMARY

All tissues (connective, muscular, nervous, and vascular) undergo predictable changes when force is applied. All tissues will eventually rupture under excessive tensile force. The amount of damage depends on such factors as the degree of force, the speed with which the force is applied, and the length of time the force is applied.

Elastic, or recoverable, elongation is optimized by high-force, short-duration stretching at normal or colder-than-normal temperatures. Plastic or permanent lengthening is more likely to be produced by low-force, long-duration stretching at elevated temperatures, followed by tissue cooling before release of tension. In addition, minimal structural weakening is associated with low-force stretching combined with high therapeutic temperatures, whereas maximal structural weakening is associated with higher forces and lower temperatures.

Therefore, the ideal stretching program to optimize increase in tissue length without damage should increase tissue temperature before stretch (by exercise or therapeutic modalities that increase body core temperature), apply low-intensity force, maintain stretching force for a prolonged period of time, and cool the tissue to normal temperature before releasing the stretching force.

Blood vessels and peripheral nerves are capable of elongation. Applications of stretch to blood vessels result in decreased blood flow. Excessive stretching of nerves impairs function and eventually results in mechanical failure. Several features protect peripheral nerves from physical deformation via elongation: slackness, path, elasticity, and extensibility.

2

CLINICAL CONSIDERATIONS

Neuroscience
of Flexibility

The nervous system constitutes one of the main communication systems of the body. Consequently, it plays a significant role in determining the quality and quantity of movement available to the body. The nervous system comprises the CNS (the brain and spinal cord) and the peripheral nervous system (the cranial and peripheral nerves). This chapter concentrates on aspects of the nervous system most related to flexibility and stretching.

SENSORY RECEPTORS RELATED TO STRETCHING

The three major receptors that have implications for stretching and maintaining optimal ROM are the muscle spindles, Golgi tendon organs (GTOs), and articular (joint) mechanoreceptors. In the following sections, their structure, function, and relationship to stretching are reviewed.

Muscle Spindles

Muscle spindles are the primary stretch receptors in muscle and are the most widely studied proprioceptors (receptors located in muscles, joints, tendons, and the vestibule of the ear). They are located in various numbers in most skeletal muscles of the body and are particularly numerous in the small, delicate muscles of the hand and eye.

The typical mammalian spindle consists of six tiny muscle fibers, encased in a connective tissue capsule. The muscle fibers inside the capsule, which provide sensory information about muscle length, are called *intrafusal* fibers. The fibers outside the capsule, the regular contractile units of the muscle, are called *extrafusal* fibers. The spindles attach at both ends to the extrafusal fibers and are therefore parallel to them Therefore, when the whole muscle is elongated, the spindle is also stretched (see figure 6.1).

Spindle Intrafusal Muscle Fibers

Two types of intrafusal fibers termed *nuclear bag fibers* and *nuclear chain* fibers are typically present in mammalian muscle spindles. This nomenclature reflects both the arrangement of myonuclei at the midportion of each of these fibers and the sequence of their formation (Walro and Kucera 1999). The nuclear bag fibers contain an abundance of sarcoplasm and cell nuclei in a dilated, swollen, baglike structure. This noncontractile structure is located in the center, or equatorial, region of the intrafusal fiber. At the distal, or polar, ends of the nuclear bag fiber are striated contractile filaments, near where the spindles attach to the extrafusal fibers. Two subtypes of nuclear bag fiber are termed nuclear bag$_1$ and nuclear bag$_2$.

The nuclear chain fibers are thinner and shorter than the nuclear bag fibers. They contain only a single row of nuclei, which are spread out in a chainlike structure through the noncontractile equatorial region. Like the nuclear bag fibers, the polar ends of the nuclear chain fibers are also composed of striated contractile filaments. Their ends often connect to the nuclear bag fibers, which in turn attach to the endomysium of extrafusal fibers.

Spindle Sensory Neurons

The *primary* and *secondary* endings are the two types of sensory (afferent) endings in each spindle. The primary endings terminate as a spiral wrap around the central region of a nuclear bag fiber and as a side branch to all nuclear chain fibers. Afferent axons of primary endings belong to the large group I fibers. To distinguish these sensory nerves from others in the group I size category, large spindle afferents are known as group Ia fibers.

Primary endings have a very low threshold to stretch and are thus easily excited (see figure 6.2a). They have both a phasic (dynamic) and a tonic response to stretch. The phasic response measures the rate, or velocity, of the stretch by changing the neuron impulse frequency

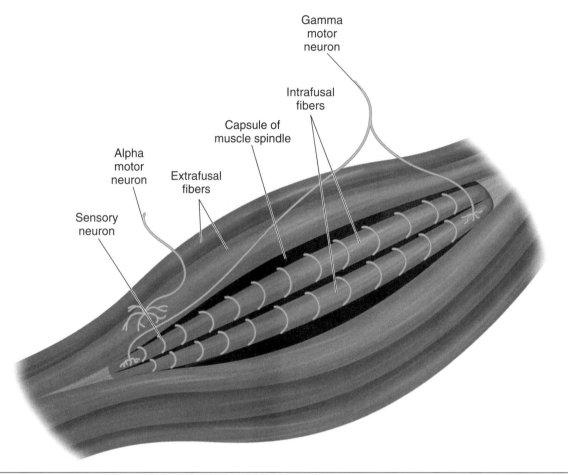

Figure 6.1 The muscle spindle.
Reprinted from Wilmore and Costill 1999.

during the stretch. Specifically, the frequency of discharge increases rapidly with the initial stretch. Then, when the stretch reaches its new length, the frequency of discharge drops to a constant level appropriate to the new tonic length (see figure 6.26). Hence, a tonic response measures the length of a muscle. In other words, the primary endings measure length plus velocity of stretch.

Secondary endings form branched or flower-spray-shaped endings. They are restricted almost entirely to the juxtaequatorial segment (near the equator) of the nuclear chain fibers. Axons of the secondary endings belong to the smaller group II afferent fibers. In contrast to the primary endings, secondary endings measure only tonic muscle length. These motor neurons cause contraction of the muscle filaments in the polar ends of the intrafusal muscle fibers. When the ends shorten, passive stretch occurs at the center equatorial region, where the sensory neuron receptors are located. Thus, activation of gamma motor neurons by the CNS can increase the amount of stretch perceived by the sensory endings (Banker 1980).

Liu et al. (2002) examined in detail the myosin heavy chain composition of intrafusal fibers from 36 spindles of human biceps brachii muscle. Virtually each muscle spindle had a different number of nuclear bag$_1$, nuclear

bag$_2$, and nuclear chain fibers. Liu et al. (2002) suggested that each muscle spindle in the human biceps has a unique identity.

Spindle Motor Neurons

The gamma efferent neurons, which make up the fusimotor system, innervate each intrafusal muscle fiber. These motor neurons cause contraction of the muscle filaments in the polar ends of the intrafusal muscle fibers. When these ends shorten, passive stretch occurs at the center equatorial region, where the sensory neuron receptors are located. Significantly, activation of gamma efferent neurons by the CNS can increase the amount of stretch perceived by the sensory nerve endings (Banker 1980) (see figure 6.3).

The two types of gamma motor axons are classified on the basis of their effects on the sensitivity of the primary and secondary sensory nerve endings. Stimulation of the *static gamma* axon can increase the length sensitivity of a primary sensory nerve ending with little or no effect on its velocity sensitivity. In contrast, *dynamic gamma* axons can markedly enhance the velocity sensitivity of a primary sensory nerve ending with little or no alteration in its length sensitivity.

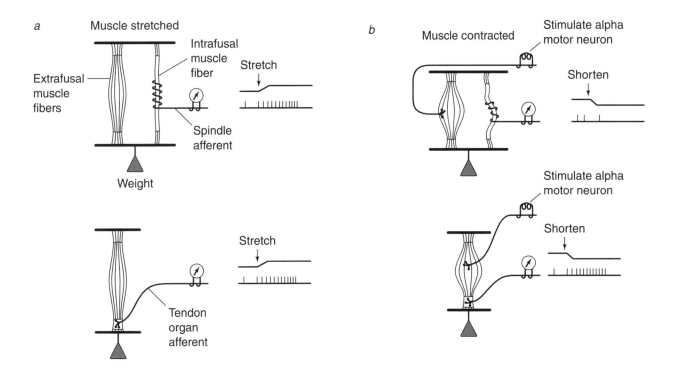

Figure 6.2 Muscle spindle and GTOs. The muscle spindle and Golgi tendon organ have different responses to muscle stretch and muscle contraction. Both afferents discharge when the muscle is stretched (*a*), the Golgi tendon organ much less than the spindle. However, when the muscle contracts (*b*), the spindle is unloaded and therefore goes silent, whereas, the tendon organ firing rates increase. (*a*) Stretching of the muscle elongates the intrafusal fibers, stretching the sensory endings in the spindle and leading to increased firing. In tendon organs, however, the collagen fibers from the tendon are stiffer than the muscle fibers with which they are in series. Therefore, most of the stretch is taken up by the more compliant muscle fibers and little direct mechanical deformation of the tendon organ takes place. (*b*) When the muscle contracts, the muscle fibers themselves pull directly on the collagen fibers and transmit the stretch to the tendon organ more effectively. As a result, tendon organs always respond more robustly to contraction than to stretch of the muscle. Spindles, in contrast, decrease their firing rates when the muscle contracts because, as the extrafusal fibers shorten with contraction, the parallel intrafusal fibers are unloaded.

Reprinted from Kandel, Schwartz, and Jessell 1995.

The *gamma system* controls spindle sensitivity to stretch. Activation of gamma motor neurons (by higher-brain motor centers) results in contraction or shortening of the intrafusal muscle fibers at their polar regions. When intrafusal fibers contract, the equatorial bag region is stretched, just as if the main muscle had been extended. This central stretch deforms the primary sensory nerve endings, thereby increasing the rate of firing of the group Ia fibers. The increase in activity of dynamic gamma motor neurons has no influence on the secondary sensory nerve endings (Pearson and Gordon 2000).

The second function of gamma motor neurons is to maintain spindle sensitivity during shortening contractions of the whole muscle (see figure 6.3). When muscles shorten, the parallel spindle is also passively shortened. This passive approximation of the spindle's two ends removes the tension on its primary sensory nerve endings (*spindle unloading*) as well as its secondary sensory nerve endings. This unloading thereby deprives the brain of information from the spindle about the muscle length changes, as well as eliminates stretch reflex input to the spinal cord. To prevent this spindle unloading, gamma motor neurons are activated to adjust the spindle sensitivity.

The neural connections of the intrafusal (and extrafusal) fibers are also important because these fibers synthesize different heavy chain subunits of myosin (MyHCs) in mammalian limb muscles (Walro and Kucera 1999). This development raises an intriguing question: What is responsible for the diversity of MyHC isoforms found in intrafusal fibers? Neural innervations are speculated to be a regulating factor of intrafusal's myosin expression. A second question arises: Does stretching modify myosin isoforms in intrafusal fibers of ballerinas, gymnasts, and long-time practitioners of yoga? Plasticity of the CNS has been demonstrated by Wolpaw (see Plasticity of the Spinal Cord Neural Circuits, p. 83).

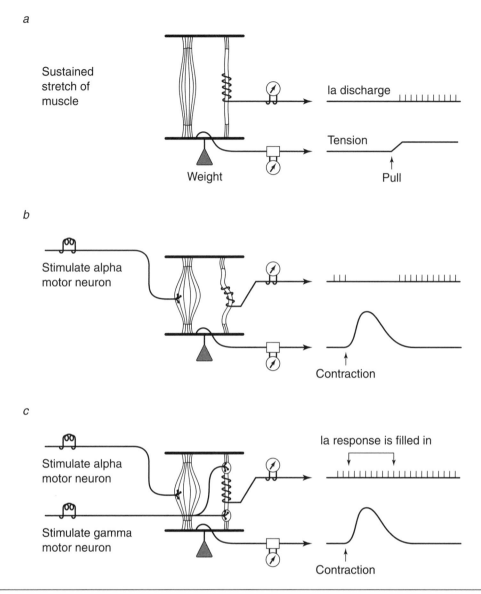

Figure 6.3   The muscle spindles do not slacken during active contractions because the tension of the intrafusal fibers is maintained by γ motor neurons. (*a*) Under normal conditions sustained tension elicits steady firing of the afferent (Ia) fibers in the muscle spindle. (*b*) If the α motor unit alone is stimulated electrically, the afferent fibers stop firing when the muscle contracts. The firing stops because the spindle is relaxed by the contraction. (*c*) If both the α and γ motor neurons are stimulated together, the spindle does not slacken during the contraction and the pause in firing of the afferent is "filled in."

Reprinted from Kandel, Schwartz, and Jessell 1995.

Golgi Tendon Organs

GTOs are contraction-sensitive mechanoreceptors of mammalian skeletal muscles innervated by large-diameter, fast-conducting group Ib afferent nerve fibers (Jami 1992). GTOs were first identified and described by Golgi in 1903. Initially, Golgi called these structures *musculotendinous end-organs*. In 1913, Nusbaum officially introduced the term Golgi apparatus. Later, in 1956 Dalton and Felix designated the structures as the "Golgi complex" (Bentivoglio 1998). Because of technical dif-

ficulties, GTOs have not been studied as much as muscle spindles. Nonetheless, their importance to stretching and flexibility cannot be overemphasized.

Location and Structure

GTOs are located almost exclusively at the *aponeuroses*, or muscle-tendon junctions. The work of Pang (quoted by Barker [1974]), which is the largest such study ever conducted, showed that 92.4% of 1,337 receptors from different portions of cat muscles were located at musculo-tendinous junctions, versus only 7.6% located within the tendon proper. The function of these purely tendinous receptors are not known (Jami 1992).

Nonmammalian GTOs are unencapsulated receptors located along the length of the tendon fascicles (collagen fiber bundles). Conversely, mammalian GTOs are encapsulated and, as previously mentioned, located at the musculotendinous or musculoaponeurotic junctions. The significance of these differences is twofold. First, encapsulated organs are possibly more sensitive to stimuli and more precise in localizing and relaying information to the CNS. Second, the location of the encapsulated GTOs enables these receptors to be extremely sensitive to change in tension in the individual muscle fibers to which they are attached (Moore 1984).

GTOs lie directly in line with the transmission of force from muscle to bone and so are said to be in series with the muscle. This arrangement is in direct contrast to the muscle spindles, which are parallel to the muscle fibers. Stretching of the tendon organ straightens the collagen fibers, thus compressing the nerve endings and causing them to fire (Pearson and Gordon 2000). In the Pang sample (Barker 1974), the number of muscle fibers attached in series with a GTO varied from 3 to 50. Each GTO is usually innervated by a single fast-conducting group Ib afferent nerve fiber (Jami 1992).

GTO Function

Currently, the multidimensional function of GTOs is only partially understood. However, this receptor is known to be more complex than was originally thought (Moore 1984). GTOs monitor all degrees of muscle tension. However, they are most sensitive to tension forces generated by muscle contraction (i.e., active tension as opposed to passive stretch tension [see figure 6.2b]). GTOs may contribute to conscious sensations. This belief is based on the fact that input from the GTOs reaches the cerebral cortex, the portion of the brain that interprets the sensory activity of the body (Roland and Ladegaard-Pedersen 1977).

As tension builds in a group of muscle fibers, the GTOs and their group Ib afferents send an increasing number of signals to the CNS. Sensory nerves of the CNS terminate in the spinal cord, on small interneurons, which then inhibit the motor neuron cell bodies that are activating the contracting muscle. This process is called *autogenic inhibition*, because the muscle's contraction is inhibited by its own receptors. The resulting reduction in muscle force decreases activation of the GTOs and the amount of inhibitory feedback being received by the CNS. This momentary inhibition in feedback enables more tension to develop in these muscles.

"Further studies are needed to fully understand the cooperation of information from GTOs and other muscle, skin, and joint receptors in feedback control of muscle contraction and in conscious proprioception" (Jami 1992, p. 658).

Misconceptions About GTOs

Numerous misconceptions about GTOs have developed and persist. One example is the relationship between GTOs and measuring stretching forces. GTOs have been called "stretch receptors." Unfortunately, this term implies that passive tension accompanying muscle stretch might also represent an adequate stimulus for the GTOs. Although GTOs can be activated by passive tension, their threshold for this kind of stimulus is very high. Therefore, extremely intense stretch is necessary to activate GTOs (Houk et al. 1971). Also, GTO discharge rarely persists during muscle stretch.

Another misconception is that GTOs lack sensitivity to active (contractile) tension. GTOs display a very low threshold and an appreciable *dynamic sensitivity*. Thus, they are capable of signaling very small and rapid changes in contractile forces (Houk and Henneman 1967; Houk et al. 1971; Jami 1992).

The function of GTOs was once postulated to be autogenic inhibition (i.e., inhibition of agonists and synergists and facilitation of antagonists). Autogenic inhibition is just one of many functions of the GTOs (Pearson and Gordon 2000) and they are assisted in this task by low-threshold joint capsule receptors and low-threshold cutaneous receptors (Moore 1984). The purpose of this autogenic inhibition is related to "protective functions." For example, if forces of muscle contraction together with external forces reach a point of potential musculotendinous damage, the GTOs "shut off" the agonist contraction and stimulate the antagonist muscle. Consequently, this process helps prevent injury in the associated muscles, tendons, ligaments, and joints.

However, this mechanism is not obligatory. The effects of the GTOs can be counterbalanced by signals from higher centers. In this case, the GTO is prevented from exerting its usual inhibitory effect on the agonist muscle. Brooks and Fahey (1987) point out that part of athletic training appears to be overriding the usual inhibitory effect on the agonist. Consequently, in some highly motivated individuals, the combination of active muscle contraction plus tension exerted by an opposing athlete can exceed the strength of tissues and result in injury.

Articular Mechanoreceptors (Joint Receptors)

All the synovial joints (including the apophyseal joints of the vertebral column) have four varieties of receptor nerve endings. These joint receptors sense mechanical forces on joints, such as stretch pressure and distension. Hence, they are called *articular mechanoreceptors*. These receptors are classified as types I to IV (see table 6.1). This classification is based on the respective morphological and behavioral characteristics of the nerve endings. In the following sections, the four types of articular mechanoreceptors will be discussed.

Table 6.1   Characteristics of Articular Receptor System

Type	Morphology	Location	Parent-nerve fibers	Behavioral characteristics
I	Thinly encapsulated globular corpuscles (100μm × 40μm), in tridimensional clusters of 3-8 corpuscles	Fibrous capsules of joints (in superficial layers)	Small myelinated (6-9 μm)	Static and dynamic mechanoreceptors: low-threshold, slowly adapting
II	Thickly encapsulated conical corpuscles (280 μm × 120 μm), individual or in clusters of 2-4 corpuscles	Fibrous capsules of joints (in deeper subsynovial layers). Articular fat pads	Medium myelinated (9-12 μm)	Dynamic mechanoreceptors: low-threshold, rapidly adapting
III	Thinly encapsulated fusiform corpuscles (600 μm × 100 μm), individual or in clusters of 2-3 corpuscles	Applied to surfaces of joint ligaments (collateral and intrinsic)	Large myelinated (13-17 μm)	Dynamic mechanoreceptors: high-threshold, slowly adapting
IV	(a) Tridimensional plexuses of unmyelinated nerve fibers (b) Free unmyelinated nerve endings	Fibrous capsules of joints. Articular fat pads. Adventitial sheaths of articular blood vessels Joint ligaments (collateral and intrinsic)	Very small myelinated (2-5 μm) and unmyelinated (<2μm)	Nociceptive receptors: very high-threshold, nonadapting. Chemosensitive (to abnormal tissue metabolites) nociceptive receptors

Reprinted, by permission, from B.D. Wyke, 1985, "Articular neurology and manipulative therapy". In *Aspects of manipulative therapy*, edited by E.F. Glasgow, L.T. Twomey, E.R. Scull, and A.M. Kleynhaw (London: Churchill Livingstone), 73.

This material was culled from Wyke (1967, 1972, 1979, 1985).

Type I Joint Receptors

Type I receptors are clusters of thinly encapsulated globular corpuscles, located mainly in the external (i.e., superficial) layers of the fibrous joint capsule. Each cluster consists of up to eight corpuscles. Furthermore, each member of a cluster is supplied from a single group II myelinated fiber (6 to 9 μm in diameter). Type I receptors are more numerous in the proximal (e.g., hip) joints than in more distal (e.g., ankle) joints.

Physiologically, the type I corpuscles behave as low-threshold, slow-adapting receptors. Consequently, they respond to very small mechanical stresses, and they continue to fire nerve impulses throughout the duration of mechanical stimulus. A force of approximately 3 g is sufficient to stimulate them. Furthermore, some of these lowest-threshold receptors are always active in the joint, even when it is immobile. Their resting discharge frequency is usually 10 to 20 Hz (impulses per second).

Type I receptors have several functions, including signaling the direction, amplitude, and velocity of joint movements produced actively or passively; regulating joint pressure changes; contributing significantly to postural and kinesthetic sensation; facilitating CNS regulation of postural muscle tone and muscle tone during joint movement; and producing an inhibitory effect on the flow of nociceptive (pain-sensing) afferent activity from the type IV articular receptor system. Type I receptors may be categorized as either static or dynamic mechanoreceptors.

Type II Joint Receptors

Type II receptors are larger, thickly encapsulated, conical corpuscles. They are located in the fibrous joint capsule, but in its deeper layers and in articular fat pads. Each cluster usually consists of two to four corpuscles. In addition, each member of the cluster is innervated by a branch of group II myelinated articular nerve fibers (9 to 12 μm in diameter). Type II receptors are also more numerous in the distal joints (e.g., the ankles) than in the proximal joints (e.g., the hip).

Like the type I receptors, type II receptors have a low threshold. However, they behave as rapidly adapting mechanoreceptors and do not fire at rest. Hence, they are totally inactive in immobile joints. Type II receptors have no static discharge, because their firing is velocity dependent. Consequently, they are acceleration or dynamic mechanoreceptors. When stimulated, each cluster emits a brief, high-frequency burst of impulses for less than 1 second, and very often less than 0.5 second. Their primary function is to measure sudden changes in movement, such as acceleration and deceleration.

Type III Joint Receptors

Type III receptors are thinly encapsulated corpuscles confined to the intrinsic (inside the joint capsule) and extrinsic (outside the joint capsule) ligaments of most joints. They are not found in the ligaments of the vertebral column. Type III receptors are the largest of the articular corpuscles and, like the Golgi tendon organs, are high-threshold, slowly adapting mechanoreceptors. They are serviced by large group I myelinated afferent axons that may be up to 17 μm in diameter.

Joint ligament mechanoreceptors have a high threshold and become active toward the extremes of joint movement. Therefore, type III receptors are completely inactive in immobile joints and respond only when high tensions are generated in joint ligaments. Stimulated type III receptors emit a discharge frequency that is a continuous function of the magnitude of that tension. Because these receptors are slow adapting, the discharge will decrease only very slowly (i.e., over many seconds) if the extreme joint displacement or joint traction is maintained.

Type III receptors appear to have two basic functions (although others are possible). Their primary function is to monitor the direction of movement. Their secondary function is to produce profound reflex inhibition of activity in some of the muscles operating over the joint. Thus, they may act with a reflex effect to produce a braking mechanism against overstress of the joint.

Type IV Joint Receptors

Unlike the other three mechanoreceptors, type IV receptors are unencapsulated. They are subdivided into two types. Type IVa receptors are latticelike plexuses found in joint fat pads and throughout the entire thickness of the joint capsule. However, they are entirely absent from synovial tissue, intraarticular menisci, and articular cartilage. The type IVb receptors are free nerve endings with a bare nerve and no associated specialized structures. They are sparse and confined largely to the intrinsic and extrinsic ligaments. These terminations are derived from the smallest (group III) afferent fibers in the articular nerves. Those group III nerve fibers that are thinly myelinated range between 2 and 5 μm in diameter.

Both type IVa and type IVb receptors constitute the pain receptor system of the articular tissues. Often referred to as nociceptors, these receptors are of major importance to those health-care practitioners (i.e., medical doctors, osteopaths, chiropractors, and physical therapists) who endeavor to relieve pain. Under normal conditions, type IV receptors are entirely inactive. However, they become active when the articular tissues are subjected to marked mechanical deformation or chemical irritation from such agents as bradykinin, prostaglandin-E, lactic acid, potassium ions, polypeptides, and histamines. These substances are secreted during conditions of ischemia (lack of blood) and hypoxia (lack of oxygen) and are constituents of inflammatory exudates. For individuals who are considering surgery to relieve certain types of pain, Wyke (1972) states

> Type IV category of receptors is entirely absent from the synovial lining of every joint that has been examined, and is also lacking from the menisci present in the knee and temporomandibular joints, and from the intervertebral disks. There is no mechanism, then, whereby articular pain can arise directly from the synovial tissue or menisci in any joint, and surgical removal of synovial tissue or joint menisci likewise does not involve removal of pain-sensitive articular tissues per se. (p. 97)

Thus, this type of surgery will not stop the pain.

REFLEXES AND OTHER SPINAL NEURAL CIRCUITS

A reflex is a response to a stimulus, It requires a neuron circuit consisting of a sensory neuron, an internuncial or communicating neuron, and a motor neuron with its effector. A stimulus is applied to the receptor ending. An impulse is initiated, which passes along the afferent process to the spinal cord, where it synapses with a connecting neuron. Finally, a motor neuron is excited, and the nerve impulse is conducted down the efferent fiber to a muscle or gland cell.

Myotatic or Stretch Reflex

According to the classical description of the stretch reflex, stretching a muscle lengthens both the extrafusal muscle fibers and the muscle spindles (i.e., the intrafusal fibers). The consequent deformation within the muscle spindles activates the primary and secondary sensory nerve endings, which results in action potentials in their group Ia and II sensory neurons. These neurons extend to the spinal cord, where they terminate on the cell bodies of alpha (large) motor neurons. If the sensory afferents produce enough depolarization in the motor neuron, it will fire action potentials. Its axon will transmit an impulse to the skeletal muscle, resulting in a reflex contraction.

The stretch reflex has a *phasic* and a *tonic* component. The phasic response is an initial burst of action potentials that results in a rapid rise of muscle tension, proportional to the velocity of the stretch. The tonic response is a later phase of slow (low-frequency) firing, lasting for the duration of the stretch, which is proportional to the amount of stretch.

The classic example of the phasic response is the knee jerk or *patellar reflex*. When the patellar tendon (located below the knee) is given a light tap, the muscle spindles parallel with the muscle fibers in the quadriceps (front thigh muscles) are stretched, creating a deformation in its muscle spindles. As a result, the firing of the group Ia muscle spindle afferents is increased. (The primary sensory nerve ending is excited more than is the secondary sensory nerve ending because the former is located on the more extensible central region of the spindle intrafusal muscle fiber, whereas the latter is located on the less extensible juxtaequatorial area.) The message is then sent to the spinal cord (via the dorsal root) and to the brain. The spinal cord sends an efferent nerve impulse to the quadriceps muscles and causes them to briefly contract, thus shortening the muscle and taking the tension off the muscle spindles. Nakazawa et al. (2001) demonstrated that stretch reflex sensitivity of the human elbow flexor and extensor muscles are not equal. Stretch reflex sensitivity is significantly greater in the elbow extensors than in the flexors. Stretch reflex sensitivity in other parts of the body remains to be examined.

In addition to detecting change in length, the stretch reflex may have other important functions. Based on the work on cat soleus muscle, Lin and Rymer (1993) have postulated that "stretch reflex compensation changes the basic form of the muscle's mechanical stiffness from one dominated by viscouslike behavior to one dominated by elastic behavior" (p. 997).

In this tonic reflex response, the stimulus is a maintained stretch, and the response is a corresponding maintained muscle contraction. The tonic response results in part from the effect of the group II afferents. A common example may be found in the postural reaction to stretch, exemplified by the contracting of the gastrocnemius (calf) muscle to correct an excess forward shifting of one's weight while standing.

Reciprocal Innervation

Muscles usually operate in pairs, and when one set of muscles, the *agonists*, are contracting, the opposing set, the *antagonists*, are relaxing. For example, when the arm is flexed at the elbow, by contraction of the biceps brachii, the triceps brachii muscle, which normally extends the arm at the elbow, must relax. This system of coordinated and opposing agonist and antagonist muscles is called *reciprocal innervation*. If not for this arrangement, a pair of muscles would pull against each other and no movement would occur.

In summary, when the motor neurons to one muscle receive excitatory impulses that cause it to contract, the motor neurons to the opposite muscle receive neural signals that make them less likely to fire and produce muscle contraction. The antagonist is therefore inhibited at nearly the same instant that the agonist contracts. Reflex *inhibition* is controlled by a small inhibitory neuron

(located in the spinal cord) to the motor neurons innervating the antagonistic muscle of the reciprocal pair. Conversely, if the antagonist muscle were similarly stretched, the agonist muscle would show reciprocal inhibition by the same process. Without this reciprocal innervation, coordinated muscular activity would be impossible.

COACTIVATION/COCONTRACTION

Coactivation or *cocontraction* refers to simultaneous contraction of the agonist and the antagonist at a variable level, with dominance of the former producing external motion. In 1909, Sherrington pointed out that antagonist muscles may be in contraction concurrently. He attributed it to *double reciprocal innervation*. Tilney and Pike (1925) concluded that, "muscular coordination depends primarily on the synchronous cocontractive relation in the antagonistic muscle groups" (p. 333). Eventually, Levine and Kabat (1952) stated that, in a human's normal voluntary movement, there was insufficient evidence of the assumption that reciprocal innervation plays the dominant role in the coordination of the contraction of antagonist muscles. Furthermore, "cocontraction seems to be the rule rather than the exception" (p. 118). Today, the central and peripheral control of agonist-antagonist coactivation has been established for various types of joint movement (DeLuca 1985; Kudina 1980; Rao 1965).

What is the purpose of cocontraction? One advantage is that it makes a joint stiffer and more difficult to perturb (Baratta et al. 1988; Enoka 2002; Kornecki 1992; Solomonow and D'Ambrosia 1991). Because coactivation increases the stiffness and hence stability of a joint, it seems like a useful property for learning novel tasks or for performing movements that requires a high degree of accuracy (Enoka 2002). Additional reasons that coactivation might be useful for various tasks have been suggested by Enoka (2002).

- During movements that involve changes in direction, modulating the level of tonic activity in an agonist-antagonist set of muscles is more economical than alternately turning them on and off (Hasan 1986).
- The ability to increase stiffness and joint stability may be desirable for lifting heavy or questionable loads (Cholewicki and McGill 1995; Lavender et al. 1989; Marras et al. 1987).
- Complex patterns of coactivation facilitate fine movements of the fingers (Sanes et al. 1995; Schieber 1995).

Autogenic Inhibition (Inverse Myotatic Reflex)

Up to a point, the harder a muscle is stretched, the stronger the resistance to the movement. The increase in resistance is the myotatic stretch reflex. However, after a certain limit is reached, the resistance suddenly yields, collapsing like the folding blade of a pocket knife. Consequently, this phenomenon is often called the *clasp-knife response*. Its physiologic name is the *lengthening reaction*. This phenomenon was originally thought to be mediated solely by the GTOs, but that view has been disproved (Jami 1992). The lengthening reaction is now believed to be the result of afferent input from group II nerve fibers coming from the muscle spindles and perhaps from thinly myelinated fibers subserving pain sensation from the joints (Moore 1984). However, additional research is needed to substantiate this view.

PLASTICITY OF THE SPINAL CORD NEURAL CIRCUITS

The mechanisms of memory, or long-term adaptive change, in the CNS have long been of interest. According to Wolpaw and Carp (1990),

> The spinal cord in general, and spinal reflexes in particular, were widely viewed as fixed and inflexible, responding in a stereotyped manner to inputs from periphery or from supraspinal areas. This common perception is not correct. Spinal cord neurons and synapses, like those of cerebral cortex and other supraspinal structures, change in the course of development and in response to trauma. (p. 138)

Neuronal activity can produce persistent changes in the CNS. These *plastic changes*, which can be as striking as the sprouting of new synaptic connections or as subtle as modification in specific membrane ionic conductances, are thought to be responsible for subsequent changes in CNS activity that are expressed as altered behavior (Wolpaw and Lee 1989). To investigate this phenomenon, several experimental tasks must be undertaken. First, the neuronal and synaptic substrates, or memory traces, of learned changes in behavior must be defined. Second, these substrates must be precisely located. Third, the characteristic memory trace—the change in the CNS that is responsible for a particular change in behavior—must be described. In other words, it is necessary to describe learning, the process that creates the trace.

Method of Plasticity Research and Findings

Since the early 1980s, researchers have examined the capability of nonhuman primates to alter the magnitude (size) of the *spinal stretch reflex* (SSR) as part of a systematic study of the anatomical and physiological substrates

governing memory. The SSR, also called the *tendon jerk* or M1, is the initial response to sudden muscle stretch. The SSR is the simplest action of which the vertebrate CNS is capable.

In a series of experiments, the biceps brachii and triceps surae muscles in monkeys were operantly conditioned through the use of an implanted electromyograph electrode biofeedback device and liquid juice reward. Monkeys were subjected to a conditioning task that required prolonged change in neuronal activity influencing the SSR pathway and that was thus likely to produce a memory trace located in this pathway (Wolpaw 1983; Wolpaw et al. 1983). Over a span of 250 days, the monkeys showed the ability to increase (uptrain) or decrease (downtrain) the magnitude of the SSR and H-reflex. The monkeys could even be trained to reverse the changed response, thereby demonstrating an adaptive plasticity (see figure 6.4). Perhaps the most important finding was that, even after total spinal cord transection above the lumbosacral site of the SSR pathway (which eliminated the influence of the brain), the animals previously subjected to the operant conditioning still displayed their trained reflex. This study substantiated the hypothesis that altered reflex activity eventually modifies the spinal cord (Wolpaw et al. 1991).

Site of the Plastic Changes

Three possible locations of the spinal cord memory traces responsible for change in SSR size have been hypothesized. The most likely site is the Ia afferent terminal on the motor neuron (see figure 6.5a). Transmission through the Ia synapse is inhibited by presynaptic inputs from several supraspinal sites (Baldissera et al. 1981; Burke and Rudomin 1978). Furthermore, studies suggest that short-term changes in presynaptic inhibitions are important in motor behavior (Capaday and Stein 1987a, 1987b). Thus, chronic alterations or long-term change in this inhibition might modify the Ia terminal. Wolpaw and Carp (1990) suggest that presynaptic inhibition may affect depolarization-induced calcium entry and transmitter release and thereby alter the size of the excitatory postsynaptic potential (EPSP) produced in the motor neuron when the Ia sensory afferent is stimulated.

A second possible location is a memory trace produced by prolonged change in the motor neuron that alters its response to any input (see figure 6.5). For example, motor neuron membrane properties that control resting potential and input resistance, such as ion permeability, could be altered. Needless to say, a modification in a motor neuron membrane's properties would have widespread effects on motor neuron function and would help determine the response of the motor neuron to any input (see figure 6.5b). However, Wolpaw and Carp (1990) and Wolpaw et al. (1991) believe that generalized membrane modifications present a less likely and more complex explanation for the reflex change.

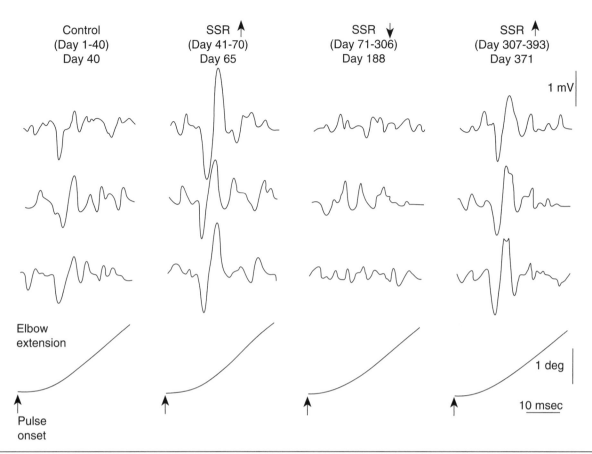

Figure 6.4 Series of individual trials of raw EMG from a monkey under the control mode (left side), after initial SSR (up) exposure, after SSR (down) exposure, and, finally, after SSR (up) reexposure (right side). Each series is made up of consecutive trials. Pulse onset is indicated by the arrows, and the average course of pulse-induced extension is shown by the bottom trace. Background EMG, represented here by the 10 ms immediately after pulse onset, and pulse-induced extension are stable across the four series. In contrast, SSR amplitude increases well above control with minimal SSR (up) exposure, decreases well below control with subsequent SSR (down) exposure, and increases again with SSR (up) reexposure.

Reprinted from Wolpaw 1983.

A third location is a very localized postsynaptic modification (see figure 6.5). This process could perhaps be manifest as a change of receptor sensitivity or dendritic architecture. However, pathways capable of producing such a selective modification are not known at present (see figure 6.5c). Carp et al. (2001) have also found "that conditioning mode-specific change in motoneuron firing patterns causes activity-dependent change in muscle properties" (p. 382).

Implications of Neural Plasticity

The confirmation that the spinal cord can be altered (i.e., spinal cord plasticity) has highly significant implications for understanding the mechanism by which neurological insults affect the body, the means to optimally rehabilitate the injured part, and the acquisition and maintenance of normal motor learning (Wolpaw and Tennissen 2001), particularly developing flexibility.

Clinical Perspectives on Neural Plasticity

From a clinical perspective, an interesting question is whether human SSRs can be experimentally conditioned and, if so, whether hyperactive SSRs (found in spastic muscles) might be downtrained or hypoactive SSRs (in flaccid muscles) uptrained more easily than in nonhuman primates. According to Wolf and Segal (1990), the data of several researchers suggest that the human nervous system can be conditioned by monitoring and feedback of the SSR (Evatt et al. 1989; Neilsen and Lance 1978).

Relationship of Neural Plasticity to the Development of Flexibility

Individuals striving to increase their flexibility (ROM) should modify the excitability of their stretch reflex if this action does not impair safety and performance. Specifically, individuals should seek to make their stretch reflex less excitable, thereby permitting their muscle to

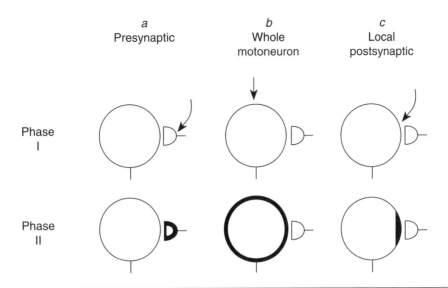

Figure 6.5 Possible locations of the spinal cord memory traces responsible for change in SSR, or H-reflex, amplitude. In each case, phase I change in descending influence on a site in the SSR pathway (indicated by the arrow) eventually produces phase II change (that is, the memory trace at the site). (*a*) The most likely site is the Ia afferent terminal on the motor neuron. A memory trace here could be produced by prolonged change in presynaptic inhibition. (*b*) The memory trace could be a generalized change in the motor neuron that alters its response to any input. However, such a modification would have widespread effects on motor neuron function. (*c*) The trace could be a very localized modification in the postsynaptic membrane, such as a change in receptor sensitivity or dendritic architecture.

Reprinted from Wolpaw and Carp 1990.

elongate further before firing. For individuals concerned with increasing their ROM, research regarding plasticity of the spinal cord may explain why static stretching has been used so effectively by practitioners of yoga. Static stretching held for a given period of time may modify the stretch reflex excitability and thereby reduce the muscle's resistance to stretch. If a controlled test could be designed, determining which technique of stretching (i.e., ballistic versus static) most facilitates beneficial plastic changes of the spinal cord would make a fascinating study.

Relationship of Neural Plasticity to Motor Learning

Changes in the SSR appear to occur throughout one's life. In children, gradual changes in the SSR occur with acquisition of fundamental motor skills (Myklebust et al. 1986). Wolpaw et al. (1991) and Wolpaw and Tennissen (2001) suggest that comparable changes seem to take place later in life during learning of such skills as ballet (Goode and Van Hoven 1982; Nielsen et al. 1993) and aerobic versus anaerobic activities (Rochcongar et al. 1979). Thus, "slow activity-driven changes in the spinal cord and elsewhere in the CNS may account for much learning, and serve to explain why acquisition of many skills depends on prolonged practice" (Wolpaw et al. 1991, p. 344). This observation has major implications in such fields as athletics, the performing arts, ergonomics, medicine, chiropractic, and physical therapy.

In sports medicine, the discovery of plasticity of the spinal cord has additional implications. For example, abnormal gait patterns after an injury may cause foot, knee, hip, and back pain (Day and Wildermuth 1988). Furthermore, these changes could result in plastic changes in the spinal cord that could further complicate and delay full recovery. Up to 33% of the patients suffering acute sprains will have residual symptoms long after their rehabilitation programs have ended (Bosien et al. 1955; Evans et al. 1984; Itay et al. 1982). The subsequent functional instability may result from lost and unrecovered joint, limb, and body proprioception (Freeman et al. 1965). This loss may be, in part, a consequence of plastic changes to the spinal cord.

Effects of Stretching Techniques on Neural Plasticity

Because insults to the body can result in plastic changes to the spinal cord, significant questions need to be investigated. What clinical techniques, either alone or in combination, can most efficiently, effectively, and rapidly correct the physical alteration to the spinal cord? Should therapy consist of a chiropractic adjustment or osteopathic manipulation, various stretching techniques (e.g., muscle energy, proprioceptive neuromuscular facilitation [PNF], static, or ballistic), mobilization, traction, or employment of physical modalities? Would the use of medications that are commonly employed as an adjunct to therapy actually facilitate or impede this process?

Relationship of Neural Plasticity to Athletics and Sport Rehabilitation

An old sports adage is that twice as much time is needed to correct something that was incorrectly learned. Thus, when an incorrect technique is learned, mastered, and ingrained, the neuromuscular pathways become "grooved," and subsequent neural plastic changes may take place. During the relearning phase, the undesired motor pattern must be "unlearned." This process necessitates not only unlearning the "grooving" of the neuromuscular pathways but also proper modification of the plastic changes that occurred during the initial learning.

NEUROLOGICAL AND OTHER FACTORS OF FLEXIBILITY TRAINING

Gains in muscle strength are believed to result from two principal factors: (1) hypertrophy and (2) hyperplasia and neural recruitment. Whereas muscle hypertrophy (i.e., an increase in size) occurs in the later stages of training (Enoka 2002; Komi 1986; McDonagh and Davies 1984; Sale 1986), strength gains achieved during the first weeks of training reflect an increased ability to activate motor neurons and therefore appear to be neural in origin. Abundant evidence demonstrates that neural changes occur soon after strength training begins. Voluntary strength increases rapidly before muscles exhibit hypertrophy (Ikai and Fukunaga 1970; Jones and Rutherford 1987; Liberson and Asa 1959; Moritani and de Vries 1979; Rose et al. 1957; Tesch et al. 1983) and before increases in electrically evoked tension occur (Davies and Young 1983; McDonagh et al. 1983). These early strength increases are accompanied by increased integrated electromyographic (Komi 1986; Sale 1986) and increased reflex amplifications (Milner-Brown et al. 1975; Sale et al. 1982; Sale, MacDougall et al. 1983; Sale, Upton et al. 1983; Upton and Radford 1975).

Extrapolating to flexibility training: What is responsible for the initial increase of flexibility during the first weeks of training versus many months of training? Also, does the type of training (e.g., ballistic, static, or PNF) influence the nature of these changes? Certain reflexes are modified in dancers as compared with the untrained (Goode and Van Hoven 1982; Koceja et al. 1991; Nielsen et al. 1993). Two such examples were the findings of Nielsen et al. (1993) that both the H-reflex and the disynaptic reciprocal inhibition were lowest in ballet dancers. Noting that muscle cocontraction/coactivation is accompanied by increased presynaptic inhibition and decreased reciprocal inhibition, the investigators speculated that the prolonged cocontractions required by the classical ballet postures lead to persistent decreases in synaptic transmission at the Ia synapses and thereby account for the reductions in H-reflexes and reciprocal inhibition. "Viewed from the perspective of performance, the decreased direct peripheral influence on motor neurons indicated by the smaller reflexes may increase cortical control and allow more precise movement" (p. 823).

Nonneural factors may also be involved. Koceja et al. (1991) suggest that the difference between the two groups in their previous studies is their relative tissue compliance. They argue that long-term training can change the composition of the connecting tendon and that these changes might result in less loading on the muscle spindle apparatus, given equal tendon-tap force. Byrd (1973) demonstrated that endurance training produced less tension per unit of cross-sectional area in the tail tendons of rat. This evidence suggested a greater fraction of soluble collagen. Viidik (1973) demonstrated that stretched tendon exhibits a tendency to remain in a stretched state. Consequently, any subsequent loading on the tendon will result in less force being transmitted to the muscle.

However, three additional factors could explain the altered reflex sensitivity of long-time practitioners of yoga or those involved in dance. (1) Repeated and prolonged long-term stretching modifies the titin in the intrafusal fibers. If this happens, the direct effect is reduced intrafusal contraction force (Avela et al. 1999). No investigation has demonstrated titin modification in the intrafusal fibers. (2) Stretching somehow modifies the myosin heavy chain (MyHC) isoforms in the intrafusal fibers. Walro and Kucera (1999) discussed the possibility that "slow shortening velocities that are characteristic of developmental MyHcs might be adaptive for precise calibration of muscle spindles as sense organs" (p. 180). (3) Sustained passive stretching could modify titin isoforms and cause some irregularities of filament overlapping within the extrafusal fibers. Consequently, this condition could lead to increased compliance of the sarcomere and a decrease in the number of attached cross-bridges, which, in turn, would lead to "a reduced external force response to stretch and, therefore, a decrease in the mechanical effect on the muscle spindles" (Avela et al. 1999, p. 1290). Thus, the modified titin isoforms would eventually cause altered reflex sensitivity.

Stevens et al. (1974) also alluded to altered reflex sensitivity in some subjects. They tested 232 physical education students, identifying the 15 supplest subjects and the 15 stiffest subjects in the hamstring muscle group. They found a stronger electromyographic activation in the stretch patterns of the hamstrings and other muscles and an earlier onset (the last 40° of the stretch movement) and a longer duration of stretch reflex muscle activity in the stiff subjects than in the supple subjects. In contrast, the supple subjects showed stretch reflex activation in the last 20° of the stretch movement. These data "encouraged the hypothesis of a stronger sensitivity of the muscle spindles (fusimotor bias) as well as a stronger excitability of the circuit downstream from the spindles or an enhanced gamma activity among stiff subjects" (p. 496).

In a follow-up study, Stevens et al. (1977) applied a vibration (to elicit the tonic vibration reflex) to the tendon of the biceps femoris for 2 minutes, followed by stretch. The mean integrated electromyographic activity did not significantly differ in the two groups. However,

> It was only in the stiff subjects that repeated stretch movements provoked a decreasing gradient of the maximum angle and the point at which the stretching activity started (i.e., the stretch reflex started later as a function of the repeated stretch movements). (p. 508)

In the opinion of the researchers, these findings "may suggest the hypothesis that viscoelastic components of a stiff muscle changes by stretching while the neurological component remains constant" (p. 509). In contrast, these tendencies were not found in the supple subjects.

Two studies challenge the previous results. Vujnovich and Dawson (1994) demonstrated a significant effect of passive muscle stretch on decreasing the activity of neurons within the L5-S1 spinal segment by both static and ballistic stretch, which correlates with increased flexibility. Halbertsma and Göeken (1994) investigated whether stretching exercises lengthened the hamstrings by changing the elasticity of the muscles and showed that a slight but significant increase in the extensibility of the hamstrings was accompanied by a significant increase of the stretching (moment) force tolerated by the passive hamstring muscles. However, the elasticity remained the same. They concluded, "stretching exercises do not make short hamstrings any longer or less stiff, but only influence the stretch tolerance" (p. 976).

Are neural influences more or less important than other factors in flexibility training? The question needs to be further investigated. The application of therapeutic stretch increases ROM. Two simple explanations for the increased ROM are (1) the mechanical elongation of muscle and intervening connective tissue and (2) the reduction of neuronal excitability. Additional research is needed to quantify how therapeutic stretching modifies the viscoelastic component of soft tissues and neural response among different populations—the healthy and those with disorders—and to establish the most efficient technique to achieve the desired outcome.

SUMMARY

The structural and functional unit of the nervous system is the neuron. Two significant mechanoreceptors are the muscle spindles and GTOs. The primary stretch receptors in muscle are the muscle spindles. In contrast, the GTOs are primary contraction-sensitive mechanoreceptors. Receptors that sense mechanical forces on joints, such as stretch pressure and distention, are called articular mechanoreceptors. These nerve endings may be classified as type I to type IV based on morphological and behavioral criteria.

The nervous system operates through a complex set of interactions called reflexes, three of which are the stretch reflex, reciprocal inhibition, and the inverse myotatic reflex. In addition, coactivation/cocontraction has been established during various types of joint movement. Neuronal activity can produce persistent changes in the CNS called plastic changes. These changes have implications for rehabilitation, motor learning, and developing flexibility in particular.

7

Hypermobility of the Joint

Hypermobility, or joint laxity, has long been a curiosity and a source of entertainment. The earliest known clinical description of hypermobility is attributed to Hippocrates who, in his *Airs, Waters and Places*, drew attention to a race of people called Scythians. According to Hippocrates, the Scythians' elbows were so lax they could not effectively draw their bows to shoot arrows! The old German diagnosis of *konstitutionelle Bindegewebenschwache* (connective tissue weakness) brought awareness of this condition into twentieth century, after which it received only scant attention in standard textbooks (Rose 1985). In the 1880s, a series of articles on contortionists appeared in several leading British medical journals ("The American Contortionist" 1882; "A Contortionist" 1882; Owen 1882; "Voluntary Power" 1882). The book *Anomalies and Curiosities of Medicine* by Gould and Pyle (1896, pp. 473-475) briefly dealt with the subject. Finkelstein (1916) and Key (1927) presented the first detailed reports on joint hypermobility. Wiles (1935) used radiography to perform a detailed analysis of the lumbar vertebrae of two extremely flexible professional acrobats.

During the 1950s and 1960s, the importance of generalized joint laxity in the pathogenesis of joint dislocation was recognized (Bowker and Thompson 1964; Carter and Sweetnam 1958, 1960; Carter and Wilkinson 1964; Massie and Howarth 1951). Kirk et al. (1967) finally described the terms *hypermobility syndrome* (HMS) and *hypermobility* in the medical literature. The former was defined as joint laxity associated with musculoskeletal complaints. Buckingham et al. (1991) employed the term *hypermobile joint syndrome*. In recent years, the term *benign joint hypermobility syndrome* (BJHS) has been used more widely (Grahame 1999; Grahame and Bird 2001, p. 559; Magnusson, Julsgaard et al. 2001, p. 2720; Mishra et al. 1996, p. 861). The term BJHS is preferred because it stresses the absence of life-threatening complications (Grahame 2000). In contrast, *generalized hypermobility* is said to be present when the joints are unduly lax and ROM is in excess of the accepted norm in most of the joints.

Beighton et al. (1988) identified this syndrome as "familial articular hypermobility syndrome." They excluded genetic diseases that include joint hypermobility as an associated finding, such as Ehlers-Danlos syndrome, osteogenesis imperfecta, and Marfan syndrome. Ehlers-Danlos syndrome will be discussed later in the chapter.

TERMINOLOGY

Numerous papers have been published with reference to an excessive ROM in joints. This characteristic is popularly referred to as being "double jointed." Among health professionals excessive ROM has been variously described as *ligamentous laxity* (Grana and Moretz 1978), *loose jointed* (Lichtor 1972), *joint hypertonia* (Finkelstein 1916; Jahss 1919), *joint looseness* (Marshall et al. 1980), *joint laxity* (Balaftsalis 1982-1983; Barrack et al. 1983; Bird 1979; Bird et al. 1980; Brodie et al. 1982; Cheng et al. 1991) and *hypermobility* (Ansell 1972; Child 1986; Grahame and Jenkins 1972; Gustavsen 1985; Key 1927; Kirk et al. 1967; Klemp and Learmonth 1984; Klemp et al. 1984; Rose 1985). Beighton et al. (1999) wrote an entire text (currently in its third edition) devoted to this topic, which adopted the term *hypermobility*. The reason for its adoption was as follows:

> It has been argued that the word "hypermobility" is inaccurate in its medical context and that it should be replaced by "hyperlaxity" or "hyperextensibility." However, for the sake of clarity we have adhered to the terminology used in previous publications and have employed these terms interchangeably. (Beighton et al. 1983, p. xi)

ASSESSMENT OF JOINT HYPERMOBILITY

Many different systems of measuring hypermobility, or joint laxity, have been devised, including simple clinical tests (Carter and Wilkinson 1964), a modified system (Beighton et al. 1973), a global index (Bird et al. 1979), radiologic assessment (Bird et al. 1980; Harris and Joseph 1949), photographic techniques (Troup et al. 1968), a pendulum machine (Barnett 1971), and a fixed torque measuring device (Silman et al. 1986).

Carter and Wilkinson (1964) devised the first scoring system that established the criteria for hypermobility. It assessed the following joint movements:

- Passive opposition of the thumb to the flexor aspect ("front side") of the forearm
- Passive extension of the fingers so that they lie parallel with the extensor aspect (backside) of the forearm
- The ability to hyperextend the elbows more than 10°
- The ability to hyperextend the knees more than 10°
- An excessive range of passive dorsiflexion of the ankle and eversion of the foot

Carter and Wilkinson (1964) defined generalized joint laxity as being present when three of the five movement tests were positive and both upper and lower limbs were involved.

Kirk et al. (1967) suggested a more complex assessment. However, this procedure proved to be too time consuming for routine use. Beighton and Horan (1969) revised the test to measure joint laxity in people with Ehlers-Danlos syndrome (EDS), an inherited connective tissue disorder. Because passive extension of the fingers was too severe, it was replaced by passive extension of just the little finger beyond 90° with the forearm flat on a table. The range of ankle movement was replaced by forward flexion of the trunk with the hands flat on the floor and with the knees fully extended (i.e., legs kept straight). Test subjects were then given a score between 0 and 5.

Because many of the study subjects were ballet dancers, Grahame and Jenkins (1972) further modified the system to include passive dorsiflexion of the ankle to beyond 15° past the right angle. Therefore, six movements were evaluated in this test. Beighton et al. (1973) slightly amended the procedure by utilizing a rapid and easily applied screening test. In this test, which is scored from 0 to 9 the highest score denotes maximum joint laxity. However, the number of points necessary for a classification of generalized hypermobility has not been agreed upon. According to Child (1986), a score of 4 or more out of 9 indicates generalized hypermobility of the joints. However, Rose (1985) states that a score of 6 or more allows definite identification of the syndrome.

The following are the movement tests used in this 9-point scoring system:

- Passive dorsiflexion and hyperextension of the fifth metacarpophalangeal (MCP) joint (i.e., the little finger) beyond 90° (1 point for each hand, 2 points for both)
- Passive apposition of the thumb to the flexor aspect of the forearm (1 point for each thumb, 2 points for both)
- Hyperextension of the elbow beyond 10° (1 point for each elbow, 2 points for both)
- Hyperextension of the knee beyond 10° (1 point for each knee, 2 points for both)
- Forward flexion of the trunk with the knees fully extended so that the palms of the hands rest flat on the floor (1 point)

Rotés (1983), cited by Russek (1999), proposed an 11-point scale.

In addition to the assessment tools that examine multiple joints, several other methods measure joint laxity using a single joint. A hyperextensometer method was developed that used passive extension of the fifth MCP joint and a goniometer (a device for measuring joint motion) to measure the ROM. Because this procedure is relatively imprecise, Grahame and Jenkins (1972) employed a predetermined force of 0.91 kg (2 lb) to standardize the test. Jobbins et al. (1979) constructed a device that measured torque (joint movement force). A torque of 2.6 kg/cm was found to be of most use in the detection of hyperlaxity in a Caucasian population.

Brodie et al. (1982) derived the *global index* by using goniometry to assess the ROM at almost all joints in the body and summating the measured arcs of movement. The result is then divided by 100.

DETERMINING FACTORS OF HYPERMOBILITY

The prevalence of hypermobility in the general population is 4% to 7% (Carter and Wilkinson 1964; Jesse et al. 1980; Scott et al. 1979). In contrast, Klemp et al. (1984) found a 9.5% rate among 377 ballet dancers. What factors contribute to joint hypermobility, or joint laxity, and how can it be altered? ROM is multifaceted and is discussed throughout this text. Generally, it is affected by such things as skin tension, muscle tone, muscle fiber length (sarcomere number), various connective tissues (e.g., fascia, ligament, and tendon), and joint structure. ROM can also be affected by such things as training, hormonal variations, temperature, gender, and genetic predisposition.

Gender, Ethnic, and Racial Differences

If either generalized hypermobility or HMS is hereditary, the question then arises about gender, ethnic, and racial variations (Ansell 1972; Beighton 1971; Bird 1979; Child 1986; Wood 1971). HMS is more prevalent among females than among males (Al-Rawi et al. 1985; Beighton et al. 1973; Biro et al. 1983; Decoster et al. 1997; Jesse et al. 1980; Larsson et al. 1987; Rikken-Bultman et al. 1997; Wordsworth et al. 1987). Wood (1971) found no difference between 81 Caucasian and 45 black subjects in Buffalo, New York. However, most research has demonstrated that true ethnic differences exist.

People of Asian Indian origin have more hyperextension of the thumb than do people of African origin, who in turn have greater hyperextension than people of European descent (Harris and Joseph 1949; Wordsworth et al. 1987). Similar results were obtained by comparing the finger joints of different racial groups in Southern Africa (Schweitzer 1970) and among Iraqis (Al-Rawi et al. 1985). Specifically, Al-Rawi et al. (1985) found that the prevalence of hypermobility was 25.4% in males and 38.5% in females. This prevalence is compared with 43% in Nigerians (Birrell et al. 1994).

Pountain (1992) determined that the flexibility scores in 16-year-old to 25-year-old residents of Oman were considerably lower than those reported in the 20-year-old to 24-year-old Iraqi students previously cited. Cheng et al. (1991) found that Chinese children were more lax than both African children and adults measured by Beighton et al. (1973). Klemp et al. (2002) found the 6.2% prevalence of hypermobility in Maori similar to that in European New Zealanders and Caucasians elsewhere.

Genetic and Biochemical Defects That Influence Joint Hypermobility

Three important factors of joint hypermobility and laxity include (1) the anatomical structures of the joints that normally restrict movements, (2) the contribution of muscular tone to restricting joint movement, and (3) the role of the extracellular matrix components in the mechanical properties of joint connective tissues. The third factor is most important. Therefore the discussion here is limited to hypermobility caused primarily by an alteration in collagen.

Connective tissue cells synthesize collagen according to instructions carried in the genes of their DNA. Any abnormality collagen synthesis can result in weakened and therefore distensible connective tissue. An increased understanding of the basic biology (biochemistry, molecular biology, and developmental biology) made possible the identification of the mutations in the COL5A1 and COL5A2 genes that cause EDS types I, II, and VII. In contrast, EDS type VIIA is caused by exon 6 skipping mutations in the COL1A1 gene of type I procollagen (Kadler and Wallis 1999).

Magnusson, Julsgaard et al. (2001) investigated the viscoelastic properties and flexibility of the human muscle-tendon unit in the hamstring muscle of subjects with BJHS. The main findings were the following. (1) The viscoelastic stress relaxation and the passive energy absorption for a given common joint angle of the hamstring muscle group were comparable in patients with BJHS and age-matched control subjects. (2) BJHS patients displayed a greater subjective tolerance to stretching loads, which may explain the greater flexibility. (3) The increased flexibility in BJHS cannot be explained on the basis of altered passive properties.

CONSEQUENCES OF HYPERMOBILITY

Generalized hypermobility may benefit dancers, musicians, some athletes (Beighton et al. 1999; Grahame 1999, 2000; Larsson et al. 1993), circus clowns, and contortionists. Violinists, flautists, and pianists (of all ages) with lax finger joints suffer less pain than their less-flexible peers (Larsson et al. 1993). However, negative consequences are possible both for those with HMS and for those with generalized hypermobility. "People with HMS may have an increased incidence of nerve compression disorders, although data are scant" (Russek 1999, p. 595). People with generalized hypermobility may experience impaired proprioceptive acuity (Barrack et al. 1983; Mallik et al. 1994), increased risk of joint trauma (such as sprains), recurrent dislocation, effusions, and premature osteoarthrosis (Beighton et al. 1999; el-Shahaly and el-Sherif 1991; Finsterbush and Pogrund 1982; Grahame 1971). The degree of the negative consequences depends on factors such as the degree of hypermobility or joint laxity, the physical condition of the individual, and the individual's vocation and avocation (Beighton et al. 1999; Larsson et al. 1993; Stanitski 1995).

Several researchers (Adair and Hecht 1993; Westling et al. 1992; Westling and Mattiasson 1992) have also found a correlation between temporomandibular dysfunction and HMS. They also "showed that the general hypermobility seemed to have an important role in developing TMJ pain and dysfunction, even in young people" (p. 89). Al-Rawi et al. (1985) also reported that complaints of flat feet and easy bruising correlated well with joint hypermobility. People with HMS are also more likely (69.3%) to have anxiety disorders than are comparison groups with rheumatological conditions (22.0%) (Bulbena et al. 1993) or groups with other chronic medical conditions (21.3%) (Wells et al. 1988). Russek (1999) suggests "anxiety may also be due to the perception of joint instability and frequent pain and injury without understandable antecedent" (p. 595).

GENERAL MANAGEMENT OF HYPERMOBILITY

A short-term and long-term management plan must be developed for each hypermobile patient. However, the management of these patients can be complex and time consuming (Grahame 2000). General treatment for HMS (i.e., joint laxity and musculoskeletal complaints) depends on a number of variables, including the degree or grade of hypermobility, the presence of any other medical conditions (e.g., EDS, rheumatoid arthritis, Marfan syndrome, or dislocation injury), the degree and quality of pain, and the individual's vocation and avocation. The course of treatment will be ultimately based on a trained health-care practitioner's professional knowledge and experience.

Conservative Management of Hypermobility

The most conservative treatment is used for individuals with the lowest grade of HMS. The premanagement stage entails determining the patient's history and the clinical evaluation. The management of such cases begins with an assurance of the absence of serious disease (Biro et al. 1983; Kirk et al. 1967). Next, the patient is counseled about the nature of the condition and how to live with it (Rose 1985). At this stage the most aggravating and relieving factors are explored with the patient and suggestions for modifying the pattern of daily living are made (Child 1986). This modification may entail avoidance of strenuous sports, a change of occupation, or alteration of the manner in which a particular job is performed (Beighton et al. 1999; Russek 1999). Whenever practical, education about joint protection should be facilitated (Child 1986; Rose 1985; Russek 1999). Another rationale is that "helping patients with HMS understand their disorder may help them cope with the pain they experience" (Russek 1999, p. 596).

Exercise represents another conservative strategy. Practitioners have encouraged moderate exercise to keep body weight low and muscular and ligamentous support maximal (Child 1986; Magnusson, Julsgaard et al. 2001), and they should provide correct postural training (Rose 1985). Swimming is recommended because it involves less joint stress than weight-bearing activities such as jogging (Child 1986; Kirk et al. 1967). Russek (1999) suggests advising individuals with HMS to use stretching exercises cautiously, distinguishing between stretching muscles and stretching joints. The former may be beneficial, but the latter may be harmful.

Exercise will not increase stiffness of the lax ligaments of patients with HMS (Russek 1999). However, in both animal and human models resistance training increased passive muscle-tendon stiffness (Klinge et al. 1997; Reich et al. 2000). On the other hand, whether resistance training may also assist in reducing excessive joint motion and the progression of joint pain in BJHS has not been established (Magnusson, Julsgaard et al. 2001). Significantly, although many authors recommend exercise for HMS patients, "few have any data on which to base that recommendation" (Russek 1999, p. 597).

The utilization of braces, support splints, and surgical corsets further enhances joint protection (Beighton et al. 1999; Rose 1985). However, these strategies warrant further research (Russek 1999). More aggressive treatment by health practitioners may include manual physical therapy techniques or modalities, including massage, gentle mobilization (Beighton et al. 1999), or gentle manipulation (Child 1986). However, Beighton et al. (1999) advise caution when forceful manipulation is used in hypermobile patients, as joint subluxation may result from overenthusiasm.

For many patients, symptomatic pain relief may be achieved by hydrotherapeutic exercises performed in a pool heated to 35° C (95° F) (Beighton et al. 1999). Other modalities such as acupuncture, transcutaneous electrical nerve stimulation (TENS), ultrasound and other types of electrical stimulation, may also be of use in the presence of pain.

Moderate Management

Topical, oral, or intravenous medication is another treatment available to some allied health practitioners (chiropractors and massage therapists cannot dispense medication or inject patients). Medication may help relieve mild musculoskeletal pain, reduce inflammation, or facilitate the healing process. The more common medications are NSAIDs (nonsteroidal anti-inflammatory drugs, such as aspirin), analgesics (pain-relieving compounds, such as acetaminophen), and corticosteroids (hormones produced by the adrenal gland) (Beighton et al. 1999; Child 1986; Rose 1985). However, some authors (Child 1986; Gedalia and Brewer 1993; Russek 1999) report that these agents are neither practical nor effective. Almekinders (1993) reminds us that "many questions regarding the exact effects and roles of NSAIDs remain unanswered" (p. 141) and that "choice of NSAIDs, timing and dosage schedules also remain unclear" (p. 141). The potentially negative consequences of the use of drugs or other compounds should be obvious to practitioners and are increasingly recognized by an informed public. The risk of side effects must be carefully weighed against the potential benefits to the patient. Therefore, practitioners should be judicious in the use of medications and discontinue them as soon as feasible.

Radical Management

In severe cases, radical management, including major invasive techniques such as surgery, may be employed as a last resort after conservative and moderate treatments have failed. Conditions that might require surgery are soft-tissue lesions (such as sprains), persistent synovitis (inflammation of the tissue layer lining the interior of the joint capsule), recurrent dislocation, spinal instability, and advanced cases of both rheumatoid arthritis and osteoarthritis (Beighton et al. 1999).

INHERITED SYNDROMES

A number of genetic syndromes are associated with joint laxity. Perhaps the most well known is Ehlers-Danlos syndrome, an inherited connective tissue disorder characterized by articular hypermobility, dermal (skin) extension, and cutaneous scarring. The extent to which individuals may be affected by EDS varies considerably. The disease has been divided into at least nine subtypes based on clinical, genetic, and other grounds. EDS affects as many as 1 in 5,000 individuals (Pyeritz 2000a, 2000b; Steinmann et al. 1993).

The first written reports of EDS appeared in 1657, in Latin, by a surgeon called Van Meerken. Van Meerken describes the hyperelastic skin of a Spanish sailor and the joint laxity of a professional contortionist whom Van Meerken presented to a group of senior physicians at the Academy of Leiden. More than 100 years ago, a Russian dermatologist published a report detailing a patient with scars, hyperextensibility, and joint laxity (Tschernogubow 1892). Nine years later, Edvard Ehlers, a Danish dermatologist, presented a case in which a patient had joint laxity and hyperextensible skin (Ehlers 1901). Later, Henri-Alexandre Danlos, a French dermatologist, highlighted a similar case (Danlos 1908). The eponym Ehlers-Danlos syndrome was first suggested by Poumeau-Delille and Soulie (1934). As a result of an article published in the *British Journal of Dermatology* by Frederich Parkes Weber in 1936, the joint eponymous title Ehlers-Danlos syndrome was formally proposed and ultimately accepted. Over time, EDS was divided into 11 subgroups according to clinical phenotype. However, in 1988, the *International Nosology of Heritable Disorders of Connective Tissue* (Beighton et al. 1988) refined EDS into subtypes I to VIII and X. Beighton et al. (1997) proposed a new classification scheme of six major types of EDS.

Familial undifferentiated hypermobility syndromes are a heterogeneous group of disorders associated with excessive ROM. Generalized joint laxity is the primary clinical manifestation (Beighton et al. 1999). Some of the earliest descriptions of familial hypermobility were those of Finkelstein (1916), Key (1927), and Sturkie (1941). Carter and Sweetnam (1958, 1960) and Carter and Wilkinson (1964) showed a close association between familial joint laxity and the incidence of dislocations in close relatives. Beighton and Horan (1970) described two families in which joint laxity was transmitted as an autosomal (i.e., genetic) dominant trait.

Joint laxity is present in a number of other inherited disorders such as Marfan syndrome, Osteogenesis imperfecta (OI), Larsen syndrome, and several inherited skeletal dysplasias (malformations) in which dwarfism is the major feature. (See Beighton et al. 1999.)

RESEARCH PERSPECTIVES IN HERITABLE DISORDERS OF CONNECTIVE TISSUE

The term *heritable disorders of connective tissue* became established in the medical literature with the publication of the 1956 book of the same name by Victor McKusick. Since that time, more than 200 distinct disorders have been identified. Currently, clinical manifestations are found in patients with more than 1,000 mutations thus far characterized in 22 genes for 12 of the more than 20 types of collagen (Myllyharju and Kivirikko 2001). For more complete reviews of collagen biochemistry and clinical aspects of EDS, see Burrows (1999), Byers (1995), Mao and Bristow (2001), Myllyharju and Kivirikko (2001), Pope and Burrows (1997), and Pyeritz (2000a, 2000b).

Many of these disorders not only influence ROM but also affect the patients' well-being. In addition, these disorders have major financial costs for patients and for society. Thus, the following research priorities were identified by Byers, Pyeritz, and Uitto (1992).

1. Identify and characterize genetic mutations in all disease phenotypes.
2. Determine structure-function relationships of normal connective tissue matrix molecules.
3. Describe developmental regulations of matrix formation.
4. Perform multidisciplinary analysis of disease mechanisms.
5. Design clinical studies of natural history and clinical trials in the treatment of genetic diseases.
6. Establish disease registries.
7. Provide periodic workshops, and include disease studies in major symposia on matrix biology.
8. Identify and study existing animal models of genetic diseases, and create animal models by transgenic technologies to identify phenotypes produced by mutations in specific genes.
9. Apply genetic linkage strategies to heritable disorders of connective tissue.
10. Pursue the molecular basis of common disease analogs of specific heritable disorders of connective tissue.

During the past decade, many of the molecular components of the extracellular matrix have been identified. Researchers have isolated and characterized the genes that encode these proteins, identified and characterized the biosynthetic pathways of most matrix proteins, defined interactions among these proteins, and characterized mutations in genes that produce a limited variety of these disorders.

Currently, three fundamental mechanisms of disease are known to produce EDS: deficiency of collagen-processing enzymes, dominant-negative effects of mutant collagen α-chains, and haploinsufficiency. Mao and Bristow (2001) detailed these mechanisms.

> The two known examples of deficient enzyme activity leading to EDS are lysyl-hydroxylase deficiency and procollagen peptidase deficiency. In the first case, the inability to hydroxylate lysine residues precludes normal inter-molecular cross-linking of collagen trimers, and in the second instance, absence of procollagen peptidase prevents normal proteolytic cleavage of the NH_2-terminus of procollagen chains. In both circumstances, the morphology and strength of the collagen fibril is compromised. (p. 1063)

Dominant-negative mutations are either exon-skipping mutations or missense mutations that disrupt the collagen triple helix. Here, it is thought dominant-negative mutations in [the genes] COLSA1 and COL5A2 alter fibril assembly. However, the precise mechanism is still unknown. In the opinion of Mao and Bristow (2001),

> It seems highly likely that genes other than the fibrillar collagens and their known modifying enzymes participate in the complex process of collagen fibrillogenesis and establishment of matrix architecture. Given that much of EDS is still unexplained, it seems equally likely that other noncollagen genes will be discovered to cause disease in some fraction of EDS patients. (p. 1068)

Perhaps future researchers will have a more complete understanding of the factors that affect connective tissue and ultimately determine one's ROM.

ADDITIONAL ISSUES

Complaints and complications associated with EDS depend upon the specific category. Among the complaints and complications associated with classical EDS are sprains, dislocations, subluxations, pes planus, muscle hypotonia (muscle weakness), delayed gross motor developments, fragile tissues, and easy bruising (Beighton et al. 1998).

Martín-Santos et al. (1998) investigated the relationship of joint hypermobility syndrome to anxiety disorder (panic disorder, agoraphobia, or both) in 99 diagnosed patients. Joint hypermobility syndrome was found in 67.7% of patients with anxiety disorder. Furthermore, "on the basis of statistical analysis, patients with anxiety disorder were over 16 times more likely than control subjects to have joint laxity" (p. 1578). The investigators determined that "intermediate variables such as early life stressors, fear experiences, and separation anxiety may also be important in the development of panic" (pp. 1581-1582). Future research must elucidate, "whether joint hypermobility syndrome is in any way associated with neurotransmitter dysfunction, autonomic dysregulation, or a physical genetic locus" (p. 1582).

CONTORTIONISM

Contortionism is the art of manipulating the body parts in feats of extreme suppleness and skill. The art was present in virtually all ancient civilizations. The earliest recordings of contortionists, in the form of sculpture, painting, and literature, show that contortionism was connected with dance and tumbling, the most fundamental art of the people. Evidence is seen in pictographs found in Egyptian tombs. According to Toepfer (1999), during the twentieth century, the 1930s and 1940s were perhaps the most glamorous era for contortionism. After World War II, the appreciation of contortionism declined in North America. A regeneration of the discipline in North America can be attributed to several factors. First, the directors of Cirque du Soleil, a circus that emphasizes performance art and theatre, rather than animal acts, made the strategic decision to make contortionists an integral part of the 1991 American tour (Nouvelle Experience). The Cirque du Soleil has also been seen on television by millions of viewers. Second, the Internet has also helped to revive interest in the art of contortionism (Young 2002). One Web site, Stretchmagazine.com, is of the opinion that Tige Young has done probably more to further the popularity of contortion than any other person through the creation of the Contortion Home Page.

Nicknames and Terminology

Contortionists have a number of popular nicknames, including "Posturers," "Limber Jims," "Pretzels," "Benders," "Frogs," "Kinkers," "Boneless Wonders," "India-Rubber Men," and "Elastic Incomprehensibles." (Kattenberg 1952; Louis n.d.; Speaight 1980). Within the profession, contortionists are usually classified as "legs," who can perform unusual acts of flexibility about the hips; "front benders," who bend forward from the waist; "back benders," who actually bend their trunk backward; and "dislocationists," who can dislocate major articulations of their body, including the neck. An "elastic person" is one whose skin can be stretched several inches and, on release, immediately returns to its former position. Such individuals have EDS (see figures 7.1-7.4).

Contortionists can be categorized into two subgroups: shockers and artistic. Viewing audiences may consider

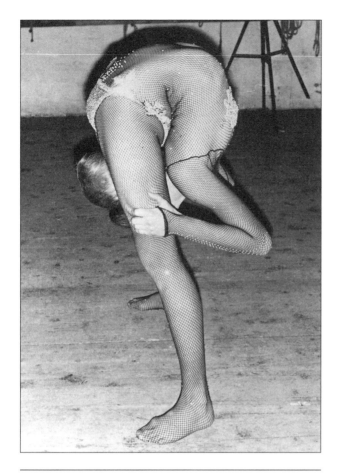

Figure 7.1 "Back bender" Diane Bennett, hair pin.
M. Louis. Reprinted with permission.

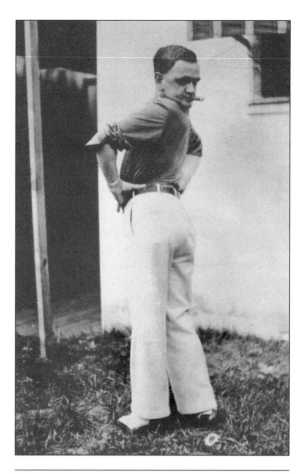

Figure 7.2 "Dislocationist" Martin Laurello.
Reprinted with permission. Circus World Museum Library.

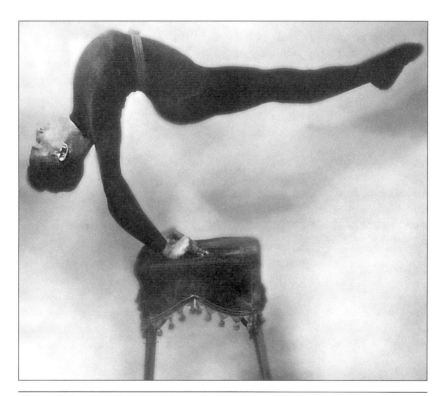

Figure 7.3 Oreval performing an inverted planche.
M. Louis. Reprinted by permission.

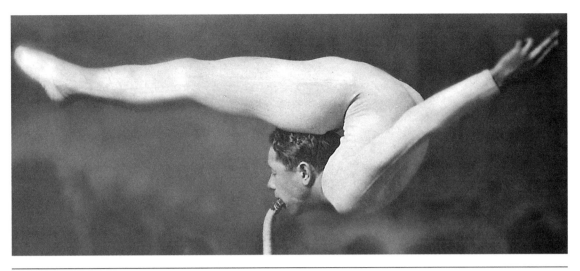

Figure 7.4 Ben Dova performing a Marinelli mouth piece balance.
M. Louis. Reprinted by permission.

shockers to be anatomical wonders, curiosities, freakish, or, at the extreme, grotesque. Many dislocationalists are in this category. Some of these performers may have an actual deformity or abnormal physical appearance. Artistic contortionists present graceful routines; however, they display amazing flexibility (ROM) without dislocating their joints (Young 2002). Audiences can be captivated by their style, choreography, costumes, makeup, execution of difficult technical feats, mastery of technical devices (props), or buffoonery (in the case of clowns).

Training Versus Nature

An age-old question is whether contortionists are born or created. Some contortionists are undeniably graced with inherent articular laxity. These performers require very little training or warm-up. According to Beighton et al. (1999), a number of well-known circus performing families possess an autosomal dominant trait that explains their natural suppleness. However, biographies of current performers on the Internet reveal that most contortionists develop their skills by years of rigorous training. They must practice several hours each day and require a long warm-up period before a performance. Furthermore, even a few days of inactivity results in a marked stiffening of the joints. Thus, the difference between these two groups is the difference between the gifted and the merely talented: channeled effort, focus, and hard work.

Young (2002) believes that successful contortionists are probably the result of three factors: (1) inherent higher-than-average extensibility and joint laxity, (2) initiation into flexibility training at a very young age, and (3) many years of consistent, diligent, and hard training. Two additional factors deserve careful consideration. First, extreme flexibility (ROM) associated with those who have connective tissue syndromes does not guarantee their success as contortionists. Extreme joint laxity may

make them unable to perform skills requiring strength, balance, and coordination. Second, extreme flexibility has "no" correlation to artistic presentation, which is necessary for success (Young 2002).

Contortionism of Today

Contortionism can be seen in many arts and disciplines, especially in circus and variety show acts. Hatha yoga, because it incorporates countless *asanas*, or postures, many of which include extreme degrees of flexibility, is perhaps the best-known discipline that features "contortionism." However, obtaining an extreme ROM is "not" the ultimate goal in yoga. In ballet and some other types of dance (classical, avante-garde, and erotic), extreme degrees of suppleness are displayed. Similarly, gymnastics and figure skating have in recent years shown a trend toward displaying extreme ROM. Rhythmic gymnastics and acrobatics are two specific disciplines that display "artistic contortionism" as a substantial requisite of their code of points. Other disciplines known for developing high degrees of flexibility include circus performing (e.g., by acrobats, aerialists, clowns, hula hoopers, and jugglers), cheerleading, fitness modeling, and martial arts (e.g., karate and kung fu). Thus, many artistic disciplines are available for youngsters who are graced with natural flexibility or who desire to work hard to attain extreme, yet aesthetic and functional, ROMs. Interested persons should contact the appropriate federations or governing bodies or search the contortionhomepage.com on the Internet.

Misconceptions

Several misconceptions exist regarding contortionists. They are thought to be "double-jointed," but, technically, no such condition exists. Rather, contortionists are loose-jointed as a result of extensive training or a joint laxity syndrome. Male contortionists are commonly perceived as lacking masculinity. However, over 3,000 records gathered by Kattenberg (1963) indicated that many of these performers were married and had children. Contortionists are believed to have short life expectancies, but many are documented to have attained a ripe old age (Kattenberg 1963). However, many contortionists who have the extreme varieties of EDS or miscellaneous joint laxity syndromes (e.g., Marfan syndrome) do in fact die early. The cause of death is usually spontaneous rupture of large arteries (Beighton et al. 1999). Beighton (1971) suggested that the secret of contortionists' (i.e., those without life-threatening joint laxity syndromes) continuing health is perhaps their good nature and readiness to please other people.

SUMMARY

Joint hypermobility and laxity has been recognized since antiquity, and numerous systems have been developed to quantify these conditions. Furthermore, extensive research related to its predisposing factors has been conducted. Various types of medical management can be employed in treating hypermobility syndrome. Therapy is determined by the extent of the symptoms. With advances in biology, identifying the specific gene responsible for several types of EDS deficiencies has become possible.

Contortionism is the art of manipulating the body parts in feats of suppleness and skill. It is an ancient and widespread practice. In recent years, this art has experienced a renaissance among those endowed with extraordinary flexibility or who are willing to work long, hard hours to develop their flexibility.

Relaxation

Many articles and books have been written on the topic of *relaxation*. What is relaxation, and why is it so important in the development of flexibility? First, we must define relaxation before addressing this question and other crucial questions.

DEFINING RELAXATION

"Relaxation is a familiar, commonly used term, yet a clear definition in the context of therapeutic relaxation appears to be elusive" (Kerr 2000, p. 52). For example, Zahourek (1988) stated that relaxation is defined by *what it is not*—the absence of tension. The concept of relaxation has a long and varied history, reflecting its complexity (Kerr 2000). Thus, relaxation may be defined in several ways. For motor learning, it is "the ability to control muscle activity such that muscles not specifically required for a task are quiet, and those which are required are fired at the minimal level needed to achieve the desired results" (Coville 1979, p. 178). Accordingly, relaxation "can be considered as a motor skill in itself because the ability to reduce muscle firing is as important to motor control as is generation of firing" (p. 177). Consequently, relaxation potentially determines optimal performance.

In skilled performance, movement is characterized by an appearance of ease, smoothness of motion, coordination, grace, self-control, and total freedom. It may also be characterized by beauty, harmony, precision, and virtuosity. Thus, in motor learning, relaxation is the absence of anxiety, inhibition, tension, and extraneous motion.

Relaxation is economical energy consumption and resistance to fatigue involving a minimal expenditure of energy consistent with desired ends (Basmajian 1998). When more muscle fibers than necessary are activated, inefficient energy expenditure compensates for the shortfall of oxygen and energy. The cardiovascular system is taxed that much more, and the unnecessary expenditure of energy may actually interfere with the execution of the task at hand. More significantly, it may help to bring on fatigue more quickly.

Relaxation can help reduce the risk of injury. When one is less fatigued, one is less prone to injury. In contrast, awkward movements and psychological tension increase the frequency of accidents.

Although muscular relaxation is important, our concern is with flexibility (i.e., ROM) and stretching. How does relaxation affect flexibility, and why should a muscle be relaxed before stretching? Theoretically, passive stretching should begin when a muscle is in a completely relaxed state to maximize the potential benefits of stretching (Mohr et al. 1998). That is, a minimal amount of tension should be developed by the contractile components to minimize active resistance. This reduced internal tension should permit the individual to most effectively and efficiently stretch out the connective tissue, which truly limits extensibility. Each muscle cell is capable of at least a 50% increase in length, accomplished by the longitudinal sliding of the actin and myosin filaments that leaves at least one cross-bridge maintained (see chapter 3). Usually, muscle lengthening (the stretching phase) is performed slowly or at a constant rate, thus reducing the likelihood of activating the stretch reflex and ultimately the muscular contractile components. However, in an investigation of proprioceptive neuromuscular inhibitory techniques (PNF), Moore (1979) found that complete relaxation was not a requisite for effective stretching. This topic is investigated in chapter 14.

MEASURING RELAXATION

Relaxation can be measured by galvanic skin responses, electroencephalography (EEG), and electromyography (EMG), depending on which physiological response is to be analyzed. Physiological responses that can be evaluated include oxygen consumption, respiratory rate, heart rate, blood pressure, skin temperature, muscle tension, and alpha brain waves. EMG is probably the best method for measuring muscle tension via a muscle's action potential. In contrast, researchers in sleep laboratories are more concerned with brain wave patterns recorded during sleep and would thus utilize an EEG.

METHODOLOGIES OF FACILITATING MUSCULAR RELAXATION

According to Hertling and Jones (1996), types of relaxation training and related techniques are difficult to classify because they employ a combination of strategies and methodologies. Kerr (2000) loosely classified relaxation techniques as physical and nonphysical. Earlier, Payne (1995) had developed more elaborate classifications of physical approaches (passive muscular relaxation, behavioral relaxation training, differential relaxation, and stretching) and nonphysical ("mental") approaches (self-awareness, imagery, goal-directed visualization, autogenic training, and meditation). Additional representative categories of strategies and techniques are

- the somatic, or physical, approach, which uses special breathing and movement, special stretching techniques, massage and acupressure, or adjustment and manipulation;
- physiological therapeutic modalities, which use cold, heat, needles, lasers, or traction;
- cognitive, mental, and mind-controlling techniques;
- sophisticated technology, such as biofeedback; and
- drugs or medications.

To determine whether a plan of action is cost-effective and efficient, one should consider the safety of the plan, the need for special assistance or instruction, the need for special equipment and ergogenic aids (i.e., anything that enhances performance), the amount of time required, and the financial cost. Ideally, a plan of action should be implemented only after thoughtful consideration of these issues.

Somatic Approach

Somatic, or physical, strategies are either *passive distraction* or *active distraction*. The former strategies include progressive relaxation, massage, and certain respiratory techniques. The latter strategies include techniques such as Alexander, Feldenkrais, and tai chi chuan. Interested readers should see the summaries of Hertling and Jones (1996).

Breathing Techniques

Various breathing techniques are known to facilitate relaxation. A classic example is found in hatha yoga. Many relaxation techniques employ specific breathing patterns in conjunction with specific physical and mental strategies. In sports medicine, the close relationship between respiration and the motor system has been termed *respiratory synkinesis*, which occurs when a certain type of movement is linked either with inspiration or with expiration (Lewit 1999). Researchers have investigated the relationship of breathing cycles and the Valsalva phenomenon (an expiratory effort against a closed glottis that results in an impeded blood flow to the heart and a fall in arterial pressure) among weight lifters. Other areas of research have involved the relationship between the respiratory pattern and the movements in specific activities such as bicycling (Bechbache and Duffin 1977), golf (Kawashima et al. 1994), gymnastics (Mironov 1969a, 1969b), rowing (Clark et al. 1983; Maclennan et al. 1994; Mahler et al. 1991; Steinacker et al. 1993), running (Pechinski 1966); singing (Cleveland 1998a, 1998b, 1998c; Freed 1994), swimming (Holmer and Gullstrand 1980; Keskinen and Komi 1991; Lerda and Cardelli 2003), and walking (Hill et al. 1988). The following section is an attempt to integrate the anecdotal, empirical, and experimental literature of breathing as it relates to stretching, flexibility, and performance.

How Can Proper Breathing Facilitate Stretching?

Theoretically, coupling correct breathing patterns with specific movements can facilitate movement itself. This effect can be explained neurophysiologically, mechanically, and experientially or subjectively using forward flexion of the vertebral column as an example.

Neurophysiologically, during forward flexion of the trunk, the musculature of the lower back is put under passive tension. The greater this tension, the more difficult flexing the upper torso toward the thighs becomes. The tension in these muscles must be minimized. A deep inspiration with the chest expanded and the abdominal muscles drawn in is accompanied by active contraction of the erector spinae muscles (muscles of the lower back) (Campbell 1970; Roaf 1977). However, contraction of the erector spinae is undesirable because contraction of these muscles will further increase resistance to forward flexion and initiate extension of the lower torso, which is a motion counter to the desired trunk flexion. Hence, to deeply inhale during forward flexion is usually self-defeating. The appropriate course, in most cases, is to slowly exhale to facilitate a relaxation of the erector spinae. Thus, relaxation can be achieved by a gentle expiratory effort. (Campbell [1970] has also shown that in some instances, a maximum expiration can result in activity of the sacrospinalis muscles of the lower back.)

Mechanically, to facilitate stretching, one can incorporate gravity and appropriate breathing. During inspiration the lungs become inflated. Thus, inhalation creates a "lifting" or "rising" effect (see figure 8.1). However, during forward flexion of the trunk, the objective is to descend and to lower the upper torso, not to raise it. The lifting effect of inflated lungs counters the desired direction of movement. When the lungs are deflated, this lifting force

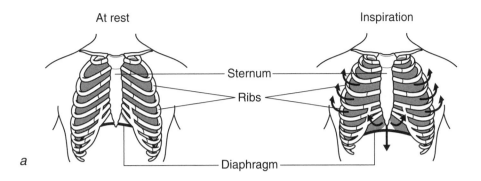

At rest   Inspiration

Sternum

Ribs

Diaphragm

a

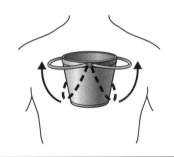

Ribs move like a bucket handle, expanding the side-to-side dimensions.

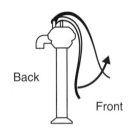

Sternum moves forward and up like a pump handle, expanding the front-to-back dimensions (viewed from the side).

Back

Front

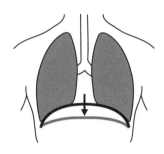

Diaphragm flattens down, increasing the top-to-bottom dimension.

b

Figure 8.1 The different ways in which capacity of thoracic cavity is increased during inspiration.

Reprinted, by permission, from J.H. Wilmore and D.L. Costill, 1999, *Physiology of sport and exercise, Second Edition* (Champaign, IL: Human Kinetics), 248.

is absent, and nothing counters the effect of gravity acting to lower the upper torso to the thighs. Hence, exhalation during stretches involving forward flexion of the upper torso toward the lower limbs (e.g., the modified hurdler's stretch) is usually advantageous. In contrast, inhaling or holding the breath is usually best when returning the torso to the upright position. The rationale for permitting breath holding is discussed below.

During forward flexion, most of the spinal flexion occurs by the time the trunk is inclined 45° forward. The remainder of the spinal flexion occurs via forward rotation (anterior tilt) of the pelvis. The pelvis rotates around the fulcrum of the hip joints. X-ray studies by Mitchell and Pruzzo (1971) documented that the sacral apex (inferior tip) moves posteriorly during exhalation, so that the opposite, top end moves forward. Hence, exhalation facilitates pelvic tilt and trunk flexion.

In the upright posture, the diaphragm has an inspiratory action on the lower rib cage, whereas in the supine posture, the diaphragm has an expiratory action on the lower rib cage (De Troyer and Loring 1986). With trunk flexion, the diaphragm is gradually elevated. In part, this action is facilitated by gravity, simulating the action of exhalation.

As the diaphragm rises in the chest with exhalation, it pushes up against the heart and slows down the heart rate.

Therefore, slow breathing, with the exhalation longer than the inhalation, decreases heart rate and blood pressure. Furthermore, exhalation decreases stress and tension on the ribs, intercostal muscles, abdominal wall, and related musculature and fascia. This decrease in muscle tension is transmitted by the appropriate muscle spindles and other proprioceptors, resulting in a subjective perception of less stress and greater relaxation. In contrast, inhalation is associated with increases in the heart rate, blood pressure, and stress on various structures of the body.

Coordinating Breathing and Eye Positioning With Mobilization

As a general rule, muscular activity is facilitated during inspiration and inhibited during expiration. However, this statement is an oversimplification. In actuality, several important exceptions to the rule with regard to exhalation exist. For example, Lewit (1999) points out the close connection among looking up, inspiration, and straightening of the body, and among looking down, expiration, and stooping. However, this connection applies only to the cervical and lumbar spine (which are decisive in view of their great mobility) and not to the thoracic spine. In contrast, in the thoracic spine, the following relationship applies.

Here it is maximum inhalation that facilitates flexion in a kyphotic position and maximum exhalation that facilitates extension in a lordotic position, i.e., the thoracic erector spinae contracts, and this to such an extent that deep inhalation is probably the most effective method of mobilizing the thoracic spine into flexion, and maximum exhalation most effective for extension. (p. 27)

Furthermore, Lewit (1999), citing the work of Gaymans (1980), points out an alternating facilitation and inhibition of individual segments of the spinal column during side bending.

It can be regularly shown that during side-bending resistance increases in the cervical as well as in the thoracic spine in the even segments (occiput-atlas, C2, etc., and again in T2, T4, etc.) during inhalation; during exhalation we obtain a mobilizing effect in these segments. Conversely, resistance increases in the odd segments (C1, C3, T3, T5, etc.) during exhalation, while we obtain mobilization during inhalation. There is a "neutral" zone between C7 and T1. An important feature of the atlas-occiput segment is that here inhalation increases resistance not only against side-bending but in all directions, while exhalation facilitates mobility. This effect is most marked at the craniocervical junction and decreases in a caudal direction; in particular, the mobilizing effect of inhalation (in the odd segments) diminishes in the lower thoracic region. (p. 27)

What, then, does the research show regarding the coordination of eye position and breathing to enhance ROM? Fellabaum (1993) investigated the effect of eye position on flexibility during lumbar flexion. Thirty subjects were tested using a set of specially prepared eyeglasses. The lenses were painted, except for a clear circle about 0.5 cm in diameter placed in the midline vertical plane at "12 o'clock" (up) on one pair and "6 o'clock" (down) on another pair. Half of the subjects started with the downward-viewing glasses, and the other half started with the upward-viewing glasses. The flexibility of subjects was then measured in centimeters from the tip of the subject's fist to the floor on the fourth attempt at forward flexion. "The findings suggested that eye positioning in the vertical plane does significantly affect forward flexion, with downward gaze enhancing forward flexion" (p. 15). Sachse and Berger (1989) investigated the efficacy of cervical mobilization induced by eye movement and fixed to a respiratory phase. Their research demonstrated the efficacy of linking eye movements, breathing, and body movement by use of cervicomotograms.

Facilitating Inhalations and Exhalations During Manual Therapy

These findings have practical implications for practitioners of mobilization and manipulative techniques, such as chiropractors, osteopaths, and physical therapists. The importance of reducing arousal and tension is paramount for those practitioners in particular who utilize thrusting techniques, because the more the patient is aroused, tense, or resistive, the greater the force that must be applied to overcome such resistance. Greater external force increases the risk of trauma produced by the manual technique. The perfect technique offers the body the least amount of energy needed to achieve the desired objectives (Gold 1987). Manual techniques require a unique interaction between the patient and doctor or therapist. This interaction can only take place when the patient is totally relaxed and receptive to therapy. No wonder the thrust is usually timed to coincide with the exhalation and subsequent "release" of the patient. This timing is especially important when working on the spine, because exhalations decrease *pneumatic* resistance and tend to relax the long extensors as well as flexors of the body (Hellig 1969). To achieve this end (i.e., facilitating relaxation) appropriate breathing and related strategies should be employed.

Holding the Breath to Facilitate Stretching

Virtually every textbook or magazine article that deals with the topic of stretching will categorically state that one should *never* hold one's breath or inhale during the stretching procedure. Is holding one's breath or inhaling ever advantageous during the stretching procedure? Lewit (1999) writes:

A well-known yet no less striking phenomenon is, that we breathe in and hold our breath in situations in which maximum muscle activity is desired, for instance when delivering a blow, lifting a heavy weight or sprinting; that is, when oxygen consumption can be expected to be very high. If we have no time to take a breath, as when we are forced to brake suddenly while driving, we hold our breath without breathing in . . . He therefore rightly described the diaphragm as a 'respiratory muscle with a postural function' and the abdominal muscles as 'postural muscles with a respiratory function'. The significance of holding the breath during maximal muscle activity (the Valsalva manoeuver) lies in the fact that postural stability is achieved at the cost of the vital function of respiration, which is (momentarily) sacrificed to it. A significant but frequently neglected role is also played by the pelvic diaphragm. (pp. 27-28)

Yogic Breathing

Yogic breathing is receiving increasing attention in the popular media. The basis of all yogic breathing is rhythmic breathing. "In the yogic model, breathing functions as an intermediary between the mind and body. It is affected by soma and psyche, but ultimately exerts influence over both" (Sovik 2000, p. 495). According to the yoga tradition, the optimal breathing pattern is diaphragmatic, nasal (exhalation and inhalation), deep, smooth, even, quiet, and free of pauses. For detailed descriptions of the theory and practice of yogic breathing techniques see Coulter (2001). "If, as yogis suggest, breathing patterns have an important effect on physiological and psychological functioning, and if they can be integrated consciously as a new substrate of behavior, then it may be possible to provide inexpensive training that is both ameliorative and preventive in nature" (Sovik 2000, p. 503). Clearly, additional clinical research is necessary to examine the impact of all aspects of optimal breathing.

Stretching

Stretching can facilitate relaxation. The two strategies employed to induce muscle relaxation, based on spinal reflex physiology, are the static stretch and proprioceptive neuromuscular facilitation.

Static Stretch

Static stretching involves stretching the muscle to the point where further movement is limited by the muscle's own tension. At this point, the stretch is held and maintained for a time, during which relaxation and reduction of tension occur. This relaxation phenomenon has three possible explanations: (1) The muscle's stretch receptors (i.e., muscle spindles) become desensitized and subsequently *adapt* to stretch. Hence, the stretch reflex is reduced. (2) If the passive tension from the stretch is great enough, GTO and joint receptors (see chapter 6) will be activated, thus initiating the *autogenic inhibition reflex*. In turn, this reflex will inhibit the motor neuron of the muscle under stretch. Consequently, the muscle's tension will decrease, thereby facilitating relaxation. Thigpen (1984) demonstrated that short bouts of static stretching reduce electrical activity within the muscle. Similarly, Etnyre and Abraham (1984, 1986b) found that static stretching produced a slight depression of the motor pool excitability throughout stretching of the human soleus muscle. (3) Muscle and connective tissue possess time-dependent mechanical properties. That is, when a constant force is applied, *creep*, or a progressive change in length, occurs along with *stress-relaxation*, a progressive reduction in tension.

Proprioceptive Neuromuscular Facilitation

Proprioceptive neuromuscular facilitation (PNF) is a strategy that can induce relaxation of a muscle. It is based in part on the physiology of the muscle spindles and GTOs. Using the *hold-relax* technique, a limb or muscle is stretched to the point where further motion in the desired direction is prevented by the tension in muscle being stretched (antagonistic muscle). At this point, the antagonistic muscle gradually exerts a near-maximal isometric contraction for 5 to 10 seconds. Theoretically, this contraction will cause the GTOs to fire, consequently initiating the autogenic inhibition and relaxing the stretched muscle.

A modified PNF technique is believed to employ the strategy of reciprocal innervation (see chapter 6). Once again, a muscle is stretched to the point where further motion is prevented by the tension in the muscle. However, at this point either an isometric or isotonic contraction of the opposite muscle (the agonist) can be employed. The tension in the antagonistic muscle should be reduced via reciprocal innervation.

Massage

Massage is the systematic manipulation of body tissues for the purpose of affecting the nervous and muscular systems and general circulation (Knapp 1990). The effects of massage may be classified as *reflex effects* and *mechanical effects*. By reflex action, the sensory nerves in the skin produce sensations of pleasure or relaxation, which cause the muscles to relax and blood vessels to dilate (Dubrovskii 1990; Longworth 1982). Massage may possibly release endorphins and create a sensation of well-being or promote a feeling of well-being through decreased arousal levels (Hemmings et al. 2000). Another reflex effect is sedative, reducing mental tension (Yates 1990). Motor neuron excitability can be reduced by massage of the triceps surae (calf muscles [Morelli et al. 1989]) if the massage is given in a monotonously repetitive manner (Knapp 1990).

The mechanical effects of massage consist of stimulating circulation of venous blood and flow of lymph through or from an area; stimulating metabolism in an area, thus increasing removal of waste or fatigue products; and stretching adhesions between muscle fibers. Several studies have found massage to be an effective means of increasing ROM (Crosman et al. 1984; Nordschow and Bierman 1962). In the latter study, the effect of Swedish massage was a statistically significant improvement in muscle relaxation in normal subjects (as measured by trunk flexion). In contrast, Wiktorsson-Möller and colleagues (1983) found that stretching resulted in a significantly increased ROM in all muscle groups tested, whereas only one muscle group was influenced by massage, warming up, or a combination of the two. Preyde (2000) also verified that patients with subacute low-back pain benefited from massage therapy.

The three basic types of massage hand movements are *stroking, compression,* and *percussion*. Stroking, or *effleurage*, may be superficial or deep. The movements must be slow, rhythmic, and gentle. This technique improves the movement of venous blood and lymph flow. Compression, or *petrissage*, includes kneading, squeezing, and friction. This method limits or eliminates adhesions. Percussion, or *tapotement*, employs hacking, clapping, or beating and produces stimulation.

Massage is contraindicated with the slightest suspicion of local malignancy (cancer), sepsis (infection), or thrombosis (blood clot). Nor should massage be used in the presence of skin irritations or in inflammatory disease of the joints. Corbett (1972) believes that under certain conditions, massage may be psychologically harmful because "tense muscles are often the symptom of anxiety or depression and, while stroking away the evil humours is temporarily effective, the long-term effect is often to make the patients dependent on it or even addicted to it" (p. 137). Massage is an effective tool when utilized properly.

Manipulation and Chiropractic Adjustment

Manipulation is a form of manual medicine in which passive movement is used to restore ROM and decrease joint pain. Its use dates back to antiquity. Shambaugh (1987) found an average 25% reduction in muscle activity and muscle tension as a result of a chiropractic adjustment. Pain reduction via manipulation has been documented by several studies (Kokjohn et al. 1992; Terrett and Vernon 1984). Manipulation performed on an experimental group of young males under very controlled and artificial conditions resulted in a small but statistically significant elevation in levels of plasma γ-endorphin (an opioidlike substance found in the brain and other tissues that produces, among other things, analgesia, or pain relief [Vernon et al. 1986]). In contrast, Sanders et al. (1990) found a significant reduction in pain via manipulation but with no significant accompanying change in the plasma γ-endorphin concentration. Earlier, Christian et al. (1988) also failed to identify any differences in endorphin levels after spinal manipulative therapy.

Currently, the mechanisms by which manipulation or chiropractic adjustment decreases muscle tension and pain are not fully understood, although numerous theories have been proposed. What is known is that in many patients, manipulation has been effective in improving muscular relaxation, which is an important component in stretching.

Physiological Therapeutic Modalities

In the following sections, a variety of methods to facilitate or induce relaxation are discussed, ranging from the simple to the complex and from the safe to the potentially dangerous. Theoretically, the facilitated or induced relaxation should enhance stretching and ultimately increase ROM. Regardless of the technique employed, application of increased knowledge will make the treatment more effective, efficient, and safe.

Heat

The application of heat is probably one of the oldest and most common methods of relieving pain and muscular tension. Heat facilitates relaxation either as an analgesic or as a sedative. The exact mechanisms and effects of heat in these two areas, however, are poorly understood. Henricson et al. (1984) point out that heat is used in therapy because of its effect on the physical properties on connective tissue and muscle, including increased extensibility of collagen, decreased joint stiffness, relieved muscle spasm, and relieved pain. The increased blood flow and superficial rise in temperature may also create a feeling of warmth and relaxation and may produce a positive attitude toward stretching (Halvorson 1990; Minton 1993).

What method of heating should be employed? In the opinion of Hardy and Woodall (1998), "the most important variable to consider in choosing a modality for administering heat is the depth of temperature penetration required to reach the restricted tissue" (p. 153). In what dosage should heat be used? These questions are a matter of clinical judgment and should be answered by a physician, therapist, or athletic trainer.

Superficial Heat.

One of the most common methods of applying heat is the use of hot water bottles or wet packs. Agitated water baths, which stir heated water in a whirlpool or Jacuzzi-type device, may also be used. Because the temperature usually ranges from 40° to 43° C (104° to 110° F), caution must be used to avoid burning oneself, inducing mild fever, or falling asleep in the bath or tub. In most instances, however, a simple hot bath or shower should more than adequately fulfill one's needs. Hot water immersion does temporarily enhance ROM (Sechrist and Stull 1969). Similarly, Sawyer et al. (2003) found that moist heat application did not significantly affect hamstring muscle flexibility. In contrast (Lentell et al. 1992), a study of 92 male volunteers ages 19 to 36 years found that "applying heat [via hot packs for 10 minutes] in conjunction with a low-load prolonged stretch to a nonpathologic shoulder is a clinically superior method of improving flexibility compared with a low-load prolonged stretch alone" (p. 200).

Electric heating pads offer another simple method of applying heat. They have the advantage of different levels of intensity and steadily maintained temperature. Because the temperature is maintained, however, one is more likely to be burned if not careful. Wrapping an electric heating pad around a wet hot pack must be avoided to prevent electric shock. Henricson et al. (1984) demonstrated that

20 minutes of heat applied to a thigh by an electric heating pad at 43° C (110° F) did not increase ROM of flexion, abduction, or external rotation either immediately after treatment or 30 minutes after treatment. In contrast, heat followed by stretching significantly increased the flexion and abduction ROM immediately after treatment, and flexion was still increased 30 minutes after treatment. However, the combination of heat and stretching did not significantly increase the ROM compared with stretching alone.

Contradictions to the use of superficial heats include (Hardy and Woodall 1998):

- impaired areas of sensation;
- impaired areas of circulation;
- phlebitis, infections, and gangrene;
- capillary fragility as seen in hemophilia, long-term steroid therapy, and postacute trauma;
- repaired or deinnervated blood vessels because of their poor dilation-constriction ability; and
- malignancy.

Deep Heat, or Diathermy.

Another method to induce muscle relaxation and facilitate stretching is diathermy. Generally, three types of diathermic modalities are used for therapeutic purposes: shortwave, microwave, and ultrasound.

Shortwave diathermy works on the principle that energy is transferred into deep tissue by a high-frequency current. Such currents employ energy generated electromagnetic radiation having frequencies greater than a million Hz (cycles per second). Muscles heated with pulsed shortwave diathermy retain their heat three times longer than muscles heated with ultrasound (Draper et al. 1999). This feature is a major benefit to the clinician who wants to heat tissue before stretching or joint mobilizations. Muscles heated with pulsed shortwave diathermy before stretching gain more flexibility and maintain that flexibility longer than muscles heated with ultrasound. How long the flexibility is maintained depends on the subject, the duration of the stretch, and how often the area was treated (Peres et al. 2001). Microwaves are also generated by means of electromagnetic radiation and have a shorter wavelength than shortwaves. Ultrasound utilizes a high-frequency sound wave capable of penetrating into the deeper tissue layers. Here, too, frequencies in the neighborhood of a million Hz are used to produce mechanical vibration of deep tissues. Wessling et al. (1987) demonstrated that ultrasound combined with static stretch in the triceps surae (calf muscles) of human subjects significantly increased ROM more than did static stretching alone. The rate of tissue cooling after continuous ultrasound application at both 1 MHz and 3 MHz frequencies has been investigated through use of

thermistor probes inserted 1.2 cm below the skin's surface (Draper et al. 1993). After the temperature was raised 5.3° C (41.5° F) by the 3 MHz frequency, the temperature remained in the vigorous heating phase for 3.3 minutes. This period of greatest extensibility and elongation is the *stretching window* (Draper et al. 1993). Regardless of heating methodology, stretching, massage, or joint mobilization should be performed as soon as possible before the stretching window is closed.

The immediate effect of any form of diatherapy is a rise in temperature in the heated tissue. The degree and extent of the treatment effect varies in relation to the source of heating, its intensity, the length of application, and in direct proportion to the resistance of the tissue (Lehmann and de Lateur 1990; Prentice et al. 1999). Such heating can act as either a sedative or an irritant on sensory and motor nerves. The sedative action explains the relief given by diathermy, which is thought to lessen nerve sensitivity somewhat. Among other effects are increased blood flow, dilation of the blood vessels, increased filtration and diffusion through the different membranes, an initial increase in tissue metabolism, a decrease in muscle spindle sensitivity to stretch, muscular relaxation, decreased joint stiffness, and tissue that yields more readily to stretch (Lehmann and de Lateur 1990; Prentice et al 1999).

Diathermy must be used prudently. Each modality must be prescribed by a physician, physical therapist, or athletic trainer for a precise purpose.

Cryotherapy

Cryotherapy is the therapeutic use of cold. A complete text, *Cryotherapy in Sport Injury Management*, has been written on this subject by Knight (1995). The major advantages of cryotherapy are similar to the advantages of heat in that it acts as an anesthetic and can effectively promote muscular relaxation. The application of cold can improve ROM. Newton (1985), found six applications of 5 seconds each of a fluorimethane spray in combination of stretching increased passive hip flexion 8.78°. However, healthy subjects had no significant improvement in passive hip flexion. Cornelius and Jackson (1984) similarly reported greater ROM gains when cryotherapy is used before PNF exercises. Brodowicz et al. (1996) found supine hamstring flexibility after stretching with ice was greater than both stretching with heat and stretching alone. However, the previous results were contrary to other investigations (Cornelius 1984; Minton 1993; Rosenberg et al. 1990; Sechrist and Stull 1969). Burke et al. (2001) compared the changes in hamstring length resulting from modified PNF flexibility training in combination with 10 minute cold-water immersion, 10 minute hot-water immersion, and stretching alone in 45 subjects. "No advantage was apparent in using complete hot or cold immersion to increase hamstring length in healthy subjects" (p. 16).

Similarly, Lentell et al. (1992) found "the additional use of an ice pack to cool the area during the end stages of the stretch did not substantially improve the short-term outcome" (p. 205). Differences in protocols, subjects, joints, treatments, and data analysis hamper comparisons. For example, superficial ice massage or an ice pack to cool specific musculature may cause physiologic reactions that apparently improve ROM. However, cold-water immersion might restrict blood flow to all peripheral sites to regulate core temperature. Consequently, this vascular change could be responsible for the discrepancy found in other studies (Burke et al. 2001).

Cryotherapy should be used when the therapeutic goal is to tear connective tissue (such as breaking adhesions) rather than to stretch it, when no other ROM therapy can be attempted because of pain, or when muscle spasticity significantly interferes with the proper ROM therapy (Sapega et al. 1981). Using cold to decrease pain is also beneficial because it allows the patient to become more active (Halvorson 1990; Hardy and Woodall 1998), and more effective stretching is tolerated. Additional advantages of cold include decreasing swelling or effusion, decreasing inflammation, and increasing subsequent blood flow. Brodowicz et al. (1996) and Knight (1995) advise that after cooling, proper warm-up should be done to minimize stress-induced muscle tears.

How does cold reduce and relieve pain? A summary of theories are presented by Knight (1995):

- Cold decreases nervous transmission in pain fibers.
- Cold decreases excitability of nerve endings.
- Cold reduces metabolism in tissue to relieve the deleterious effects of ischemia.
- Cold causes asynchronous transmission in pain fibers.
- Cold raises the pain threshold.
- Cold acts as a counterirritant.
- Cold causes a release of endorphins.
- Cold inhibits spinal neurons. (p. 163)

Prentice (1982) found cold followed by static stretching superior to heat combined with stretching in reducing delayed muscle pain. The use of cold spray to relieve muscle spasm and pain and temporarily increase muscle length by mobilization has been documented (Harvey et al. 1983). Cold used to relieve pain is thought to send impulses to the spinal cord that compete with pain-producing impulses conveyed by much slower fibers. Thus, cold does not produce anesthesia, but rather counterirritation. This counterirritant theory is basically Melzak Wall's gate theory of cutaneous afferent impulses (cold) blocking transmission of the pain signal (Halvorson 1990; Hardy and Woodall 1998).

Because cryotherapy is relatively simple, one may treat oneself at home under the directions of a physi-

cian, therapist, or trainer. Self-treaters should be aware of the danger of freezing tissue, which can result in frostbite, but this phenomenon occurs only if ice is left directly and continuously on the body part. When ice is applied to a surface, the area goes through various stages of sensations. Initial coldness is followed by a sensation of burning, stinging, or intense aching, a partial loss of sensation, and finally numbness.

Contraindications to the use of cold include (Bell and Prentice 1999; Hardy and Woodall 1998)

- Raynaud's phenomenon,
- cold hypersensitivity with urticaria, itching, puffy, eyelids, and respiratory distress,
- cold allergy with histamine release as the allergic response,
- areas with compromised circulation,
- cryoglobulinemia (a rare condition in rheumatoid arthritis, systemic lupus erythematosis, leukemia, and multiple myeloma),
- infection, and
- open wounds or skin conditions.

The fear that *cold-induced vasodilation* after 15 minutes or more of exposure will contribute to further swelling is unfounded because the diameter of the vessel remains less than its normal, precooling diameter (Knight 1995).

Meridian Trigger Points

For thousands of years, techniques to stimulate specific sites on the skin have been utilized. Perhaps the best-known technique is the Chinese system of acupuncture. The earliest known text on acupuncture is the *Nei Ching*, or *Classic of Internal Medicine*. This work is traditionally ascribed to the legendary Yellow Emperor, Huang Ti, who supposedly lived from 2697 to 2596 BCE. Acupuncture is the science and art of inserting thin needles into specific points on the body (commonly referred to as meridians) for treating certain painful conditions, relieving various dysfunctions, and producing regional anesthesia. In the past 30 years, comprehensive studies of acupuncture have taken place involving neurophysiological, neuropharmacological, neurobiochemical and neuromorphological methods. Although numerous theories have been proposed to explain how acupuncture works, its exact mechanism of operation is still unknown. However, meridian therapy with needles has been suggested to work by blocking pain signals in or to the brain by projecting inhibitory impulses to the thalamus, cerebral cortex, or both and ultimately to the spinal cord. Finally, it blocks noxious stimuli through the pathophysiological reflex and thus produces muscular relaxation. Other theories discuss the activation of neuropeptides, opioid peptides, and neurotransmitters (Cao 2002; Debreceni 1993; Han 2003). Needles are not always needed to produce meridian stimulation. It can also be done by using finger or thumb pressure (shiatsu), a specially designed blunt instrument (teishin or a T-bar–like device used in massage therapy), and electrical stimulation modalities. Chiropractic management of trigger points was extensively studied by Nimmo (1958), who developed the *receptor tonus* technique. This technique is a method of locating and dissipating neurofascial and tendinous points in the body, which are generative points of noxious nerve circuits that disrupt function and produce pain, referred or otherwise.

A recent addition to the health-care armamentarium is the *laser* (*l*ight *a*mplification by *s*timulated *e*mission of *r*adiation). Since their development in the 1960s, an ever-growing body of data supports the effectiveness of lasers in a large number of fields. Various types of lasers enhance relaxation, reduce pain, and facilitate the healing of open lesions. "It works, but exactly how is one of the modern medical mysteries which is in the process of being systematically and scientifically unraveled" (Ohshiro 1991, p. 18).

Traction

Traction uses a manual or mechanical distraction (separating) force on specific targets of the body. It is commonly employed to stretch tissues and separate joints. It can also facilitate relaxation and decrease pain resulting from muscle guarding—a muscle contracting to stabilize a joint—and spasm.

Cognitive Approaches

The cognitive approach utilizes mental or mind-control techniques. However, many techniques employ a combination of both the cognitive and somatic approaches. Cognitive strategies include such procedures as meditation, sensory awareness techniques, autogenic training, and sentic cycles. A brief review of a number of these techniques is found in Hertling and Jones (1996). Below, two popular cognitive approaches are discussed.

Progressive Deep-Muscle Relaxation Training

Progressive deep-muscle relaxation (PDMR), developed by Edmund Jacobson (1929), seeks to relax the voluntary skeletal muscles by conscious control. The technique is practiced in a quiet setting and with a passive attitude. A muscle is contracted tightly and then suddenly relaxed. As a result, the individual becomes aware of the contrast between the feelings of tension and relaxation. Then, the individual systematically relaxes one muscle group at a time from foot to head or head to foot. Gradually, the entire body is relaxed progressively. With careful and dedicated practice, one can learn to recognize the minutest contractions and avoid them, thus achieving the deepest degree of relaxation possible (Jacobson 1938).

PDMR was modified by Wolpe (1958) and by Bernstein and Borkovec (1973). The term *relaxation training* (RT) is commonly used interchangeably for PDMR. Relaxation training may represent an effective and viable adjunctive treatment for some individuals with psychophysiological ailments (Michelson 1987). In particular, PDMR may serve as an adjunct to standard pharmacological and psychiatric therapeutics (Fried 1987, p. 90). However, some controversy has arisen regarding the specific action of relaxation training procedures in producing physiological effects (Borkovec and Sides 1979; King 1980; Lehrer and Woolfolk 1984). According to Michelson (1987), methodological issues account, in large part, for many of the equivocal findings. Various forms of PDMR have long been employed by students of yoga.

Relaxation Response

The *relaxation response* was discovered and publicized by Dr. Herbert Benson (1980) of the Harvard Medical School. Based on techniques that have been practiced for centuries by numerous cultures and cults, Benson identifies four basic components necessary to bring forth the relaxation response:

1. A *quiet environment*. Quiet allows one to "turn off" both internal stimuli and external distractions, as if inside a mental and emotional decompression chamber.
2. A *mental device*, or object, to dwell on. This stimulus should be constant. It may involve word repetition (e.g., *relax* or *stretch*), gazing at an object (e.g., mentally reaching for one's toes), or concentrating on a particular feeling (e.g., imaging the muscles "oozing out" or feeling the connective tissue untwining).
3. A *passive attitude*. In the opinion of Benson (1980), this attitude "appears to be the most essential factor in eliciting the relaxation response" (p. 111) and is accomplished by emptying all thoughts and distractions from one's mind.
4. A *comfortable position*. A comfortable posture eliminates any "undue muscular tension" (p. 161) and allows one to remain in the same position for an extended period of time.

Contraindications of Cognitive Approaches

Until rather recently, the clinical use of the relaxation response was assumed to be a totally harmless therapeutic intervention. However, Everly (1989) points out that other data contradict this position. Therefore, practitioners who incorporate various techniques to facilitate a relaxation response in conjunction with a stretching regimen must be aware of potential undesirable side effects. Based on the research of Luthe (1969), Emmons (1978), Stroebel (1979), and Everly (1989), Everly et al. (1987) identified five major areas of concern in the elicitation of the relaxation response:

1. *Loss of reality contact.* This problem includes such manifestations as dissociative states, hallucinations, delusions, and perhaps paresthesia (abnormal skin sensations).

2. *Drug reactions.* The relaxation response may actually intensify the effects of some medications or other chemical substances. Particular caution should be implemented with patients taking insulin, sedatives, or hypnotics or cardiovascular medications.

3. *Panic states.* These psychological reactions are characterized by high levels of anxiety concerning the loss of control and by insecurity.

4. *Premature freeing of repressed ideation.* Repressed thoughts and emotions are sometimes released in the deeply relaxed state. This response could have negative consequences if such reactions are unexpected or are too intense.

5. *Excessive trophotropic states.* Relaxation techniques may sometimes induce an excessively lowered state of psychophysiological functioning. Among the potential side effects are a temporary hypotensive state (low blood pressure), a temporary hypoglycemic state (low blood sugar), and fatigue.

Biofeedback

Biofeedback can promote relaxation and can serve as an adjunct to therapeutic exercise. Basmajian (1998) and Wolf (1994) describe biofeedback as a technique that uses electronic equipment to reveal instantaneously to patients and therapists certain internal physiologic events by means of meters, banks of lights, and various auditing devices. Through this feedback, humans can learn to voluntarily manipulate otherwise unsensed events by concentrating on either increasing or decreasing the electronic signals that indicate the level of physiologic activity (Basmajian 1998). Appropriate biofeedback techniques can control even individual motor units (Basmajian 1963, 1967, 1972; Basmajian et al. 1965; Simard and Basmajian 1967). In a clinical setting, Levin and Wolf (1987) demonstrated that biofeedback could be used to downtrain (reduce the amplitude of) the triceps surae SSR of stroke patients who displayed increased tone in ankle extensor muscles. In brief, the proponents of biofeedback believe that by recognizing a biological function, one can gain control of the function.

Induced psychological stress can lead to an increase in EMG (Larsson et al. 1995; Lundberg et al 1994; Westgaard and Björklund 1987). In the field of music, performance-related anxiety has been hypothesized to develop and maintain chronic musculoskeletal pain in some individuals. Consequently, the use of EMG biofeedback has been suggested as one of the prophylactic measures to alleviate chronic neck-shoulder pain among violin and viola players (Berque and Gray 1995). Palmerud et al. (1998) demonstrated that healthy subjects could, by

means of visual feedback, voluntarily reduce the EMG activity of the trapezius muscle by 33% during an arm elevation task and distribute the load to other muscles. Additional clinical research is needed to substantiate the practical implications of these findings.

In athletics and similar disciplines (e.g., dance and the martial arts), biofeedback has been suggested as a means that can supposedly treat muscle pain induced by eccentric contractions, facilitate stretching and flexibility. McGlynn et al. (1979) found that subjects who used biofeedback for 3 days after exhaustive exercise had significantly less perceived pain in the quadriceps muscle group than control subjects who rested. Contradictory to these findings, McGlynn and Laughlin (1980) found that perceived pain among the biofeedback group had significantly more perceived pain than subjects in static stretching and control groups. McGlynn and Laughlin (1980) offered two potential explanations for the contradictory results. (1) The biofeedback group may have been more conscious or sensitive to pain in their biceps brachii because the biofeedback treatment had them focus on this muscle group and perceived pain is a subjective measure. (2) Perhaps the biceps is less susceptible to biofeedback therapy than other muscle groups.

Wilson and Bird (1981) found a significant improvement in hip flexion was produced in male gymnasts in both the biofeedback and relaxation groups, with the biofeedback group improving more quickly across trials. For the female gymnasts, a significant improvement in hip flexion was noted for the control group, the relaxation group, and the relaxation plus biofeedback group. Cummings et al. (1984) determined that relaxation or biofeedback training had beneficial effects upon flexibility of sprinters only in the retention period. Because of the paucity of research, additional studies are needed to determine the effectiveness of biofeedback on flexibility.

Medications

Medication is another potential way to reduce tension and facilitate relaxation. We are constantly inundated by advertisements from the pharmacological industry proselytizing and instilling the belief that many problems can be eliminated simply by the use of a specific medication. These supposed "magic bullets" have numerous potential risks. Today's health-conscious public and medical practitioners should employ greater discretion in the dispensing and application of popular, over-the-counter medications. Failure to do so may exacerbate a major drug problem facing the world.

Analgesics and Counterirritant Balms and Liniments

Analgesics and counterirritants are among the most extensively used aids for the treatment of athletic or everyday muscular aches and sores caused by overexertion. The Food and Drug Administration has classified counterirritants as a category I drug, which means they are considered safe and effective in the treatment of muscle soreness. Analgesic balm products are a $150 million industry with almost 60 million adults in America using them at some time (Barone 1989). "However, despite their usage, the efficacy and mechanism of action of analgesic balms have been poorly studied, and have remained mainly the subject of speculation" (Ichiyama et al. 2002, p. 1440). Haynes and Perrin (1992) suggested that "counterirritants may be an effective means of treating pain and restricted range of motion associated with delayed onset muscle soreness" (p. 13).

The effectiveness of analgesics and counterirritants as a warm-up is at best questionable (Barone 1989). An effective warm-up must reach all the tissues, especially the deep muscles. The warming effect of analgesics is only superficial. Furthermore, a true warm-up increases muscle temperature and enhances the physiologic properties of the tissues. Thus, athletes and recreational players are encouraged not to substitute analgesics or counterirritants as a substitute for warm-up.

The effectiveness of the analgesic balms depends on a variety of factors, most importantly, the composition of the product and the individual to whom the product is applied. The most common ingredients of analgesic balms are eucalyptus oil, oil of wintergreen (methyl salicylate), peppermint (menthol), camphor, capsaicin (capsicum), red pepper, trolamine salicylate, and turpentine oil (Barone 1989). Analgesic balms are thought to penetrate the skin and create a mild irritant that counters or masks the sensation of pain. Besides creating a slight degree of local anesthesia, they cause the muscle fibers surrounding the blood vessels to relax and consequently cause the blood vessels to dilate. Increased circulation helps promote the absorption of inflammatory products and brings more blood and nutrients to the applied area.

A summary of potential modes of action of analgesic balms is provided by Ichiyama et al. (2002):

- Inhibition of the formation of algesic substances found in inflammation processes.
- Blocking of nerve fiber.
- Depletion of transmitter substances.
- Rubbing that accompanies application may increase the activity of large-diameter afferent fibers and engage the "gate control" mechanism.

- The analgesic effect may relate to the accompanying application of superficial heating modalities.
- The analgesic effect is a result of a placebo effect (power of suggestion).

Paraphrasing Ichiyama et al. (2002), clinical trials should investigate and attempt to elucidate the actual neuronal processes underlying the proposed theories of operation of analgesic balms, including the extent of direct penetration effects on receptors or nerve fibers and complex interactions within the central nervous system.

Muscle-Relaxant Drugs

Muscle-relaxant drugs are either *nonprescription* (over-the-counter) or *prescription*. The precise mechanism of many of these drugs is not fully understood. The therapeutic action may be related to analgesic or sedative properties. These drugs either block nerve impulses to skeletal muscles at the neuromuscular junction or act as general CNS depressants. These drugs are often indicated as an adjunct to rest, physical therapy, and other measures for the relief of discomfort associated with acutely painful musculoskeletal conditions. The potentially negative side effects of some of these drugs, include depression, allergies, dizziness, headaches, irritability, light-headedness, nausea, cardiorespiratory depression, coma, and death. Pregnant women or nursing mothers should be especially aware of potential risks. As a rule, prescription drugs should be taken only as a last resort and used according to recommended directions. Medication should be discontinued as soon as possible.

SUMMARY

Theoretically, relaxation, or the absence of muscular tension, should exist before stretching is begun. Reduced internal tension can aid in effectively and efficiently stretching out muscle and connective tissues, which substantially limit extensibility. Muscular relaxation can be induced or facilitated by the somatic, or physical, approach; physiological therapeutic modalities; cognitive, mental, and mind-controlling techniques; sophisticated instrumentation, such as biofeedback; and the use of drugs and medications. Consideration must be given to which is the safest, most effective, and most efficient means to achieve the desired goal.

Muscular Injury and Soreness: Etiology and Consequences

Sport, exercise, and stretching may result in varying degrees of discomfort, soreness, stiffness, or pain of two general kinds: (1) that occurring during and immediately after the activity and persisting for several hours and (2) that usually occurring 24 to 48 hours after the activity. Not infrequently, some injuries result in chronic pain and, perhaps more importantly, have a tendency to recur (Best et al. 1998b). This chapter examines the two general kinds of pain and the inflammation and remodeling response to injuries.

Five basic hypotheses, at one time or another, have attempted to explain the nature of muscular soreness:

1. Damaged or torn muscle
2. Damaged connective tissue
3. Metabolic accumulation or osmotic pressure and swelling
4. Lactic acid accumulation
5. Localized spasm of motor units

Although these possible causes are reviewed separately, they can occur together. Also, muscular soreness can have other causes.

DAMAGED OR TORN MUSCLE HYPOTHESIS

Hough (1902) first suggested that muscular soreness originates in a rupture within the muscle itself, that it is a direct result of muscle injury from microscopic tearing of muscle fibers. However, de Vries (1961a, 1961b, 1962, 1966) originally believed that such injury occurs much less frequently than is thought by athletes, coaches, and laypeople. He argued that "it is somewhat illogical to postulate that a tissue has been structurally damaged by the very function for which it is specifically differentiated" (de Vries 1966, p. 119). Nonetheless, de Vries reminds us that some types of activity are more likely to result in sore muscles than others, including the following:

- Vigorous contractions while the muscle is in a shortened position
- Muscle contractions involving jerky or uncoordinated movements (Some fibers in the muscle may be temporarily overloaded when a full load is placed on the muscle before a sufficient number of motor units have been recruited.)
- Activity involving repetition of the same movement over a long period of time
- Bouncing movements (At the end of a ballistic motion, the movement is stopped by the muscle and its connective tissues, bringing about reflex contractions at the same time the muscle is being forcefully elongated.)

However, since the writings of de Vries substantial improvements have been made in technology that can be used to substantiate the hypothesis that tearing of muscle fibers is the most probable cause of delayed-onset muscle soreness (DOMS). The first clear evidence of the morphological damage in muscle as a result of eccentric contraction was provided by Fridén et al. (1981). Since then, numerous photographs have clearly shown damage to the internal structure of the sarcomere after exercise (see figure 9.1). These photographs (Armstrong et al. 1983; Fridén 1984a, 1984b; Fridén and Lieber 1992; Fridén, Seger et al. 1988; Fridén et al. 1983; Kuipers et al. 1983; Newham, McPhail et al. 1983; Newham, Mills et al. 1982, 1983; Waterman-Storer 1991) clearly show mechanical disruptions of the Z-lines, referred to as *Z-disk streaming*. Theses findings indicated that during overloading, the Z-lines constitute a potential weak link in the myofibrillar contractile chain.

The damaged or torn muscle hypothesis also takes into account such events as damage to the sarcoplasmic reticulum (Byrd 1992; McCutcheon et al. 1992; Newham, Mills et al. 1983; Nimmo and Snow 1982) and the T-tubules (Stauber 1989). These disruptions also interfere with normal calcium metabolism in muscle cells.

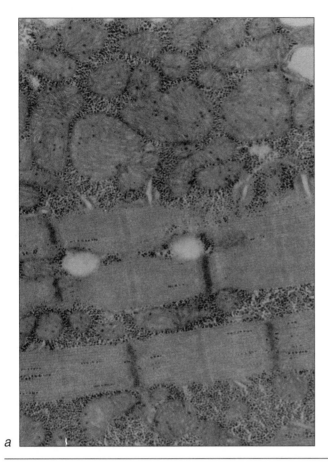 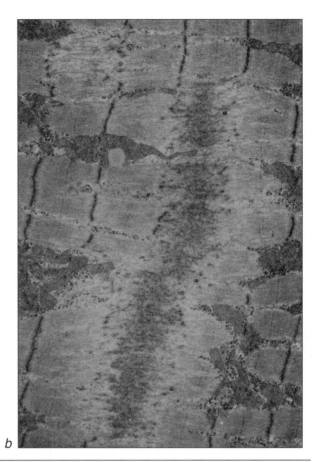

a

b

Figure 9.1 *(a)* An electron micrograph showing normal arrangement of the actin and myosin filaments and Z-disk configuration in the muscle of a runner before a marathon. *(b)* A muscle sample taken immediately after a marathon race shows a damaged sarcomere.

Reprinted, by permission, from J.H. Wilmore and D.L. Costill, 2004, *Physiology of sport and exercise, Third Edition* (Champaign, IL: Human Kinetics), 101.

The damaged or torn muscle hypothesis may be verifiable by biochemical testing. Abraham (1977, 1979) investigated the relationship between DOMS and urinary excretion of myoglobin. Myoglobin is thought to be released by the muscle into the vascular system during muscle injury and thus is indicative of muscle fiber trauma. Abraham's findings were inconclusive. The enzyme creatine kinase (CK) is another potential indicator of muscle damage. Byrnes et al. (1985) demonstrated that the concentration of CK increases after exercise, thus potentially substantiating the hypothesis. However, whereas CK may be related to soreness, it cannot actually cause DOMS because of a mismatch between the time courses of the muscle damage, the pain, and the peak enzyme efflux, which is delayed relative to the pain (Cleak and Eston 1992; Jones, Newham, Obletter et al. 1987). That is, peak CK concentrations occur as the soreness is resolving (Newham 1988).

However, Malm (2001) has raised concerns regarding the exercise-induced changes in muscle, suggesting that the paradigm of exercise-induced muscle inflammation in fact is "fiction." Malm (2001) argues that many studies employ faulty design and methodology.

- Many studies were performed on cage-raised animals and thus lack relevance to trained athletes.
- Studies that employed electrically stimulated animal muscle to replicate muscle contraction can never be considered to accurately describe voluntary physical exercise in humans.
- The use of presumable markers (e.g., leucocytosis and creatine kinase) for cell damage in blood has been criticized for lack of relevance.
- Only a few studies have used nonexercise control groups.
- Invasive procedures during biopsy inflict muscle damage on the very tissues examined.

Malm has suggested a model to serve as a possible guide for further research. It entails the "possibility that exercise-induced, inflammation-related changes observed in blood and muscle are manifestations not of muscle inflammation, but adaptive processes involving immunological events" (pp. 233-234).

Fridén and Lieber (2001) suggest that "[it] may be a misnomer to propose that exercise results in muscle injury.

Rather, it may be more appropriate to conclude that intense exercise initiates a muscle remodeling process that enables skeletal muscle to hypertrophy" (p. 325). The researchers theorize that the earliest events in muscle injury are mechanical in nature. These events are followed by an inflammation process, which may occur secondary to the initial injury. The eventual by-product of this inflammation process is an adaptation that could make the components of the sarcomere more resistant to stress and strain.

DAMAGED CONNECTIVE TISSUE HYPOTHESIS

In addition to damage to muscle contractile tissue, damage can potentially occur to the connective tissues. Selective damage to the series elastic component (SEC), which is composed of the epimysium, perimysium, endomysium, fascia, and tendons, is also widely supported. Abraham (1977, 1979) supports the hypothesis that DOMS is most closely linked to irritation of the muscle's connective tissue. His investigations revealed a significant positive correlation between urinary excretion of hydroxyproline (OHP) and subjective incidence of muscle soreness. OHP is a marker of the breakdown of connective tissue and is an indicator of collagen metabolism. Tullson and Armstrong (1968, 1981) provide additional support for the relationship between muscle soreness and connective tissue irritation or damage. Their belief is based on the finding that the connective tissues are damaged to a greater extent after eccentric contraction because of a greater passive tension on them (Sutton 1984).

HYPOTHESIS OF METABOLIC ACCUMULATION OR OSMOTIC PRESSURE AND SWELLING

DOMS possibly results from the accumulation of muscle metabolic by-products (including lactic acid, a by-product of anaerobic metabolism), extracellular potassium, and an excess of other metabolites that causes an increased osmotic pressure inside and outside muscle fibers, leading to retained excess water that in turn causes edema and pressure on sensory nerves (Asmussen 1956; Bobbert et al. 1986; Brendstrup 1962). Swelling of the muscle causes it to become shorter, thicker, and more resistant to stretching (Howell et al. 1985; Jones, Newham, and Clarkson 1987). This swelling causes stiffness when the muscle is stretched during the contraction of the antagonistic muscles.

Stauber (1989) suggested that the discomfort and swelling associated with DOMS resembles a minicompartment syndrome and that the extracellular space may be a major contributing factor. Studies by Fridén et al. (1986), Fridén, Sfakianos et al. (1988), and Wallensten and Eklund (1983) found elevated tissue fluid pressure in muscles exercised eccentrically (in which the muscle elongates as it contracts). According to Fridén, Sfakianos

et al. (1988), "eccentric muscle averaged ~3% more water content than did the concentric muscle" (p. 497). Howell et al. (1985) proposed an analogy comparing the muscle with a water balloon stuffed inside a nylon stocking. "The presence of the balloon would prevent the nylon stocking from being stretched to its full length. Similarly, water of edema within the three-dimensional matrix of the endomysium, perimysium, and epimysium would limit their extension" (p. 1718). The increased volume of fluid produces passive tension effects throughout the stocking. Associated with this tension are pain, swelling, and stiffness. Howell et al. (1985) suggested that slow extension occurring beyond the initial stiffness barrier may "represent squeezing of water out of the perimuscular connective tissue matrix into interfascial planes" (p. 1718).

However, these explanations present several problems. Muscle soreness is usually greater after exercise consisting of eccentric work (in which muscle elongates as it contracts) as opposed to concentric work (in which muscle shortens as it contracts). Eccentric contractions are less demanding in their energy requirements or oxygen consumption (Armstrong 1984; Armstrong et al. 1991; Bigland-Ritchie and Woods 1976; Davies and Barnes 1972; Dick and Cavanagh 1987; Knuttgen et al. 1982; Newham, Mills et al. 1983). Several studies (Asmussen 1953; Gibala et al. 1995; Seliger et al. 1980) have substantiated a higher electromyographic (EMG) activity for concentric work of a given resistance load than for eccentric contractions. Jones, Newham, Obletter et al. (1987) believe that increased intramuscular pressure is not likely the cause of pain, because during isometric contractions the intramuscular pressure can rise to several hundred mmHg (Hill 1948). However, this pressure is not perceived as painful in the same way as muscle tenderness is. Furthermore, even in already tender muscle, isometric contractions do not aggravate the pain. Nonetheless, stretching and cool-down after exercise is strongly encouraged to allow the muscles time to promote the removal of accumulated waste products.

LACTIC ACID ACCUMULATION HYPOTHESIS

Although lactic acid accumulation is one of the most popular explanations for DOMS, lactic acid is a by-product of anaerobic metabolism and can only form in the absence of oxygen. Therefore, lactic acid accumulates when the blood supply to the muscles is insufficient. Consequently, lactic acid must not be a factor in pain after passive exercise and most static stretching programs.

HYPOTHESIS OF LOCALIZED SPASM OF MOTOR UNITS

As postulated in numerous works by de Vries (1961a, 1961b, 1962, 1966), the delayed localized soreness that occurs after unaccustomed exercise is caused by tonic, localized spasm of motor units whose number varies with the severity of pain:

- Exercise beyond a minimal level causes some degree of ischemia (i.e., temporary lack of blood supply) in active muscle.

- Ischemia causes muscle pain. This pain probably occurs by means of the transfer of P-substance (some particular pain substance) across the muscle cell membrane into the tissue fluid, from which location it gains access to pain endings.

- The resulting pain consequently brings about a protective, reflexive, tonic muscle contraction.

- The tonic contraction then brings about localized areas of ischemia in the muscle tissue, and a vicious cycle begins, which results in a local, tonic muscle spasm.

Using specially developed EMG equipment, de Vries (1961a, 1966) quantitatively demonstrated muscular pain. He found a positive relationship between the severity of exercise-induced pain and the level of muscular electrical activity. More importantly, he found that static stretching furnished symptomatic relief and also caused a significant decrease in the electrical activity of the painful muscles. Thus, de Vries contends that some degree of control can be exerted over the prevention and relief of soreness.

However, when Abraham (1977) attempted to duplicate the EMG experiment, he was unable to find significant EMG changes as a result of induced muscle soreness. Similarly, Talag (1973), Torgan (1985), and Newham, Mills et al. (1983) were unable to substantiate the findings of de Vries. This discrepancy was probably related to the choice of recording electrodes (de Vries 1986; Francis 1983). However, Bobbert et al. (1986) have also been unable to find evidence to support de Vries' argument. Furthermore, data has raised doubts about the presence of increased EMG activity in relaxed sore muscles (Lund et al. 1991). This negative opinion is also held by Francis (1983) and Jones et al. (1987). Additional research is needed to resolve these discrepancies.

PREDISPOSING FACTORS OF DELAYED-ONSET MUSCLE SORENESS

The predisposing factors of DOMS are unknown. However, numerous factors have been proposed. Among them are eccentric contractions, state of training, and insufficient warm-up.

Eccentric Contractions

Given that eccentric contractions result in muscle damage, what factors determine the magnitude of muscle damage? Muscle damage increases with the number of eccentric contractions (McCully and Faulkner 1986; Warren et al. 1993) and with the length of stretch (Brooks et al. 1995;

Lieber and Fridén 1993). In contrast, shortening over the same range generally produces little damage (Balnave et al. 1997; McCully and Faulkner 1985). Stretching of relaxed muscle also produces little damage (Jones et al. 1989; Newman et al. 1988), and velocity of the stretch is not critical (McCully and Faulkner 1986; Warren et al. 1993). Why, then, do eccentric contractions cause more damage than concentric or isometric contractions? Possible answers to this question are discussed below.

Two additional factors have received attention of investigators. One factor deals with the force developed during the stretch, and the other factor relates to the characteristics of the length change, such as the starting length or final length (Allen 2001). Studies have shown a correlation between the degree of damage and the maximum force during the stretch (McCully and Faulkner 1986; Warren et al. 1993). However, data interpreted by Lieber and Fridén (1993) indicated "that it was *not* high force per se causes muscle damage after eccentric contraction but the magnitude of the active strain (i.e., strain during active lengthening)" (p. 520). Summarizing several studies, Allen (2001) writes

> Talbot and Morgan (1998) used toad sartorius muscle for this reason and varied starting length, stretch size and velocity. Damage was assessed by reduction in force and shift in the peak of the force-length curve. The results showed strong correlations between damage and initial length and amplitude of stretch and weak or negligible correlations with velocity, force before stretch and peak force during stretch. This result is supported by other animal studies (Lieber and Fridén 1993) and by human studies in which the extent of DOMS depended on the starting length (Newham et al. 1988). (p. 313)

DOMS might be related to the nature of the tension that develops in the tissues during elongation or stretching. When a muscle contracts *concentrically*, the muscle fibers shorten actively and *positive* work is performed. As the muscle continually shortens, its tension output decreases. To maintain tension production, a greater number of fibers take part in the contraction, so the pull exerted by each individual muscle fiber on its connective tissue is reduced. The workload is thus shared by a greater mass of muscle cells, and each is spared excessive stress and tension, and the tissue escapes injury.

During elongation, individual muscle fibers are capable of contracting. This process is called an *eccentric* contraction and produces *negative* work. Like concentric contractions, eccentric contractions produce active tension that is transmitted via connective tissues. The degree of muscle excitation is related to the number and discharge frequency of active motor units. An active motor unit consists of one motor neuron and the muscle cells supplied by its axon branches. Dean (1988) found that EMG activity has been "reported to be reduced in eccentric muscle contraction compared with concentric muscle contraction at comparable force and speed of contraction (Bigland-Ritchie and Woods 1976). This finding suggests that fewer motor units may be recruited in an eccentric contraction compared with a concentric contraction" (Dean 1988, p. 233). However, the potential recruitment pattern on EMG patterns during negative work has not been well established (Aura and Komi 1986).

The number of active motor units decreases because connective tissue passive tension, which increases with length, compensates for the decline in active tension, resulting in increased elastic tension. Faulkner et al. (1993) suggest that lengthening contraction also reflects an increased strain on individual cross-bridges. "The tension per active unit will consequently be greater in negative work than in positive, and so the chances of strain or damage to parts [i.e., connective tissue and contractile components] of the muscles" (Asmussen 1956, p. 113). However, contradictory research has been reported regarding which type of contraction produces maximal forces. For example, Doss and Karpovich (1965) and Seliger et al. (1980) reported higher eccentric forces in comparison to isometric forces. However, Singh and Karpovich (1966) reported that at certain angles of elbow extension, the maximum isometric force was significantly greater than the maximum eccentric force. Wilson et al. (1994) also found that maximum forces exerted in isometric contractions were greater than maximum forces produced during eccentric contractions.

Initially, the structural disturbances were also suggested to be secondary, resulting from an activation of lysosomal enzymes, bringing about a concomitant inflammation (Fridén et al. 1981). However, the assumption that the inflammatory process is secondary to myofibrillar damage has not been supported by other research (Armstrong et al. 1983; Fridén, Sjöström, and Ekblom 1983).

Another possible mechanism of eccentric muscle damage is sarcomere inhomogenity (Allen 2001; Morgan 1990; Morgan and Allen 1999). Not all sarcomeres are equal. Some are shorter or intrinsically stronger than others. The shortest sarcomeres are concentrated at the ends of a fiber, whereas the weakest sarcomeres are scattered throughout most of the length (Gordon et al. 1966a). A slow stretch applied to a muscle fiber possibly lengthens the weakest sarcomeres more rapidly than others. Consequently, they will become even weaker and stretch more rapidly. The shorter and stronger sarcomeres also lengthen, but only slightly. Therefore, the weakest sarcomeres are the main source of elongation in the muscle. Eventually, the lengthening is limited only by very small inertial or passive viscous forces until its passive tension brings it to a stop. This rapid uncontrolled lengthening of the sarcomere from an unstable situation to a stable one stretched beyond the thick and thin filament overlap is known as "popping" (Black and Stevens 2001; Morgan 1990, 1994) (see figure 9.2). Mathematically, popping works as follows (Morgan 1994):

1. Assume all sarcomeres in a given muscle fiber start at a length of 2.5 μm.

2. Apply a tensile force of 10% to the muscle fiber.

3. If the tensile force is distributed uniformly, all the sarcomeres within the muscle fiber have a final length of 2.75 μm.

4. If, however, the sarcomeres are *not* equal in length or strength, the lengthening is taken up by the weakest sarcomeres first.

5. The weakest sarcomeres are stretched to the length at which their tension again equals the tension of the other sarcomeres.

6. Calculations indicate that 3.95 μm generates the same tension as 2.5 μm.

7. Further estimates indicate the 10% imposed length change requires that 17% of the sarcomeres be at this length.

8. At the end of the stretch, sarcomeres exist at two lengths, 2.5 μm and 3.95 μm, with equal isometric tensions.

How, then, does the popping hypothesis explain the muscular force deficit associated with muscle soreness after eccentric training? When muscles are stretched, many sarcomeres may pop. Some recover normal interdigitation and others are permanently damaged or disrupted. The impaired sarcomeres regain filament overlap with subsequent contractions and resume force production. This recovery can occur in a few minutes. However, the irreversibly damaged sarcomeres do not regain filament overlap. Consequently, muscular force deficit cannot be made up until the damaged sarcomeres are replaced, which takes several days. Hence, potential force output is not regained until several days posteccentric exercise. After the muscle relaxes, the overstretched sarcomeres reinterdigitate. However, after repeated eccentric contractions, the thick and thin filaments in some sarcomeres fail to reinterdigitate correctly. Talbot and Morgan (1996) have provided direct evidence to support this hypothesis. These sarcomeres either remain extended or produce less force. Therefore, they extend rapidly in a new contraction. With repeated eccentric contractions, the number of permanently weakened or overstretched stretched sarcomeres increases (Talbot and Morgan 1996). The key point is that damage only occurs when the stretch extends beyond the peak of the force-length relation (Allen 2001). Hesselink et al. (1996) have also shown that the decline in muscular performance after negative work is not solely related to myofibrillar damage. Significantly, the popping hypothesis explains why stretching may not provide protection from muscle injury.

State of Training

A popular theory is that the degree of muscular pain, soreness, or stiffness corresponds to the state of training of the tissues involved. People with unexercised and tight muscles show a markedly higher reaction when subjected to a variety of physical stresses. Consequently, fibers and connective tissues are more susceptible to strain and rupture. Thus, "stiffness is a disease of the unfit" (Williams and Sperryn

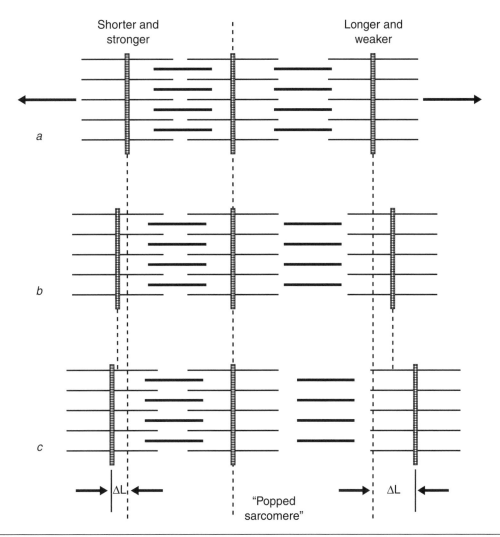

Figure 9.2   Popping sarcomere hypothesis. Schematic representation of the process of sarcomere "popping." Two adjacent sarcomeres are illustrated that are of slightly different strengths. *(a)* Sarcomeres are slightly different strengths due to differences in sarcomere length or due to intrinsic strength differences. *(b)* As the muscle is lengthened, the sarcomeres lengthen different amounts due to different strengths, and one (on the right side) reaches the sarcomere length where no myofilament overlap occurs. *(c)* The sarcomere without myofilament overlap "pops" to a longer length where the tension is born by passive muscle elements (not shown). Notice that, overall, the length change in each sarcomere (ΔL) is not equal. This nonuniformity of sarcomere length is the fundamental idea behind the "popping sarcomere" hypothesis.

Based on ideas presented in D.L. Morgan, 1990, "New insights into the behavior of muscle during active lengthening," *Biophysical Journal* 57, 209-221. Reprinted, by permission, from R.L. Lieber, 2002, *Skeletal muscle structure, function, & plasticity*, 2nd ed. (Philadelphia: Lippincott Williams & Wilkins), 327.

1976, p. 301). Substantiating this assumption, Evans et al. (1985) and Fridén et al. (1981) point out that delayed muscle soreness is much more apparent in untrained subjects than in persons accustomed to regular exercise.

A number of studies of the attempts to reduce or eliminate DOMS by training have been conducted. Cleak and Eston (1992) identified several studies that documented the alleviation of the soreness response, along with reduced morphological changes, enhanced performance, and decreased CK concentration in the blood (Byrnes and Clarkson 1986; Byrnes et al. 1985; Clarkson et al. 1987; Clarkson and Tremblay 1988; Fridén, Seger et al. 1983; Jones and Newham 1985; Knuttgen 1986; Komi and Bus-

kirk 1972; Miller et al. 1988; Schwane and Armstrong 1983; Schwane et al. 1987). The protective effects of training are suggested to last from 6 weeks (Byrnes et al. 1985) to 10 weeks (Clarkson et al. 1992; Jones and Newham 1985). Studies show that the required length of training may vary from many weeks (Fridén et al. 1983; Komi and Buskirk 1972) down to a single intense exercise bout (Armstrong et al. 1983; Byrnes et al. 1985; Clarkson et al. 1987; Clarkson and Tremblay 1988; Ebbeling and Clarkson 1989).

Insufficient Warm-Up

A long-held opinion popular among coaches and athletes is that muscle soreness results from failing to warm up before exercising or stretching. de Vries (1966) stated that very little experimental evidence with human subjects exist to support this theory, probably because no researcher cares to set up an experiment in which the subjects may be injured. However, research using animal surrogates has demonstrated that "cold" muscles and tendons have a greater tendency toward strains and ruptures than do properly warmed-up ones because they can absorb less energy (Garrett 1996; Noonan et al. 1993). Thus, everything that is known about muscle physiology supports the need for warm-up as a prudent protective measure. Warming up is discussed at greater length in chapter 10.

TRAUMA AND OVERLOAD INJURY TO THE MUSCULATURE AND CONNECTIVE TISSUES

All tissues have mechanical limits beyond which intrinsic damage occurs. Causes of insult to the body vary, but consequences are nonetheless significant in terms of joint dysfunction. In general, musculoskeletal *trauma* falls into two major categories: (1) chronic, or *overload*, injuries and (2) acute, or sudden, *tear* or *blow* injuries. An overload injury occurs when a muscle is forced to perform work of unaccustomed intensity or duration, often, with repeated forced lengthening of the muscle-tendon unit. The resulting histological picture within the muscle tissue resembles that of a necrotic inflammation, with disruption and swelling of muscle fibers and infiltration of the extracellular space by inflammatory cells such as white blood cells (Round et al. 1987). A tear or blow injury results from strong mechanical forces acting briefly on muscle tissues, disrupting blood vessels and muscle fibers. Groin and hamstring injuries are two such acute stretch injuries.

Tissue stretched beyond certain limits experiences a *sprain* (for ligamentous and capsular tissues) or a *strain* (for muscle and tendon tissue). Sprains and strains are classified according to their severity:

- *Mild (first-degree):* a tear of a few muscle fibers; minor swelling and discomfort with no or only minimal loss of strength and restriction of the movements.

- *Moderate (second-degree):* a greater damage of muscle with a clear loss of strength.

- *Severe (third-degree):* a tear extending across the whole muscle belly, resulting in a total loss of muscle function.

Mild sprains or strains may result in a little hemorrhage with disruption of a few fibers and a mild inflammatory reaction. In contrast, severe sprains or strains, result in considerable hemorrhage, with partial or complete tear of the muscle or its connective tissue. In either case, the response to injury follows an orderly and well-defined but overlapping sequence of events: injury, inflammation, repair, and remodeling. In the following sections, the inflammatory responses and consequences are reviewed.

Best et al. (1998b) addressed several major problems in studying any form of muscle damage:

- Difficulty of creating a reproducible injury to the muscle using normal pathologic joint movements and muscle contraction

- The significance of experimental models (e.g., employing highly invasive procedures, including surgical detachment and reattachment to bone of muscle-tendon units that are stretched and injured) and their similarity to in vivo muscle-tendon injury

- The lack of a unique definition for injury

Best et al. (1998b) point out that "The majority of previous studies on acute muscle stretch damage have defined injury based on mechanical data where a force decline with increasing tissue deformation constitutes injury" (pp. 201-202). However, this definition is being challenged. Best et al. (1996) have demonstrated a decline in force with increasing deformation simultaneously with total muscle-tendon separation. However, total muscle rupture is a rare event. Furthermore, Hasselman et al. (1995) have demonstrated that the contractile elements are damaged before the connective tissue structures in muscle stretch injury. Therefore, "a muscle's loss of contractile ability may be a more sensitive measure of injury than the traditional biomechanical measures of the tissue's structural properties" (Best et al. 1998b, p. 201).

Inflammatory Response

Inflammation is the initial biologic reaction to virtually all injuries. The degree of inflammation is proportional to the amount or degree of tissue damage. It is a dynamic and continuous vascular and cellular response that promotes repair and recovery. The gross features of inflammation were identified some 2,000 years ago by five cardinal signs: *rubor* (redness), *tumor* (swelling), *calor* (heat), *dolor* (pain), and *functio laesa* (altered or loss of function). In general, the increased blood flow to the region causes the warmth and redness. Swelling is a result of the outpouring of fluid into the tissue. Pain may be produced by various noxious stimuli, including chemical, mechanical, and thermal agents. A severe consequence of inflammation is a self-perpetuating pain cycle and altered function (figure 9.3).

Postinflammation Repair and Remodeling

Repair and *remodeling* are the next major pathological phases after inflammation. Repair is associated with proliferation of capillaries and fibroblasts (cells that synthesize collagen fibers). Hence, the repair phase is known as *fibroplasia*. The exact mechanisms by which the fibroblasts begin synthesizing scar tissue, primarily collagen, and protein polysaccharides, are still debated. The new collagen fibers are randomly oriented and highly soluble;

thus, the connection established is fragile. During remodeling and maturation, collagen synthesis continues along with a reorientation of the collagen fibrils in the direction of loading and the formation of normal cross-links between fibrils. Thus, the weave, or architecture, of the collagen fibers becomes more organized. If the damage is relatively severe, considerable scarring may occur. The extent to which a scar remodels varies among individuals and within the same individual, depending on age at the time of injury. Ultimately, the strength and plastic characteristics of scar tissue depend on the formation and density of intermolecular covalent bonds and on the orientation and weave of the individual collagen fibers.

Although scarring represents the lesser evil compared with having an open or unhealed injury, it also presents potential problems, which are most evident when scarring is extensive, as with a severe strain or rupture. Muscle regains strength slowly, and the rate for tendon injuries is even slower because of poorer blood supply. Despite strength gains, some injured muscles rarely, if ever, regain their full strength. Strength is not the only important physical parameter affected by scars. Scar tissue often converts an elastic, pliable tissue into an inelastic, brittle

mass. As Arnheim and Prentice (2000) point out, scarring can produce consequences that are more serious for some people, especially athletes (who often return to practice and competition before healing), because strains have a tendency to recur in already brittle scar tissue. The higher the incidence of strains at a particular muscle site, the greater the amount of scar tissue and the greater the potential for recurrent injuries. Worse yet, the fear of another "pull" may become an obsession that is more handicapping than the injury itself.

MEDICAL MANAGEMENT OF ACUTE SOFT-TISSUE INJURIES

The three phases of medical management coincide with the three phases of micropathological change.

Treatment During the Acute Inflammatory Phase

The acute inflammatory phase may last up to 72 hours, depending on the severity of the injury. The primary

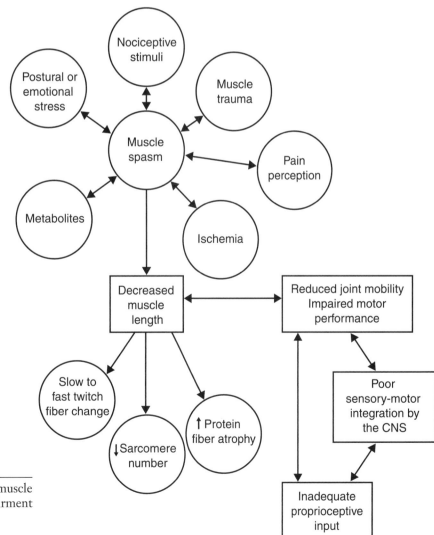

Figure 9.3 Self-perpetuating pain–muscle spasm–pain cycle and eventual impairment in motor control.

Reprinted from Vujnovich 1995.

objective at this phase is to minimize the hemorrhaging and swelling to prevent the formation of a large hematoma, which has a direct impact on the size of scar tissue at the end of the regeneration (Järvinen et al. 2000). Accordingly, the principles of management of acute soft-tissue injuries have been embodied in the well-known acronym *RICE.*

R = Rest the injured soft tissues.

I = Ice applied for 20 to 30 minutes at hourly intervals for 4 hours postinjury.

C = Compression and bandaging, continuously applied for at least 48 hours.

E = Elevated to enhance venous return.

Oakes (1981) emphasizes two important "don'ts." First, do not apply heat for at least 48 to 72 hours, because heat increases bleeding and thus increases edema formation. Therefore, muscle stimulators, ultrasound, and similar modalities should not be used in the acute phase. Second, do not drink alcohol, because it is a potent vasodilator. Oakes (1981) and Kellett (1986) also warn that the use of exogenous steroids may delay collagen repair and should be avoided.

Ice therapy is widely used. However, MacAuley (2001) has criticized the lack of guidance and other aspects of its utilization in standard textbooks. His review of 45 general sports medicine texts found 17 with "no guidance on the duration, frequency, or length of ice treatments or on the use of barriers between ice and skin" (p. 67). Furthermore, he found "considerable variation in recommended duration and frequency of advised treatments" (p. 67). Additional research is needed to determine the most effective use of ice in soft-tissue injuries.

Treatment During the Repair Phase

The repair phase may last from 48 hours to 6 weeks. In the opinion of Oakes (1981), this phase is the most difficult to manage because it requires a balance between setting optimal conditions for collagenous, injured muscle, and ligamentous repair and satisfying the needs of athletes, coaches, and management for a rapid return to competition. In particular, injury repair must be encouraged and facilitated through local mobility while maintaining cardiovascular fitness through body movement. The athlete must not return prematurely to competition. Otherwise, the injured muscle or ligament may retear, and a vicious circle is repeated (Garrett 1996).

Opinions differ regarding usage of anti-inflammatory medication. This treatment is largely empirical because no study has demonstrated the efficacy of nonsteriodal anti-inflammatory drugs (NSAIDs) (Drezner 2003; Garrett 1996). In contrast, Järvinen et al. (2000) recommend NSAIDs as a part of early treatment that should be started immediately after the injury to decrease the inflammatory cell reaction. According to Järvinen et al. (2000),

NSAIDs cause no adverse effects on tensile or contractile properties of injured muscles. However, glucocorticoids are contraindicated because they cause a delayed elimination of hematoma and necrotic tissue as well as retarded muscle regeneration. Garrett (1996) points out the concern regarding long-term treatment with nonsteroidal anti-inflammatory agents "because of the delay in the repair process seen histologically" (p. S-7).

Hyperbaric oxygen therapy is the inhalation of 100% oxygen while the treatment chamber is pressurized at more than 1 atmosphere absolute (AOSSM Research Committee 1998). In theory, this therapy will optimize the environment for the injured tissues. This treatment strategy has received attention as a potential tool for sports-related soft-tissue injuries. (AOSSM Research Committee 1998; Best et al. 1998a; Webster et al. 2002). However, clinical studies to prove the efficacy of hyperbaric oxygen therapy for soft-tissue sports injuries are still lacking. In an editorial published in *The American Journal of Sports Medicine*, the AOSSM Research Committee (1998) wrote:

> Currently, there are no accepted studies to justify the use of hyperbaric oxygen in the treatment of soft tissue injuries incurred in sports. The gap between the knowledge gleaned from laboratory and severely traumatized patients, and the application of hyperbaric oxygen to the athlete in the locker room remains vast. The benefit from hyperbaric oxygen, as a very expensive therapeutic modality in the treatment of soft tissue injury, remains unproven, while the risks—such as tympanic membrane perforation—are significant. (p. 490)

Treatment During the Remodeling Phase

The remodeling phase may last from 3 weeks to a year, and during this phase, collagen is remodeled to increase functional capabilities so that it can withstand the stresses imposed on it. The distinction between repair and remodeling is largely that the *quantity* of collagen is increased during the repair phase and that *quality* (orientation and tensile strength) of collagen is improved during the remodeling phase. Such a clear-cut distinction is, however, artificial because the two phases merge to a large degree.

EFFECTS OF MECHANICAL STRESS ON ELASTICITY AND STRENGTH OF COLLAGEN IN SCAR TISSUE

Applying a tensile force can affect the remodeling of damaged (scar) tissue so as to enhance the optimal regaining of elasticity and strength. Stress and motion stimulates a more functional alignment of collagen fibers, maximizing healing by developing the correct type of connective tissue and minimizing the development of scar tissue adhesions (Cummings and Tillman 1992). Current theory suggests that exercise or therapeutic stress can decrease the number of collagen cross-links by increasing the collagen turnover rate. The strength of collagen (and of scar tissue) appears to be in part the result of the intramolecular cross-linking between the α_1 and α_2 chains of the collagen molecule and of the intermolecular cross-linking between the collagen fibrils, filaments, and fibers (see chapter 4). The modifications of adhesions and scars are probably related to the formation or dissolution of cross-links between collagen units. This process is called *collagen turnover*, continuous and simultaneous collagen production and breakdown. If the rate of breakdown exceeds production, the scar becomes softer and less bulky. If, the rate of production exceeds breakdown, the opposite effect occurs. (The collagen in debilitating adhesions and scars is thought to be shorter and more compactly organized.) Thus, if exercise can in fact decrease the number of collagen cross-links by increasing the collagen turnover rate, stretching could possibly determine the ultimate degree of extensibility, elasticity, and strength of the remodeled tissues.

Collagen and Scarring

Another factor that places the emphasis of rehabilitation programs on ROM and flexibility is tissue healing. As collagen becomes mature during the proliferative and remodeling phases, its structure becomes more permanent. ROM and flexibility can be improved during the initial period of these phases, but as the forming structures become more mature, improvement is less likely. Young scars are easier to affect mechanically than older scars. Because new scar tissue has larger amounts of GAG and water content, the collagen cross-linkages are fewer, permitting an extraneous force to have more impact on tissue lengthening. As collagen tissue matures, however, the cross-linkages become stronger and more numerous, making stretching the structure more difficult (Houglum 1992, p. 31).

Currently, two theories, the *induction* theory and the *tension* theory, attempt to explain the force that directs fiber orientation. The induction theory suggests that the healing tissue induces the collagen weave to produce a scar that mimics the characteristics of the tissue. In contrast, the tension theory maintains that internal and external forces acting on the tissue as it heals influence the type of collagen weave produced (McGongile and Matley 1994).

According to Cummings and Tillman (1992), "time must be given for connective tissue to remodel in proportion with the increased demands of the new situation" (p. 47). The effect of stress on strength of new scar tissue is a function of the intensity and duration of stress applied. If excessive stress is applied to newly formed and weak scar tissue, the scar is pulled apart.

Stretching scar tissue can be particular dangerous because not only the remodeling connective tissue but also the vascular bed might tear, resulting in more bleeding. Consequently, inflammation will increase, and rehabilitation will be prolonged. Furthermore, inflammation may result in pain and muscle spasms, thus limiting ROM. The new collagen has not yet matured with increased quantity, cross-linkages, and fiber diameter and is thus susceptible to new injury (Ciullo and Zarins 1983). Thus, Tillman and Cummings (1992) caution:

> For the therapist who is physically stressing scar to bring about remodeling, it is important to visualize the highly cellular, fragile structure of new scar. Use of stress to "stretch" scar tissue at this stage will cause elongation of the scar by one of only two mechanisms: disruption of cell membranes and cell death, in response to high or sudden loads, or cell migration, in response to gentle and prolonged loads. (p. 29)

SUMMARY

Two types of muscle soreness can develop after exercise: immediate soreness and delayed localized soreness. Delayed-onset muscle soreness appears 24 to 48 hours after activity. Currently, muscular soreness is explained by at least five possible mechanisms that may work together or independently: the damaged or torn muscle hypothesis, the damaged connective tissue hypothesis, the hypothesis of metabolic accumulation or osmotic pressure and swelling, the lactic acid accumulation hypothesis, and the hypothesis of localized spasm of motor units. Regardless of the causes of muscle soreness, everything that is known of muscle physiology tends to support the need for warm-up, cool-down, and stretching as prudent preventive measures.

10

Special Factors in Flexibility

Besides those factors previously discussed, a number of additional factors can affect one's flexibility and suppleness, including age, gender, body build, laterality (handedness), training, and circadian rhythms. All of these factors are discussed in this chapter.

CHILDREN AND FLEXIBILITY DEVELOPMENT

Data concerning the relationship between age and flexibility are conflicting, especially data on the increase or decrease of flexibility during the growing years. The complexity is compounded because studies often focus on specific joints or specific populations involved in various athletic disciplines. Also, lack of standardized testing procedures makes comparing the various studies difficult. Consequently, the literature must be read carefully and completely. Generally, the research seems to indicate that small children are quite supple and that during the school years, flexibility decreases until about puberty, then increases throughout adolescence. After adolescence, however, flexibility levels off and then decreases. Although flexibility decreases with age, the loss appears to be minimized in individuals who remain active.

Flexibility Changes in Young Children

Gurewitsch and O'Neill (1944) carried out one of the earliest studies on flexibility and found gradual declines in flexibility from ages 6 to 12 years and then increases through age 18. Kendall and Kendall (1948) administered two flexibility tests to some 4,500 children from kindergarten to 12th grade. The tests were toe touching and touching the forehead to the knees in a long-sitting position. They found that at age 5 years, 98% of the boys and 86% of the girls could perform the toe-touch test.

Beginning at age 6, these percentages declined sharply, so that by age 12, only 30% of both sexes could perform this test. After about age 13, the percentages that were successful gradually increased each year through age 17. At age 5 years, only 15% of the girls and 5% of the boys could touch their foreheads to their knees. This percentage did not change appreciably in either group through age 17.

Hupprich and Sigerseth (1950) investigated a group of girls 9 to 15 years of age and reported no significant differences among them in six different flexibility test items. However, shoulder, knee, and hip flexion appeared to decrease from ages 12 through 15 years. Leighton (1956) measured the flexibility characteristics of boys 10 to 18 years of age and found decreases in flexibility during adolescence. Buxton (1957) found decreases in both girls and boys from age 6 to 12 and then increases through age 15. Burley et al. (1961) reported no significant age group differences in several flexibility measures among 7th-grade through 9th-grade girls. Clarke (1975) reported flexibility decreases beginning at age 10 for males and age 12 for females. Milne et al. (1976) found significant decreases in flexibility between kindergarten and 2nd-grade children. Krahenbuhl and Martin (1977) found a decrease in shoulder, knee, and hip flexibility between the ages of 10 and 14 years. A study of shoulder flexibility by Germain and Blair (1983) indicated an increase at 5 to 10 years of age and then a steady decrease with age thereafter. Docherty and Bell (1985) found a significant decrease in trunk and neck extension, shoulder and wrist elevation, and sit-and-reach flexibility between 6 and 15 years of age. Koslow (1987) investigated 320 males and females ranging in age from 9 to 21 years. Shoulder flexion-extension was greater in the 13-year-old males and females than in the 9-year-old males and females. Males and females ages 17 and 21 years were significantly more flexible than 9-year-old and 13-year-old males and females using the modified sit-and-reach test to evaluate lower-extremity flexibility. A decrease in flexibility was even found between 5-year-olds and 6-year-olds (Gabbard and Tandy 1988).

A study by Mellin and Poussa (1992) of spinal mobility in 294 male and female subjects 8 to 16 years of age found no age differences in forward flexion of the lumbar spine. This result differed from earlier reports of a decrease between the ages of 10 and 15 years (Moran et al. 1979; Salminen 1984). Lateral flexion increased with age in both genders, with greater mobility among the girls (Moran et al. 1979). Moll et al. (1972) also confirmed that lateral flexion is greater in females than in males, which continued into the eighth decade.

According to Sermeev (1966), flexibility develops unequally in various age periods and for various movements. Nonetheless, Harris (1969b) believes that one age is as good as another for studying the structure of flexibility as long as the study is kept within the specific age range. However, Corbin and Noble (1980) suggest that when evaluating the flexibility of children and adolescents, growth (especially individual differences in growth) should be considered. Pratt (1989) found that maturational age as measured by Tanner staging was better correlated with strength and flexibility for the lower extremity than was chronological age.

One's degree of flexibility depends on many interacting factors. In athletics and dance, flexibility relates to the level of preparation and training (Alexander 1991; Chatfield et al. 1990; Klemp et al. 1984; Nelson et al. 1983; Sermeev 1966). The higher the qualification requirements for many sports and events, the greater the mobility of the athlete. For laypeople, the quality and quantity of one's activities, both occupational and avocational, is of chief importance (Salminen et al. 1993). Although flexibility does decrease with age, the loss appears to be minimized in those individuals who remain active.

Increased Tightness of Children Growing Into Adolescence

Several explanations have been offered for the decline in flexibility experienced by children growing into adolescence. One explanation is that during periods of rapid growth, bones grow much faster than the muscles stretch. As a result, muscle-tendon tightness about a joint increases (Bachrach 1987; Kendall and Kendall 1948; Leard 1984; Micheli 1983). According to Feldman et al. (1999), "growth could not cause a decrease in flexibility, but rather is only associated with it" (p. 28). The controversy regarding growth spurts and flexibility is discussed in chapter 2.

Another explanation is that the decrease in flexibility, especially in the hamstrings, is directly related to the prolonged sitting position in school (Milne and Mierau 1979; Milne et al. 1981; Feldman et al. 1999). The mechanics of sitting have been investigated by Pheasant (1991, 1996). In brief, most people are comfortable when sitting with a backward rotation of the pelvis so that the superior iliac spine lies well behind the pubis. Palpation of the hamstring tendon (just behind the knee), will reveal that they are slack. Sitting up straight tightens them. Consequently, over an extended period of time, the hamstrings will shorten to take up the slack. Decreased flexibility and increased tightness could be the result of a less physically active population that is instead watching television, talking on the telephone, playing computer games, and working at desks.

Critical Periods of Flexibility Development

Does a *critical period* exist during which stretching is most effective in developing flexibility? A critical period is the time after the age when one becomes capable of performing a particular function effectively, when changes are most likely to occur at rapid or optimal rates. Flexibility can be developed at any age, given the appropriate training. However, the rate of improvement will not be the same at every age, nor will the potential for improvement.

Sermeev (1966) studied hip-joint mobility in 1,440 athletes, 10 to 30 years of age, of both sexes, and 3,000 children and adults not participating in sports. He demonstrated that hip-joint mobility is not developed identically at various ages and not equally for various movements. Specifically, the greatest improvement occurs between the ages of 7 and 11 years. By 15 years of age, the indices of mobility in the hip joint are maximal, and in later years, that amount decreases.

This information does not mean that a stretching program has no benefit after the critical period has passed or that one critical period determines all potential. Can the effects of the lack of stretching and consequent tightness during the critical period (i.e., the growing years) be counteracted by engaging in stretching programs after the critical period has passed? This question is relevant for older adolescents and adults.

Evidence suggests that even senior adults benefit from exercise programs for developing ROM (Barrett and Smerdely 2002; Bell and Hoshizaki 1981; Dummer et al. 1985; Frekany and Leslie 1975; Germain and Blair 1983; Hong et al. 2000; Hopkins et al. 1990; Lan et al. 1996; Morey et al. 1989; Rider and Daly 1991; Rikli and Busch 1986; Van Deusen and Harlowe 1987). Maintained or increased use of full joint range could help maintain ROM and offset some of its age-related loss (Bassey et al. 1989). In general, however, the longer one waits to start some type of flexibility program after adolescence, the less likelihood of absolute improvement.

GENDER DIFFERENCES IN FLEXIBILITY

Evidence suggests that, generally, females are more flexible than males (Allander et al. 1974; Gabbard and Tandy 1988; Haley et al. 1986; Jones et al. 1986). Although conclusive evidence is lacking, several factors, including anatomical and physiological differences, may account for the difference in flexibility between the sexes. Other factors could be smaller muscle mass, joint geometry, and gender-specific collagenous muscle structure (McHugh et al. 1992).

Anatomical Gender Differences

The pelvic regions of men and women allow the female human body a greater range of flexibility. Men's pelvic bones are generally heavier and rougher; the brim is not as rounded; the cavity is less spacious; the sacrosciatic notch, pubic arch, and sacrum are narrower; and the acetabula are closer together than women's. Generally, most women have broader and shallower hips than men and therefore a greater ROM in the pelvic region. In particular, the shallowness of the female pelvis permits a greater degree of joint play.

However, even among women, pelvic types vary, and each has its own influence on ROM. The most commonly used pelvic classification system was developed by Caldwell and Moloy (1933). It describes four main groups based on the shape of the pelvic brim.

1. The *gynecoid* pelvis is the most common type, occurring in 50% of all women. This pelvic type permits the easiest vaginal birth and is characterized by a round or slightly oval pelvic inlet. The subpubic angle, or the pubic arch, is almost 90°.

2. The *android* pelvis resembles the male pelvis and is found in about 20% of women. It is characterized by a heart-shaped brim, a wedge-shaped pelvic inlet, and a subpubic angle between 60° and 75°. This pelvis shape, also called the "funnel" pelvis, produces difficulty in delivery because the baby's head frequently becomes arrested transversely in the midpelvis.

3. The *platypelloid* or *flat* pelvis is the least common among men and women. It is found in less than 5% of those examined and has a kidney-shaped brim and a narrow anteroposterior diameter. During labor, rotation of the baby's head may be restricted, and deep transverse flattening of the head may occur.

4. The *anthropoid* pelvis is found in about 20% of women. It has an oval brim, a larger anteroposterior diameter, and a smaller transverse diameter compared with the other types of pelvises. Generally, the pelvis is so large that labor is easy.

Women usually have a greater range of extension in the elbow. Hyperextension may sometimes be linked to the presence of a supratrochlear foramen, an aperture linking the cornoid and olecranon fossae (Amis and Miller 1982). This ability is the result of women having a shorter upper curve of the olecranon process of the elbow than men.

Hormonal Effects of Pregnancy on Flexibility

Pregnancy affects flexibility by increasing joint laxity (Abramson et al. 1934; Bird et al. 1981; Brewer and Hinson 1978). According to McNitt-Gray (1991), the changes in the pelvic joint during late pregnancy may have both local and systemic causes. Local causes include the weight of the uterus on the pelvic brim and biomechanical factors such as modifications in the center of mass and changes on mechanical loading. Systemic causes are presumably circulating hormones the most commonly of which is *relaxin*. After childbirth, the production of relaxin decreases, and the ligaments tighten up again. Additional research is required to quantify relaxin-induced changes that occur throughout the body.

Relaxin

Relaxin is a polypeptide hormone structurally related to insulin. It is secreted by the corpus luteum. Three main biological actions have been identified with relaxin: inhibition of uterine contraction, elongation of the interpubic ligament, and softening of the cervix. During pregnancy, the cervix undergoes modifications that allow sufficient dilation for the passage of the fetus at birth. Relaxin was thought to cause joint laxity in pregnant women, but some studies found that increased joint laxity in pregnant women is not associated with serum relaxin levels (Blecher and Richmond 1998; Samuel et al. 1996). Relaxin levels were not associated with human cervical ripening (Eppel et al. 1999) nor with symphyseal distention or pelvic pain in pregnancy (Bjökrlund et al. 2000). The hormonal influences that bring about softening of the cervix are still poorly understood.

Hormone Effects on Newborns

The limited literature on the relationship between estrogen and joints in newborns deals with congenital dislocation of the hip. Andren and Borglin (1961) suggested that congenital dislocation of the hip could be the consequence of abnormal estrogen metabolism in the fetus during the perinatal period. However, Aarskog et al. (1966) criticized the work of Andren and Borglin (1961) and found no supporting data in their study. Thieme et al. (1968) also determined that this hypothesis was not supported.

Other Effects of Pregnancy on Flexibility

The biological changes that occur in pregnant women have significance for various specialized health-care providers, such as podiatrists, orthodontists, chiropractors, osteopaths, medical doctors specializing in orthopedics, and physical therapists. Peripheral joints, such as the feet, fingers, and knees experience increases in joint laxity during pregnancy (Alvarez et al. 1988; Block et al. 1985; Calguneri et al. 1982; Danforth 1967). Ligament laxity in the lower back and pelvis has been linked with sacroiliac dysfunction (DonTigny 1985) and changes in the pubic symphysis (DonTigny 1985; Mikawa et al. 1988). Regarding potential cause and treatment, Williams et al. (1995) write

> During pregnancy, the pelvic joints and ligaments relax, while movements increase. Relaxation renders the sacroiliac locking mechanism less effective, permitting greater rotation and perhaps allowing alterations in pelvic diameters at childbirth, although the effect is probably small. The impaired locking mechanism diverts the strain of weight-bearing to the ligaments, with frequent sacroiliac strain after pregnancy. After childbirth the ligaments tighten and the locking mechanism improves; but this may occur in a position adopted during pregnancy. Such sacroliac 'subluxation' causes pain by unusual ligamentous tension; reduction by forcible manipulation may be attempted. The most common position in this condition of subluxation is believed to be backward rotation of the innominate bone relative to the sacrum; usually unilateral, it is on occasion bilateral. (p. 678)

Effects of Oral Contraceptives

Oral contraceptives are administered to female athletes for a variety of therapeutic reasons (Lebrun 1993). Bennell et al. (1999b) identified several benefits from this use of oral contraceptives: It is a reliable and reversible form of contraception. It decreases the risk of iron deficiency anemia by decreasing menstrual blood loss. It allows manipulation of the menstrual cycle for travel, training, and competition commitments. However, several researchers have published papers lending credence to a hormonal influence on ligamentous laxity and anterior cruciate ligament (ACL) injury. Oral contraceptives may induce structural changes in the metabolism of ACL fibroblasts, resulting in structural and compositional changes. These changes, in turn, could reduce strength of the ACL, predisposing female athletes to ligament injury (Liu et al. 1997). Oral contraceptives may also have significant influences on factors such as neuromuscular coordination and muscular strength (Bennell et al. 1999b; Hewett 2000). Möller-Nielsen and Hammar (1989) found that women using oral contraceptives had a lower injury rate than women not using oral contraceptives. The investigators suggested oral contraceptives might "ame-

liorate some symptoms of the premenstrual and menstrual period which might also affect coordination and hence the risk of injury" (p. 126).

However, several investigators have raised awareness that oral contraceptives could possibly increase the risk of ligament injury (Baker 1998; Bennell et al. 1999b; Hewett 2000; Liu et al. 1997; Liu et al. 1996). Pokorny et al. (2000) found that "self-reported oral contraceptive use was not associated with peripheral joint laxity with the knee, fifth finger distal interphalangeal joint and second finger of the proximal interphalangeal joint" (p. 687). However, the researchers cautioned, "another possibility is that oral contraceptives do affect joint laxity, although not in the 3 joints examined" (p. 687). Clearly, additional clinical studies are needed to evaluate the effect of the oral contraceptives on joint and muscle structure.

BODY BUILD AND FLEXIBILITY

Attempts to relate flexibility to factors such as body proportions, body surface area, skinfold thickness (obesity), and weight have yielded inconsistent results. What is almost unanimously agreed upon is that flexibility is specific (American College of Sports Medicine 2000; Dickenson 1968; Harris 1969a, 1969b). Thus, ROM in the shoulder is not correlated with ROM in the hip, and ROM in one hip or shoulder may not be highly related to ROM in the same joint on the opposite side. Furthermore, flexibility is not only specific to the joints but is also specific to individual joint movements because different musculature, bone structure, and connective tissue are involved in different joint movements. Therefore, no evidence confirms that flexibility exists as a single general characteristic of the human body. Thus, no single composite test or joint action measure can give a satisfactory index of the flexibility characteristics of an individual (American College of Sports Medicine 2000; Harris 1969a, 1969b).

Body Segment Lengths and Flexibility

Several investigators have found that body build as determined by segmental length is not significantly correlated with toe-touch flexibility (Broer and Gales 1958; Harvey and Scott 1967; Mathews et al. 1957; Mathews et al. 1959). In contrast, Broer and Gales (1958) and Wear (1963) found that people with a longer trunk-plus-arm measurement and relatively short legs have an advantage in the toe-touch test over those with long legs and relatively short trunk-plus-arm measurements. The ability to touch the toes with the fingertips may be considered normal for young children; however, between the ages of 11 and 14 years, many young adolescents who show no signs of muscle or joint tightness are unable to complete this movement. Thus, apparently limited flexibility occurs gradually over the same period of years during which the legs become proportionally longer in relation to the trunk (Kendall and Kendall 1948; Kendall et al. 1970; Kendall et al. 1971). However, Harvey and Scott (1967) found no significant difference between means of the best bend-and-reach scores and excess upper body length (trunk-plus-arm length minus leg length) or the ratio of the trunk-plus-arm length to leg length. When prone back extension and supine back extension were compared with trunk length, no significant correlation was found (Wear 1963).

Questions persist regarding bias for individuals with extreme arm-leg length differences and other extreme body dimensions. Jackson and Baker (1986) investigated the validity of the sit-and-reach test. They found moderate support ($r = .64$) for the test as a measure of hamstring flexibility and less support ($r = .28$) for the test as a measure of low-back flexibility. Jackson and Langford (1989) found good support ($r = .89$ for males and $r = .70$ for females) for the sit-and-reach test as a measure of hamstring flexibility. In contrast, support ($r = .59$ for males and $r = .12$ for females) for the test as a measure of low-back flexibility was less. Liemohn et al. (1994) found the sit-and-reach test "does not have criterion related validity [$r = .29$ to $.40$, ns] as a field test of low-back flexion ROM" (p. 93).

Cornbleet and Woolsey (1996) have criticized the standard sit-and-reach test as not being a valid measure of back motion. They contend, "more attention needs to be given to the final position of the hip joint rather than measuring the final position of the finger tips" (p. 854). Therefore, an inclinometer should be placed vertically on the sacrum to measure the hip-joint angle during the sit-and-reach test. Safety concerns are another reason some have attempted to modify the sit-and-reach test. The *back saver sit-and-reach test* (BSR) is a modified version that stretches one hamstring at a time while the other leg is flexed. The rationale "emanates from the work of Cailliet (1988) who suggested that simultaneously stretching both hamstrings may result in excessive posterior disc compression due to the anterior portion of the vertebrae being pressed together" (Patterson et al. 1996). Patterson et al. (1996) found the BSR test similar to the sit-and-reach and modified sit-and-reach test of Hoeger et al. (1990) as a test of hamstring flexibility. Another improvisation is the chair sit-and-reach test (CSR). This test was designed for many older people who, because of their medical conditions or functional limitations, cannot get down and up from the floor positions. The CSR required "participants to sit near the front edge of a chair, extending one leg straight out in front of the hip, with the other leg bent and slightly off to the side" (Jones et al. 1998, p. 339). The CSR test results for both male and female participants were reasonable accurate ($r = .76$ and $.81$, respectively).

One possible confounding factor is the difference in individual scapular abduction during the sit-and-reach test. Scapular abduction may account for an estimated 3 to 5 cm of variation in the final sit-and-reach score (Hopkins 1981). Consequently, Hopkins (1981) and Hopkins and Hoeger (1986) have proposed a modified sit-and-reach (MSR) test to negate the effects of shoulder girdle mobility and proportional differences between arms and legs. The MSR test establishes a zero point for each individual on the finger-to-box distance (FBD) based on proportional differences in limb lengths (see figure 10.1). Hoeger et al. (1990) and Hoeger and Hopkins (1992) found that the MSR test does help control for disparities. Normative data and flexibility fitness categories for the MSR test have been reported (Hoeger 1991; Hoeger et al. 1991).

Gatton and Pearcy (1999) suggest that taller subjects have a larger range of spinal flexion than shorter subjects, based on the assumption that ligament strain is the limiting factor in spinal flexion. Because taller people in general are expected to have slightly longer torsos compared with shorter people, taller people are therefore reasonably expected to have longer ligament lengths. Elaborating, they write

> We can investigate the effect of subject height change in a mathematical model of the lumbar spine simply by adjusting the initial height of the intervertebral discs. A 10 mm change in subject height approximately represents a 0.45 mm change in height of the lumbar spine. Spreading this change equally over the joints of the lumbar spine results in an increase in trunk rotation of 0.8 degrees. This change in *[sic]* comparable to the observed relationship between height and range of spinal rotation where a 1 cm height change results in a 0.72 degree increase in spinal flexion.

The relationship between subject height and range of spinal flexion raises some interesting questions in relation to apparent differences in range of spinal flexion between males and females. This study reported a significantly larger range of spinal flexion for males than females. Taking into account that the mean height of males is 0.11 m larger than that for females, one must ask whether the difference in range of spinal flexion between the sexes is not, at least partially, a remnant of the height difference (p. 381).

Body Weight and Somatotype Effects on Flexibility

Weight, somatotype, skinfold thickness, and body surface area have all been investigated for their possible relationships to flexibility. McCue (1963) found very few significant relationships between overweight and

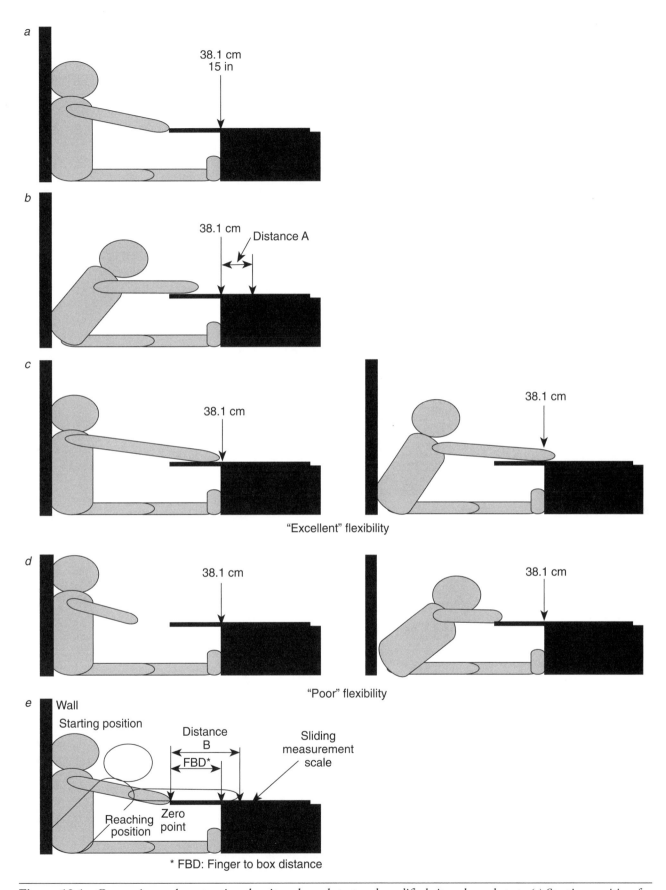

a

38.1 cm
15 in

b

38.1 cm   Distance A

c

38.1 cm

38.1 cm

"Excellent" flexibility

d

38.1 cm

38.1 cm

"Poor" flexibility

e   Wall
Starting position

Distance
B

Sliding
measurement
scale

FBD*

Reaching
position

Zero
point

* FBD: Finger to box distance

Figure 10.1   Comparing and contrasting the sit-and-reach test and modified sit-and-reach test. (*a*) Starting position for the sit-and-reach test. (*b*) The standard sit-and-reach test. (*c*) "Excellent" flexibility on the standard sit-and-reach test. (*d*) "Poor" flexibility on the standard sit-and-reach test. (*e*) The modified sit-and-reach test.

Reprinted from Hoeger and Hopkins 1992.

underweight body builds and flexibility. Tyrance (1958) found few significant relationships between flexibility and three extremes in body build: thinnest underweight, fattest overweight, and most muscular. Correlations between flexibility and somatotype are also insignificant (Laubach and McConville 1966a, 1966b). A misconception is that very large individuals (in excess of 300 pounds, or 150 kg) have limited flexibility. Size may be a factor where the extra accumulation of either fat or muscle serves as a wedge (e.g., a large midsection impeding a sit-and-reach test). However, the ability of sumo wrestlers weighing 200 kg to master a complete straddle split eliminates any doubt that size is necessarily a limiting factor in flexibility.

In terms of lean body mass as calculated by skinfold measurements, flexibility differences were again found to be insignificant (Laubach and McConville 1966a). Krahenbuhl and Martin (1977) found that relationship between body surface area and flexibility was significantly inversely related or not related at all, depending upon the body parts tested. Gabbard and Tandy (1988) examined the relationship of body fatness to the performance of 5-year-old and 6-year-old males and females on the sit-and-reach flexibility test. The data suggested that body fat at four measured sites had little to do with flexibility in either sex. Kettunen et al. (2000) found former elite athletes aged 45 to 68 years with a high body mass index (BMI) had lower ROM than subjects with low BMI.

Passive stiffness is significantly correlated to body mass and muscle thickness (Kubo, Kanehisa, and Fukunaga 2001a). Furthermore, Magnusson et al. (1997) reported that the cross-sectional area of the lateral hamstrings was positively related to the passive torque offered by the hamstrings during a stretch maneuver. Women have less resistance to stretch than men, which is attributed to their muscle mass (Gajdosik et al. 1990). Women also have less collagen in their connective tissue.

RACIAL DIFFERENCES IN FLEXIBILITY

The literature reveals that the properties of skeletal muscle and connective tissue *are* related to physical performance, and these also differ among certain racial groups (Suminski et al. 2002). The term *race* implies membership in a group in which substantial genetic similarities exist among individuals (Malina 1988). Milne et al. (1976) compared 553 black and white children in kindergarten, 1st grade, and 2nd grade. The grade-race interaction effect indicated that white children were generally more flexible than black children, but the only significant difference ($p < .01$) was at the 2nd-grade level. Jones et al. (1986) tested 2,546 black and white children in grades 2, 4, and 6. Racial differences in flexibility across sexes and grades were not substantiated. Elbow hyperextension has also been reported to be greater in blacks than in whites (Amis and Miller 1982).

The relationship between genetics, race, and viscoelastic characteristics of muscles has not received much attention. Fukashiro et al. (2002) investigated the viscoelastic properties of the triceps surae muscle group. They compared 44 college athletes (black: $n = 22$; white: $n = 22$; female: $n = 11$; male: $n = 11$). Black athletes were found to have significantly greater muscle viscosity and elasticity than white athletes. Thus, muscle stiffness was greater among black athletes. The researchers speculated that the "greater muscle stiffness could contribute to greater sprint/jump performance among black athletes, compared with white athletes" (p. 183).

A decisive conclusion regarding the relationship between racial origin and flexibility or muscle stiffness cannot be rendered without detailed and controlled studies. The obstacles to such studies are extremely challenging: "This could be a difficult task given the methodological issues facing such studies, for example, confounding factors (e.g., influence of environmental factors), genetic heterogeneity, and the need to use a longitudinal study design" (Suminski et al. 2002, p. 671).

GENETICS AND FLEXIBILITY

Researchers have documented a genetic factor among some contortionist families. Inherited connective tissue syndromes such as EDS clearly have a genetic component. What does the research indicate regarding flexibility values for biological relatives? Unfortunately, research in this area is limited. A review of the literature was carried out by Bouchard et al. (1997).

> Estimated heritability for lower-back flexibility in a sample of male twins 11 to 15 years old was 0.69 (Kovar 1981a), while heritabilities in a combined sample of male and female twins 12 to 17 years old were .84, .70, and .91 for trunk, hip, and shoulder flexibility, respectively (Kovar 1981b). In contrast, estimated heritability of the sit-and-reach in Indian twins of both sexes 10 to 27 years of age was only .18; controlling for age and several anthropometric indicators of body size raised the estimated heritability to .50 (Chatterjee and Das 1995).

Correlations for lower-back flexibility in biological siblings and parent-offspring pairs were, respectively, .43 and .29 in a Mennonite community (Devor and Crawford 1984) and .36 and .26 in a nationally represented sample of the Canadian population (Pérusse, Leblanc, and Bouchard 1988). Interestingly, among the Mennonite community, grandparent-grandchild and uncle/aunt-nephew/niece correlations were of similar magnitude, .37 and .30, respectively (Devor and Crawford 1984). Although the data are limited, the preceding findings may suggest somewhat more genetic influence in flexibility than in strength and motor tasks. In addition, spouse resemblance in lower-back flexibility is quite low, −.99 in the Mennonite (Devor and Crawford 1984) and .10 in the Canadian samples (Pérusse, Leblanc, and Bouchard 1988).

DOMINANT LATERALITY AND FLEXIBILITY

Human handedness has been a source of curiosity for centuries. One of the earliest mentions of handedness is found in the Bible (*Judges* 20:16), which states that the 26,700-man army of Benjamin had 700 left-handed soldiers. Many people tend to favor a dominant side in their chosen sports or activities. Consequently, they often possess greater strength, coordination, balance, and proprioceptive awareness on one side. Reasons for unilateral development are unknown, although theories exist.

Lateralization Versus Mixed Dominance

Sometimes dominance may be mixed (i.e., no clear hand preference exists). For example, a baseball player may bat left-handed and throw right-handed, or a right-handed diver may twist to the right side (right-handed people normally twist to the left side because the dominant right arm is used to thrust or wrap across the body). Occasionally, some athletes exhibit bilateral skills, despite the unilateral nature of their activities. A baseball switch-hitter, for example, can bat from either side of the plate. In some disciplines, bilateral skills are possible (e.g., dribbling a basketball, leg kicks in the martial arts, and dribbling and kicking in soccer), and in others they are required (e.g., swimming and power lifting).

Studies have provided evidence of the effect of dominant laterality on the normal musculoskeletal system. Hand grips are stronger on the dominant side (Haywood 1980; Lunde et al. 1972), and bone density is reportedly greater on the dominant side in the lower radius (Ekman et al. 1970) and in the os calcis (Webber and Garnett 1976). Dobeln (personal communication, cited in Allander et al. 1974) found that the radioulnar width in 434 males aged 16 to 27 years (including 307 subjects aged 19 to 21 years) was greater in the right side (*p* = .001). Muscles of the leg and forearm on the dominant side tend to be larger, more dense on computer tomographic scans, and stronger than on the nondominant side of normal people (Merletti et al. 1986; Murray and Sepic 1968). Furthermore, bone density and muscle mass are also greater in the dominant arm of tennis players (Chinn et al. 1974).

Mysorekar and Nandedkar (1986) observed that human beings have a tendency to incline their heads predominantly to one side or the other. They investigated whether dominance in the atlantooccipital articulations would account for this phenomenon. They found that the right side has a tendency to have larger facets or condyles. Because the difference was not statistically significant, a clear right-side dominance could not be identified.

The relationship between dominant laterality and ROM has received attention, but only a few studies have involved general populations. Allander et al. (1974) found reduced mobility in the right wrist in comparison with the left in both sexes. The researchers believed that this observation was "in accordance with the higher level of exposure to trauma of the right hand in a predominantly right-handed population" (p. 259). Their study also found restriction of movement in the rotation of the left hip joint compared with the right (*p* = .001 for males; *p* = .05 for females). This observation might be relevant to the position of the body at work. Kronberg et al. (1990) determined that the average angle for humeral head retroversion was 33° on the dominant side and 29° on the nondominant side in 50 healthy subjects, regardless of gender. A larger retroversion angle was consistent with an increased range of shoulder external rotation. Nonetheless, the study found only slight ROM differences between the dominant and nondominant shoulders. Moseley et al. (2001) measured passive ankle plantarflexion-dorsiflexion flexibility obtained from 300 able-bodied volunteers aged 15 to 34 years. Flexibility variables did not differ between the left and right ankles nor between the dominant and nondominant legs. The symmetry "may be a response to the relatively equal demands placed on both lower limbs during locomotion" (p. 517).

Effect of Lateralized Athletic Skills on Flexibility

Most of the research regarding ROM and laterality pertains to athletes. Chandler et al. (1990) found that tennis players' internal shoulder rotation was significantly tighter on the dominant side than on the nondominant side, and that their range of external shoulder rotation was significantly greater on the dominant side than on the nondominant side. Chinn et al. (1974) substantiated that both male and female tennis players displayed significant decreases in flexibility in internal shoulder rotation of the playing arm. Both sexes also had significant decreases in radioulnar pronation and supination of the playing arm.

Gurry et al. (1985) found no significant differences in the flexibility of the right and left sides among baseball players. In contrast, Tippett (1986) found a significantly greater hip flexion on the kick leg than on the stance leg and a greater internal hip rotation of the stance leg than of the kick leg of baseball pitchers. According to Tippett (1986), "the results appear to be products of the pitching mechanism or the pitcher himself, just as specific upper extremity motion, strength, and anatomical characteristics have been found specific to pitchers" (p. 14).

Koslow (1987) tested 320 male and female students of specific ages (i.e., 9, 13, 17, and 21 years) for bilateral flexibility of shoulder flexion-extension and of the lower extremity (by a modified sit-and-reach test). Little difference was found between the dominant and nondominant shoulders of the 13-year-old, 17-year-old, and 21-year-old females. In contrast, shoulder range measurements for the males significantly decreased for the same age groups. Dominant shoulder joint flexibility measures of the 17-year-old and 21-year-old females were significantly greater than those of the 17-year-old and 21-year-old males. Males' decrease in dominant shoulder flexibility with age may relate to their activity patterns in such a way as to inhibit increases in flexibility. Specifically, males may exhibit a more forceful and mature (effective) throwing pattern as compared with females across all ages. Flexibility measures of the nondominant lower extremity of the 17-year-old and 21-year-old males were significantly greater than the same measures of the dominant lower extremity. For the females, a very small and insignificant increase of flexibility in the nondominant leg was found for all the age groups except the 9-year-olds.

In another study (Bonci et al. 1986) of static and dynamic range of the glenohumeral joint of male and female athletes, the dominant arm had approximately 5% more motion compared with the nondominant arm in both sexes. Dynamic ROM averaged 25° more than static motion. An analysis of the effect of a modified Bristow surgical procedure for recurrent dislocation or subluxation of the shoulder demonstrated that static and dynamic ROM were significantly reduced by surgery. Henry (1986, p. 17), commenting on the paper of Bonci et al. (1986), stated that the main point is "postoperative range of motion in the dominant shoulder compared to the range of motion in the nondominant side can be misleading due to the increased range of motion of the dominant shoulder prior to surgery."

WARMING UP AND COOLING DOWN

Warm-up is a group of exercises performed immediately before an activity to provide a period of adjustment between rest and exercise. Warm-up improves performance and reduces the chance of injury by mobilizing the individual mentally as well as physically (Sweet 2001). Analogous to warm-up is cool-down (also called warmdown). *Cool-down* is a group of exercises performed immediately after an activity to provide a period of adjustment between exercise and rest. Stretching is often utilized as an adjunct to warm-up or cool-down. However, stretching is not a warm-up activity. Stretching before warm-up increases the risk of injury.

Warming Up

Warm-up is either *passive* or *active*. Passive warm-up incorporates the use of an outside agent or modality (e.g., hot baths, infrared light, or ultrasound). Active warm-up is self-initiated and can be further divided into *formal* and *general* warm-up. Formal warm-up includes movements that either mimic or are employed in the actual performance activity (e.g., a baseball player will throw a ball or swing a bat to warm up). General warm-up consists of movements not directly related to those employed in the activity itself (e.g., light calisthenics, jogging, or stationary bicycling). The nature of the warm-up depends on the individual's needs. It should be intense enough to increase the body core temperature and cause some sweating but not so intense as to cause fatigue (Hagerman 2001; Karvonen 1992; Kulund and Töttössy 1983; Shellock and Prentice 1985; Stewart and Sleivert 1998). The effects of warm-up will ultimately wear off (Whelan et al. 1999), but how soon depends on a number of factors such as clothing, exercise intensity, and specificity of the warm-up. Hardy et al. (1983) found that passive warm-up was significantly more effective in increasing hip flexion than active warm-up. Whelan et al. (1999) also found warm-up significantly increased flexibility as measured by the sit-and-reach test in downhill skiers. Stewart and Sleivert (1998) found that warm-up improved ROM in ankle dorsiflexion and hip extension, but knee flexion did not change.

The benefits of warm-up are possibly more psychological than physiological (Harmer 1991; Karvonen 1992; Kulund and Töttössy 1983; Miller 2002; Shellock and Prentice 1985; Sweet 2001; Tiidus and Shoemaker 1995). Explanations depend upon specific circumstances and methodologies. Conventional warm-up may help athletes become more mentally prepared, "if they use a specific method of warm-up which provides them with a rehearsal of the event" (Shellock and Prentice 1985, p. 271). The time before the athletic competition may be a time of frustration for certain athletes. Warm-up routines may provide a suitable constructive outlet channel for athletes to vent their anxieties. An athlete's level of arousal influences performance. As explained by Karvonen (1992), "complex performances are enhanced if arousal can be alleviated, while simple performances are improved when arousal is increased. Perhaps warm-up could be used either to alleviate or to enhance arousal depending on the type of performance to follow" (p. 197). Consequently, performance is enhanced.

A clear distinction should be made between *warm-up exercises* and *flexibility exercises*. Flexibility exercises are used to increase the ROM of a joint or set of joints progressively and permanently. Flexibility exercises should always be *preceded* by a set of mild warm-up exercises because the increase in the tissue temperature produced by the warm-up exercises makes the flexibility exercises both safer and more productive (Sapega et al. 1981).

However, an increase in temperature causes a reduction in tensile strength of connective tissue, and thus more ruptures might be expected after warming up, but increased temperature seems to cause an increase in extensibility, which may be the reason warming up does indeed prevent ruptures (Troels 1973). Despite the widely held belief that warm-up reduces the risk of injury and improves performance, compliance of athletes and nonathletes has been found inadequate among golfers (Fradkin et al. 2001) and college students (Simon 1992). Furthermore, contrary to popular belief, warm-up performed "without" stretching does not increase ROM (Shrier and Gossal 2000).

Benefits associated with warming up include the following (Bishop 2003; Goats 1994; Hemmings et al. 2000; Karvonen 1992; Whelan et al. 1999; Verkhoshansky and Siff 1993):

- Increased body and tissue temperature
- Increased blood flow through active muscles by reducing vascular bed resistance
- Increased heart rate, which will prepare the cardiovascular system for work
- Increased metabolic rate
- Increases in the Bohr effect, which facilitates the exchange of oxygen from hemoglobin
- Increased speed at which nerve impulses travel, and thereby facilitation of body movements
- Increased efficiency of reciprocal innervation (thus allowing opposing muscles to contract and relax faster and more efficiently)
- Increased physical working capacity
- Decreased viscosity (or resistance) of connective tissue and muscle
- Decreased muscular tension (improved muscle relaxation)
- Enhanced connective tissue and muscular extensibility
- Enhanced psychological performance

Kopell (1962) believes that some fatalities associated with exercise may have been avoided if adequate warm-up had occurred. Barnard et al. (1973a, 1973b) have suggested that warm-up also prevents ST segment depression (an electrocardiographic abnormality). This abnormality is sometimes seen in healthy people at the beginning of fast running performances.

Viscosity Effects

Viscosity is resistance to flow, or an apparent force that prevents fluids from flowing easily. Connective tissue and muscular viscosity might be partially responsible for restricting movement. Viscosity has no long-term effect on the improvement of one's flexibility. Rather, its effects

relate to various physiological factors that exist at the moment stretch is developed. Temperature has an inverse effect on viscosity; that is, as the temperature increases, fluid viscosity decreases, and vice versa. Reduced viscosity facilitates relaxation of collagenous tissues (Sapega et al. 1981). The mechanism behind this thermal transition is still unknown. However, the collagen intermolecular bonding possibly becomes partially destabilized, enhancing the flow properties of collagenous tissue (Mason and Rigby 1963; Rigby et al. 1959). This reduced viscosity in turn decreases resistance to movement and increases flexibility.

The most common method of elevating body temperature and reducing tissue viscosity is warm-up exercise. Other methods include superficial heat (heat packs, hot showers) and deep heat (diathermy and ultrasound). The effectiveness of a heat pad applied to the back of the thigh did not affect the ROM in the hip joint. However, when combined with stretching, hip flexion increased further but not significantly (Henricson et al. 1984). Heating pads raise temperature in superficial muscles only a few degrees. The subcutaneous fat and natural vascular cooling system possibly prevent further increases in temperature of the muscles and the connecting tissues of the hip joint (Lehmann et al. 1966; Prentice 1982).

Continuous ultrasound can effectively increase temperatures in human muscle and tendon (Draper et al. 1995; Draper et al. 1991) to therapeutic levels. However, Draper et al. (1998), Draper and Ricard (1995) and Rose et al. (1996) found tissue temperatures remain at therapeutic levels for only 2 to 4 minutes. Therefore, stretch must immediately follow treatment to take advantage of these higher temperatures (Draper et al. 1998). Draper et al. (1998) found the increased ROM associated with ultrasound heat "is not maintained over the long term and is not more than the range of motion gained from stretching alone" (p. 141).

Effect of Warm-Up on Injury Rates

Several studies have raised questions about the ability of warm-up exercise to increase flexibility and reduce injury. Williford et al. (1986) investigated the effects of warming up the joints by jogging and then stretching on increasing joint flexibility. Their results did not support the claim that warming up the muscle by jogging before stretching results in significant increases for all the joint motion angles evaluated. The Ontario cohort study of 1,680 runners found that runners who say they never warm up have less risk of injury than those who do, and runners who use stretching "sometimes" are at apparently higher risk of injury than those who usually or never use stretching (Walter et al. 1989). However, Grana cautioned in an interview by Finkelstein and Roos (1990), that the study's findings probably reflect "the terrible number of variables that you can't control" (p. 49) in such a study.

van Mechelen et al. (1993) conducted a 16-week study of 316 subjects randomly split into an intervention group (159 subjects) and a control group (167 subjects). Injury incidences for control and intervention subjects were 4.9 and 5.5 running injuries, respectively, per 1,000 hours of running exposure. Therefore, warm-up, cool-down, and stretching exercises did not reduce the running injury incidence.

Further confounding the controversy regarding the benefits of warm-up was a study by Strickler et al. (1990) investigating the effects of passive warming on biomechanical properties of the musculotendinous unit of rabbit hindlimbs heated to 35° C (95° F) and 39° C (102° F) and then subjected to controlled strain injury. The force at failure was greater at 35° C than at 39° C, and the difference in energy absorbed by the muscles before rupture was not statistically significant. Obviously, the relationship among warm-up, stretching, flexibility, and injury is extremely complex, and additional research is needed to resolve these uncertainties.

Murphy (1986) points out a dangerous misconception about the order of stretching and warm-up in an exercise program:

> Some health clubs and fitness instructors have encouraged athletes to stretch *before* warming up. Their reasoning: Cold muscles, they claim, are like plastic, and stretching them results in a more permanent stretch, as opposed to stretching the muscles when they are warm and pliable like a rubber band. (p. 45)

This method is *not* supported by any research. It is an invitation to probable injury. Stretching should *always* be preceded by warm-up.

Cooling Down

Cool-down is a group of exercises performed immediately after an activity to provide a period of adjustment between exercise and rest. Although cool-down may serve as an additional effort to improve flexibility, its main objective is to facilitate muscular relaxation, promote the removal of muscular waste products by the blood, reduce muscular soreness, and allow the cardiovascular system to adjust to lowered demand. Stretching should be incorporated immediately after the main part of a workout and cool-down period, because tissue temperatures are highest (Sapega et al. 1981).

Karvonen (1992) has suggested that cool-down is also important in reaching an emotional balance after the possible disappointment of a poor performance. In particular, when the next competition or performance soon follows, preparation for it can begin during the cool-down from the initial performance. Furthermore, the cool-down period may be the most beneficial time for the coach to give feedback.

STRENGTH TRAINING AND FLEXIBILITY

Numerous misconceptions and stereotypes exist about the relationship between strength training and flexibility (Prentice 2001). Many coaches and athletes believe that strength gains may limit flexibility or hinder suppleness or, conversely, that substantial gains in flexibility may have a deleterious effect on strength (Hebbelinck 1988). Some research has demonstrated that "strength increases are accompanied by increases in the stiffness of the muscle-tendon unit" (Klinge et al. 1997, p. 715). A common term used to describe well-developed and inflexible athletes is "muscle-bound." Brainum (2000) claims the true definition of muscle-bound "involves a chronic shortening of muscle, which would be induced by partial-rep training" (p. 123).

Todd (1985) identified several individuals who helped contribute to the myth of "muscle-bound lifter." Mac-Fadden (1912) wrote: "In taking up weight lifting, it would always be well to take some exercise for speed and flexibility to counteract the tendency to become slow. Weightlifting alone has a tendency to make the muscles slow" (p. 847). UCLA track coach Dean Cromwell (1941) commented: "The athlete . . . should not be a glutton for muscular development . . . If one goes too far . . . he can defeat his purpose by becoming muscle-bound and consequently a tense, tied-up athlete in competition" (p. 236). However, the belief that weight training causes a "muscle-bound" condition is false.

Arthur Jones (1975), the developer of Nautilus® equipment, points out several possible reasons why such beliefs persist: Certain individuals with large muscles lack a degree of flexibility; large muscles can be developed while doing absolutely nothing to improve one's flexibility; and activities that build large muscles can produce a loss of flexibility. However, the size of a person's muscle has very little or nothing to do with flexibility, and if strength training is properly conducted, it can in fact increase flexibility. This last point deserves special attention. Several investigators (Leighton 1956; Massey and Chaudet 1956; Schmitt et al. 1998; Wickstrom 1963; Wilmore et al. 1978) demonstrate that weight training does not decrease flexibility and in some instances actually improves it. However, an investigation (Barlow et al. 2002) that compared the flexibility of 29 male bodybuilders and 25 male non-bodybuilders revealed a significantly decreased internal rotation ROM (–11°) of the shoulder compared with the control group. No rationale was presented to explain the difference. Nevertheless, the investigators emphasized the importance of proper education and instruction on maintaining appropriate shoulder ROM and selection of proper resistance exercise to minimize the risk of shoulder pathology.

Bodybuilders and Decreased Internal Rotation

What causes the decreased internal rotation in the bodybuilders? Several causes are hypothetically possible. The body might be adapting to undue stresses that are imposed on the external rotators, the posterior shoulder muscular (i.e., the posterior deltoid, middle deltoid, teres minor, and infraspinatus), associated connective tissue, and joint capsule. Therefore, years of training might cause calcium deposits, adaptive shortening, and scar injury. Perhaps modification of the titin isoforms of the shoulder musculature occurs.

The external rotators resist glenohumeral joint distraction and help control and stabilize the scapula (i.e., these muscles communicate the shoulder joint to "come back"). Specifically, the bodybuilder's external shoulder rotators are at increased risk for injury because they contract eccentrically to resist glenohumeral joint distraction (either as prime synergists or stabilizers) during various exercises: the recovery (elongating or lowering) phase of double-arm cable rowing, straight-leg dead lifts, morning exercises, and one-arm dumbbell rows. The external rotators also probably play a role in stabilizing the scapula during the lowering phase of standing biceps curls. Therefore, decreased internal rotation may be the body's adaptive response to the lesser of two evils: the distraction of the humeral head out of the glenoid or undesirable movement of the scapula.

Many bodybuilders perform a wide variety of exercises to strengthen the major muscles associated with the shoulder (latissimus dorsi, the trapezius, the pectoralis major, and the posterior deltoids). However, very few perform exercises to strengthen the rotator cuff muscles (subscapularis, teres minor, supraspinatus, or infraspinatus). Many bodybuilders are perhaps obsessed with developing big showy muscles and concentrate disproportionately on these large muscles, which are often the area of focus when posing. They often neglect or ignore the important, yet relatively smaller, rotator cuff muscles such as those that externally rotate the shoulders. However, "the reverse of any action to contract a given muscle group becomes a stretch for that same muscle group" (Siff and Verkhoshansky 1999). Therefore, to stretch the internal rotator muscles, exercises must be performed that work the external muscle rotator group (i.e., the teres minor, supraspinatus, and infraspinatus). Excessive concentration on the internal rotator muscles can result in stronger, larger, and even shortened muscles and associated connective tissues.

Perhaps bodybuilders spend insufficient time stretching the muscles and connective tissues that restrict internal shoulder rotation. Bodybuilders might unknowingly employ training errors that promoted muscle imbalance and reduced ROM in the shoulder. Ways to increase internal shoulder rotation include (1) stretching the entire shoulder region, especially the external rotators; (2) strengthening the external rotators; and (3) eliminating faulty biomechanical or training errors.

In certain unique cases, a large increase in muscle bulk may affect ROM. For example, an athlete with large biceps and deltoids may experience difficulty in stretching the triceps. Holcomb (2000) points out that altering an athlete's training program can decrease muscle bulk. However, this change may not be advisable for power athletes such as shot-putters or offensive linemen in football. Therefore, Holcomb cautions strength and conditioning professionals to "keep the requirements of the athlete's sport in mind; the need for large muscles may supersede the need for extreme joint mobility" (p. 323).

Resistance training could have an adverse effect on the muscular stretching parameters (Wiemann and Hahn 1997). This hypothesis is based on the research of Suzuki and Hutton (1976) who found a postcontractile motor neural discharge produced by muscle afferent activation. Accordingly, a muscle should display an increased resting tension and decreased flexibility after resistance training. Consequently, a muscle should be stretched after each resistance-training workout to counteract the shortening effect of strength training (p. 340). However, Wiemann and Hahn (1997) found no change in resting tension as a result of resistance training. They also found no sign of any decrease in muscle-resting tension through short-term stretching. Elaborating on the study, they write: "Thus the risk of getting hypertensed muscles after resistance training seems to be rather unlikely. Consequently, the recommendation to perform stretching exercises especially after resistance training to avoid shortened muscles is questionable" (p. 345). Additional research is required to determine whether resistance training is followed by reduced or enhanced resting tension.

Only a few studies investigate the effects of strength training on flexibility in older subjects. Girouard and Hurley (1995) compared 31 untrained men between the ages of 50 and 74 years. Subjects were divided into three groups: strength and flexibility training, flexibility only training, and no training. Strength and flexibility training did significantly increase ROM in shoulder abduction and shoulder flexion (both $p < .01$), but none of these changes was significantly different from those in the inactive control group. "The implications of these results are that clinicians and instructors who are involved in exercise prescription should not assume that strength training alone will increase range of motion beyond a normal variability simply by selecting balance muscle use and going through the full range of motion" (p. 1448). Barbosa et al. (2002) determined that weight training without stretching exercises increased flexibility in elderly women between 62 and 78 years of age. Similarly, Fatouros et al. (2002) in a study of 32 inactive older men (65 to 78 years of age) found that "resistance training may be able to increase range of motion of a number of joints of inactive older individuals possibly due to an improvement in muscle strength" (p. 112). Thus, with proper training, one can improve overall strength and flexibility as long as the training is technically correct.

Developing flexibility with resistance techniques involves two key principles. (1) The entire muscle or muscle group must be worked through its full ROM, and (2) the emphasis on the negative phase of work must be gradual. *Negative work*, or *eccentric contraction*, takes place when a muscle is stretched (i.e., elongated) while it is contracting. This eccentric contraction is associated with the lowering phase of a resistance exercise.

During negative work, the number of contracting muscle fibers decreases. Because the workload is shared by a smaller number of muscle contractile components, the tension in each component increases. Consequently, the excessive stress and tension produces a greater stretch on the involved fibers, resulting in enhanced flexibility. However, eccentric training is also associated with muscle soreness.

CIRCADIAN VARIATIONS AND FLEXIBILITY

The quantitative study of biological phenomena that fluctuate periodically over time is called *chronobiology*. The term *diurnal* is frequently used for a rhythm whose period is 1 day. Conroy and Mills (1970) prefer *circadian* to indicate a period of approximately 24 hours. The term is derived from the Latin (*circa* = about; *dies* = day). Most physiological functions exhibit circadian rhythmicity: maximum and minimum functions occur at specific times of day. In humans, circadian rhythms are expressed by oscillations in various physiological systems, including blood pressure, body temperature, heart rate, hormone levels, and tremors. In addition, alertness and responsiveness to either internal stimuli (e.g., neurotransmitters, electrolytes, or metabolic substrates) or external stimuli (e.g., environmental factors, drugs, or food) oscillate as a function of circadian rhythms (Winget et al. 1985). Individuals commonly recall periods of stiffness related to specific times of the day as well as stiffness after activ-

ity or inactivity (Gifford 1987, Reilly 1998). Stiffness increases as body temperature decreases. Consequently, the increased stiffness commonly experienced toward the end of the day may reflect the fall in body temperature (Reilly 1998). This section discusses the interrelationship of time of day or night to flexibility.

Research Regarding the Diurnal Rhythm of Flexibility

Saying that people perceive greater stiffness after sleeping or at different times during the day is one thing, but determining whether a quantifiable decrease in ROM occurs is another. An early observation that flexibility varies with the time of day was reported by Osolin (1952, 1971) and cited by Dick (1980) and Bompa (1990). The highest amplitude of movement seems to be available between 1000 and 1100 hours and between 1600 and 1700 hours, whereas the lowest amplitude likely occurs earlier in the morning. According to Osolin (1971), the reason "seems to lie with the continuous biological changes (CNS and muscle's tonus) which occur during the day." Gifford (1987), citing the work of Stockton et al. (1980), found the greatest improvement of suppleness was between 0800 and 1200 hours. However, no details were given.

O'Driscoll and Tomenson (1982) measured cervical movements at 0700 and 1900 hours and recorded greater ranges in the evening than in the morning. Baxter and Reilly (1983) reported a "time of day" effect for trunk flexibility in 14 young swimmers, best at 1330 hours and poorest at 0630 hours. Gifford (1987) investigated the circadian flexibility in five different areas taken every 2 hours over a 24-hour period using 25 normal subjects between 25 and 32 years of age. The ability to bring the fingertip to the floor while standing on a wooden platform revealed that maximum stiffness occurred in the morning at or before rising from bed. Maximum flexibility occurred between midday and midnight. Maximum stiffness for lumbar flexion was recorded during the hours of sleep, with flexibility increasing from 0600 hours through the day. Lumbar extension displayed a rise from maximum stiffness during the early hours to maximum flexibility around 1400 hours, before gradually stiffening again toward evening. With the passive straight-leg raising test, minimal scores occurred when the majority of the subjects were either recumbent or relatively inactive (2200 to 0800 hours). Glenohumeral lateral rotation indicated an overall rise in ROM through the day and a decrease during the early hours of the morning. Russell et al. (1992) conducted a study of 10 young adults who were tested every 2 hours over a 24-hour period. The results showed a significant decrease in flexion, extension, and lateral bend for the lumbar spine after sleep and a significant increase in the afternoon compared with measurements taken between 0200 and 0730 hours. A report by Wing et al. (1992) on 12 volunteers found a decrease of lumbar flexion by 12 mm ($p < .005$) in the morning. The researchers speculated that the decreased flexibility may have been "due either to the overnight expansion of the intervertebral discs (inability of the discs to be compressed at the anterior border), or to stiffness of soft tissues resulting from overnight rest" (p. 765). Ensink et al. (1996) found that mean lumbar ROM in 29 patients with LBP rose from 54.30° in the morning to 68.30° in the evening. Mean flexion rose from 11.10°, whereas extension increased only 2.90° during the day.

Circadian Variation in Human Stature and Disk Height

The stature or height of the human body fluctuates throughout the day. These bodily fluctuations are important because of their potential influence on posture, mechanical efficiency, risk of injury, low-back pain, perception of stiffness, and flexibility. Fluctuation in bodily stature are the effects of posture, occupation, movement, vibration, load, gravity, age, disease, trauma, and nutritional status of the vertebral disks.

Factors That Influence Recovery of Stature

Recovery from spinal shrinkage occurs with bed rest. Can recovery be facilitated more quickly or effectively? Goode and Theodore (1983) demonstrated that a group of female subjects could adjust their height upward between 7 and 36 mm when standing tall compared with relaxed standing. Theoretically, applying a tensile force on the spinal column should enhance recovery from spinal shrinkage (Boocock et al. 1988, 1990; Kane et al. 1985; Nosse 1978). Badtke et al. (1993) demonstrated that positioning subjects in a specially developed extension apparatus produces in 8 minutes the same gain in spinal column length as 2 hours bed rest. In contrast, Pope and Klingenstierna (1986) reported that the increase in height is greater with lying down quietly than with traction. Recovery of height can also be achieved by adopting the Fowler position (i.e., supine with legs on a stool and with hips and knees flexed to achieve minimal spinal loading). Wilby et al. (1987) found that 20 minutes reclining in the Fowler position resulted in a 4.5 mm and 3.4 mm gain in body length in the morning and evening, respectively. Magnusson and Pope (1996) had 12 subjects loaded with 10 kg on the shoulders for 5 minutes. They experienced an average 6.33 mm loss of height. One group averaged a gain of 1.12 mm during the intervening unloaded sitting period. Those sitting unloaded and stretching for 15 seconds every minute for 5 minutes by hyperextensions experienced an average height gain of 5.05 mm. The researchers speculated that hyperextension "may be a means of temporarily shifting loads from the disc to the

facet" (p. 238). In addition, stretching "may be a way in which disc hydration can temporarily increase with a concomitant improvement of disc nutrition" (p. 238). Previously, Magnusson, Pope, and Hansson (1995) had also demonstrated that passive hyperextension for 20 minutes gave a significantly increased height recovery compared with the prone posture. Beynon and Reilly (2001) and Eklund and Corlett (1984) also substantiated that if short periods of unloading of the spine are allowed in a heavy job, a substantial recovery can take place during these rest pauses. Consequently, the total shrinkage or disk compression is diminished. Implementing appropriate rest pauses in occupational or athletic situations may potentially serve to reduce the risk of injury.

Influence of Sleep on Flexibility

People often feel stiff after sleeping. The following sections explore possible causes for this phenomenon.

Influence of Sleep on Increased Sensitivity

One possible explanation for waking with stiffness is a temporary change in the sensitivity of the Pacinian corpuscles, joint mechanoreceptors, muscle spindles, or Golgi tendon organs during sleep. Specifically, the respective receptors' sensitivity settings might be temporarily *reset* during the period of inactivity or sleep. Lee and Kleitman (1923) and Tuttle (1924) demonstrated a reduction of the amplitude of the patellar tendon reflex (knee jerk) in humans during sleep. Hormone effects may also influence spinal processes, as suggested by Tyrer and Bond (1974), who demonstrated diurnal variation in physiological tremor, which they hypothesized to be primarily the result of changes in circulating catecholamines among other possible explanations. Wolpaw et al. (1984) and Wolpaw and Seegal (1982) documented that the amplitude of the spinal stretch reflex in monkeys is subject to diurnal rhythm (i.e., altered excitability function by time of day). Winget et al. (1985) cite a dissertation (Freivalds 1979) that determined the minimum Achilles tendon reflex sensitivity (ms) as occurring between 2138 and 0845 hours. Additional research is required to determine whether the decreased body temperature during sleep can influence the various proprioceptors' stretch response thresholds.

The relationship between sleep, body temperature, and stiffness upon awakening has not been thoroughly investigated. Gillberg and Åkerstedt (1982) and Barrett et al. 1993) demonstrated that "deep body temperature shows a strong circadian rhythm, with a usual range variation of about 1° C" (Barrett et al. 1993, p. 93). Body temperature shows the greatest fall during the onset of sleep (Barrett et al. 1993; Gillberg and Åkerstedt 1982). Barrett et al. (1993) found sleeping temperatures were lower than corresponding waking temperatures by a mean of 0.31° C (32.5° F). In contrast, "waking up was accompanied by a slower transition, as temperatures tended to remain lower in the first hour after waking" (Barrett et al. 1993, p. 98). Can a difference of only 0.31° C influence tissue extensibility and perceived stiffness or influence joint receptors and muscle spindles? Additional research is required to answer this question.

Influence of Sleep on Vertebral Disks

During sleep, the spine is only lightly loaded and the disks swell by uptaking the body's tissue fluid. Consequently, total body length increases, and the fibers of the disk are under more tension (Botsford et al. 1994). However, throughout the normal activities of the day, the extra fluid is rapidly expelled from the disk. Adams et al. (1987) have identified three significant implications of diurnal variations in the stresses on the lumbar spine: (1) this swelling accounts for the increased stiffness in the spine during lumbar flexion upon awakening; (2) lumbar disks and ligaments are at greater risk for injury in the early morning; and (3) ROM increases later in the day.

As explained by Adams et al. (1987), creep loading reduces the disk height and brings the vertebrae closer together throughout the day (see figures 10.2 and 10.3; table 10.1). In turn, this disk compression produces slack in the annulus fibrosus, in the intervertebral ligaments of the neural arch, and in the back muscles and lumbar fascia. This slackening explains the small amount of extra flexion (5%) in the afternoon. However, during sleep, disks swell, increasing disk height and spreading the vertebrae. Consequently, this swelling causes increased stiffness in the morning. Furthermore, this change in fluid content of the disks affects the strain on the fibers of the annulus and may affect the likelihood of injury in the postsupine state.

Arthritis and Morning Stiffness

Morning stiffness is a frequent complaint among patients with rheumatoid arthritis (RA). Morning stiffness is used in clinical trials of RA to help determine disease activity and responses to treatment, and to differentiate *inflammatory* from *noninflammatory* arthritic conditions (Yazici et al. 2001). The American Rheumatism Association (ARA) also uses morning stiffness for a diagnosis of RA. In 1987, the ARA defined morning stiffness in terms of duration: "morning stiffness in and around the joints lasting at least one hour before maximal improvement, present for at least six weeks" (Lineker et al. 1999, p. 1056). The current definition of morning stiffness has been called inadequate because it lacks precise wording and therefore does not provide reliable findings for classification, prognosis, or outcomes. Lineker et al. (1999) have suggested adopting the term *gelling*. However, this description was criticized for its shortfalls (Edworthy 1999).

Several explanations have been put forward to explain morning stiffness. Perhaps the most plausible is an accumulation of fluid in and around joints during sleep (Wright and Johns 1960). However, one study of

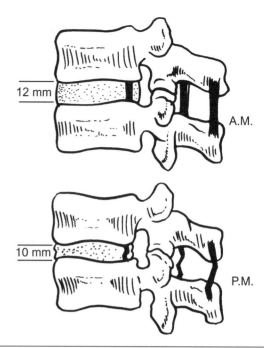

Figure 10.2   (A.M.) Motion segment with three bands or ties representing the structures that resist forward-bending movements; these are (from left to right) the annulus fibrosus, the intervertebral ligaments of the neural arch, and the back muscles and lumbodorsal fascia. (P.M.) Creep loading reduces disk height and gives slack to the three ties. The annulus is affected most because it is the shortest tie; the muscles and fascia are affected least because they are the longest tie. Thus, creep loading reduces the motion segment's resistance to bending and transfers bending stresses from the disk (especially) and intervertebral ligaments onto the back muscles and fascia.

Reprinted from Adams, Dolan, and Hutton 1987.

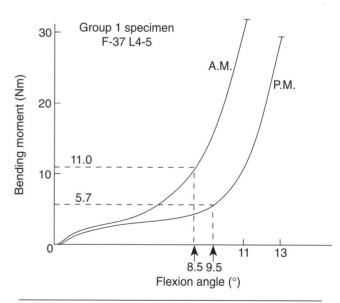

Figure 10.3   Bending stiffness curves for a typical motion segment before (A.M.) and after (P.M.) creep loading.

Reprinted from Adams, Dolan, and Hutton 1987.

Table 10.1 How Bending Stresses on Disk and Ligaments Decrease in Live Subjects in Course of a Day

| | Bending moment resisted (Nm) | | | | % reduction | |
| | A.M. | | P.M. | | | |
Specimen no.	Disk	Ligaments	Disk	Ligaments	Disk	Ligaments
1	2.8	7.0	0.7	3.4	76	52
2	4.9	11.8	1.6	7.3	67	39
3	3.9	9.7	0.8	6.0	81	37
4	3.2	7.8	0.8	4.9	75	37
5	6.7	16.4	1.6	9.8	76	40
6	4.4	10.9	0.4	2.7	92	75
7	3.9	9.7	1.0	5.5	75	44
8	4.5	11.0	1.2	5.9	73	46
9	2.1	5.0	0.4	3.6	79	29
Averages	4.0	9.9	0.9	5.5	77	44
	(±1.3)	(±3.3)	(±0.4)	(±2.1)	(±7)	(±13)

Reprinted, by permission, from M.A. Adams, P. Dolan, and W.C. Hutton, 1987, "Diurnal variations in the stresses on the lumbar spine," *Spine* 12(2), 136.

the effect of a diuretic on morning stiffness failed to find any difference in either the severity or duration of stiffness (Magder et al. 1986). Additional research is needed to identify the actual cause(s) of morning stiffness and find effective treatments for the cause and not the symptom.

SUMMARY

Numerous factors can affect one's potential degree of flexibility, including age, gender, body proportions, weight, dominant laterality, warm-up, activities, and time of day. Flexibility is specific to each joint. In general, flexibility can be developed at any age, given the appropriate training; however, the rate of development and potential for improvement varies with age.

Females are generally more flexible in the pelvic region. ROM is also affected by relaxation of the ligaments during pregnancy. The effects of body segment lengths, body weight, somatotype, race, laterality, warm-up and cool-down, strength training, and circadian variations on flexibility have also been investigated. Through a proper understanding of these relationships, misconceptions, myths, and stereotypes can be eliminated, along with their potential deleterious consequences.

11

Social Facilitation and Psychology in Developing Flexibility

The discipline of *psychology* attempts to describe, explain, and predict behavior. According to Sage (1984), "social facilitation examines the consequences upon individual behavior of the sheer presence of others" (p. 352). The field of *social psychology* is concerned with how and why the behavior of any person affects the behavior of another. This chapter explores four issues related to the influence of psychology on the development or reversal of flexibility and ROM: effects of an audience, mental concentration, psychosomatic conditions, and compliance with prescribed stretching programs.

EFFECTS OF AN AUDIENCE ON DEVELOPING FLEXIBILITY THROUGH STRETCHING

No matter how often an athlete claims not to pay attention to the audience or to the opinions of teammates, at times the athlete cannot escape the influence of others. The same holds true for someone working out with a friend or for a patient rehabilitating with a health-care practitioner.

Many athletes, gymnasts, swimmers, and track and field athletes, perform alone for all practical purposes. Nevertheless, these athletes are involved in dynamic social relationships with coaches, teammates, opponents, and frequently with fans and spectators. For participants in activities such as cheerleading, dancing, and team sports, interactions with comrades and the audience are obvious. These social factors may well affect the development of flexibility and ultimately the performance itself.

Because the people who may influence the athlete—friends, parents, peers, strangers, and authority figures—have different relationships to the athlete, their potential for affecting the athlete's behavior and psychological state varies. They may be perceived as positive, neutral, or negative influences, depending on the athlete's past experiences with them.

Ramifications of Social Facilitation

The audience may be passive and do nothing to encourage or discourage the performer, or it may be active and verbal, either giving encouraging or making disparaging remarks. Research on the effects of a passive audience performance has yielded contradictory results. In some studies performance was impaired, whereas in others it was improved. However, Zajonc (1965), after an analysis of research findings, uncovered a subtle consistency. In general, performance is enhanced but learning is impaired by the presence of spectators.

The motivational effects induced by spectators may be learned, for they are likely a function of positive or negative experiences associated with being observed or evaluated. The anxiety level of the individual must also be considered in such instances. Cottrell et al. (1968) indicates that the level of a person's anxiety parallels the level of perceived stress in a given situation.

How does social facilitation with an audience affect potential development of flexibility? Misconceptions and stereotypes regarding extreme flexibility in men are one example of the negative effect of social facilitation. For example, a man's ability to perform a split or some other feat of extreme suppleness may be perceived negatively by an audience. For very young children, such a situation may present a very real source of anxiety and psychological stress. Boys who wish to participate in dance may be discouraged from doing so. Toufexis (1974) states that potential boy dancers "must surmount not only physical difficulties but psychological ones" (p. 47). Male dancers often confront stereotypes about their sexuality (Schnitt and Schnitt 1987; Toufexis 1974). However, Schnitt and Schnitt (1987) state that changes in the public perception of sex roles may be responsible for males entering the dance field in larger numbers and at earlier ages.

Social facilitation affects people's decisions to continue participating in sports. Smith (1986) proposed a theoretical framework to explain the process of withdrawal from children's sports. Reviewing Smith's framework, Gould

(1987) distinguish between sport burnout and sport dropout: "Burnout-induced withdrawal is defined as the psychological, emotional, and physical withdrawal resulting from chronic stress, whereas dropping out results from a change of interests and/or value reorientation" (p. 71). Based on the works of others, Gould (1987) explains the process of dropping out:

> The decision to participate and persist in sport is a function of costs (e.g., time and effort, anxiety, disapproval of others) and benefits (e.g., trophies, feelings of competence) with the athlete constantly trying to maximize benefits and minimize costs. Thus, interest and participation is maintained when the benefits outweigh the costs, and withdrawal occurs when costs outweigh benefits. However, behavior is not fully explained by a simple rewards-minus-costs formula. The decision to participate and persist is mediated by the athlete's minimum comparison level (the lowest criteria one uses to judge something as satisfying or unsatisfying) and the comparison level of alternative activities. Consequently, someone may choose to stay involved in sport even if costs are exceeded by rewards because no alternative opportunities are available. Similarly, an athlete who perceives that the rewards outweigh costs in a program may discontinue involvement because a more desirable alternative activity is available. (p. 72)

The key to the question of how an audience affects development of flexibility is how much the individual values the approval of others over personal goals. To avoid the potentially negative effects, practice sessions during the early stages of learning may be best conducted in privacy. In this way, pressure from either an active or a passive audience can be eliminated. The instructor's explanation of the factors that determine one's flexibility may mitigate the influence of negative audience perceptions. Instilling into students an understanding and appreciation of the rewards in partaking in the chosen discipline may also be helpful.

Effects of Coaction in Developing Flexibility Through Stretching

Coaction with teammates, that is, engaging in the same activity or task while in view of one another can be a definite aid in the development of flexibility. When teammates (or coactors) stretch and warm up together, they often provide each other with learning cues and thus serve as guides or models for one another. They can reinforce correct responses to achieve optimum flexibility.

Coaction can also elicit the desired response through negative means. Social pressure may be imposed, requiring participants to capitulate or face ostracism. Such an example is the *hurt-pain-agony* approach employed in swimming (Counsilman 1968). Unless one is willing to tolerate the highest levels of discomfort, one is not likely to excel in the sport. Pride is fostered when swimmers push themselves hard during the agony phase of exertion. Furthermore, other team members will develop contempt for a laggard or one who does not "put out" in practice.

If pain or discomfort becomes an everyday experience shared by all members of the team, the aversion to it subsides. Consequently, the more the athletes engage in unemotional talk about their discomfort, the more acceptable it becomes. Thus, they develop mental as well as physical callousness to pain. They come to accept some degree of pain as a natural and necessary part of attaining their goals. Such an approach may be practical for such competitive disciplines as bodybuilding, swimming, and running, but it is not practical for developing flexibility.

THEORETICAL ASPECTS OF MENTAL TRAINING

Mental training includes psychological methods to improve performance. In flexibility training the targeted muscles must relax during the stretching phase and the body segments must move through the desired ROM at the desired velocity with the desired accuracy. *Imagery*, or *visualization*, and *self-hypnosis* are two mental training techniques that may be employed for both tension management and performance enhancement. Mental training can theoretically facilitate the development of flexibility on two levels: decreased motor neuron activation, resulting in greater relaxation, and altered programming levels of the motor system. The most illustrative research on the relationship between mental training and stretching is in the area of biofeedback.

CYBERNETIC STRETCH

One psychological approach to the development of flexibility is the *cybernetic stretch*, a technique adapted by Bates (1976) from Dr. Maxwell Maltz's highly recommended book *Psycho-Cybernetics* (1970). The basic approach of cybernetic stretch is "mind over matter." In the preface, Maltz states, "The 'self image' sets the boundaries of individual accomplishment. It defines what you can and cannot do. Expand the self image and you expand the area of the possible" (p. ix).

The psycho-cybernetic method consists of learning, practicing, and experiencing new ways of thinking, imaging, remembering, and acting to bring about happiness and success in achieving particular goals. Psycho-cybernetics holds that the human brain, nervous system, and muscular system are a highly complex "servomechanism" used and directed by the mind.

According to *Psycho-Cybernetics*, experiencing success is the key to functioning successfully. Confidence is built upon the experience of success. When we begin any new undertaking, we have little confidence because we have not yet learned from experience that we can succeed. Because the nervous system cannot tell the difference between an imagined experience and a real experience, visualizing successful performance can build confidence and help enhance actual performance.

As described by Bates (1976), cybernetic stretch consists of a mental practice step and a direct practice step. Following Maltz's guidelines, the first task is to select a specific goal. To facilitate visualizing the goal, the "creative automatic mechanism" must be provided with facts. "Physiologically, a 50 percent increase in muscle length is possible if no inhibitions to stretch are operative; therefore your goal of 'making it flat' in the side split exists" (p. 240). Of course, this assumes the absence of any structural limitations. Knowing that the goal is attainable and practical is essential.

Next, by the use of imagination, one sets up mental images that one's "servomechanism" will work to fulfill. A mental practice period of 30 minutes each day for at least 21 days is recommended. The setting should be quiet, comfortable, and relaxing. The key to the mental practice step is making the image as real as possible. As Bates (1976) points out, "It is most important that you see yourself successfully and ideally completing the flexibility action" (p. 241).

The final step is direct practice. Bates (1976) writes

Skill learning of any kind is accomplished by trial and error, mentally correcting aim after an error, until a successful motion is achieved. Your servo-mechanism achieves its goal in the same manner, it remembers the successful responses and forgets the past errors. Stretch slowly, keeping spindle firing to a minimum, up to the point of pain; ease off slightly, causing spindles to stop firing briefly and allowing the muscle to relax. The servo-mechanism remembers that position and the absence of muscle contraction that opposes holding that relaxed position, if you are supplying it with the "end result" or goal.

Relax while you maintain your held position; you must allow your servo-mechanism to work rather than force it to work. Connections exist on both alpha and gamma motor neurons from higher centers such that sensory information to these motor neurons may be offset by information from the higher brain centers. While relaxing, your servo-mechanism is finding the pathway and the degree of inhibition to maintain in order to achieve your goal.

Proceed further forward when you have learned to reduce the tension at your present level. As increased stretch positions are achieved it is helpful to have a partner maintain your position, after you have eased off slightly . . . In fact, it is often advisable in the very beginning for the partner to passively assist in increasing the range of motion, allowing for the easing off, and then maintain the subject's position. (pp. 240-241)

IDEOKINETIC IMAGERY

Another method that integrates principles from both science and somatics into a stretching protocol was developed by Batson (1994). The somatic learning method emphasizes that the body learns improved movement organization and quality by consciously directing sensory awareness while moving or thinking about moving. Batson's premise is that "While science provides the intellectual foundations for safe and effective stretching based on the behavior of muscle and connective tissue, somatics cultivates sensory responsivity, enhancing our awareness and our organization of movement" (p. 39). Batson's approach incorporates blending the strategies of the Alexander Technique and Sweigard Ideokinesis. For a detailed discussion on this topic, see Batson (1993, 1994), along with the cited references.

Four possible images outlined by Batson (1994, p. 51) for stretching the hamstrings include

- "melting" the head of the femur into the "black hole" of the socket (i.e., approximating the hip joint and neurally inhibiting the larger muscles of the thigh (Sullivan et al. 1982) (see figure 11.1a);
- "scraping" the femoral shaft with an imaginary spatula down the condyles, and the tibial condyles down toward the midshaft to release the superficial muscles (see figure 11.1b);
- visualizing the bone as a "spacer" (Pierce 1983, 1984) that "lengthens" within the muscle sleeve (the anatomical axis is the line of movement) (see figure 11.1c); and

Stress

Under extreme duress, the body secretes stress hormones (adrenaline, noradrenaline, and cortisol) that switch the body into high alert. Bodily functions that are not involved are put on hold, causing a range of problems from sudden nausea to bone loss. In general, symptoms of stress are either cognitive problems that create worry and disrupt attention or somatic problems that increase physiological arousal, leading to muscle tension and poor motor coordination and flexibility. The end result is a higher rate of injuries.

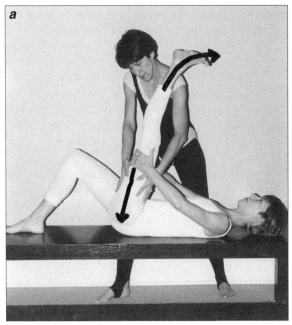

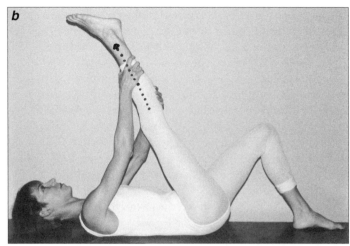

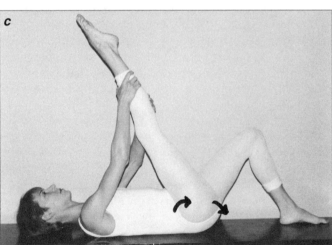

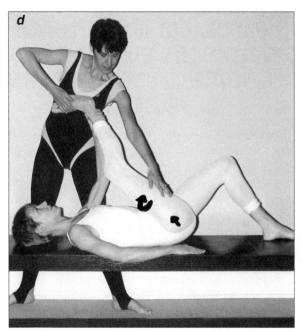

Figure 11.1   (*a*) Image: sinking the femur into the "black hole" of the thigh socket (downward arrow). Image: projecting the line of movement out the heel and toes (upward arrow). (*b*) Image: scraping the soft tissue down the shaft of the tibia with a sculpting tool (the dancer gives herself tactile feedback). (*c*) Image: counterrotating the ASIS of the pelvis toward the femur (hip flexion, anterior tilt) while reaching with the sitz bone down to the ground (hip extension, posterior tilt) to stretch the fibers closer to the ischial tuberosity. (*d*) Image: the "eyeball" on the femoral head scouting out the hip joint (looking inward and downward) as the dancer performs flexion-adduction external rotation of the hip joint to selectively stretch the lateral hamstrings and iliotibial band.

Reprinted from Batson 1994.

- counterrotating the ASIS of the pelvis toward the femur (enhancing hip flexion) as the leg extends over the chest while keeping the sitz bone as parallel to the floor as possible (activating the psoas/rectus to release the hamstring by reciprocal innervation) (see figure 11.1d).

Appropriate images and pictures sometimes help the relaxation mindset. For example, imagine that your legs are the ends of a rope spread apart as you perform a split. Visualizing heat is very helpful. Mentally wrap the spot with the most muscular tension with a hot towel in a few layers. As the hot application heats up, the muscle softens up and relaxes. (Tsatsouline 2001a, p. 25)

PSYCHOSOMATIC FACTORS

The idea that certain ailments and diseases may have psychosomatic causes has been recognized for thousands of years. In the Bible we read, "A soft heart is the life of the flesh: but envy is the rottenness of the bones"

(*Proverbs* 14:30) and "A merry heart doth good like medicine: but a broken spirit drieth the bones" (*Proverbs* 17:22). In recent times, psychosomatic disorders, which are physical disorders of the body caused or complicated by psychological factors, have become more recognized and accepted. Two physical disorders of presumably psychogenic origin that potentially affect ROM are myofascial trigger points (small nodules of spastic or degenerative muscle tissue that serve as focal points for referred pain and other noxious reflexes) and arthritis (Asterita 1985; McFarlane et al. 1987). The growing recognition of the importance of this area is evident by the number of publications that deal exclusively with this topic, including the *Journal of Psychosomatic Research*, the *Journal of Psychosomatic Medicine*, and *Psychosomatics*.

PSYCHOLOGY OF COMPLIANCE IN FLEXIBILITY TRAINING, INJURY PREVENTION, AND REHABILITATION PROGRAMS

Patient compliance problems date back at least 2,500 years to Hippocrates, who reported that patients often lied about taking their medicines and that, when treatment then failed, the physician was blamed by patients and their families (Ulmer 1989). In the following sections, attention is primarily devoted to athletes and nonathletes recovering from injury and in need of rehabilitation. However, compliance for the healthy individual is equally important in the maintenance of good health. Compliance is an economic concern for individuals and for corporations. For the ill and the healthy, it is also a matter of potential longevity and quality of life (Hilyer et al. 1990; Locke 1983).

Definition of Compliance

Webster's Dictionary defines *compliance* as "acquiescence to a wish, request, or demand" or "a disposition or tendency to yield to the will of others." Compliant behavior may be defined as a class behavior resulting from a specific set of cues and consequences (Ice 1985). The term compliance has been criticized for its connotation that health-care providers dictate what patients should do (Chen et al. 1999). Researchers have substituted a number of other terms for this concept: adherence, obedience, cooperation, concordance, collaboration, maintenance, patient cooperation, and therapeutic alliance (Chen et al. 1999; DiMatteo and DiNicola 1982).

Importance of Compliance

At the economic level, client and patient compliance is vital to the financial success and livelihood of the proprietors and employees of health-care providers and institutions, fitness and health clubs, yoga schools, and allied institutions. Without client or patient compliance (e.g., registering or signing up for classes, attending appointments, and receiving services), no income is earned. Thus, providers have an ulterior financial motive when telling the client or patient to adhere to a given practice or recommendation. Awareness of the financial motive may be one reason many clients do not completely trust the provider and hence fail in compliance.

Compliance and noncompliance affect patients, the health-care providers, and society as a whole. When patients fail to carry out their instructions and programs, the health-care provider's experience and expertise are nullified (Fisher et al. 1988). Noncompliance interferes with the health-care provider's therapeutic efforts. Failure to adhere to directions can exacerbate the condition of the patient. Consequently, the practitioner may needlessly order a renewed round of diagnostic evaluations or prescribe a second-choice treatment regimen. Most important, the patient may take longer to recover (DiMatteo and DiNicola 1982; Fisher et al. 1988; Johnson 1991). Conversely, when patients comply, treatment outcomes improve dramatically. Compliance is very important in preventive measures, particularly those that seek to forestall, reduce the severity of, or prevent the occurrence of undesired consequences.

Noncompliance may result in ongoing disability and lead to decreased labor production and loss of wages (Kirwan et al. 2002). Failure to follow directions adds to society's costs through lost work time, productivity, and income. It increases expenses to insurance companies, which in turn pass on costs in the form of increased insurance premiums to the public. Failure to keep medical appointments is expensive because clinician and clerical staff time is wasted (Sackett and Snow 1979). If patients drop out of treatment, their histories, physical examinations, and tests must be repeated when they seek care in another medical setting (DiMatteo et al. 1979; Kasteler et al. 1976). If treatment fails or diagnoses are delayed, the question may arise as to who was responsible for the failure. Too often, this confusion results in malpractice issues (Ulmer 1989).

Noncompliance in clinical trials has implications for both efficacy and safety. Obviously, noncompliance can compromise the validity of results in even the most well-designed trial (Sereika and Davis 2001). Also, when volunteers in a study do not follow prescribed directions, interpretation of trial results is imprecise, and the amount or extent of effectiveness may be obscured. Therefore, the effectiveness may be underestimated for full compliers, and the expected outcome may be overestimated for poor compliers (Peck 1999). Significantly, in some clinical studies, noncompliance could lead to underreporting of adverse effects (Friedman et al. 1998; Sereika and Davis 2001).

Statistics Related to Compliance

Estimates of client and patient compliance are difficult to make. However, knowing what criteria are being used to make the determination is important (Meichenbaum and Turk 1987). Estimates vary greatly, depending on a number of factors, including method of measurement, age, and definition of compliance (Groth and Wulf 1995). Elaborating on the last, several writers (Perkins and Epstein 1988; Sluijs et al. 1993; Turk 1993) point out that compliance is not all-or-nothing, but rather a matter of gradation. However, Hansson (2002) states, "At its broadest, non-compliance indicates any deviation from the prescribed therapy" (p. 192). Rates of compliance with exercise regimens range from 40% to 55% (Feinberg 1988). Of 1,178 patients who were instructed to perform home exercises prescribed by physiotherapists, 35% reported that they fully adhered, 41% reported that they partly adhered (exercising "now and then"), and 22% reported that they were totally nonadherent (Sluijs et al. 1993). Dishman (1988), in summarizing his review of the adherence literature, stated that among adults who start exercise programs, the dropout rate is 50% or greater within the first 6 to 12 months.

Factors Contributing to Compliance and Noncompliance

In a landmark publication, Haynes et al. (1979) developed 13 categorical tables of factors (pp. 454-474) studied in relation to compliance. Within these 13 tables, more than 200 factors were identified. Their research and the work of others (Ice 1985; Ley 1977; Milberg and Clark 1988; G. Miller et al. 1977; Sluijs et al. 1998) identified numerous compliance variables. Several of these variables were age, intelligence, medical knowledge, state of anxiety, mood, social support, self-motivation, economic factors, perceived exertion, disease features, discomfort or pain tolerance, difficulty in changing lifestyle, available time, patient-therapist interaction, features of the therapeutic regimen, and compliance strategies. Meichenbaum and Turk (1987) reduced this list to five general categories: (1) characteristics of the patient, (2) characteristics of the treatment regimen, (3) features of the disease, (4) the relationship between the health-care provider and the patient, and (5) the clinical setting (p. 41).

Another important compliance factor is a patient's ability to remember advice dispensed by health practitioners. Patients cannot be expected to comply with advice or information that they cannot remember (Ice 1985). Jette et al. (1998) reduced existing literature about adoption and maintenance of exercise behaviors in adults into three categories: (1) psychological state, (2) physical characteristics, and (3) sociodemographic background of the individual. Sluijs et al. (1993) found three main factors relating noncompliance with exercise regimens during physical therapy: (1) the barriers patients perceive and encounter, (2) the lack of positive feedback, and (3) the degree of helplessness. Campbell et al. (2001) found "a necessary precondition for continued compliance was the perception that the physiotherapy was effective in ameliorating unpleasant symptoms" (p. 132). Yet, perceptions of compliance to home exercise programs differ greatly between health-care providers and patients (Kirwan et al. 2002).

Given that recall is vital for optimal compliance, how can it be facilitated? The way in which medical information is presented to a patient may affect recall (Ice 1985). Ley (1977) found that recall after oral, visual, or written presentation was not significantly different. However, the information given earliest in the presentation was retained better than that provided later. "In clinical practice, this research suggests placing instructions and advice first and stressing their importance will reduce forgetfulness and increase recall" (Ice 1985, p. 1833).

Sluijs et al. (1993) found preventative exercises usually have less meaning to patients than curative exercises. Jette et al. (1998) studied 102 sedentary, functionally limited, community-dwelling adults, aged 60 to 94 years, who participated in a home-based resistance-training program. They determined that "it was the psychological factors that were most important to adherence to this home-based program" (p. 16).

Compliance: A Matter of Faithfulness

What does one actually desire when compliance is sought from another? The answer is an act of faithfulness! *Belief* is a state or habit of mind in which trust or confidence is placed in some person or thing. We may define compliance as an action based upon a belief. All the belief that one holds is useless unless action follows. This statement is true for almost any situation in which the compliance of another is sought. Doctors, therapists, athletic trainers, teachers, and even baby-sitters all want the same thing: action and not just words. Thus, compliance and faithfulness is when the "rubber meets the road" with patient acceptance and action. However, to gain a patient's compliance, a health-care provider must gain that patient's trust.

Practical Strategies for Securing Compliance

Numerous practitioners and researchers have proposed various strategies to improve compliance. Although no method guarantees compliance, several important dos and don'ts must be observed by health-care providers. Three obvious things to keep in mind are that the so-called average person does not exist, no two people are alike, and compliance is a two-way process. Meichenbaum and Turk (1987) state, "Because of the complexity and multidetermined nature of treatment nonadherence and the heterogeneity of the patient population, there is an increasing recognition that integrative interventions are required" (p. 235). Table 11.1 presents one example of a summary of suggestions for improving communication with patients. In contrast, table 11.2 summarizes and presents commonly employed examples of a variety of compliance gaining strategies. These strategies run the spectrum from positive to negative.

Overcompliance

Noncompliance can also take the form of *overcompliance*. In athletics and the performing arts, overcompliance is a real issue. Overcompliance related to flexibility training or flexibility rehabilitation is typified by individuals going above and beyond the prescribed physical protocols and ignoring recommended limits (Greenberg 2001; Heil and O'Connor 2001). "In some cases this leads to faster rehabilitation—and if so, all the better. However, some may

Table 11.1 Suggestions for Improving Communication With Patients

Satisfaction	Short waiting time
	Be friendly rather than businesslike
	Some talk about nonmedical topics
	Listen to patient
	Find out what worries are
	Find out what expectations are; if not to be met, say why
Selecting content	What does patient want to know
	What are the patient's health beliefs: Vulnerability Seriousness Effectiveness Costs and barriers
	What do you want the patient to know
	What motivating communications help
Understanding and memory	Avoid jargon
	Use short words and short sentences (simplification)
	Encourage feedback
	Increase recall Primacy Stressed importance Explicit categorization Specific rather than general Repetition
	Written back-up Readability Physical format: letter size, color, quality of print and paper

Reprinted, by permission, from P. Ley, 1988, *Communicating with patients: Improving communication, satisfaction, and compliance* (London: Croom Helm), 180.

Table 11.2 Sixteen Compliance-Gaining Techniques With Reference to Athletes

1. *Promise:* If you comply, I will reward you.	You offer to reduce the number of laps required to run after practice if the athlete stretches at the specified time.
2. *Threat:* If you do not comply, I will punish you.	You threaten the athlete to increase the number of laps required to run after practice if he/she does not stretch at the specified time.
3. *Expertise (Positive):* If you comply, you will be rewarded because of the "nature of things."	You point out that if the athlete stretches before the workout, he/she will be able to improve performance with lower running times.
4. *Expertise (Negative):* If you do not comply, you will be punished because of the "nature of things."	You point out that if the athlete does not stretch at the specified time, he/she will pull a hamstring.
5. *Like:* Actor is friendly and helpful to get the target in "good frame of mind."	You try to be as friendly and pleasant as possible to the athlete in the "right frame of mind" by asking him/her to stretch at the specified time.
6. *Pre-Giving:* Actor rewards the target before requesting compliance.	You have the athlete lead the stretching or warm-up session before the start of the workout.
7. *Aversive Stimulation:* Actor continuously punishes the target making cessation contingent on compliance.	You forbid the athlete to participate in the practice session until he/she has adequately stretched at the specified time.
8. *Debt:* You owe me compliance because of past favors.	You point out that he/she owes it to the coach/trainer to stretch at the specified time because the coach/trainer has provided tutoring in school and transportation after school for the athlete.
9. *Moral Appeal:* You are immoral if you do not comply.	You tell the athlete that it is morally wrong for a person who is blessed and talented not to take advantage of what he/she has been blessed with. Therefore he/she should stretch and warm up diligently at the specified time to guarantee an optimal performance.
10. *Self-Feeling (Positive):* You will feel better about yourself if you comply.	You tell the athlete that he/she will feel better about himself/herself by following the team rules about stretching at the specified time.
11. *Self-Feeling (Negative):* You will feel worse about yourself if you do not comply.	You tell the athlete he/she should feel ashamed for not stretching and warming up before practice and therefore having a bad performance and costing the team a victory.
12. *Altercasting (Positive):* A person with "good" qualities would comply.	You tell the athlete that since he/she is mature and intelligent; he/she will naturally want to stretch and warm up more before practice to improve his/her performance.
13. *Altercasting (Negative):* Only a person with "bad" qualities would not comply.	You tell the athlete that only a self-consumed person would not stretch and warm up before practice and potentially let the team down.
14. *Altruism:* I need your compliance very badly, so do it for me.	You tell the athlete that you want very badly for him to get a scholarship and get into a good college and that you wish he/she would stretch and warm up more before each practice as a personal favor to you.
15. *Esteem (Positive):* People you value will think better of you if you comply.	You tell the athlete that the whole team will be very proud if he/she stretches before practice and has an improved performance.
16. *Esteem (Negative):* People you value will think worse of you if you do not comply.	You tell the athlete that the whole team will be very disappointed in him/her if he/she does not follow the team rules about stretching and warming up before practice.

Modified from "Dimensions of compliance-gaining behavior: An empirical analysis" by G. Maxwell and D. Schmitt, 1967, *Sociometry* 30(4), 357-358. Copyright 1967. Adapted by permission.

push their recuperative ability beyond physical limits while increasing the risk of injury. When this happens, it can also lead to treatment setbacks and reinjury" (Heil 1993, p. 201). A practical example is overzealous stretching of healing tissues (sprained ankle or strained hamstring). Such stretching could rupture these already weakened tissues and blood vessels, cascading into additional inflammation and scar tissue. In the other extreme, a healthy athlete taking part in flexibility training goes that extra inch of stretch and either sprains (ligament) or strains (muscle) various tissues.

Coaches, trainers, and therapists must understand the various psychological motivation for overcompliance. Some individuals are strongly motivated because they love what they are doing. Others may be motivated because their self-identities are overly dependent on sports participation (Taylor and Taylor 1997). Another group may believe that more is better and results in a faster and more efficient recovery. "In other words, if two sets of an exercise are good, then four sets will be more beneficial" (p. 48). For others, the prime motivation may be the pressure from coaches and teammates to return to play quickly (Greenberg 2001; Heil 1993). In dance, "any time away from training may lead to loss of standing for the individual dancer in a company or class" (Hald 1992, p. 393). For the professional athlete, a fast recovery could determine one's starting assignment and impact his or her financial livelihood.

The following list contains guidelines for managing persistent overcompliance problems (Heil 1993, p. 202):

- Educate the athlete about the mechanisms of injury and rehabilitation.
- Emphasize that the prescribed amount of activity is the best amount and that overdoing prescribed activity may aggravate injury and slow recovery.
- Present the goal as a bull's-eye, a target to be hit with precision. This imagery counters the notion that a goal is a line to be crossed, the further the better.
- Support consistency and accuracy in a goal attainment.
- Consider having the athlete use the Rating of Perceived Exertion Scale (Borg 1998) to identify and maintain appropriate levels of effort during rehabilitation.
- Develop a flare-up plan for helping the athlete cope with treatment setbacks.
- Redirect the athlete's desire and energy for more work at rehabilitation into mental training.

Psychological Factors When Treating Victims of Abuse

Every year thousands of victims are subjected to physical and mental abuse. Furthermore, thousands of others are subjected to torture. According to Amnesty International (2001), torture continues to be practiced systematically in more than 120 countries. The current estimate of the number of refugees is 35 million worldwide. In 2000, the U.S. Department of Justice (Rennison 2001) reported 260,950 victims were raped or sexually assaulted. As the number of victims continues to increase, health-care providers (physicians, chiropractors, osteopaths); allied healthcare providers (massage therapist, occupational specialists, physical therapists); and coaches, instructors, and trainers (for athletes, the performing arts, and yoga) are more likely to encounter such clients and patients. Lack of awareness and lack of training on the part of providers are likely to affect such clients and patients in a direct way (Moreno and Grodin 2002). Providers who lack training or awareness may even retraumatize a victim during a professional encounter (Moreno et al. 2001).

Moreno and Grodin (2002) have suggested a meaningful and successful clinical approach to survivors of physical, mental, and sexual abuse. This interaction includes "avoiding retraumatization, building trust, spelling out any limits on confidentiality, and above any other, establishing empathy with the patient" (p. 220). Additional strategies culled from various sources (Physicians for Human Rights 2001; Piwowarczyk et al. 2000; Weinstein et al. 1996) include having the health-care provider do the following:

- Introduce himself or herself to the client or patient.
- Explain to the client or patient the purpose of the treatment.
- Inform the client or patient when and where he or she will be touched.
- Give the client or patient a sense of control.
- Allow the client or patient the right to terminate the interview, examination, or treatment at any time.

SUMMARY

The mind sets the boundaries of individual accomplishment and defines what one can and cannot do. Accordingly, if one can expand the self-image and mind, one can expand the "area of the possible." However, being social in nature, we are affected by the presence of people around us. This influence may be positive, neutral, or negative.

A major determining factor of the success of a flexibility-training program or a rehabilitative program is the compliance of the patient or athlete. Compliance is based upon belief. Both undercompliance and overcompliance can produce negative consequences. Numerous theories have been proposed to explain the nature of compliance and potential strategies that facilitate it.

3

PRINCIPLES
OF STRETCHING

CHAPTER

12

Stretching Concepts

Why do people have difficulty motivating themselves to stretch regularly? Perhaps a primary reason is time constraints (Hedricks 1993). Another reason is people lack knowledge about proper stretching, how it should be done, and its potential benefits. This chapter addresses several of these issues by examining a variety of concepts related to stretching.

HOMEOSTASIS

Homeostasis is the maintenance of a steady state. Organisms have means of maintaining steady states in their internal environments and also in their external environments. Stressful environmental factors (such as overwork) may alter the steady state of an organism. When an organism's ability to maintain homeostatic control is exceeded, injury or death may result.

The concept of homeostasis can be extended to the cellular and even subcellular level. Thus, within certain limits, the cell is capable of adjusting to varying demands. However, like the organism as a whole, its adaptive capability may be exceeded, and cellular injury or death may follow.

One's response to stress depends in part on one's ability to adapt oneself to new conditions. During or after stress, the functioning of the homeostatic mechanism may change, and the individual may enter a new state. This process is called *adaptation*. Adaptive responses for increased flexibility involve both functional and structural changes. Consequently, quantitative as well as qualitative improvement in performance can be achieved. However, for such changes to occur, one's homeostatic state must be overloaded.

OVERSTRETCHING PRINCIPLE

Doherty (1985) suggests, "If we accept the word *overloading* as related to building strength in muscles, then overstretching should be acceptable in building flexibility" (p. 425). This *overstretching principle* is the physiological principle on which flexibility development depends. According to this principle, when the body is regularly stimulated by an increasingly intense stretching program beyond the homeostatic level, it will respond with an increased ability to stretch. Conversely, a decrease in the intensity of a stretching program lowers the ability to stretch. Therefore, the body adapts to the increasing demands placed on it. "Overstretching" in this context does "not" mean stretching body parts that exceed their safety limits and result in injury and impairment in function.

Flexibility is simply a result of stretching. No other factor is more important in the development of flexibility in a healthy person. Stretching may be applied either manually (i.e., by oneself or a partner) or by machine. Increased flexibility is achieved by implementing a movement that exceeds the existing range of possible motion (Jones 1975). Consequently, flexibility is best acquired by stretching up to the edge of discomfort. However, discomfort is a subjective matter and will vary from person to person.

FLEXIBILITY-TRAINING METHODS

All flexibility-training methods that strive to develop optimum functional flexibility depend on two dominant factors, namely structural conditioning and functional (central nervous and neuromuscular) conditioning. Consequently, flexibility training may be categorized according to its major structural and functional aims relative to the importance of nervous system training method. Table 12.1 is a simple chart demonstrating these aims.

RETENTION OF FLEXIBILITY

A significant issue for concern is the retention of functional adaptation for a given period after training has ceased. This topic is especially significant for therapists who give a home exercise program following discharge from therapy (Willy et al. 2001). Unfortunately, the question of what happens to flexibility gains when a stretching

Table 12.1   Major Aims of a Flexibility or Rehabilitation Training Program

Structural			Functional		
Connective tissue	Muscle tissue	Neuromechano-receptors	Passive ROM	Stiffness, damping, elasticity, extensibility	Active ROM
Isoforms	Isoforms	Isoforms?			Flexibility: strength
Matrix	Sarcomere	Muscle spindles			Flexibility: endurance
Fluids	Numbers of sarcomeres	Numbers of nuclear bag$_1$, nuclear bag$_2$, and nuclear chain fibers			Flexibility: speed

program ceases has not received the attention that other aspects of stretching programs have received (Depino et al. 2000; Spernoga et al. 2001; Zebas and Rivera 1985). Even less research has investigated the decreased training effect on stiffness and damping capacity of various tissues. Stretching produces increases in joint ROM that are still evident 1 day or more after cessation of treatment in people without clinically significant contractures (Harvey et al. 2002). However, these results should be interpreted with caution because no studies of "high" quality have been conducted. Compounding matters, "it is possible that both 'moderate' and 'poor' quality studies exaggerate the real size of the treatment effect" (p. 11).

Research in the area of retained flexibility falls into two categories: multiple-day stretching programs and single, same-day acute stretches. Möller, Ekstrand et al. (1985) compared the retention of flexibility in several treated muscle groups 0, 30, 60, and 90 minutes after the stretching procedure. The increased flexibility remained for 90 minutes for most of the muscle groups. Möller, Öberg et al. (1985, p. 52) subsequently found "the effect of stretching done at the start of the session persists over the training session and up to 24 hours." Another study by Hubley et al. (1984) determined that "Fifteen minutes of cycling or inactivity did not result in significant differences ($p < .05$) from the initial gains resulting from the [static] stretching" (p. 104). Toft et al. (1989) investigated the use of contract-relax stretching performed twice a day for 3 weeks. The stretches were repeated five times and measurements taken 90 minutes later. "There was no correlation between: (1) flexibility and short-term effect of stretching, (2) flexibility and the long-term effect of stretching, or (3) the short-term and long-term effects of stretching" (p. 489). However, a reduction of passive tension occurred after 3 weeks.

Magnusson et al. (1996a) applied a single 80-second stretch maneuver to the hamstrings of 10 male volun-

teers. The experiment produced an 18% to 21% decline in passive torque. However, 1 hour later no measurable effect was seen. Zito et al. (1997) investigated the lasting effects of one bout of two 15-second passive stretches on ankle dorsiflexion ROM in 19 healthy volunteers. The study "found no statistically significant length gains using a single bout of two 15-second stretches." Furthermore, the data of the study "did not provide evidence of lasting lengthening at this duration" (p. 214).

DePino et al. (2000) investigated the duration of maintained flexibility gains in knee-joint ROM after same-day static hamstring stretching. Subjects were warmed up and then performed four 30-second static stretches separated by 15-second rests. In contrast, they reported gains in stretching ability as a result of static stretching are transient, lasting for only 3 minutes after cessation of the stretching protocol and then decreasing with time. The ROM gains returned to the baseline by 6 minutes after stretching. The significance of their findings was that "athletes who statically stretch and then wait longer than 3 minutes before entering a game or practice can expect to lose the range of motion gained" (p. 59). This discovery has implications for athletes who statically stretch and then attend a team meeting or sit on the sideline for 30 minutes. The investigators recommend that future research should

- determine whether intermittent stretching or activity alone is sufficient to maintain temporary increases in ROM obtained from acute stretching bouts;
- determine the most efficient type of acute stretching to effect same-day ROM increases;
- determine the optimal duration of stretch to produce long-term or permanent changes; and
- perform comparisons between men and women, across age groups, and between subjects with

range restriction greater than 20° and less than 20° to determine whether these findings generalize beyond young men with a 20° or greater restriction.

Spernoga et al. (2001) investigated the duration of hamstring flexibility gains after a one-time modified hold-relax stretching protocol. Thirty male military cadets volunteered for the study. All subjects performed six warm-up active knee extensions. The control group received in addition five modified hold-relax stretches. The findings suggested, "that a sequence of five modified hold-relax stretches produced significantly increased hamstring flexibility that lasted 6 minutes after the stretching protocol ended" (p. 44).

In a review of the literature, Zebas and Rivera (1985) and Depino et al. (2000) determined that a number of studies have primarily been focused on the hip joint, and in all cases, a significant amount of flexibility was retained in the hip joint. Specifically, hip flexibility was retained after 3 weeks (Long 1971), 4 weeks (Tweitmeyer 1974), 8 weeks (McCue 1963), and several months (Riddle 1956). Other significant flexibility retention was found in the neck joint (McCue 1963; Turner 1977) and back (McCue 1963). A retention of flexibility 4 weeks after cessation was also found by Zebas and Rivera (1985). However, they point out, "even though flexibility was retained from the pretesting period through the retention period, there were significant losses of flexibility from the posttesting period to 2 weeks after the cessation of exercise" (pp. 188-189). They also addressed one major limitation of such longitudinal measures: The activities outside of the class could not be monitored or controlled. However, Wallin et al. (1985) suggested that stretching once a week is frequent enough to maintain ROM gained through a stretching program.

Willy et al. (2001) conducted a study to determine the effects of cessation and resumption of a hamstring muscle stretching protocol on knee ROM. Eighteen subjects participated in a 16-week study. The first 6 weeks consisted of the initial stretching period followed by 4 weeks of nonstretching and an additional 6 weeks of stretching. The initial 6-week hamstring static stretching regimen resulted in a significant gain in knee ROM. The ROM returned to the baseline after the 4 weeks cessation period. Therefore, the gained ROM was not retained. The resumption of stretching resulted in a significant gain in ROM. Thus, "the benefits of the stretching exercise will be lost relatively quickly if stretching is not continued" (p. 143).

Why do individuals, both men and women, with very tight hamstring muscles have a greater ROM gain after a stretching treatment than do individuals with just tight hamstring muscles? Starring et al. (1988) speculate that differences lie in the connective tissue composition. A very "tight" (limited ROM) muscle may have more connective tissue, and one of the main functions of connective tissue is to prevent muscle from being overstretched. However, a shortened muscle requires even more protection to prevent even normal ROM. Furthermore, the increased connective tissue results in a decrease in the elasticity and extensibility of the muscle tissue. With prolonged stretching, plastic deformation of the soft tissue occurs, resulting in an increased ROM that is maintained after 1 week of treatment. However, "in the individual with 'less tight' muscles, more elastic elements are present, and the muscle tissue will return more easily to the original length" (p. 318).

REQUISITE KNOWLEDGE FOR STRETCHING

The methods of stretching employed in athletics, dance, physical therapy, and yoga can vary considerably. However, certain knowledge is required in all of these disciplines. A basic knowledge of the normal neuromuscular mechanism, including motor development, anatomy, neuroscience, and kinesiology is very helpful, if not essential. Furthermore, whatever the method of stretching used, one should be thoroughly familiar with the structure and function of the joint in question. One should know not only the degree of limitation of motion but also which tissues are responsible for the limitations.

POTENTIAL FACTORS INFLUENCING FLEXIBILITY (ROM)

ROM is restricted or impaired by a variety of factors:

- Lack of elasticity of connective tissues in muscles or joints
- Skin disorder, including scleroderma or scarring from burns
- Muscle tension
- Contractures
- Reflexes
- Lack of coordination and strength in the case of active movement
- Limitations imposed by other synergistic muscles
- Paralysis
- Spasticity
- Length of ligaments and tendons
- Bone and joint structure limitations
- Gender (e.g., pelvic structure)
- Hormones (e.g., relaxin)
- Pregnancy (e.g., sit-and-reach test)
- Body fat/obesity (e.g., sit-and-reach test) (acting as a wedge between two lever arms)
- Postural malalignment, such as scoliosis or kyphosis

- Inflammation and effusion
- Pain (stretch threshold or tolerance)
- Fear
- Immobilization in a cast or splint
- The presence of any simultaneous movement in another direction
- Body mass (large biceps limit flexion)
- Temperature
- Age
- Ethnic origin
- Training
- Circadian variations (time of day)
- Personal activity patterns (e.g., poor posture sitting)
- Vocation
- Medications
- A full bladder
- Warm-up

In general, to increase ROM at a joint, stretching and ancillary procedures must do at least one of four things (when appropriate): (1) increase the extensibility of connective tissues in muscles or joints, (2) reduce muscular tension and thus produce relaxation, (3) increase the coordination of the body segments and the strength of the agonistic muscle group (see table 12.2), or (4) reduce inflammation, effusion, and pain. The caveat, "when appropriate" is determined by the stretching technique employed. Loss of motion because of abnormal bone and joint structure is beyond the scope of traditional stretching procedures.

ADDITIONAL PRINCIPLES OF STRETCHING

A diversity of opinion concerning parameters and protocols in evaluating and developing optimum ROM and stiffness may be attributed to the various disciplines and professions involved (e.g., athletics, contortionists, dance, laypersons, rehabilitation, yoga). Therefore, guidelines should be tempered with a balance of philosophy, science, and clinical experience. Following are some principles that should be observed when developing flexibility. These principles are not necessarily the final word but do represent some of the more important points to remember when undertaking a flexibility-training program.

Safety

Safety always comes first. The primary objective of any instructor or health-care provider is to locate, analyze, and correct a student's or patient's stiffness or lack of optimal flexibility in the safest and most efficient manner. Although the instructor or health-care provider is ultimately responsible for the safety of those in their charge,

Table 12.2   Theoretical Model of Approaches and Courses of Action to Improve Range of Motion

Approach	Physiological conditions	Courses of action	
		Physical	**Psychological**
Decrease resistance of target area	Lengthen connective tissue	(a) Prolonged stretch	?
		(b) Contract target area while under stretch	?
	Relax myotatic reflex	(a) Reciprocal inhibition	(a) Mind-set (gamma bias)
		(b) Accommodation	(b) Biofeedback (monitored inhibition)
		(c) Heat, ice, massage, exercise, fatigue, etc.	(c) Relaxation training
Increase strength of opposing muscles	Muscle loading of opposing muscles	(a) Isometric	(a) Motivation
		(b) Concentric	
		(c) Eccentric	
	Facilitation techniques	(a) Successive induction (proprioceptive neuromuscular facilitation)	(a) Learning: recruitment, coordination, synchronization

Reprinted, by permission, from S.J. Hartley-O'Brien, 1980, "Six mobilization exercises for active range of hip flexion," *Research Quarterly for Exercise and Sport* 51(4), 627.

these individuals must also be involved in the prevention of injury. However, *more* than the health-care provider or instructor causing no harm assures patient or client safety. Safety is a multiple-stakeholder enterprise that is only as successful as its weakest link. Consequently, safety requires attitudes, skills, and knowledge about the control of potential hazards. The American Alliance for Health, Physical Education, and Recreation (1968) advocates a simple four-step approach to safety issues: (1) know the hazards, (2) remove the hazards when feasible, (3) control the hazards that cannot be removed, and (4) create no additional hazards.

Medical Examination

Ideally, a history should be obtained and a medical examination (assessment) should be performed before undertaking any exercise program. Only by eliciting information relative to a person's health status can an instructor or health-care provider formulate an appropriate protocol to achieve the desired goals. A case history is necessary

- To determine the overall health status of the athlete or patient
- To develop a better understanding of the individual's concerns
- To detect any condition that may limit an athlete's participation
- To detect conditions that may predispose an athlete to injury during competition, such as past or untreated injuries or illnesses, congenital or developmental problems, or lack of physical conditioning
- To meet legal or insurance requirements (Hunter 1994)

A medical examination may reveal that certain types of stretching exercises are contraindicated. An examination may also lead the instructor or health-care provider to modify his or her stretching regimen to ensure safety. A list of contraindications for therapeutic muscle stretching (TMS) (i.e., specific muscle stretching performed, instructed, or supervised by a therapist in patients with dysfunctions of the musculoskeletal system) has been developed by Mühlemann and Cimino (1990):

- Lack of stability. TMS is contraindicated if joint integrity or stability is jeopardized or decreased by any (pathologic) process.
- Endangered vascular integrity. Pathologic processes or drugs (e.g., anticoagulants) can endanger vascular integrity or facilitate bleeding.
- Inflammation or infection in and around the involved structures.
- Acute injury to the soft tissues and muscles. If performed without sufficient time for healing, TMS

must be postponed until scar formation is sufficient for moderate tensile loads to be tolerated.

- Diseases of the soft tissues and muscles. Contraindications can be relative (i.e., TMS can or cannot be administered, depending on the actual condition of the tissue, the operator's skills, the patient's cooperation, and so forth) or absolute (as in conditions such as myositis ossificans).
- Lack of patient compliance and excessive pain or reaction. Any therapeutic maneuver is contraindicated if the patient cannot or does not want to tolerate its application. If the pain during TMS is not tolerated even though TMS is administered as skillfully and painlessly as possible, then TMS maneuvers should not be used. Patients may be taught self-stretching exercises instead, the performance of which should be supervised, and, later, controlled periodically.
- When common sense says "No." (p. 255)

Additional contraindications to the use of stretch include uncontrolled muscle cramping that occurs when attempting to stretch, arterial insufficiency, local hematoma as a result of an overstretch injury, tendon repair, Dupuytren's contracture, contracture (desired functional shortening) requiring stability to a joint capsule or ligament, or intentional contracture to improve function (e.g., tenodesis of finger flexors to allow grasp in an individual with quadriplegia) (Fredette 2001; Hardy and Woodall 1998; Kisner and Colby 2000).

Identifiable Goals

One should establish his or her goals before beginning a flexibility program and have an idea of how much time is required to reach the desired degree of flexibility. For example, the goal may be the ability to place the palms flat on the floor with legs straight after 6 weeks of stretching. Whatever the goals are, they should be realistic.

Individualized Program

Ideally, all exercises should be designed to fit an individual's specific needs. However, one is often expected to fit into a group or team in a flexibility-training program. Should a coach, instructor, or trainer insist that a given stretch be held for a specific time or encourage each athlete to sustain the stretch until his or her individual threshold or objective is fulfilled?

The answer to this question depends on a number of factors. Ideally, one should have already warmed up and stretched on one's own before participating in the team stretch. However, doing so is not always possible or even desirable if the individual does not have the knowledge to warm up and stretch safely. The team approach is usually the most appropriate course to follow. At least some stretching is guaranteed if one participates in a group, and a team program fosters camaraderie and team spirit. At the end of the team workout, each individual can concentrate on those muscles that need additional stretching.

However, if one is stretching in a class at a fitness or health club, one should listen to one's own body and either participate with the class or hold the stretch as individually appropriate. Such a class may have a wider range of abilities, and stretching beyond one's safety limit is a real possibility, especially for beginners. Instructors should educate class members about which and to what degree exercises should be attempted. In addition, instructors should tell their students that stopping and resting in the middle of a class session or modifying an exercise is allowed. Adaptation is particularly appropriate in the case of fatigue, pain, or excessive difficulty with a given exercise. The instructor must constantly monitor all members of the class during the workout for potential complications.

Keep Accurate Records

A well-planned program is also a recorded one. Records should include the date and time of exercise; types of exercises performed; exercise intensity, duration, and frequency; and self-evaluation before, during, and after the program. A variety of devices are available for measuring and evaluating ROM, ranging from the sophisticated and expensive to the simple and inexpensive. They include radiography, photography, videofluroscopy, schematography, spine motion analyzers, grids, outline tracing, goniometers or protractors, electrogoniometers, single/double inclinometers (mechanical, electronic, or fluid-filled), tape measures, performance charts, and visual observations. Regardless of the method chosen for measuring ROM, a standardized procedure for warm-up before testing should be established (Maud and Cortez-Cooper 1995).

Record keeping is prudent for a variety of reasons (American Medical Association 1993; Hubley-Kozey 1991; Protas 2001; Rondinelli and Katz 2000). (1) Analytical information can be gained concerning the ROM. (2) Information may reveal positive or negative patterns in the training program. (3) Recorded evaluations could also identify areas that may be associated with poor performance of a skill or with possible risk of injury. (4) Collected data could assess the rehabilitation procedure after injury and assist in determining the suitability of the individual to return to play. (5) The accumulation of normative values for various populations could enhance the interpretation of flexibility testing. (6) Record keeping can serve as a motivational tool and (7) can also provide valuable information in the event of legal challenges to the care provided.

Measuring and evaluating pain or stiffness is a specific concern for physical therapists, rheumatologists and heath-care providers, either primary or allied. Joint stiffness can be evaluated on a subjective basis. However, these evaluations may be unreliable. Wright and Johns (1960) developed a technique (arthrography) that permitted quantitative and qualitative measurements of joint stiffness in precise physical terms (Lung et al. 1996). Since then, several pressure gauge methods of objectively assessing soft-tissue consistency or compliance have been developed. Pressure-pain threshold measurement is referred to as *algometry*. Regardless of the methodology, measuring the rheological properties of joints or soft tissues presents many challenges (Bovens et al. 1990; Gifford 1994; Helliwell 1993) such as age, gender, circadian variations, anti-inflammatory drugs, disease, and stiffness. Measurements must be made in reference to the equilibrium point of the joint.

The reliability of ROM measurements is subject to a host of factors (intraobserver reliability, instrument reliability, subject cooperation and effort). According to Rondelli and Katz (2000), "these conditions can make it quite easy for measurements to vary by 5° or more, which could have a significant effect on an impairment rating" (p. 56). Thus, one may diligently record the measured results; however, this diligence does not guarantee the measured results are in fact accurate. Accordingly, Gajdosik and Bohannon (1987) advise, "As a rule, ROM of measurements are just that, not measurements of muscle 'tightness,' the length of specific structures, or other factors that may affect ROM" (p. 1872). Technology and research continue to progress at a rapid rate. Therefore, those concerned with measuring ROM or stiffness should keep abreast of the newest innovations that can afford optimum means for gaining this information.

Expect Gradual Progress

The development of flexibility takes time. Therefore, set realistic goals and begin with easy exercises before advancing to more difficult ones. Plateaus, or periods of no apparent progress, are part of the learning process.

Comparing and Competing

Do not compare yourself with others. Improvement and progress are important, not competition with someone who may be at a different level of ability. No two people are alike: Some may develop flexibility rapidly; others may take longer to reach the same level (see figure 12.1).

Clothing and Positioning

Wear loose and comfortable clothes when working out. Because a warmed muscle is believed to be more flexible and pliant, people often wear sweat suits and wool socks. Position yourself as comfortably as possible to reduce muscle tension and make the stretching more enjoyable.

Attitude and Mind-Set

A positive mental attitude is important. The mental, physical, and spiritual aspects of life are inseparable from

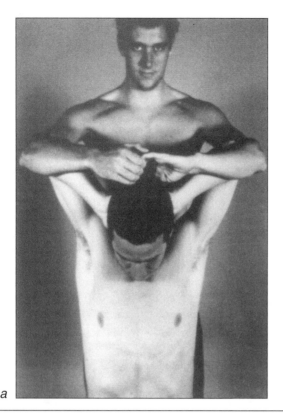 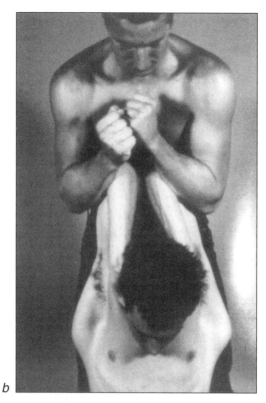

a   b

Figure 12.1 Comparing degrees of flexibility in different individuals. Each swimmer was able to perform at peak efficiency. If the individual in *(a)* tried to equal the limits of flexibility of the individual in *(b)*, he may have overstretched musculotendinous units beyond their effective ranges. *(a)* An NCAA division II gold-medal winner in the 100-yard freestyle. *(b)* An NCAA division II gold-medal winner in the 200-yard butterfly.

Photo courtesy of J.V. Ciullo, MD.

one another. Without a positive mind-set, the best of all possible results will never be achieved. Another important and deleterious consideration is that some athletes and performers believe perfection of their discipline takes precedence over their physical condition (Weisler et al. 1996). This attitude can potentially result in chronic or acute injuries. An example is a ballet dancer who attempts to force the turn-out position by employing the dangerous technique called "screwing the knee."

Relaxation

In certain types of stretching exercises (passive stretching) relaxation may be beneficial. On the other hand, in specific types of stretching exercises (functional stretching; PNF) developing or maintaining a certain amount of tension might in fact be safer and more efficient. Relaxation is the opposite of tension. Inappropriate tension originating in contracted muscles can result in inflexibility, an insufficient oxygen supply, and fatigue. Therefore, the ability to relax can be important because it decreases tension and its negative consequences, thus allowing one to function more effectively and efficiently. In general, stretching slowly and exhaling gently at the moment of maximum stretch can often facilitate stretch-

ing. However, exhaling during the stretching phases of a movement is not always beneficial or conducive for safe and efficient stretching.

Breathing

Most publications devoted to stretching, athletic training, physical therapy, and rehabilitation recommend that participants should either never hold their breath when stretching or exhale during the effort phase. Siff and Verkhoshansky (1999), in their text *Supertraining*, warn not to follow this popular advice as applied to resistance or strength training. Can this advice be expanded to include stretching exercises? Their argument is that during resistance or strength training, "breath-holding plays a vital role in increasing the intra-abdominal pressure to support and stabilise the lumbar spine during heavy lifting" and "exhalation during lifting increases the risk of lumbar injury" (p. 170). Thus, without breath-holding, far greater pressure is exerted on vulnerable structures of the lumbar spine, in particular the intervertebral discs and ligaments.

Obviously, in cases of passive stretching or static stretching where maximal force and spinal stabilization are not produced, exhalation is often advantageous. Many of the advantages of exhalation were explored in chapter 8. However, two specific situations bear special consideration. During several types of PNF maneuvers, holding breath and not exhaling may in fact be highly advantageous for stabilizing the body and facilitating maximal or near maximal contractions. During active or functional stretching, the constant interplay of mobility and stability must not be lost. If for example, when a ballerina or gymnast is training to master a technique that must be maintained for several seconds, exhalation may in fact make lifting and holding the leg in the desired position more difficult. Clearly, ideal training must include neuromuscular interactions in the execution of all skills. Thus, "appropriate techniques of breathing should always be combined with all phases of movement to enhance mobility, stability and relaxation" (Siff and Verkhoshansky 1999, p. 186).

Warm-Up and Cool-Down

Warm-up and cool-down exercises improve performance and reduce the chances of injury. The most important advantages of both active and passive warm-ups are increased muscle temperature, reduced muscular viscosity, decreased muscular tension, and more extensible tissue. A stretching program is used as an adjunct to warm-up or cool-down to increase flexibility. Stretching is *not* a warm-up procedure. See chapter 11 for more information about warm-up and cool-down.

Isolate the Muscle and Connective Tissues

Ten important caveats must be kept in mind when attempting to "isolate" a muscle, muscle group, or its respective connective tissues. First, "the real function of muscles/muscle groups must always be taken into account" (Evjenth and Hamberg 1989, p. 7). Second, a targeted muscle or muscle group cannot be truly isolated. Adapting the words (in reference to strength training) of Siff and Verkhoshansky (1999, p. 407), the concept of muscle isolation training when stretching incorrectly implies that only one specific muscle group is being stretched by a given procedure. This idea is very misleading. Movements of parts of the human body are interconnected and not isolated from the whole. In the case of active stretching or functional flexibility (ROM), movements are a combined result of the appropriate contribution of agonists (prime movers), antagonists, stabilizers, synergists, and neutralizers. "This is why it is vital to remember that all human movement involves the intricate orchestration of concurrent and sequential contractions of movers and stabilizers" (p. 407). Third, as a joint progresses through a ROM (i.e., during nonstatic stretching) different portions of muscle groups and their respective connective tissues are stressed more than other portions at each joint position as a consequence of simple

geometry (Martin et al. 1998). Therefore, once again, the concept of "isolation" is in fact a misnomer. Fourth, muscles often cross more than one joint. Consequently, using just one single stretch may not result in an optimum stretch or "isolation". Fifth, several important functional ROMs are not limited to a single joint, but result from a combination of movements by multiple joints (Protas 2001). For example, the ability to bend over and tie one's shoe requires adequate ROM in the trunk, hip, and shoulders. Sixth, in the case of active stretching with large loads (i.e., a resistance as in PNF stretching), isolation becomes virtually impossible because stabilizing muscles become involved to ensure that the body or specific joints remain stable, while the prime movers attempt to cope with the load (Siff and Verkhoshansky 1999, p. 241). Seventh, when attempting to identify a specific stretch for a specific muscle or muscle group, "the reverse of any action to contract a given muscle group becomes a stretch for that same muscle group" (Siff and Verkhoshansky 1999, p. 186). For instance, the biceps brachii flexes the elbow and supinates the forearm. Therefore, elbow extension and pronation result in stretch to that muscle. Eighth, for stretching to be most beneficial, the proper muscle group and its respective connective tissues must be the target to develop the optimum tensile force. Undesired compensation by other muscles and structures (e.g., the spine) may facilitate a reduction in the desired tensile force. For example, the anterior tilt position is more important than stretching technique (PNF or static stretching) for increasing hamstring muscle length (Sullivan et al. 1992). Ninth, if two stretching procedures result in significant gains in flexibility, the safest and most effective procedure should be the one employed. Tenth, the concept of multidirectional stretching may at first appear contradictory to the idea of isolating the muscle. "Multi-directional stretching is important, since the structural orientation of the fibers is different for the different collagenous tissues and is specifically suited to the functions of each tissue" (Siff 1993b, p. 128).

Starting Position

For stretching to be safe and effective, the starting position must be stable. That is, you can "support, control and relieve your muscles throughout the exercise" (Evjenth and Hamberg 1989, p. 11). Caution must be observed when attempting stretches balanced on one leg, sitting on a chair, or employing a raised platform. Additional stabilization may be provided by the use of equipment such as belts or splints. These devices may help avoid substitute motions when stretching or assist in maintaining support and control. Another important factor when stretching is the stabilization of one attachment site of the muscle (usually proximal) or limb during stretching (Brody 1999). For example, to optimally stretch the hamstrings, the pelvis must be tilted. "Failure to stabilize proximally results in lumbar spine flexion, posterior pelvic tilt, and movement of the hamstring origin closer to the insertion, thereby minimizing the stretch" (p. 100).

Application of the SAID Principle

According to Wallis and Logan (1964), strength, endurance, and flexibility training should be based on the principle of *specific adaptation to imposed demands* (SAID). That is, one should stretch at a velocity not less than 75% of the maximum velocity through the exact plane of motion, through the exact ROM, and at the precise joint angles used while performing skills in a specific activity (e.g., high leg kicks emulate punting a football). For movements performed at rapid velocity, a slow stretch should precede the application of the SAID principle.

Application of the "Overstretching" Principle: Stretching Duration, Frequency, Timing, and Intensity

The physiological principle on which strength development depends is the *overload principle*. Its analogue for flexibility is the *"overstretching" principle*. The difference between the two is that the latter uses stretch, whereas the former uses resistance, usually weight. Many individuals seek an established number of exercises to perform similar to the recommended dietary allowance for vitamins and minerals (Shrier and Gossal 2000) or a universal stretching dosage or recipe. Individuals want to know the exact duration, frequency, timing, nature, and intensity of the stretch to achieve their desired goal. Unfortunately, recommendations for these variables have sparked much debate and little consensus. Stretching protocols need to take into consideration variations and differences between healthy and injured tissues. Perhaps, the most important consideration is the purpose of the flexibility-training session. Specifically, is the purpose of the program development, maintenance, or rehabilitation of flexibility (Alter 1998)?

Stretching Duration

The utilization of specific stretching procedures such as static, dynamic, or PNF in part determines the duration of a stretch. Many programs recommend holding each stretch for 6 to 12 seconds. However, 10 to 30 seconds is also commonly recommended. The problem with holding stretches for longer than 30 seconds is that stretching programs might last longer than many workouts (Alter 1998). Magnusson, Aagaard, and Nielson (2000) reiterate, "multiple repetitions of sustained static stretches for a single muscle group can be very rigorous, time consuming, and hence an unrealistic stretching program" (p. 1160). Several impinging determinants for the time to maintain each stretch include the number of muscle groups or joints targeted and the number of repetitions

and sets of each stretch (Alter 1998; Brody 1999; Knudson 1998). According to Prentice (1999), stretches lasting for longer than 30 seconds seem to be uncomfortable for some athletes. An additional mitigating factor could include fatigue.

Bandy and Irion (1994) compared the effectiveness of 15, 30, and 60 seconds of static stretching of the hamstrings. Their study revealed that 30 and 60 seconds of stretching were more effective at increasing hamstring flexibility than stretching for 15 seconds or no stretching at all. "In addition, no significant difference existed between stretching 30 seconds and for 1 minute, indicating that 30 seconds of stretching the hamstring muscles was as effective as the longer duration of 1 minute" (p. 845). Later, this finding was again substantiated (Bandy et al. 1997). Consequently, this study reiterated the use of increased duration, and frequency beyond one 30-second stretch per day cannot be supported. Grady and Saxena (1991) also found that a 30-second stretch of the gastrocnemius is adequate to improve flexibility, with minimal additional gains when the stretch is extended to 2 or 5 minutes. Cipriani et al. (2003) found no difference between a 10-second stretch repeated six times for a total of 1 minute or a 30-second stretch repeated two times for a total of 1 minute. In both groups, stretching of the hamstrings was performed twice daily for a total of 2 minutes each day for 6 weeks.

Walter et al. (1996) determined that 30 seconds of passive stretch of the hamstrings was superior to 10 seconds at 85% and 100% intensity. The investigators suggested, a minimum threshold seems to exist for intensity and duration to be effective in improving ROM. In contrast, Madding et al. (1987) compared the effectiveness of a 15-second, 45-second, and 2-minute passive stretch to increase hip abduction ROM in 72 male subjects. No significant mean difference between the three groups was demonstrated. Based on these data, the authors concluded that it was "reasonable to stretch 15 seconds in athletic settings where immediate increases in abduction ROM are desired" (p. 416). In a study of people 65 years of age or older (Feland et al. 2001), the straight-leg-raising technique for the hamstrings was compared. Subjects were randomly assigned into groups that stretched five times per week for 6 weeks for 15, 30 and 60 seconds. Stretches were repeated four times with a 10-second rest between stretches. The 60-second stretch produced a greater rate of gains in ROM and more sustained increase in ROM. These results differed from those of Bandy and Irion (1994). The investigators speculated the longer duration of stretch "may have been more beneficial than shorter durations in overcoming the increased muscle stiffness and collagen deposition that accompany the aging process" (p. 1116).

Borms et al. (1987) compared the effects of 10, 20, and 30 seconds of active static stretching on active coxofemoral flexibility. The program consisted of two sessions per week lasting for 10 weeks. Their findings suggested that a duration of 10 seconds for static stretching is sufficient for improving hip joint flexibility. Roberts and Wilson (1999) suggested, "that holding stretches for 15 seconds, as opposed to five seconds, may result in greater improvements in active ROM" (p. 259). However, Apostolopoulos (2001) and Bates (1971) are of the opinion that 60 seconds of maintained stretch is optimal for increasing and retaining flexibility. A stretch normally takes about 30 seconds to progress from the middle of the muscle belly to the tendons. Therefore, "a token 10 [to] 15-second stretch may be beneficial to the muscle belly but will have minimal influence on the ligaments, tendons, and fascia that are largely responsible for range of motion and flexibility" (p. 54). However, Proske and Morgan (1987, 1999) point out that "when a passive muscle and its tendons are stretched, initially most of the movement is taken up by the tendon and only when tension begins to rise are the muscle fibres themselves stretched" (1999, p. 434). In contrast, the American College of Sports Medicine Position Stand (1998) proposes that static stretches should be held for 10 to 30 seconds, whereas PNF techniques should include a 6-second contraction followed by 10-second to 30-second assisted stretch. Similarly, Krivickas (1999) advocates holdings stretches for 15 to 30 seconds. Anderson (2000) suggests beginning with an easy stretch for 10 to 15 seconds followed by a "developmental" stretch for an additional 10 to 15 seconds. At the lowest end of the time spectrum, Mattes (1990) and Wharton and Wharton (1996) also promote a 1-second to 2-second lengthening strategy as an integral part of the Active Isolated Stretching protocol. Weider (1995), a world-renowned body trainer and publisher, also recommends holding each stretch for 2 seconds. His rationale is that after 2 seconds "the muscular response is to tighten up the area to prevent injury, which not only defeats the purpose of stretching but can also lead to microtrauma and soreness" (p. 139). In contrast, Brody (1999) recommends a patient or an athlete hold a stretch based on his or her perceived need or comfort level. However, "when in doubt, a stretch should be held for a longer period rather than a shorter period" (p. 103).

Another avenue to determine the optimum duration of a stretch is the use of animal models. Experiments on rabbit extensor digitorum longus and tibialis anterior muscle-tendon units by Taylor et al. (1990) suggests that the greatest amount of stress relaxation muscle elongation occurs during the first 12 to 18 seconds of a static stretch.

Given that time constraints limit ideal stretching during a workout session, athletes and performers must stretch on their own time. For some, serious stretching can be concentrated on off days, whereas others, particularly highly specialized athletes and performers, will need to stretch religiously on a daily basis. Empirical evidence would probably reveal a significant improvement in flexibility occurs when stretching is done on personal time. Later, this flexibility is transformed into finely coordinated and skilled movement.

Stretching Repetitions and Sets

Differences of opinion are apparent regarding the most effective frequency or number of repetitions (Smith 1994). Repetitions can refer to the number of times a stretch is performed within a set (i.e., the completion of one "turn" or a consecutive series or repetitions), the number of sets in a workout, the number of workouts in a session, or the number of sessions in a week. The number of sets and repetitions depends on the frequency and the number of exercises performed (Brody 1999). Their number is also determined by the objective of the stretching and one's state of health (healthy, rehabilitation for an injury). The American College of Sports Medicine (1998, 2000) recommends at least four repetitions per muscle should be completed for a minimum of 2 to 3 days a week. Weider (1995) advocates stretching for only 2 seconds but performing 3 to 4 or even more sets of microstretches for as often as needed. In contrast, Apostolopoulos (2001) recommends stretching once or twice a day three times per muscle group per session.

Taylor et al. (1990) experimented using rabbit extensor digitorum longus and tibialis anterior muscle and tendon units. The greatest change (80%) in muscle and tendon length occurred in the first four static stretches in a series of 10. Further stretching did not result in significant increases in length. In addition, "relaxation-curves of the first two stretches demonstrated statistically significant differences from the other curves. There were no significant differences in curves 4 through 10." Taylor et al. (1990) state, "the magnitude of the stretching force or the duration of hold time may have an influence on the ideal number of stretches" (p. 307). The research by Taylor et al. (1990) is admirable and commendable. However, Carborn et al. (2001) point out that "the study did not account for the added difficulty of stretching muscles that act across multiple joints, the components of functional muscle groups that present divergent sites of insertion, or the learning of proper technique" (p. 679). In addition, the development of flexibility is multifaceted, and extrapolating research carried out on animals to finely conditioned athletes has limitations.

Stretching Frequency

In general, the frequency of the stretching program is often inversely related to the intensity and duration (Brody 1999). Therefore, stretch exercises of high intensity and duration are performed less frequently and vice versa. Generally, one should stretch at least once a day for maintenance of flexibility. Such daily workouts are feasible if interest and motivation can be maintained (Rasch and Burke 1989). However, empirical evidence suggests that stretching at least twice a day is preferable. Perhaps the best time to stretch is when one feels as if one wants to.

Placement and Timing of the Stretching Program

Many texts and articles recommend stretching in the morning or in the evening. The common subjective feeling of "stiffness" or "tightness" in the lower and upper torso is caused by the change in fluid content of the vertebral disks (Adams et al. 1987). Consequently, the lumbar disks and ligaments are at greater risk for injury in the early morning (Adams et al. 1987). Another issue is the placement of stretching exercises in a workout.

Several options are possible for the placement of the stretching program within a workout. Opinions on the specific placement of stretching exercise are usually based on an intuition. Several researchers and writers have recommended stretching at the end of the workout. Their rationale is

- tissue temperatures are elevated;
- the time to perform your developmental stretching (meaning to actually increase your functional flexibility) is at the end of your workout, when you are totally warmed up and loose;
- stretching a muscle may temporarily decrease its force production capacity; and
- stretching at the beginning of the workout takes time from the overall workout.

What about stretching throughout a workout session? The recommendation that stretching should be conducted at the end of a workout should not be construed to mean that one should not stretch during a workout. To the contrary, one may in fact need to stretch during a workout, especially if a tight muscle group (i.e., hamstrings) is negatively affecting one's technique. However, most people seem careful to not go overboard and spend an excessive amount of time stretching if the total workout is short. Office workers (e.g., secretaries, people working at computer terminals, nurses) are now being advised to take small stretch breaks to reduce the risk of injury.

Cornelius et al. (1988) investigated the placement of stretching exercises in a workout and discovered that adherence to a static flexibility program will produce gains in joint ROM regardless of the placement of the flexibility routine. Their findings refute claims that specific placement of stretching exercises within a workout session makes a difference in increasing ROM. Placement is more relevant for "other objectives such as increasing tissue temperature and reducing tissue discomfort that might be affected by specific placement of stretching" (p. 236).

Stretching Intensity

The correct target intensity of stretching is extremely significant because, like any form of training, it can provide a potentially traumatic stimulus to the muscle-tendon unit (Knudson 1998). Like other forms of training, acute stretching programs can result in the structural weakening of the muscle-tendon unit and increase the risk of injury (Noonan et al. 1994; Sapega et al. 1981; Taylor et al. 1990). Stretching has also been documented in certain situations to produce a short-term strength deficit.

The intensity of stretch affects the increase in ROM (Walter et al. 1996). Their research suggested 85% to 100% intensities resulted in significantly greater flexibility than 60%. However, they cautioned "there may be an intensity that produces maximal gains in flexibility lower than 85% but greater than 60% of a maximal stretch" (p. 43). In contrast, Apostolopoulos (2001) advocates stretching should always be performed at a low-intensity level of approximately 30% to 40% of perceived exertion.

The dilemma regarding stretching intensity is threefold. First, intensity is subjective. Second, stretching intensity is most often conducted under conditions in which the intensity cannot be quantified. Third, vigorous stretching is important for optimum progress (i.e., for athletes and highly trained performers); however, stretching intensity beyond the adaptability of the respective tissues capacity could result in injury.

In general, the intensity of the stretch should also be up to you. Although stretch may produce some discomfort (especially for beginners), it should not be so great a discomfort as to cause pain. If your muscle begins to quiver and vibrate, if pain persists, or if ROM decreases, you have stretched too much, and either the force or the duration of the stretch should be decreased. Discomfort and pain are subjective matters, so no absolute answer about where to draw the line can be given. The best advice is "Train, don't strain."

Mechanics

The individual must use proper mechanics and techniques when stretching to achieve optimal results. Applying proper mechanics involves identifying and "isolating"

Postworkout Stretching

Some investigators (Anderson 2003a; Bledsoe 2003) suggest that postworkout stretching is more advantageous than preworkout stretching. They cite research by Vandenburgh and Kaufman (1983) that demonstrates stretching-related stimulation of the passage of amino acids into muscle cells, accelerate synthesis inside the cells, and inhibit protein degradation rates. Consequently, postworkout stretching should theoretically help muscle cells repair themselves and synthesize energy-producing enzymes and structures, which enhance overall fitness. Thus, these effects may be the reason athletes who stretch after workout are injured less often.

those muscle groups and tissues to be stretched and using the appropriate exercise to fulfill that goal. Correct technique reduces the risk of injury and the impairment of performance.

Reflex

A variety of reflexes can influence ROM. Perhaps, the best known and commonly cited is the stretch reflex. In general, laypeople, the sedentary, and the elderly should use slow or static methods of stretch because sudden or painful movements may elicit a stretch response, causing the muscle to simultaneously contract (see chapter 6). Therefore, ballistic stretching for these populations should be avoided, especially during the early stages of a program. On the other hand, most sports and disciplines necessitate some ballistic stretching as a part of their training program. Flexibility training encompasses both structural conditioning and functional (central nervous and neuromuscular) conditioning. Individuals engaged in those sports or activities should first warm up thoroughly, then progress from passive or static stretching to dynamic sports-related movements. Other potential reflexes impacting on ROM during stretching include reciprocal innervation and the positive support reaction reflex.

Anticipation and Communication

During passive stretching or specific PNF stretching exercises, partners should communicate with each other. The person being stretched should inform the partner when the stretch becomes unpleasant or painful. The person applying the stretch should anticipate how much overstretch should be employed. This activity is a two-way process.

Appropriate Injury Management

If injured, one should determine to the best of one's knowledge the extent of the damage. As a general rule, rest, apply ice and pressure, and elevate the injured part of the body, then seek appropriate medical care. The sooner an injury is treated, the earlier rehabilitation can begin and the faster the recovery will be. Again, use common sense.

Reversibility

Muscle and connective tissue respond to disuse and immobilization. Consequently, these tissues will "detrain" if not constantly trained toward a set goal (Bischoff and Perrin 1999). Maintenance of flexibility is a continuous process. Here, the relevant axiom is "Use it or lose it."

Enjoyment

Stretching should be enjoyable and satisfying and create a sense of well-being. Enjoyment and pleasure are a matter of satisfying one's motives. However, stretching has the potential to involve varying degrees of pleasantness or unpleasantness. When stretching ceases to be enjoyable, it can become self-defeating.

SUMMARY

Homeostasis is maintenance of a steady state. To develop flexibility, one's homeostatic state must be exceeded by added stress to enter a new state, in a process called adaptation. Overstretching is the physiological principle on which flexibility development depends: When one properly stretches regularly, the body will respond with an increased ability to stretch. For stretching to be successful, a movement must actually exceed the existing ROM. However, "overstretching" in this context does not mean stretching body parts that exceed their safety limits and result in injury and impairment in function.

Before engaging in a stretching program, one should have some knowledge about anatomy, physiology, and the structure and functions of joints. In addition, a number of important principles must be observed when developing flexibility: safety always comes first; expect gradual progress; warm-up and cool down; and use appropriate medical treatment in case of injury.

CHAPTER 13

Types and Varieties of Stretching

Coaches and teachers of specialized physical activities have long recognized the need for high flexibility in certain joints or groups of joints. To help participants achieve this flexibility, they have developed special stretching exercises and drills, which can be broadly classified into two categories: ballistic and static. In addition, a variety of stretching devices and machines have been developed to facilitate or maintain flexibility. Regardless of methodology, safety and maintaining the increased ROM (active, functional, and passive) is important in determining the effectiveness of the stretching program.

TRADITIONAL CLASSIFICATIONS OF STRETCHING

Ballistic stretching is usually associated with bobbing, bouncing, rebounding, and rhythmic motion. It imposes passive momentum that exceeds static ROM on either relaxed or contracted muscles (Siff and Verkhoshansky 1999). Ballistic stretching lacks a held end position. Often the terms *dynamic*, *fast*, *isotonic*, or *kinetic* are used to refer to ballistic stretching. *Static* stretching involves the use of a position that is held and that may or may not be repeated. Synonyms for static stretching are *isometric*, *controlled*, or *slow* stretching.

Regardless of the method employed, the possibility of stretching beyond one's safety limit depends on a variety of factors, including the intensity of the stretch, the duration of the stretch, the frequency, or number of movements performed in a given period, and the velocity or nature (e.g., eccentric or isotonic) of the stretch.

Ballistic Stretching

One of the more controversial topics in sports science is the relative value of ballistic versus static stretching for developing flexibility. The controversy is complicated by the lack of research on ballistic flexibility compared with other types of stretching regimens (e.g., PNF). One obvious problem deals with an ethical concern: Who would knowingly design a test that would injure volunteers? Ballistic stretching is more difficult to assess because of the need for elaborate equipment and technical expertise in measuring the force that is required to move the joint through its ROM at both fast and slow speeds (Stamford 1981). Zehr and Sale (1994) have recommended as a future area of research the neurophysiological mechanisms and anatomical loci underlying agonist premovement EMG depression and physiological adaptations responsible for specific neuromuscular training effects subsequent to ballistic training. Other potential topics of study include the extent to which ballistic training adaptations reflect neural adaptation and muscle-level changes such as muscle and motor unit contractile properties, changes in muscle fiber type proportions, and alterations in the force-velocity relation. Regardless of the controversy, however, a considerable amount of research indicates that both ballistic and static methods are effective in developing flexibility (Bandy et al. 1998; Corbin and Noble 1980; Logan and Egstrom 1961; Sady et al. 1982; Stamford 1981; Wallin et al. 1985).

Arguments Supporting Ballistic Stretching

Four major arguments support ballistic stretching, based on the following advantages: development of dynamic flexibility, effectiveness, team camaraderie, and interest. Ballistic training has been time-tested in various disciplines (e.g., martial arts). Most important, ballistic stretching helps to develop dynamic flexibility. Because most activities and movements are dynamic in nature, ballistic stretching permits specificity in training and warm-up. Although ballistic stretching is usually associated with bobbing, bouncing, rebounding, and rhythmic motion, it can also occur simultaneously with contraction of the same muscles.

Ballistic training may induce neural adaptions involving reflex responses (Zehr and Sale 1994). For example,

Mortimer and Webster (1983) found karate-trained (ballistically trained) subjects were able to manifest larger increases in the gain of long-latency myotatic pathways preceding movement, greater limb acceleration, and shorter rise times in initial agonist burst than untrained subjects were. Another possible advantage of ballistic training is the improvement of reflex reactions (Wallin et al. 1985).

A special type of ballistic training technique is called *plyometrics*. Plyometric training has a greater effect on the series elastic component (SEC) than static stretching (Siff 1993b). Research has conclusively demonstrated the importance of the SEC in fast movements. Consequently, this specific type of training "should not be avoided by serious athletes, since the ability to use elastic energy is vital to all high level performance" (p. 127). It must be incorporated with deliberate planning and execution to reduce the risk of injury.

Another point is raised by Shrier and Gossal (2000). They acknowledge that an increased risk of injury can be a concern. However, they add an important caveat for athletes: "ballistic is more controlled than most athletic activities. Therefore it [ballistic stretching] is likely to be much less dangerous than the sport itself if performed properly and not over aggressively" (p. 61).

Vujnovich and Dawson (1994) demonstrated that ballistic stretch after static stretch appears to be twice as effective as static stretch alone in reducing α–motor neuron pool excitability, which correlates with increased flexibility. This research "contradicts traditional opinion that therapeutically applied rapid stretch results in a reflex contraction of muscle" (Vujnovich 1995, p. 154). However, these results should be interpreted with caution considering the size of the static and ballistic stretching groups—14 and 5 people, respectively. Another practical advantage of ballistic stretching is that it can be easily practiced in unison to a beat or cadence, thus promoting team camaraderie. Finally, ballistic stretching can be less boring than static stretching (Dowsing 1978; Olcott 1980).

Arguments Against Ballistic Stretching

The major arguments against ballistic stretching cite the following disadvantages: inadequate tissue adaptation, soreness resulting from injury, initiation of the stretch reflex, inadequate neurological adaptation, and increased viscosity.

When muscle and its supporting connective tissues are rapidly stretched, they are not given adequate time to adapt. All living tissues are characterized by the presence of time-dependent mechanical properties, including *stress-relaxation* and *creep* (see chapter 5). Tissues that are stretched too rapidly allow little chance for time-dependent stress relaxation or creep to occur to reduce the tension (at a given length change) or to increase the length (for a given applied force) (Sun et al. 1995; Taylor

et al. 1990). Permanent lengthening is most effectively achieved by lower force, longer duration stretching at elevated temperatures (Laban, 1962; Light et al. 1984; Warren et al. 1971, 1976).

Opponents of ballistic stretching claim this technique should be avoided also because it generates rather large and uncontrollable amounts of angular momentum, as can be demonstrated by swinging the arms horizontally in an extended position. When the movement reaches its limit and suddenly stops, the angular momentum can often exceed the absorbing capacity of the tissues being stretched, such as with improper or uncontrolled swings in baseball and golf.

A logical extension of the argument concerning tissue adaptation is that ballistic stretching can result in soreness or injury. If a tissue is stretched too fast, it can be strained or ruptured, resulting in pain or impairment of ROM. However, if the tissue is slowly stretched through the same range, it is less likely to strain or rupture because it is not required to absorb the same amount of energy per unit of time (Taylor et al. 1990). However, if progressively stretched, all tissues will ultimately reach a point of rupture, regardless of velocity.

If a sudden stretch is applied to a muscle, the stretch reflex causes the muscle to contract. As a result, muscular tension increases, making connective tissues more difficult to stretch out and defeating the very purpose of the stretching procedure. Generally, for stretching to be safest, the contractile elements of the muscle should be totally relaxed.

Ballistic stretching does not allow adequate time for neurological adaptation to take place. Walker (1961) found that the amount of tension for a given amount of stretch is more than doubled by a quick stretch as compared with a slow stretch. Granit (1962) reported that a pull on a muscle with a given force produced an efferent impulse frequency of more than 100 impulses per second within 1 second after the stretch. However, with a slower increase in muscle length until the same force was applied, a peak volley of only 40 impulses per second was produced within 6 seconds. The reduced motor neuron firing frequency reduces the tension in the muscle.

Fast stretching results in greater viscosity and stiffness (e.g., the spine). The classic analogy is a plunger immersed in a viscous fluid. The faster one tries to move the plunger, the higher the pressure within the fluid. Fast stretching can increase passive stresses that otherwise would not develop (McGill 1998; Yingling 1997). Combined, these factors are thought to increase the risk of injury.

Implementing a Safe Ballistic Stretching Program

If ballistic movements are to be a part of a stretching program, how should they be implemented? Zachazewski (1990) recommends a *progressive velocity flexibility program*

(PVFP). As with all programs, the PVFP is preceded by a warm-up. Then, the individual goes through "a series of stretching exercises in which the velocity and range of lengthening are combined and controlled on a progressive basis" (p. 228). PVFP permits the muscle and musculotendinous junction to progressively adapt to functional ballistic movements, which reduces the risk of injury. Zachazewski (1990) briefly describes the program as follows:

> The athlete progresses from an environment of control to activity simulation, from slow-velocity methodical activity to high-velocity functional activity. After static stretching, slow short end of range (SSER) ballistic stretching is initiated. The athlete then progresses to slow full range stretching (SFR), fast short end range (FSER) and fast full range (FFR) stretching. Control and range are the responsibility of the athlete. NO outside force is exerted by anyone else. (p. 228) (See figure 13.1.)

No controlled clinical studies or research has been published on PVFP. Consequently, Bandy (2001) recommends carefully monitoring of the program upon its initiation and advises caution to make sure "that the athlete is not being overaggressive, creating pain in or damage to the muscle being stretched" (p. 40).

Static Stretching

Static stretching involves a position that is held for a period of time and that may or may not be repeated. Static stretch may be either the result of a static muscle contraction or assisted by gravity, a partner, or apparatus.

The key qualities of static stretching are maximum control, little or no movement, and minimal to no velocity of movement. The pros and cons of static stretching are reviewed in the following sections.

Arguments Supporting Static Stretching

Traditionally, static or slow stretching is preferable to ballistic stretching. Static stretching has been used for centuries by practitioners of hatha yoga and is time proven. Static stretching is scientifically based and is effective in enhancing ROM. Significantly, prolonged slow static stretching is associated with permanent viscous deformation of connective tissue (Laban 1962; Sapega et al. 1981; Warren et al. 1971, 1976). It is also comparable to cyclic stretching in reducing ankle stiffness in people with stroke (Bressel and McNair 2002).

Furthermore, static stretching is required for the optimal development of static flexibility (i.e., specificity of training). Thigpen (1984) demonstrated that short bouts of static stretching reduced electrical activity within the muscle, which theoretically facilitates stretching. In theory, a minimal EMG signal would imply muscle relaxation, thereby minimizing the active resistance to stretch and maximizing the potential benefits of stretch. This condition leads to one of the most commonly cited rationales for static stretching: the influences of the stretch reflex will be minimized.

According to de Vries (1966, 1986), static stretching requires less energy expenditure than ballistic stretching. Furthermore, static stretching probably results in less muscle soreness and provides more qualitative relief from muscular distress. Static stretching is likely a much safer stretching technique, especially for sedentary or untrained individuals (Prentice 2001). Proper static

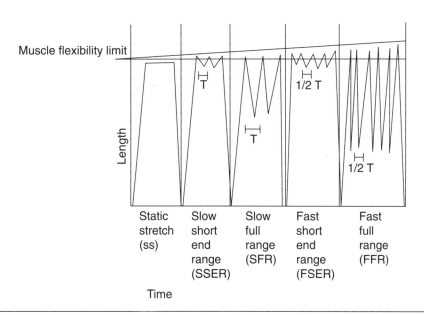

Figure 13.1 Progressive velocity flexibility program.
Reprinted from Zachazewski 1990.

stretching is safe, and it alleviates the typical constraints of limited funds, time, and space. Static stretching can be performed anywhere.

Arguments Against Static Stretching

At first glance, the arguments against static stretching do not seem as substantive as those against ballistic stretching. On a superficial level, static stretching is said to be boring. A more persuasive argument is that it may be practiced to the exclusion of ballistic exercise (Schultz 1979). Because most activities and movements are ballistic in nature, static stretching is not the optimal training technique. Stated another way, "the enhancement of static flexibility is of limited benefit to the serious athlete, since the mechanical properties of his soft tissues change dynamically during all sporting activities" (Siff 1993a, p. 32). A blending of both stretching methods is the optimal solution to this problem (Dick 1980; Schultz 1979; Stamford 1981).

Murphy (1991) reviewed studies on the shortcomings of static stretching. His investigation revealed that the supposed usefulness of static stretching usually was attributed to one of five causes: (1) it aids warm-up, (2) it aids cool-down, (3) it helps relieve postexercise delayed-onset muscle soreness, (4) it helps enhance athletic performance, and (5) it helps prevent injury. However, the literature provides very little support for these notions. In fact, clinical research as well as neuromuscular physiological principles indicate that these rationales for static stretching are incorrect.

As Murphy points out, the very nature of static stretching is passive. It cannot increase core or peripheral temperatures and thus does not aid warm-up. Again, because it is passive, it does not facilitate the redirection of blood flow away from the exercised muscles and therefore cannot aid in cool-down. The notion that static stretching relieves delayed-onset muscle soreness as originally proposed by de Vries (1961a) has not been reproduced in the studies of McGlynn et al. (1979b) and Buroker and Schwane (1989). Furthermore, Abraham (1977) found that static stretching only provided relief for 1 to 2 minutes after active exercise. No scientific studies substantiate the claim that static stretching improves athletic performance. In fact, Iashvili (1983) showed that passive flexibility as developed by static stretching has a relatively low correlation to the level of sports achievement, whereas active flexibility has a relatively high correlation. The search of the literature failed to support the notion that static stretching reduces injury. In elaborating on this point, Murphy (1991) writes:

> While it has been shown that the lack of "flexibility" is highly correlated to increased injury rate (Ekstrand and Gillquist 1982, 1983), it has never been shown that SS [static stretching] as a means of establishing flexibility does anything to prevent injury. Rather, as Iashvili (1983), Mora

(1990), and Gajda (personal communication) have pointed out, SS can actually increase chances of muscular injuries, even if it is done "properly" (Iashvili 1983). (p. 68)

Others (Evatt et al. 1989; Wolpaw 1983; Wolpaw and Tennissen 2001) have demonstrated that an individual can downtrain, or reduce the amplitude of, the stretch reflex. The stretch reflex is an important protective mechanism for the muscles and the joints that it controls (Radin 1989). With this downtraining, athletes may be prone to stretching beyond their safety limits, causing injury.

In addition to the issues posed by Murphy, one more challenge can be raised. An advantage of static stretching is its facilitation of two physical characteristics of soft tissues: stress-relaxation and creep. What is the minimum amount of time necessary for these actions to take place in a living person? Stress-relaxation and creep occur during sustained traction of 10 to 20 minutes. If stress-relaxation and creep require this amount of time to develop, then this argument for static stretching is not valid in a nonclinical setting because "compliance may decrease if durations of stretching are too long, particularly in people with muscle tightness" (Bandy and Irion 1994, p. 849). DePino et al. (2000) pointed out that increases in stretching ability resulting from static stretching are transient, lasting for only 6 minutes after administration and then decreasing with time. Their study employed four consecutive 30-second static stretches of the hamstrings. Thus, although static stretch is an effective technique when temporary gains in ROM are desired, it might not be effective in actually increasing connective-tissue extensibility for an extended period of time. Magnusson Aagaard, and Nielson (2000) employed three 45-second static stretches separated by 30 seconds that produced a 20% viscoelastic stress relaxation. The investigators suggested that the static stretching protocol used in their study "had no short-term effect on the various viscoelastic properties of human hamstring muscle group" (p. 1160).

Mohr et al. (1998) have also raised a question, perhaps underlying one of the chief neurophysiological rationales of static stretching advocates: the stretch reflex influences will be minimized. Their study examined EMG during clinically relevant stretching positions, in which 16 volunteer athletes imparted the stretch force themselves, and examined changes in EMG activity over a stretch duration up to 90 seconds. "Results of the study show there is no change in muscle activity beyond 30 seconds for a given stretch. Therefore, if the intention is to stretch while attaining as much muscle relaxation as possible, 30 seconds or perhaps less is probably sufficient" (p. 219). Furthermore, according to Taylor et al. (1990), the "static stretching, recommended by many for its reduction in reflex activity [i.e., the stretch reflex], is actually a clinical example of stretch relaxation" (p. 307).

Stopka et al. (2002) raise one more important facet. "Because static stretching has been taught in physical education classes, athletic settings, and the classroom for so long, it has been assumed that the application of a static stretch is the best way to increase overall flexibility" (p. 29). However, research does not substantiate this assumption.

ADDITIONAL CLASSIFICATIONS

Another way to classify stretching or exercises for the maintenance of ROM is based on who or what is responsible for the ROM. The movement can be further analyzed as to whether it is free or resistive. The following sections discuss the better-known categories of stretch, including passive, passive-active, active-assisted, and active.

Passive Stretching

In passive stretching, the individual makes no contribution to generating the stretching force, as in the absence of active contraction (i.e., voluntary muscular effort). Motion is performed by an outside agent (see figure 13.2a), which may be either a partner or special equipment, such as traction equipment. Pezzullo and Irrgang (2001) divide passive exercise into *physiologic* or *accessory* components. They further divide passive physiologic exercise into ROM and stretching. *Passive physiologic ROM* is motion that occurs within the unrestricted ROM, the normal ROM for a given joint. In contrast, *passive physiologic stretching* incorporates movements beyond the restricted range—the available ROM at a specific joint with restricted, or limited, motion—which are executed in an attempt to increase motion. Properly performed,

passive stretching increases passive flexibility. Passive extensibility is an important component of total muscle function because it allows maximal length of both non-activated and activated muscles (Garrett 2001).

Passive ROM can be restrained by passive mechanical forces or stretch-induced contractile responses to stretch. What percent of the restraint is attributed to each factor? McHugh et al. (1998), employing the straight-leg raise test found "seventy-nine percent of the variability to maximum SLR ROM could be explained by the passive mechanical response to stretch" (p. 928). Furthermore, the study substantiated the notion that the greater the increase in passive torque (resistance to stretch), the lower the maximum ROM (i.e., the tighter the subject). Conversely, the greater the energy absorbed over the total stretch, the looser the subject, and the higher the maximum ROM. This investigation provided "support to the concept that musculoskeletal flexibility can be explained in mechanical terms rather than by neural theories" (p. 928).

Hunter and Spriggs (2000) attempted to determine in an investigation of 20 male recruits whether measures of passive flexibility could be used to yield useful information about the active stiffness of the plantar-flexor muscles. Their results implied that "measurements of passive flexibility and active stiffness of the lower leg musculature are independent measures of components of muscle-tendon unit flexibility" (p. 600). Further research is needed to determine the relationship between passive flexibility and passive stretching as they relate to muscle-tendon unit in different age groups and sexes.

A significant relationship exists between passive flexibility measurements and running economy (Craib et al. 1996; Gleim et al. 1990; Godges et al. 1989). Additional research is necessary to explain the relationship between passive stiffness, elasticity, and running performance (see chapter 19). Understanding the relationship between passive stretching and prevention of injuries is still incomplete. Black and Stevens (2001) applied a 5% L_o strain, at a velocity of 0.5 mm/s, in the exterior digitorum longus of 22 mice in situ to determine whether the stretching protocol could prevent acute contraction-induced injury. The results did not support the belief that passive pre-stretching before exercise prevents injury.

Passive accessory motions cannot be produced by voluntary muscle contraction. They are usually performed by a health-care provider to increase joint play. They are traditionally classified as *mobilization* or *manipulation*. Mobilization involves low-velocity, medium-amplitude to high-amplitude passive movements of one or more joints, sometimes in graded oscillations. *Manipulations* use sudden, high-velocity, low-amplitude thrusting techniques at the end of the available ROM.

With the passive stretching technique, forced motion restores the normal ROM when it is limited by the loss of soft-tissue extensibility. The effect on muscle is passive lengthening of the elastic portion. The greater length

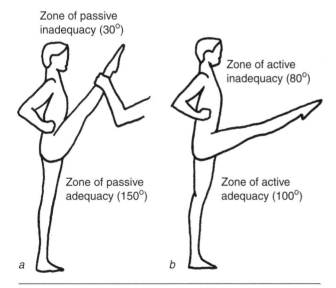

Zone of passive inadequacy (30°)

Zone of active inadequacy (80°)

Zone of passive adequacy (150°)

Zone of active adequacy (100°)

a   b

Figure 13.2 Flexibility zones. (*a*) Zone of passive inadequacy (30°). Zone of passive adequacy (150°). (*b*) Zone of active inadequacy (80°). Zone of active adequacy (100°).

Reprinted, by permission, from M.J. Alter, 1988, *Science of stretching* (Champaign, IL: Human Kinetics), 88.

then allows greater ROM in the affected joints. "During passive stretching, most of the elongation will take place in the muscle belly rather than its tendon" (Lederman 1997, p. 26). Passive stretching is indicated either because the agonist, or prime mover, is too weak to move the joint or because attempts to inhibit the antagonistic muscle are unsuccessful.

According to Dowsing (1978) and Olcott (1980), passive stretching with partners provides several additional benefits:

- Teammates counting for each other ensure that repetitions are completed. Furthermore, the individual tries harder to complete the repetitions because the partner is always watching.

- The coach is free to walk around and help with corrections. Once a correction is made, that partner can help others avoid the same mistakes.

- A greater feeling of progress exists when partners can recognize improvement in others and let them know it.

- Exercises performed with partners tend to promote the teammates' concern for one another.

- Tandem exercises are more enjoyable.

However, when implementing partner flexibility exercises, both partners must be totally familiar with each exercise. Because each partner is working the other's body, each must listen to the other's signals for stopping and holding the stretch. Just one mistake can wipe out all the benefits of a flexibility-training program.

Passive stretching may not be the optimal technique in treating tightness (Cherry 1980) or in attempting to regain muscular ROM, especially after injury (Jacobs 1976). According to Jacobs, passive stretching is contraindicated for at least four reasons. First, extreme stretch could cause the Golgi tendon organs (GTOs) to fire. Second, passive stretching can be painful. Third, flexibility is not retained, because the muscular imbalance is not eradicated by the GTO's short-lived inhibitory message. Consequently, no motor learning and no improvement in the capacity for active motion of the tight muscle or its antagonist occur. Fourth, if passive stretching occurs too rapidly, the muscle spindle complex may activate, and the resultant stretch reflex may initiate contraction of the muscle, thus defeating the very purpose of the procedure.

Passive-Active Stretching

Passive-active stretching is only slightly different from passive stretching. Initially, some outside force accomplishes the stretch. Then the individual attempts to hold the position by contracting the agonistic muscles isometrically for several seconds. This approach strengthens the weak agonist opposing the tight muscle.

Active-Assisted Stretching

Active-assisted stretching is accomplished by the initial active contraction of the agonistic group of muscles. When the limit of one's flexibility is reached, the ROM is then completed by a partner. This method can activate or strengthen the weak agonist opposing the tight muscle and help to establish the pattern for coordinated motion.

Active Stretching

Active stretching (see figure 13.2b) is accomplished by the voluntary use of one's muscles without aid. Siff and Verkhoshansky (1999) add an important component to this definition: "by non-ballistic action of muscles on the limb" (p. 184). Pezzullo and Irrgang (2001) divide active exercise into *free active* and *resistive* classes, each with its own components. Free active exercise or stretch occurs when "muscles produce movement without application of additional external resistance" (p. 108). Free active exercise comprises *ROM exercises* and *stretching*. ROM exercises "include those movements within the unrestricted available range of motion that are produced by voluntary contraction of the individual's muscles" (p. 108). ROM exercises are performed to maintain the current level of motion, whereas stretching exercises are designed to enhance or increase motion. Additional advantages of both active and active-assisted stretching exercises include

- limiting the adverse effects of immobility and maintaining contractility of muscles,

- providing sensory feedback,

- assisting in proprioception and kinesthesia,

- providing a stimulus for maintaining integrity of bone,

- increasing circulation,

- improving coordination and motor skills necessary for functional activities,

- improving strength of very weak muscles, and

- allowing incorporation of neurophysiologic principles of stretching.

Active exercises to increase flexibility can also use resistive strategies. Resistive exercises are defined by Pezzullo and Irrgang (2001, p. 108-109) as "those exercises in which the individual uses voluntary muscle contraction to move against an applied resistance" (pp. 108-109). The resistance may be mechanical, as in the case of isokinetic machines, or manual. Examples of resistive exercise to enhance ROM are PNF and muscle energy techniques (METs). Resistive exercises may include concentric or eccentric contractions.

Iashvili (1983) verified that active ROM values are lower than passive ones, but active flexibility has a higher correlation to the level of sports achievement ($r = .81$) than does passive mobility ($r = .69$). Iashvili also found that when using stretching exercises primarily, the coefficient of correlation between active and passive movements varies within the limits of .61 to .73. However, when using strength and combined exercises (active and passive), the coefficient of correlation increases to .91. Therefore, the relationship between passive and active flexibility is dependent on the training methods (Hardy 1985; Iashvili 1983; Tumanyan and Dzhanyan 1984).

Total ROM is the combination of active and passive ROMs. If passive stretching exercises are used to develop flexibility, then mainly passive flexibility is developed. Consequently, a reduction occurs in the passive inadequacy zone (see figures 13.2a and 13.2b). However, the greater the difference between a joint's ranges of active and passive movement, the greater is the likelihood of an injury (Iashvili 1983). To avoid such risks, strength exercises in the active inadequacy zone are recommended. They will reduce the passive inadequacy and increase the zone of active mobility.

Tumanyan and Dzhanyan (1984) compared four training methods. The control group in their study showed no changes in active or passive flexibility. The second group, which used stretching exercises alone, experienced approximately the same increase in active and passive flexibility. However, the difference between the active and passive flexibility remained unchanged. The third group, which used strength exercises alone, experienced only increased active flexibility. The fourth group, which used both strength and stretching exercises, had the greatest gain in active flexibility along with an increase in passive flexibility. Consequently, as active and passive flexibility increased, the difference between them decreased.

Roberts and Wilson (1999) investigated the effect of different durations of stretching (5 or 15 seconds) on active and passive ROM in the lower extremity during a 5-week flexibility-training program. Twenty-four university sports team/club members with a mean age of 20.5 years volunteered for the study. Active stretching procedures significantly increased active and passive ROM in the lower extremity. However, the most practical findings were (1) holding an active stretch for longer may not significantly influence increase in passive ROM, and (2) stretch duration may have a significant effect on improvements in active ROM.

If active stretching increases active ROM, does the duration of isometric contraction also affect flexibility? A study by Hardy (1985) found that larger gains in active flexibility were associated with longer periods of isometric contraction in the active muscle group.

Active stretching can be either ballistic or static. According to Matveyev (1981), ballistic exercises should be performed in a series, with a gradual increase in the size of the movements. The number of repetitions in a series usually ranges from 8 to 12. Repetitions should cease when the amplitude of the movements decreases because of fatigue. Well-trained athletes may perform as many as 40 or more repetitions with maximum amplitude. Static stretch training is characterized by a gradual increase in holding time from a few seconds to dozens of seconds. The amount of elastic (recoverable) or plastic (irreversible) deformation that occurs during cyclic muscle stretching is determined by the number of cycles, the rate of deformation, and duration of force per cycle (Starring et al. 1988).

Although both active and passive exercises contribute to improved flexibility, their effects on active and passive flexibility are different. When should one type of exercise be preferred over the other? Passive stretching is preferred when the elasticity of the muscles to be stretched (antagonists) restricts flexibility. Active stretching is preferred when the weakness of those muscles producing the movement (agonists) restricts flexibility. Therefore, one should know the elasticity of the antagonists and the strength of the agonists at the joints in question (Pechtl 1982).

Active Isolated Stretch (AIS)

A number of stretching systems have been vying for prominence in sport. *Active isolated stretch* (AIS) is an approach that has received much attention. AIS was developed by Aaron L. Mattes and is also referred to as the Mattes Method. Currently, AIS has had many advocates and promoters (e.g., Jim and Phil Wharton, the authors of *The Wharton's Stretch Book*) and satisfied clients. AIS operates under simple principles (Mattes 1990; PennState Sports Medicine Newsletter 1998; Wharton and Wharton 1996):

- Focus on stretching one isolated muscle at a time.
- Actively contract the muscle opposite the isolated and targeted muscle. This action will serve to relax the muscle you are trying to stretch.
- Stretch the targeted muscle gently and quickly.
- Hold the stretch for no more than 2 seconds.
- Release the stretch before the isolated muscle goes into its protective contraction and return to the starting position.
- Repeat stretch eight to 10 times with each movement exceeding the previous resistance point one by 1° to 4°.

AIS is claimed to assist lymphatic drainage and deliver greater amounts of blood, oxygen, and nutrition to specific regions than static or isometric muscle contractions. Some proponents claim with active-isolated stretching, warm-up is not necessary before stretching, as the stretching routine is actually warm-up. One just eases into each stretch, and watches as ROM increases with each stretch.

A criticism of the neurophysiological rationale supporting AIS pertains to the physiology of muscle spindles. Wharton and Wharton (1996, p. xxii) write: "If you elongate a muscle too quickly or too far, it automatically and ballistically recoils to protect itself from ripping. This compensation, called a 'myotatic reflex,' kicks in at *three seconds*" (italics by Wharton and Wharton). Do muscle spindles take 3 seconds for a "too quickly" elongated (i.e., stretched) muscle to respond? The stretch reflex in the calf muscles is elicited in 30 msec (0.030 s) or 3 hundredths of a second. Muscles that are closer to the spinal cord, such as the hamstrings, are even faster. Two seconds is an eternity in the nervous system. To think that one can "sneak up on a muscle and avoid eliciting a stretch reflex by doing a stretch for 2 seconds is ridiculous" (Moore 2003). However, the notion of slow, cyclic stretching is definitely supported in the literature and in clinical practice.

Tsatsouline (2001b) believes that AIS will make gains in passive and active flexibility. Instead, he maintains, "there are far more superior methods" (p. 63). Currently, no published studies have compared the efficacy of AIS to other stretching techniques. However, a review of the literature reveals a variety of names for "variations" of the same stretching technique if the "two second" protocol is removed:

- IA (Isometric contraction of the agonist) (Holt et al. 1970)
- Working the reciprocal group (to the hypertonic group) (Reciprocal lengthening reaction) (Waddington 1976)
- Slow Active Stretching (SS) (Turner 1977)
- Active Proprioceptive Neuromuscular Facilitation (Hogg 1978)
- 3-PI (a passive flexibility maneuver—3-second maximum voluntary isometric contraction of the agonist) (Cornelius and Hinson 1980)
- Active PNF (active only) (Hartley-O'Brien 1980)
- DROM (Dynamic ROM) (Dominguez and Gajda 1982)
- Concentric, Isometric Contractions (CI) (Turner and Frey 1984)
- AC (Agonist Contract) (Condon and Hutton 1987)
- ACR (Agonist Contract-Relax) (Osternig et al. 1990).

On a second level, AIS can be likened to a "modified PNF" technique. Perhaps, it is most closely related to the HR technique if just one phase is modified. Additional PNF techniques can also be easily modified. This modification can be demonstrated by either adding, deleting, or reversing (morphing) one phase of a respective PNF technique. The following are examples:

- CR [Contract-Relax] (isometric contraction of the antagonist, relax, followed by moving into the newly gained range). Reverse the contraction of the antagonist to a contraction of the agonist = AIS.
- HR [Hold Relax] (isometric contraction of the antagonist, relax, followed by moving into the

---

A Joint's Maximum Sustainable Active and Passive Flexibility

Coaches and athletes need to understand the importance of (1) developing both passive and active flexibility and (2) having quantified data on the limits of a joint's allowable maximum active and passive ROM. "By knowing the amount of reserve (the high rating of passive mobility) and the actual (passive and active) mobility in joints, one can determine the amount of potential increase" (Karmenov 1990, p. 200). To calculate the potential increase of maximum active flexibility, subtract the measure of maximum active flexibility from the measure of maximum passive flexibility. This difference is the *zone of active inadequacy*. Siff and Verkhoshansky (1999, p. 200) refer to this difference as the *loaded active flexibility deficit* or *flexibility deficit* (p. 184).

For example (see figure 13.2), given the amount of maximum passive adequacy (flexibility; ROM) is 150° of hip flexion with both legs kept extended, and the maximum active adequacy (flexibility; ROM) is 100°, then the potential increase in active flexibility is 30°. Thus, the greater the zone of maximum active inadequacy (flexibility deficit), the greater is the potential to increase maximum active flexibility. However greater differences between the ranges of active and passive flexibility increases the likelihood of injury (Iashvili 1983).

Determination of the potential increase in maximum passive adequacy (passive ROM) is calculated by subtracting the maximum passive adequacy from the amount of reserve mobility, (i.e., the high rating of passive mobility). This difference is the zone of passive inadequacy. For example, assume that elite gymnasts should possess 180° of hip flexion with the legs kept straight (determined by standardized test data that establish norms for related age groups). If the current zone of maximum passive adequacy is 150°, then the potential increase in passive adequacy is

$$180° - 150° = 30°$$

Such information could assist coaches and trainers in improving performance and reducing the risk of injury (modified from Alter 1998, p. 18).

newly gained range): Reverse the contraction of the antagonist to a contraction of the agonist = AIS.

- SR [Slow-Reversal] (an isotonic contraction of the antagonist, followed by an isotonic contraction of the agonist): Delete the isotonic contraction of the antagonist = AIS.
- IA-CA (isometric contraction of the agonist IA, followed by a concentric contraction of the antagonist, i.e., the CA): Delete the CA = AIS.
- CRAC (isometric contraction of the antagonist, relax, followed by an agonist contraction): Delete the initial CR = AIS.

However, each PNF technique is utilized to fulfill a specific goal and purpose.

AIS is a simple and effective stretching technique. However, superior techniques may in fact exist. Controlled clinical studies must be performed to clarify the advantages and disadvantages of all stretching protocols. In the meantime, the prudent course is to implement a personal stretching protocol that is designed for the rehabilitation, maintenance, or improvement of ROM determined by one's sport, activity, or life situation.

PROPRIOCEPTIVE NEUROMUSCULAR FACILITATION

Proprioceptive neuromuscular facilitation (PNF) is a method of "promoting or hastening the neuromuscular mechanism through stimulation of the proprioceptors" (Knott and Voss 1968, p. 4). It is a philosophy of treatment based on the belief that all human beings, including those with disabilities, have untapped existing potential (Adler et al. 2000). Herman Kabat developed PNF in the late 1940s and early 1950s. Maximal resistance throughout the ROM was emphasized, using many motion combinations related to primitive movement patterns and postural and righting reflexes (Voss et al. 1985). These motion combinations include isometric, concentric, and eccentric contractions, along with passive movement. PNF may be applied manually by oneself or an assistant or nonmanually. PNF techniques are utilized for rehabilitation and in such areas as athletic training.

Basic Neurophysiological Principles of PNF

PNF techniques are based on several important neurophysiological mechanisms, including facilitation and inhibition, resistance, irradiation, and reflexes. *Facilitation* or *facilitatory techniques* are designed to increase motor neuron excitability. Examples of facilitatory PNF techniques are any stimuli that increase the depolarization (increase the excitability) of motor neurons or cause the recruitment of additional motor neurons. In contrast, *inhibitory techniques* are designed to decrease excitability. They initiate stimuli that hyperpolarize (reduce the excitability of) motor neurons or result in a drop in the number of actively discharging motor neurons (Harris 1978; Knott and Voss 1968; Prentice 1983). Although inhibition is the opposite of facilitation, the two processes are inseparable: facilitation of the agonist simultaneously results in inhibition of the antagonist. Thus, an overlapping effect occurs on both opposing muscle groups (Knott and Voss 1968). However, inhibitory techniques are of greatest relevance to increasing flexibility. The underlying assumption is that by inhibiting motor neurons to antagonistic muscles, these muscles will be more relaxed and therefore will provide less active resistance to the intended agonist movement.

Facilitation and inhibition produce muscular *resistance* (i.e., active contractions). Originally, *maximal resistance* was defined as the greatest amount of resistance (opposing force) that can be applied to an isotonic contraction or an active contraction allowing full ROM to occur (Knott and Voss 1968). Currently, many PNF instructors consider the terms *optimal resistance* or *appropriate resistance* more accurate (Adler et al. 2000). Maximal resistance produces overflow, or *irradiation*, from stronger to weaker patterns of movement. Thus, irradiation is the spread of excitation in the CNS that causes contraction of synergistic muscles in a specific pattern (Adler et al. 2000; Holt n.d.; Surburg 1981).

The effectiveness of PNF techniques also involves the stretch reflex. The stretch reflex involves muscle spindles, which are sensitive to a change in length as well as to the rate of change in length of the muscle fiber. GTOs, which detect changes in tension, may also be activated by extremes of passive stretch. Both receptors help produce changes in the excitability of motor neurons that cause muscles to relax under specific conditions. Efforts to increase ROM by moving the joint to its physiological extreme will excite not only the muscle spindles and GTOs but also the sensory endings in the joint itself.

Basic Biomechanical Principles of PNF

PNF techniques employee active contractions. Theoretically, these contractions could improve ROM via two biomechanical methods. Increased tissue temperature is associated with decreased stiffness and increased extensibility (Sapega et al. 1981). First, in vitro research has demonstrated that a 15-second contraction, which elevated intramuscular temperature 1° C (33.8° F), increased force and length to failure (Safran et al. 1988). Thus, perhaps the elevated temperature facilitates the improved ROM. Second, Safran et al. (1998) suggested that this altered biomechanical behavior may have resulted from the force of the muscle contraction itself, which caused stress relax-

Altered Stretch Perception

In recent years, increased ROM after stretching has been suggested to be a result of increased "stretch tolerance" (Chan et al. 2001; Halbertsma and Göeken 1994; Halbertsma et al. 1996; Magnusson 1998; Magnusson et al. 2000; Magnusson et al.1996c). In contrast, Magnusson, et al. (1996a) refer to the term "altered stretch perception." "Currently, the relative contribution of improving flexibility by the 'tolerance of stretching' and the 'mechanical/ physiological' component remain unexplained" (Chan et al. 2001, p. 85). However, Proske and Morgan (1999) caution, "As often happens in science, we may have been swayed by the freshness and novelty of the new ideas" (p. 434).

Several plausible mechanisms may explain altered stretch perception, especially as they relate to active stretching or PNF techniques. Hagbarth and Nordin (1998) cite "an old observation that lifting a weight a few times leaves an after-effect making a subsequently lifted, lighter weight feel lighter than before" (Müller and Schumann 1899). Hagbarth and Nordin (1998) also describe a well-known parlor game: a volunteer is asked to stand in a doorway with his arms abducted for a while forcefully against the doorposts. After relaxing, the subject lets his arms slowly return to their initial position. At this point, he experiences a "transient sensation of lightness while the arms start to rise again due to a non-volitonal contraction of the arm abductor muscles" (p. 875). Subjects of several active or PNF stretching techniques also experience this sensation of lightness.

Hagbarth and Nordin (1998) revealed several divergent hypotheses regarding the neural mechanisms responsible for such after-contractions. One explanation is the so-called *posttetanic potentiation* of the α–motor neurons after the muscle spindle activation during largely isometric voluntary effort preceding the aftereffect. Other published reports have suggested "after-contraction phenomena are primarily caused by central excitability changes (Gilhodes et al. 1992) or to lasting after-discharge from muscle spindles (Hutton et al. 1987)" (Hagarth and Nordin 1998, p. 875). Recently, the contractions have been suggested to leave an aftereffect of increased intrafusal and extrafusal stiffness, both of which may contribute to the lightness illusions caused by thixotropic changes in the muscle spindles (Axelson and Hagbarth 2001; Hagbarth and Nordin 1998; Proske and Morgan 1999; Proske et al. 1993).

The presence or absence of slack can significantly alter the shape of the tension rise seen during stretch of a passive muscle and impact muscle spindle stretch sensitivity (Gregory et al. 1998; Hagbarath et al. 1995; Jahnke et al. 1989; Wilson et al. 1995). Elaborating on this point, Proske and Morgan (1999) write:

> Slack can be introduced at a particular test length by contracting a muscle at a longer length, letting it relax completely and then shorten it back to the test length. The slack can be removed by a contraction at the test length. (p. 437)

Slack in intrafusal fibers reduces background spindle afferent discharge and responsiveness (Proske et al. 1992, 1993; Wilson et al. 1999). The significance of intrafusal slack is that it leads to reduced strain on the sensory endings of spindles. That, in turn, lowers background levels of activity in spindles and reduces spindle stretch sensitivity" (Proske and Morgan 1999). Gregory et al. (1998) reported a voluntary contraction as weak as 10% of maximum voluntary contraction is sufficient to remove slack and sensitize muscle spindles to stretch. Consequently, collectively, the sequence of events discussed above may be responsible for an increased tolerance of stretch.

ation across the myotendinous junction. However, Magnusson et al. (1996a) are of the opinion that an isometric contraction does not alter the biomechanical response.

Benefits of PNF Techniques

People who endorse PNF techniques claim that PNF offers a wide range of benefits. The particular benefits depend on the technique employed. Regarding ROM, numerous investigators (Moore and Hutton 1980; Prentice 1983; Sady et al. 1982; Tanigawa 1972) found that PNF techniques produced the largest gains in flexibility, as compared with other forms of stretching. This effectiveness has also been claimed by other authors and researchers (Beaulieu 1981; Cherry 1980; Cornelius 1983; Cornelius and Hinson 1980; Hartley-O'Brien 1980; Hatfield 1982; Holt n.d.; Holt and Smith 1982; Holt et al. 1970; McAtee and Charland 1999; Perez and Fumasoli 1984; Sullivan et al. 1982; Surburg 1983).

Among other potential benefits of PNF are greater strength, greater balance of strength, and improved stability about a joint (Adler et al. 2000; Cherry 1980; Handel et al. 1997; Hatfield 1982; Holt n.d.; Knott and Voss 1968; Lustig et al. 1992; Moore 1979; Sullivan et al. 1982; Surburg 1981, 1983). Because flexibility without strength may predispose the individual to joint injury, specific PNF techniques may be useful in preventing athletic injuries by developing both qualities together (Moore 1979).

PNF techniques also have been claimed to improve endurance and blood circulation (Adler et al. 2000; Cailliet 1988; Knott and Voss 1968; Sullivan et al. 1982; Surburg 1981) and to enhance coordination (Adler et al. 2000; Knott and Voss 1968; Sullivan et al. 1982; Surburg 1981). Proponents further claim that PNF techniques result in superior relaxation of the muscles (Cherry 1980; Holt n.d.; Knott and Voss 1968; Prentice 1983; Sullivan et al. 1982; Tanigawa 1972). However, not all PNF techniques produce the same positive results (Adler et al. 2000; Condon 1983; Condon and Hutton 1987; Etnyre and Abraham 1984, 1986b, 1988; Moore 1979; Moore and Hutton 1980). Last, "application of PNF principles of spiral and diagonal patterns of movement (discussed later) also produces superior three-dimensional functional ROM to standard static stretches" (*Fitness and Sports Review International* 1992, p. 6).

Controversy About PNF Techniques

Although PNF techniques offer many potential benefits, they also have disadvantages. For instance, most methods require a well-motivated individual (Cornelius 1983; Moore and Hutton 1980). Cornelius (1989) and Stopka et al. (2002) pointed out that PNF stretching requires a certain amount of initial instruction and supervision. Furthermore, the assistance of a partner is often required, increasing training time. However, Stopka et al. (2002) found that PNF stretching techniques can be taught to individuals with mild to moderate mental retardation in a concise and comprehensive manner. Another drawback reported by Moore (1979), Moore and Hutton (1980), and Condon and Hutton (1987) is that certain PNF stretches are perceived as more uncomfortable and painful than static stretch. Various PNF techniques are sometimes more dangerous than static stretching because PNF stretching actually occurs with more tension in the muscle. In particular, the hold-relax technique, which employs an isometric contraction of the antagonist at its extreme range, applies an additional stretching force to the structures in series with that muscle, such as the tendon and its attachment. PNF procedures therefore must be closely monitored to minimize the chance of soft-tissue injury. Furthermore, most PNF exercises are designed as partner stretches and if done incorrectly can cause injury (Beaulieu 1981; Cornelius 1983).

Another disadvantage of PNF techniques is the possibility of the Valsalva phenomenon, which elevates systolic blood pressure (Cornelius et al. 1995) and has obvious implications for hypertensive individuals (Cornelius 1983; Cornelius and Craft-Hamm 1988; Knott and Voss 1968). The Valsalva phenomenon is an expiratory effort against a closed glottis (holding the breath and bearing down), which can occur during the performance of an isometric or heavy-resistance exercise. The process begins with a deep inspiration followed by closure of the glottis and contraction of the abdominal muscles. Consequently, intrathoracic and intraabdominal pressures increase, which leads to decreased venous blood flow to the heart and a decreased cardiac output, followed by a temporary drop in arterial blood pressure and an increase in the heart rate. When expiration finally occurs, an increase in blood pressure follows, which may reach levels of 200 mmHg or higher. Finally, a rapid venous blood flow into the heart causes a forceful heart contraction. The higher the maximum voluntary isometric contraction utilized during a PNF procedure, the greater the probability of the Valsalva phenomenon.

Cardiac patients, those who recently had abdominal surgery, or even the simplest surgery on the eye are cautioned about the dangers of the Valsalva phenomenon (Jones 1965). Another danger is herniation of abdominal contents if a weakness or defect in a muscular or fascial layer of the abdominal wall is present (Jones 1965). However, a review of the literature by Fardy (1981) indicated that the risk of the Valsalva phenomenon occurring during isometric exercise is less than has been presumed.

Cornelius and Craft-Hamm (1988) investigated the systolic blood pressure (SBP) and diastolic blood pressure (DBP) during one repetition of PNF using the hamstrings muscle group. Their findings showed no significant differences between the resting level and those obtained during the isometric phase. These findings have limited interpretability because the study only investigated subjects in the supine position. Cornelius and Craft-Hamm (1988) also emphasized the importance of knowing which medications patients are taking and their arterial blood pressure responses to PNF procedures.

Blood pressure measures vary considerably when the body assumes different postures, and many postures are used when engaging in a stretching program (Holt et al. 1995). More recently, Holt et al. (1995) demonstrated that less than maximal efforts (contractions) can produce gains in ROM similar to those from maximum efforts. The implication of this finding is that "it seems, then, that low-intensity PNF stretching can help improve range of motion and at the same time have little negative consequences on cardiovascular function" (p. 416).

Nevertheless, preventive measures should be incorporated into an exercise program to reduce potential risks. These measures include exhaling during heavy resistance exercise and breathing rhythmically during other exercises.

Experiments by Eldred et al. (1976), Suzuki and Hutton (1976), and Hutton et al. (1987) challenge some of the ideas supporting the neurophysiological basis of PNF. Specifically, these studies have found that a static contraction preceding a muscle stretch facilitates contractile activity through a lingering after-discharge of the spindles in the same muscle. Furthermore, contrary to traditional views, a muscle is initially more resistant to change in length after a static contraction (Smith et al. 1974). Supposedly, this resistance occurs because the

GTOs are only momentarily depressed after sustained contractions of muscle on stretch. These issues are dealt with in greater detail later in this chapter.

Etnyre and Lee (1987) raise questions about the difficulty of interpreting comparative data from the large number of studies utilizing various stretching methodologies. In reviewing the research, they state,

> Although it appears PNF methods produce the most favorable results, investigations to determine the efficacy of various flexibility techniques have differed greatly in methodology, experimental design, and procedures, making direct comparison difficult. Contradictions and controversies exist in the comparative literature over the effectiveness of static stretching and PNF methods. Discrepancies have been attributed to varied training programs, measurement instrument differences, and inadequate controls (Hardy 1985; Sady, Wortman, and Blanke 1982). Differences in administration of stretching methods reported in the comparative research include length of time for each session, number of sessions per week, and number of weeks of treatment (Lucas and Koslow 1984). Also, the experimental designs have varied in whether treatments were administered to the same group or separate groups. (pp. 185-186)

The need for well-designed and carefully implemented studies cannot be overemphasized.

One Plane–Single Muscle PNF Techniques

Before the development of PNF techniques, paralyzed patients had been rehabilitated using a method that emphasized one motion, one joint, and one muscle at a time (Voss et al. 1985). An example of a single-plane-of-motion stretch is manually stretching the patient's triceps brachii muscle. PNF techniques also can employ this same strategy of stretching in a single plane of motion. This technique is easier to master than the more complex spiral-diagonal technique covered in the next section. Single-plane PNF techniques are effective but not optimal. Nonetheless, excellent facilitation can be obtained by using various single-plane PNF strategies without ever using a diagonal mass movement (Kabat et al. 1959).

Spiral and Diagonal-Plane (Rotary) PNF Techniques

Normal, functional human movement is not performed in one motion, by one joint, or by one muscle at a time. Rather, movement occurs through mass movement patterns or spiral-diagonal patterns. Kabat and Knott developed techniques that use natural patterns of movement and thus stimulate the nervous system more effectively in the rehabilitative process (Houglum 2001; Voss et al.

1985). *Mass movement patterns* are defined by Voss et al. (1985) as "various combinations of motion . . . [that] require shortening and lengthening reactions of many muscles in varying degrees" (p. 1). The spiral-diagonal character of normal movement patterns arises from the design of the skeletal system and the placement of the muscles on it. The muscles spiral around the bones from origin to insertion, and, therefore, when they contract they tend to create a spiral motion.

Line of Movement

PNF techniques using a particular movement pattern assume a starting position with the major muscle components in their completely lengthened state, where the fibers of related muscles may be subjected to the maximal stretch. This starting position is the *lengthened range*, the *range of initiation*, or the *stretch range*. A pattern of motion that is optimal for a specific "chain" of muscles allows these muscles to contract from their completely lengthened state to their completely shortened state when the pattern is performed through the full ROM.

Because most muscles lie diagonally between origin and insertion points, they function optimally by contracting in a diagonal and frequently spiral direction (Kabat et al. 1959). This diagonal line of movement, or *groove*, is produced by the maximal contraction of the major components in proper sequence from their lengthened state to their shortened state (Voss et al. 1985).

Motion Components

Each diagonal or spiral pattern has three component motions or pivots of action that participate in the movement: flexion or extension, motion toward and across the midline, and motion across and away from the midline. Rotation is the third component of PNF patterns (Houglum 2001). The motion component that places the most stretch on a muscle determines its primary action component. The other components are considered secondary and tertiary action components.

PNF therapy uses two different spiral-diagonal patterns for each extremity (arm or leg) called *diagonal 1* (D1) and *diagonal 2* (D2). Figures 13.3 and 13.4 diagram the PNF patterns for the lower extremities. The patterns are named according to the proximal pivot at the hip.

Specific PNF Techniques

PNF involves a variety of techniques that promote specific results. They may combine isotonic and isometric (both concentric and eccentric) contractions. They may also involve contractions of agonistic and antagonistic muscles. The following descriptions of PNF techniques are based on the works of Adler et al. (2000), Knott and Voss (1968), Sullivan et al. (1982), and Surburg (1981).

Repeated Contractions

Repeated contractions (RC) involve contracting the agonistic muscle group until fatigue is evident (see figure 13.5a). In the less advanced form of RC, only isotonic

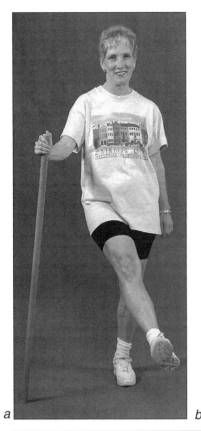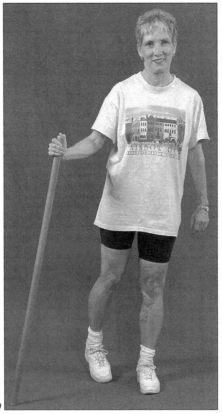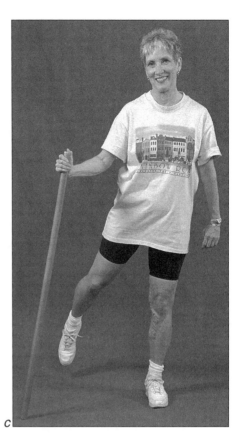

a   b   c

Figure 13.3   Free movements demonstrating PNF patterns for the lower extremity. D1 extension (toe-off): *(a)* initiation, *(b)* midphase, and *(c)* end position. D1 flexion (soccer kick): *(c)* initiation, *(b)* midphase, and *(a)* end position.
Reprinted from McAtee and Charland 1999.

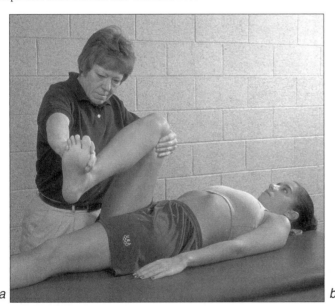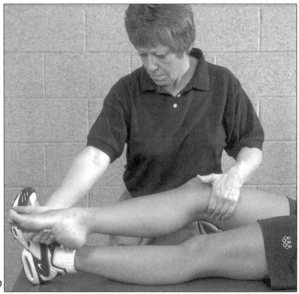

a   b

Figure 13.4   PNF patterns for the lower extremities. *(a)* D1 flexion and *(b)* D2 extension.
Reprinted from Houglum 2001.

contractions are used. RC may be preceded by an isotonic contraction of the muscles of the stronger antagonistic pattern to facilitate the weakened musculature. After an initial isotonic contraction, the more advanced form of RC is performed against resistance with resultant overflow to a weak pivot action. Then the individual holds an isometric contraction until active effort is felt to be lessening. Resistance is increased at the weakened pivot, the individual pulls again, and the isometric contraction becomes an isotonic one. RC helps to develop strength and endurance and promotes ease of impulse transmission through the central nervous pathway.

Rhythmic Initiation

Rhythmic initiation (RI) involves voluntary relaxation, passive movement, and repeated isotonic contractions of the major components of the agonistic pattern (see figure 13.5b). With this technique, passive, active-assisted, active, and resistive exercises are progressively executed. RI improves the ability to initiate movement, improves coordination and sense of motion, and aids relaxation.

Slow Reversal

Slow reversal (SR) involves an isotonic contraction of the antagonist, followed by an isotonic contraction of the agonist (see figure 13.5c). This technique improves action of the agonistic muscles, facilitates normal reversal of antagonistic muscles, and develops strength of antagonistic muscles. Resistance is always graded to allow movement through as much active range as possible.

Slow Reversal-Hold

Slow reversal-hold (SRH) involves an isotonic contraction of the antagonist, followed by an isometric contraction of the antagonist, followed by the same sequence of contractions by the agonist (see figure 13.5d). SRH may be applied to the stronger pattern because it may have a facilitatory effect on the weaker antagonistic musculature. SRH achieves the same beneficial effects as the SR technique.

Rhythmic Stabilization

Rhythmic stabilization (RS) alternates between isometric contraction of agonistic and antagonistic patterns (see figure 13.5e). The strength of the contractions is gradually increased as the ROM is progressively reduced during the entire sequence. RS improves active and passive ROM, increases holding power, increases stability and balance, improves local circulation, and aids later relaxation.

Contract-Relax

Contract-relax technique (CR) involves a maximal isotonic contraction of the antagonist against a resistance from a point of ROM limitation, followed by a period of relaxation. Next, a partner moves the limb passively through as large a range as possible until the limitation of ROM is felt (see figure 13.5f). Then the process is repeated. A similar technique, contract-relax agonist-contract (CRAC), is identical to CR except that during the final stretching phase, the agonist is concentrically contracted. CR improves passive ROM. CR may present a greater chance of injury compared with static stretching and the hold-relax technique because of the gradual increase of tension within the muscle.

Hold-Relax

Hold-relax (HR) is effective when ROM has decreased because of muscle tightness on one side of a joint. This technique employs an isometric contraction of the antagonist followed by a period of relaxation. Then the limb actively moves against minimal resistance through the newly gained range to the new point of ROM limitation (see figure 13.5g).

Slow Reversal-Hold-Relax

Slow reversal-hold-relax (SRHR) involves an isotonic contraction of the antagonist, followed by an isometric contraction of the antagonist, a brief period of voluntary relaxation, then an isotonic contraction of the agonist (see figure 13.5h). SRHR facilitates normal reversal of antagonistic muscles and develops strength in the antagonistic muscles.

Agonistic Reversal

Agonistic reversal (AR) employs movement isotonically through an ROM with a resistance. At the end of the concentric range, a slow, controlled, rhythmical sequence of eccentric and concentric contractions of the same muscle is repeated a number of times (see figure 13.5i). AR promotes both concentric and eccentric contractions of a movement pattern.

Modification of PNF Techniques

Siff and Verkhoshansky (1999) describe two types of PNF: classical and modified. The former is based on the works of Knott and Voss (1968). This technique emphasizes the use of patterns, along with verbal and nonverbal signals (e.g., contact with the hand). Modified PNF refers to "an approach which adapts certain PNF techniques and principles for application by hand or apparatus in physical conditioning" (p. 407). Siff and Verkhoshansky (1999) advocate the use of the term *functional neuromuscular conditioning* (FNC) in place of modified PNF for several reasons:

> Firstly, it is sometimes desirable to deviate from strict PNF principles to achieve a specific goal. Secondly, there are other movement disciplines such as Feldenkrais, Alexander, yoga, Tai Chi and Laban which offer invaluable additional methods of conditioning the body. Thirdly, PNF might not only involve neuromuscular processes, since contractile activity in a muscle may be facilitated by local after-discharge of the same muscle. Fourthly, the PNF repertoire includes methods which may not be classified accurately as proprioceptive, such as cognitive, perceptual and other sensory mechanisms. Finally, the term Proprioceptive Neuromuscular Facilitation is too technically daunting for the average coach or athlete. (p. 407)

Neurophysiology of PNF Techniques

Although many theories exist, much is still not completely understood about the neurophysiology of PNF techniques. PNF stretching techniques that employ "active

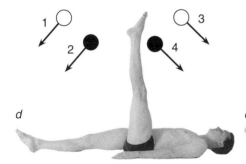

a

1. Isotonic contraction of antagonist.
2. Isotonic contraction of agonist.
3. Isometric contraction of agonist.

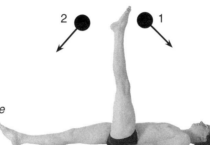

b

1. Passive stretch of antagonist.
2. Active-assistive contraction of agonist.
3. Active contraction of agonist.
4. Active-resistive contraction of agonist.

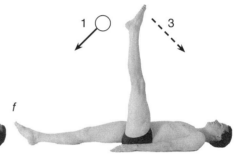

c

1. Isotonic contraction of antagonist.
2. Isotonic contraction of agonist.

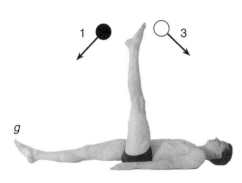

d

1. Isotonic contraction of antagonist.
2. Isometric contraction of antagonist.
3. Isotonic contraction of agonist.
4. Isometric contraction of agonist.

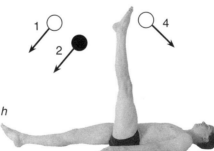

e

1. Isometric contraction of agonist.
2. Isometric contraction of antagonist.

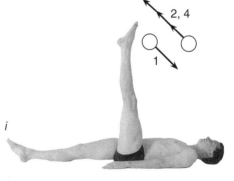

f

1. Isotonic contraction of antagonist.
2. Relaxation.
3. Passive stretch of antagonist.

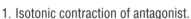

g

1. Isometric contraction of antagonist.
2. Relaxation.
3. Isotonic contraction of agonist against minimal resistance.

h

1. Isotonic contraction of antagonist.
2. Isometric contraction of antagonist.
3. Relaxation.
4. Isotonic contraction of agonist.
5. Relaxation.

i

1. Isotonic contraction of agonist.
2. Eccentric contraction of agonist.
3. Relaxation.
4. Eccentric contraction of agonist.

Figure 13.5 PNF procedures. (Isotonic contraction = open circle; isometric contraction = closed circle; passive stretch = dotted line; active stretch or contraction = solid line; eccentric contraction = line with arrows.) *(a)* Repeated contraction (RC). *(b)* Rhythmic initiation (RI). *(c)* Slow reversal (SR). *(d)* Slow reversal-hold (SRH). *(e)* Rhythmic stabilization (RS). *(f)* Contract-relax (CR). *(g)* Hold-relax (HR). *(h)* Slow reversal-hold-relax (SRHR). *(i)* Agonistic reversal (AR).

Adapted, by permission, from M.J. Alter, 1988, *Science of stretching* (Champaign, IL: Human Kinetics), 92.

muscle contractions to minimize active resistance and overcome passive resistance to stretch [are] best assessed through careful consideration of the effects of the components of the stretching procedures on neural activity and passive structures in the limb" (Condon 1983, p. 13). Because PNF stretching techniques include several components in a variety of possible combinations, these components are considered independently. The major components are static stretch, relaxation, contraction of the antagonist, and contraction of the agonist.

Static Stretch

A slow static stretch will normally result in low levels of EMG activity during most of the stretch, demonstrating lower motor neuron excitability. At the initial application of stretch, dynamic discharge of the muscle spindles in the antagonistic muscle will facilitate its α–motor neuron pool. Once the elongation phase ceases and the stretch is maintained, the dynamic portion of the muscle spindle discharge should lessen and subside (Burke et al. 1978; Condon 1983; Moore and Hutton 1980; Vallbo 1974a). During a very slow stretch, high sensitivity of Ia afferents to small increases in muscle length may be maintained through selective activation of the γ–static neurons. However, Vallbo's (1974b) studies of spindle afferents in humans have failed to demonstrate significant gamma activity during passive stretch.

Theoretically, during the maintained stretch, autogenic inhibition by the GTO could occur through the Ib pathways. However, slow passive stretch is not an optimal stimulus for GTOs (Burke et al. 1978; Houk et al. 1971). Another possible source of autogenic inhibition during stretch is small muscle afferents (Rymer et al. 1979). Because the static stretch requires no voluntary effort, supraspinal input would be expected to be minimal (Condon 1983). A subject's ability to voluntarily relax the muscle while it is being stretched could reduce the central drive to the α–motor neurons and would lower the background motor activity upon which peripheral contributions summate (Moore and Hutton 1980). Phillips is quoted in Condon (1983, p. 14) as stating, "the corticospinal tract has the potential for very potent transmission to alpha motoneurons." However, "if a person chose to resist a stretch for any number of reasons, which may include attempts to minimize pain or maintain a posture, he/she is certainly capable of overriding spinal inputs and discharging alpha motoneurons" (Condon 1983, p. 14).

Relaxation

The relaxation component can follow or precede a static stretch or contraction of an agonist. This component can be completely passive. As with the static stretch component, one can also facilitate or inhibit the relaxation component voluntarily (via supraspinal mechanisms), depending on the quality of concentration on the desired end product. Respiratory, imagery, eye movement, and gravity techniques can further assist relaxation (see chapter 8).

Contraction of the Antagonist

Originally, simple reflex theories suggested that muscle relaxation will follow a prior contraction of the same muscle. Contracting a muscle under stretch possibly causes the GTOs to begin to discharge, causing relaxation, or the Renshaw cell synaptic connections may inhibit muscle contraction (Condon 1983). Another theory is that the isometric contractions somehow alter the manner in which the muscle spindles respond to stretching conditions by decreasing the afferent flow of impulses from these proprioceptors (Holt n.d.). Consequently, this decrease in muscle spindle firing would tend to enhance greater ROM by offering less resistance to stretch.

However, these concepts have been challenged (Condon and Hutton 1987; Etnyre and Abraham 1988; Moore 1979; Moore and Hutton 1980). Although a contraction of an antagonist should theoretically facilitate relaxation or inhibit subsequent contraction of the antagonist, the opposite results are seen. That is, the contraction may instead leave the muscle in a more excitable state. A hypothesis to explain this phenomenon has been proposed, based on peripheral and central neural factors. See Condon (1983), Condon and Hutton (1987), Moore (1979), and Moore and Hutton (1980) for a detailed review of this subject.

The lingering discharge (facilitation) of a muscle being stretched resulting from a preceding contraction of the same muscle challenges a basic and fundamental concept of stretching. Spinal segmental neural circuitry and functional interactions are much more complex than commonly believed. The preceding discussion and the issues addressed in chapter 6 emphasize that simplistic notions concerning reciprocal inhibition during muscle stretch should be discarded (Moore and Hutton 1980).

These findings have several implications: Complete muscle relaxation is *not* a requisite for effective stretching; greater muscle relaxation is *not* associated with greater ROM (Osternig et al. 1990); and claims that techniques similar to CRAC promote relaxation of the muscle to be stretched should be viewed with some skepticism. If comfort, time, or learning difficulties are important considerations, static stretch may be preferred because it is more comfortable and elicits less resistive activity than the other types of stretching. Further research into the details of how these stretching techniques really work is needed (Condon 1983; Condon and Hutton 1987; Etnyre and Abraham 1988; Moore 1979; Moore and Hutton 1980).

Another relevant factor is the preference of using a static contraction or concentric contraction of the antagonist. Research has demonstrated that maximal static contractions produce more tension than maximal concentric contractions (Coyle et al. 1979). However, the output of the Golgi tendon organ is proportional to the amount of tension generated by a muscle. Therefore, "concentric contractions may not be as effective as static contractions for promoting muscle relaxation and subsequent increases in flexibility" (Lustig et al. 1992, p. 157).

Contraction of the Agonist

The effects of reciprocal innervation are used to explain an agonist contraction during stretch. Specifically, contraction of the agonistic muscles (e.g., quadriceps) is said to induce relaxation of the antagonistic muscles (e.g., hamstrings) through reciprocal inhibition. Thus, when motor neurons of the agonist muscle receive excitatory impulses from afferent nerves or from the brain motor centers, the motor neurons that supply the antagonistic muscles are inhibited (e.g., if the quadriceps contract, the hamstrings must relax). So, during an agonist-contract procedure, reciprocal Ia inhibition of the antagonist would be favored by both spinal and supraspinal inputs. Therefore, an agonist contraction theoretically produces lower levels of contractile resistance in the antagonist than occurs in a static stretch procedure (Condon 1983).

In contrast, Condon and Hutton (1987), Moore (1979), and Moore and Hutton (1980) found that an agonist contraction significantly increased EMG activity in the antagonistic muscle. Therefore, the antagonistic muscle was apparently not relaxed after contraction of its agonist. However, active reciprocal inhibition may still occur in a muscle but not be apparent. The reciprocal inhibition effects may be masked by excitatory input from other pathways, resulting in a net excitatory effect to the antagonist. Etnyre and Abraham (1988) suggested that the appearance of cocontraction between antagonistic muscles was actually a result of intermuscular electrical cross talk (i.e., cross talk between the electrodes). Therefore, the apparent electrical activity in the antagonistic muscle may actually be an artifact of the activity in the agonistic muscle (the likelihood of this situation is greater when the two opposing muscles are small and close together).

Another potential advantage of a voluntary contraction of the agonist is the reduction of discomfort arising from the muscles under stretch. Moore and Hutton (1980) interviewed subjects after their experiment utilizing the CRAC method. The subjects tended to associate the discomfort with the preliminary contraction of the antagonist while it was in the stretched position, rather than with the hamstring stretch phase during the agonist contraction. Moore and Hutton (1980) suggested that the voluntary contraction of the agonists tends to mask discomfort arising from the antagonistic muscles under stretch.

ADDITIONAL STRETCHING TECHNIQUES

In addition to PNF, several other methods facilitate muscle relaxation to enhance and restore movement. Three such methods, developed by osteopaths, are muscle energy, strain-counterstrain, and functional techniques. To paraphrase Goodridge (1981), these techniques should not be considered a panacea, but an addition to one's store of professional resources. Descriptions of these and other techniques can be found in a variety of texts (Chaitow 2002; Hammer 1999; Jones 1995).

Muscle Energy Technique

The *muscle energy technique* (MET) was developed by Fred L. Mitchell, Sr., between 1945 and 1950. MET is an osteopathic manipulative treatment in which the patient actively uses his or her muscles on request, "from a precisely controlled position in a specific direction, against a distinctly executed counterforce" (Goodridge 1981, p. 67). MET appears to be similar in many ways to the CR, HR, and AR methods of PNF. In particular, the neurophysiological basis of MET is the same as that of the PNF methods.

However, several important differences exist, one of which is the degree of force or counterforce. Pounds of force may be utilized in dealing with large muscles (e.g., the hips), but only ounces of force should be used when weaker, shorter, and smaller muscles are being treated (Goodridge 1981). Others state that no more than perhaps 20% or 25% of a patient's strength should be employed (Chaitow 1990; Stiles 1984). A second major difference is the localization of the resisting force. This factor is considered more important than the intensity of the force. In MET, "localization depends on the operator's palpatory proprioceptive perception of movement (or resistance to movement) at or about a specific articulation" (Goodridge 1981, p. 71). Last, different terminology is used, such as barrier (i.e., resistance) and localization. According to Goodridge (1981), resistance can be visualized as a gate in one of three positions: open, partially closed, or closed.

> The striking bar on a gatepost represents an end point much like that of a bony ridge in the body's skeletal system. A wet rope attached to that gate might restrain its range of motion and prevent it from closing; and when the rope has dried and is shortened, it offers further restraint to motion, somewhat resembling that of a muscle that is shortened. If the gate has springing type hinges, they will produce greater initial resistance to movement than ordinary hinges, requiring initial force to overcome the spring resistance before the gate is moved. A similar proprioceptive sensation may be perceived as one initiates passive abduction of a patient's hip. This restraint may be muscular or ligamentous and voluntary or involuntary. (p. 68)

The efficacy of MET lacks substantial verification. Schenk et al. (1994) determined a 4-week treatment period using 18 volunteers. The study indicated a significantly greater ROM for left and right cervical rotation compared with the control group. The researchers also summarized two unpublished theses (Wolfson 1991; Harris 1991). Wolfson's results indicated a significant change in lumbar flexion. However, Schenk et al. (1994, p. 150) point out, "There may have been an unconscious bias in measurements because the experimenter had knowledge of subject groupings" (p. 150). In the Harris (1991) study, six treatments were given to an experimental group of asymptomatic people over 2 weeks. This group showed a trend toward significance with the mean ROM increasing from pretest to posttest. Additional research in the efficacy of MET must employ larger samples and compare with other methods of increasing ROM.

Strain-Counterstrain

Strain-counterstrain is a technique first introduced and characterized by Lawrence Jones (Chaitow 2002; Jones 1995). Two factors commonly associated with a reduction in movement after injury are the presence of spasm and localized areas of tenderness called *trigger points*. When the position of part of the body is distorted because of muscular spasm, any attempt to stretch or elongate the muscle meets increased pain and spasm. To reduce movement, the muscle remains in a guarded state of contraction or spasm. The adjacent joint is moved to the position that maximally shortens the muscle containing the tender spot. This position creates a sense of ease or comfort.

Jones found that moving a joint further into the direction of its distortion, actually exaggerating the guarded position, facilitates an immediate release of the muscle in spasm. This action usually requires moving the opposing muscle to, or close to, a position of strain (Laxton 1990). The joint is held in this position for 90 seconds. When the muscle relaxes, the joint is very slowly returned to its neutral position. In effect, the malfunctioning agonistic muscle spindles are turned off by applying a mild strain to their antagonists, a "release by positioning." This position may mimic the position in which the original strain was experienced. In addition to this treatment technique, Jones (1995) also discovered that the tender point also vanished or was markedly reduced if it was pressed lightly while in the position of greatest ease.

Functional Technique

The functional technique was developed by Harold Hoover (1958). As with strain-counterstrain, the goal is to reduce the exaggerated muscle spindle discharge from facilitated segmental muscles. The position of spontaneous release is the same as in strain-counterstrain, and so is the direction of movement toward ease and comfort. However, the functional technique differs in that at the end position, the tensions in the tissues around the joint are equal. This position is termed *dynamic neutral* (Hoover 1958). Contraction or relaxation is indicated by checking the texture of the tissue.

One neurophysiological explanation of the cause and treatment of the movement problem after injury has been postulated by Korr (1975). When the γ–motor neuron discharge to the muscle spindle is excessive, the result is a sustained contraction of the intrafusal fibers (i.e., muscle spindles). In turn, this activity keeps the primary endings firing continuously, which maintains the extrafusal fibers (i.e., muscle) in a state of contraction, leading to high resistance to stretching. Any lengthening of the facilitated muscle causes the muscle spindle to fire and therefore creates more tension. By reducing the hyperactive spindle responses from the facilitated segmental muscles, the muscle can be stretched. This reduction is accomplished by passively positioning the facilitated muscle so that it is shortened, which reduces the afferent discharge from the primary endings of the muscle spindle. Subsequently, the central nervous system decreases the γ–motor neuron discharge.

MOBILIZATION

Mobilization involves low-velocity, medium-amplitude to high-amplitude passive movements of one or more joints. The technique is applied with an oscillatory motion or a sustained stretch, depending on the nature of the abnormal movement and the goal of the treatment (to decrease pain or increase mobility). Mobilization maneuvers are commonly passive but are under control of the patient, who may prevent them from taking place (Kranz 1988). Two well-known systems of grading dosages for mobilization are (1) Maitland's Five Grades of Movement and (2) Kaltenborn's Three Grades of Movement.

MANIPULATION AND CHIROPRACTIC ADJUSTMENT

Dorland's *Illustrated Medical Dictionary* (2000) defines manipulation as "1. Skillful or dextrous treatments, as by the hand. 2. In physical therapy, the forceful passive movement of a joint beyond its active limit of motion." However, this section will adopt the definition given by Sandoz (1976) for a chiropractic adjustment as synonymous with manipulation:

> A passive manual manoeuvre during which an articular element is suddenly carried beyond the usual, physiological limit of movement without however exceeding the boundaries of anatomical integrity. This usual but not obligate characteristic of an adjustment is the thrust which is a brief, sudden and carefully dosed impulse delivered at the end of the normal passive range of movement and which is usually accompanied by a cracking noise. (p. 91)

This description corresponds to *grade V mobilization* in Maitland's system. This definition is contradictory to many "traditional" chiropractors because manipulation is thought of as putting a bone through a hyper ROM in order to increase mobility. In contrast, a chiropractic adjustment is applied to correct a vertebral subluxation (American Chiropractic Association 1991; Federation of Straight Chiropractic Organizations n.d.; International Chiropractors Association 1993; World Chiropractic Alliance 1993).

Effects of Manipulation on Joint Mobility

According to Sandoz (1969), cracking resulted in a gain of 5° to 10° in the passive ROM of the finger metacarpophalangeal (MCP) joint in all directions (figure 13.6). The gain in amplitude was pluridirectional. The active range was also increased, but to a lesser extent. Motion at other joints can be increased by manipulation too. Gál et al. (1994) demonstrated for the first time "that relative rotations have been shown to be significant for any type of spinal manipulative therapy delivered to the human vertebral column." In addition, numerous studies have substantiated an improvement in ROM after either an adjustment (i.e., a specific force applied by a chiropractor; see figure 13.7) or a manipulation (i.e., a nonspecific force that produces a passive movement of a joint beyond its active limit of motion). Following is a brief review of a variety of these studies.

Several investigators have studied the relationship between spinal manipulation and ROM in the hip and spine. Fisk (1975) demonstrated that spinal manipulation is usually followed by an increase in the angle of straight-leg raising. Fisk and Rose (1977) demonstrated that a significant difference between the right-side and left-side hamstring tightness was eliminated by spinal manipulation. Evans et al. (1978) found significant increases in forward flexion during periods in which patients were being treated by spinal manipulation. Rasmussen (1979) reported that 12 out of 12 manipulated patients showed increased forward flexion, whereas only 6 of 12 control

subjects showed any improvement. Using a controlled clinical trial, Fisk (1979) demonstrated that selected patients with unilateral low-back pain showed substantial decreases in hamstring tightness as a result of spinal manipulation. Nwuga (1982) reported increased mobility in manipulated patients measured for spine flexion and extension and a significant increase in lateral flexion and rotation. Kim et al. (1992) investigated the effect of a single chiropractic manipulation on the sagittal mobility of the lumbar spine in 96 symptomatic patients with low-back pain in a double-blind controlled study. The study demonstrated a mean lumbar ROM increase of 0.20 cm.

Several studies have assessed the effect of manipulation in the cervical spine. Yeomans' (1992) study revealed that after spinal manipulative therapy (SMT), mobility was significantly ($p < .05$) greater than the pre-SMT data, with exception of the C1 segment of both the male ($n = 22$) and the female ($n = 36$) treatment groups. The manipulative approach was a high-velocity, low-amplitude thrust, in a specific line of drive at the end of the normal passive ROM. Cassidy et al. (1992) found a posttreatment increase in all planes of cervical ROM utilizing 21 male and 29 female patients suffering from unilateral neck pain with radiation into the trapezius muscle. The patients received a single, rotational manipulation to the same side as the pain.

In contrast to the positive findings of increased mobility via manipulation, several other investigators failed to substantiate such gains. Jayson et al. (1981), using a goniometer, and Farrell and Twomey (1982), using a spondylometer, found no effects of manipulation on forward flexion. Using another measure of forward flexion (i.e., distance from the fingers to the floor during maximal forward bending), Doran and Newell (1975) and Hoehler et al. (1981) failed to observe any effect of spinal manipulation. Hoehler and Tobis (1982) found that patients with low-back pain had diminished anterior

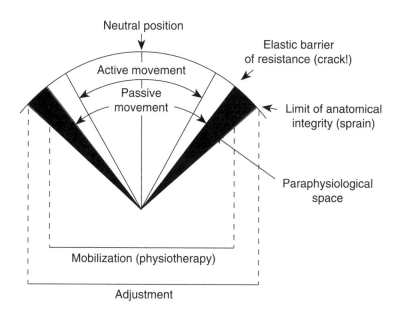

Figure 13.6 Schematic representation of the range of movement in mobilization and adjustment of a normal diarthrodial joint. In passive mobilization, the range of movement is limited by the elastic barrier of resistance. When the movement is forced beyond the elastic barrier, one enters into the paraphysiological space. At the end of this space, one encounters the barrier of anatomical integrity of the joint.

Reprinted from Sandoz (1976).

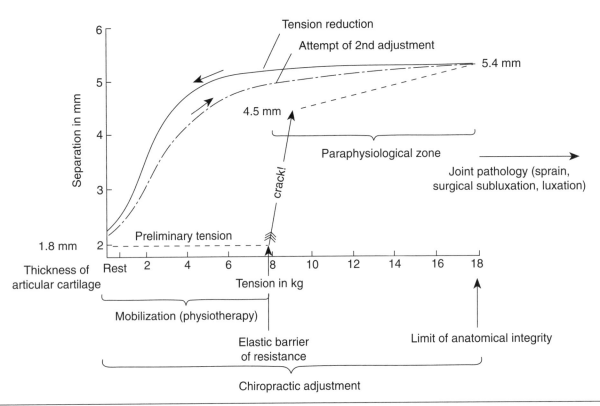

Figure 13.7　Composite graph of the effect of an adjustment of a carpometacarpal joint under axial stretch.
Reprinted from Sandoz (1976).

flexion and did not appear to be greatly affected by spinal manipulation.

Relationship Between Spinal Manipulation and Cervical Passive End-Range Capability

Spinal manipulation can increase cervical passive end-range capability. The question that has yet to be definitively answered is the exact mechanism(s) responsible for the increased ROM after an adjustment or manipulation. Nansel and Szlazak (1994) reduced various hypotheses into two general categories: structural and neuromuscular reflexogenic. Below is a summary of these hypotheses.

Structural Hypotheses

- *Meniscus Entrapment.* This theory maintains that ROM is restricted by the presence of a fatty meniscoid trapped between articular surfaces. The manipulation could dislodge and displace the meniscoid, thereby restoring full ROM.

- *Meniscus Extrapment.* This theory proposes that the meniscoid is drawn out of the joint cavity during flexion. However, with extension, the meniscoid does not reenter its proper location. Consequently, the displaced meniscoid causes capsular distension and restricts ROM. Once again, manipulation is postulated to displace and return the meniscoid to

its appropriate position and return full motion to the joint.

- *Intradiscal Nuclear Displacement.* This theory supports the idea that after flexion, a fragment of the nuclear pulposus extrudes into a radial fissure and gets trapped between the superficial laminae of the annulus fibrosus. However, with extension, a smaller fragment gets trapped. This action is likened to a bubble that would act to restrict compression and thus impede motion along that plane. The manipulation is postulated to "force the fragment circumferentially into another plane, or back along the radial fissure into its normal position among the central disk material." The result is a restoration of normal ROM.

- *Intrazygapophyseal Adhesions.* This theory suggests that ROM is limited by adhesions formed between folds of synovium, the capsule, or other connective tissues as a result of exudation. Manipulation restores the ROM by breaking down these adherent connective tissue elements.

- *Zygapophyseal Capsular Fibrosis.* This theory postulates that fibrotic changes take place over a course of time in the capsular membranes themselves. Consequently, the elastic capsule loses its elasticity, becoming rigid and limiting ROM. The manipulation then stretches or tears this elastic tissue, thus restoring ROM. However, Nansel and Szlazak

(1994) point out that manipulation does not necessarily restore normal elasticity of the capsule.

- *Fibrosis of Periarticular Tissues.* This theory suggests that fibrous adhesions form in the connective tissues surrounding the joint (ligaments, tendons, and muscle fascia), limiting ROM. Manipulation might potentially break down these adhesions or induce changes in blood flow that secondarily might influence fluid dynamics and interstitial fluid buildup. The end result is returning to the joint its normal ROM.

Reflex Hypotheses

- *Reflexes Involving Capsular Afferents.* This theory speculates that aberrant afferent signals caused by type I and II afferents might lead to inappropriate increase in muscle tone, thus restricting ROM. The manipulation might break this cycle, thereby permitting an increased ROM.
- *Reflexes Involving Muscular Afferents.* This theory maintains that restriction of ROM is caused by aberrant muscular afferents of "shunt" or perhaps other muscles. The effect of the manipulation might be similar to the "clasp-knife" muscular release mechanism via inhibitory Golgi tendon reflex pathways or related pathways.

Need for Additional Research

Manipulative therapy is a conservative and alternative method to traditional medical and surgical therapy (Kranz 1988). It is effective in many instances (Quebec Task Force on Spinal Disorders 1987). However, like many treatments, the procedure has risks. Currently, the precise reasons why an adjustment or manipulative therapy improves ROM and provides relief for many conditions have not been scientifically explained, although numerous theories exist. The Quebec Task Force on Spinal Disorders (1987) has established four categories of research priorities in the field of spinal disorders: causation (e.g., physical, physiological, and psychological factors), prevention (e.g., designing comprehensive educational and interventional measures), clinical terminology, and clinical management (e.g., identifying the safest and most efficient methods).

TRACTION

The term *traction* is derived from the Latin word *tractio*, the act of drawing or pulling. Traction is a technique in which a longitudinal tensile force is applied to a part of the body to stretch soft tissues or separate articular surfaces. Traction is a form of mobilization because it involves the passive movement of joints by mechanical or manual means (Saunders 1986). Traction is usually administered as an adjunct to other therapies, including heat, massage, various types of manipulation and mobilization, and exercises.

Traction has been used since the beginning of recorded history. Hippocrates, along with other Greek and Roman physicians, recognized the importance of traction for treating patients with spinal disorders (such as scoliosis) and fractures. Any treatment modality that has remained a viable clinical choice for several thousand years must have some successful therapeutic effect. Nonetheless, several reports have challenged the efficacy of traction as a means of therapy for neck and back pain (Van der Heijden et al. 1995; Waddell et al. 1996). Saunders (1998) challenged these negative findings on the basis that most of the studies contained significant flaws. Therefore, Saunders (1998) writes: "We must objectively oppose reports that say traction is ineffective when they are based on flawed conclusions" (p. 287). Randomized clinical trials with clearly define treatment methodologies and patient selection criteria are needed to resolve this controversy.

Types of Traction

Traction is usually categorized as mechanical or manual (in which the therapist utilizes a special belt, harness, or strap). Within these two main categories are additional subclassifications. The type of traction used depends on a number of factors, including therapeutic objectives, patient's condition, ease of use, durability and maintenance, cost, and safety. Seven types of traction are discussed in the following sections.

Self-Treatment

Self-treatment comprises a series of techniques, proposed by McKenzie (1981, 1983), employing repeated movements and sustained positions to centralize or abolish symptoms. In one technique, the patient lies supine with the head, neck, and upper torso extended over the edge of the treatment table. The patient then allows the cervical spine to extend and distract in an inverted position. Self-treatment places a major emphasis on educating the patient about proper posture to avoid aggravating and perpetuating the symptoms.

Positional Traction

Positional traction involves a particular body position, combined with rolls, sandbags, pillows, and blocks, to create a tensile force on the desired structure(s). This technique usually incorporates lateral truncal bending. Consequently, only one side of the spinal region is affected or stretched (Saunders 1986).

Manual Traction

The tensile force created with *manual traction* is directly produced by the therapist. It can be applied by direct contact with the patient or by use of special belts, harnesses, head halters, and straps. Manual traction offers several advantages as well as disadvantages when compared with mechanical traction. One advantage is that the therapist can use manual traction to assess the patient's potential response before applying mechanical traction. Another advantage is that the therapist can adjust the amount, duration, and angle of tension based on tactile feedback from contact with the patient. Some patients may have more difficulty relaxing with manual than with mechanical traction because the exact amount of manual force cannot be anticipated (Saunders 1986). For other patients, the "laying of hands" inherent in manual traction may result in greater relaxation. Unlike mechanical traction, manual traction requires the continuous concentration of the therapist. Any sudden twist or turn may exacerbate a previously existing condition. Manual traction is also more physically demanding for the therapist.

Continuous Mechanical Traction

Continuous mechanical traction, as its name suggests, is traction force applied continuously in a single direction. The duration may range from a few minutes up to several hours. With long-duration traction, only small weights are generally used. Experimental findings by Colachis and Strohm (1965) suggest that a constant pull causes no more vertebral separation after 30 or 60 seconds than it does after only 7 seconds.

Intermittent Mechanical Traction

Intermittent mechanical traction is traction force alternately applied and released over a period of time. Consequently, during the period that tensile force is not applied, the muscles can relax and thus reduce their fatigue. This technique is thought to facilitate vascular flow, lymph drainage, and mechanoreceptor stimulation and to reduce edema.

Autotraction

Autotraction is a back treatment applied on a bench of a special design. The bench consists of two sections that can be individually angled and rotated. The patient applies the traction by pulling with his or her own arms on an upper bar while the pelvis is fixed by a belt and the feet are braced or supported against a lower bar.

Gravity Traction

A popular technique available to the general public is *gravity traction*, which employs special boots or straps attached to the pelvis or to the ankles. The patient hangs from a frame in an inverted position. About 50% of the body weight exerts a tractive force on the spine. Supposedly, this force provides sufficient pull to distract or separate the lumbar vertebrae from one another.

Indications for Traction

Traction has two broad purposes: *mechanical* (e.g., to elongate tissues and separate joint spaces) and *therapeutic* (e.g., to relieve pain and muscle spasm). The most common uses of traction are to stretch the musculature, to stretch fibrotic tissues and break adhesions, to separate or stretch joints, to promote distraction and gliding of joint facets, to lessen or eliminate muscle spasm, to restore blood and lymph circulation, to dissipate edema or congestion in an area, to lessen or eliminate pain, to trigger proprioceptive reflexes, to maintain muscle tone, to reduce and immobilize fracture, to prevent fracture deformity (i.e., to regain normal alignment), to straighten spinal curves, to regain normal body or spine length, and to promote the return of a herniated disk's nucleus (Craig and Kaelin 2000; Downer 1996; Hinterbuchner 1985; Hooker 1999; Kisner and Colby 2002; Rechtien et al. 1998; Winkenwerder and Shankar 2002).

Contraindications for Traction

Contraindications to traction are in part determined by the type and degree of injury sustained by the patient. Traction has the capacity to aggravate and further complicate existing conditions and symptoms. Several of the main contraindications for traction are acute traumatic syndromes, fractures, cancer or malignancy, spinal cord compression, osteoporosis, rheumatoid arthritis, joint instability, acute inflammation, infectious diseases (e.g., tuberculosis), hernias, cardiovascular or pulmonary problems, pregnancy, claustrophobia, relative age, and any condition in which movement exacerbates the existing problem (Craig and Kaelin 2000; Downer 1996; Hinterbuchner 1985; Hooker 1999; Kisner and Colby 2002; Rechtien et al.1998; Winkenwerder and Shankar 2002).

Actions Before Implementing Traction

All forms of mobilization present a degree of risk. To reduce or eliminate such risks, a number of precautions should be taken. According to Hinterbuchner (1985), traction should not be administered until three prerequisites have been implemented: a complete medical work-up of the patient, a definitive diagnosis of the condition, and the establishment of specific indications for traction. Hinterbuchner describes a complete work-up as consisting of a careful history, physical examination, and diagnostic radiographies. With the spine in particular, the X-ray views must be anteroposterior, lateral, and oblique.

Principles of Traction

The following list of general principles for the application of traction has been culled from Craig and Kaelin (2000), Downer (1996), Harris (1978), Hinterbuchner (1985), Hooker (2002), Kisner and Colby (2002), Rechtien et al. (1998), Saunders (1986), and Winkenwerder and Shankar (2002).

- Explain to the patient what will be done during the treatment.
- Make sure sanitary factors have been addressed (i.e., the surface should be clean, disinfected, and, if necessary, sterilized).

- Traction force must be great enough to effect a structural change at the targeted area or structure.

- Place the patient in a position that will most optimally affect the final outcome.

- Secure all attachment halters, straps, or other traction connections.

- Make sure the skin has ample protection.

- The magnitude of the traction should increase and decrease slowly.

- The duration of the treatment should be tailored to the patient.

- Undertreatment is better than excessive magnitude or duration.

- Monitor the patient continuously.

- Discontinue treatment with the start of dizziness, nausea, undue discomfort, or other adverse sensory changes (e.g., numbness).

- Allow a period of transition after the treatment (i.e., time for the patient to rest).

Parameters of Traction

The application of traction has three significant parameters: magnitude, angle of pull, and duration. These parameters are discussed below.

Magnitude of Traction

Magnitude refers to the amount of tractive force that must be applied to achieve the optimal results. This force is commonly measured in weight or poundage. In general, the longer the treatment, the smaller the weight, and the shorter the treatment, the heavier the weight. Additional factors that determine magnitude include the medical condition being treated, the region of the body being treated, the physical status of the patient, and patient tolerance. Always start with a minimal tensile force to avoid exacerbating an existing condition.

Angle of Pull

The *angle of pull*, which may vary from horizontal to vertical, is determined by such things as the body region being treated (e.g., cervical versus lumbar spine), the positioning of the other parts of the body, and patient tolerance.

Duration of Traction

The *duration* of the therapy is determined by several factors, the most important of which are the medical condition being treated, the physical status of the patient (e.g., age, the presence of inflammation, or stage of healing), and patient tolerance. Other factors include the mode of traction used and the clinical expertise of the therapist. Hinterbuchner (1985)), in a review of the literature found "a great deal of variation in the magnitude and duration of the tractive force required to achieve optimal results with minimum discomfort to the patient" (p. 180).

NONTRADITIONAL STRETCHING DEVICES

This section defines *nontraditional* devices as those that are primarily targeted toward the nonmedical community. Popular fitness magazines and the Internet feature a diverse array of stretching devices. Among the targeted groups are athletes, practitioners of the martial arts and yoga, dancers, and members and staff of health and fitness gyms. However, these devices may also be utilized by the medical community in clinical or hospital settings.

Hippocrates records descriptions of various stretching devices. The function of these inventions was essentially orthopedic or therapeutic. Stretching devices have also been used as a means of torture. The earliest known description of a stretching machine was written by Noverre (1782-1783). His letter described a device called the *tourne-haunch* (i.e., hip, hindquarter) to assist the ballet dancer in improving his or her turnout:

> I avoid mentioning the tourne-haunch, a clumsy and useless invention, which, instead of producing good effect, serves only to lame those who use it, by giving a distortion to the waist, much more disagreeable than what it was intended to remove.

> The simplest and most natural means are those which reason and good sense ought to adopt; and of these, a moderate, but continual exercise is indispensible: the practice of a circular motion or turning of the legs, both inwardly and outwardly, and of boldly *beating* at full extent from the haunch, is the only certain exercise to be preferred. It insensibly gives freedom, spring, and pliancy; while the motions acquired by using the machine, have more an air of constraint, than of that liberty and ease which should find conspicuous in them . . . No more can a dancer hope to attain the perfection of his art, if for one half of his life he is confined in shackles? I repeat it again, sir, that the use of the machine, is hurtful: for natural or innate defects are not to be overcome by violence; it must be the work of time, study and application. (pp. 71-73)

Almost 60 years after Noverre's warning, the utilization of the tourne-hanche was cited by Kirstein (1939) as part of Alberic Second's *Les Petits Mystères de l'Opéra* (1844). In this opera, Gavarni, a dancer, complained, "Each morning the Master imprisoned my feet in a grooved box. There, heel to toe, and knees turned outward, my martyred feet became accustomed to remain in a parallel line. It is called 'turning oneself out' (*se tourne*)" (p. 67).

Since Noverre's writing, the need to improve ROM has become increasingly recognized and appreciated among the general population. A number of inventors and entrepreneurs have attempted to meet the demand for an "elixir" to enhance ROM. Consequently, professional instruments and training aids have proliferated in the marketplace.

Stretching Devices and Machines

Stretching machines range in technical sophistication, from simple, inexpensive equipment using balls, ropes, and sticks to complex, high-tech machines that require a substantial ($500 or more) investment of money. The more expensive machines may have power motors, special features (e.g., a modulating stretch), the capacity to produce measurements of high reliability and validity, and the ability to stretch multiple parts of the body.

Stretching machines have several potential advantages, depending upon the specifics of each machine. One obvious advantage is that exercises can be performed independently of a clinician, thus maximizing time and energy (Gribble et al. 1999; Starring et al. 1988). Additional benefits discussed by Brainum (2000) include the following:

- Stretch machines can place you in a biomechanically correct position while preventing bouncy stretch motions that are antithetical to increased ROM.

- Stretch machines can partially simulate the effects of having a partner for extended stretches.

- Stretch machines may offer the ability to calibrate stretch positions, thus providing a way to quantify flexibility gains as well as a motivation to stretch. Measurable progress is always an encouragement to keep doing something.

A major problem facing health-care providers is limited amounts of time. Using stretching machines allows patients to achieve stretching of the targeted muscles and the health-care provider to finish the sessions with assistance, saving time and energy for both clients and care providers (Burkett et al. 1998; Starring et al. 1988).

One problem with stretching devices and machines on the market is a lack of published studies to verify their efficacy and safety. Only a few studies have been published, and these are at times insufficient. Rankin et al. (1992) found using the Power Stretch Device twice a week for 6 weeks increased flexibility. However, no significant differences were found between Power Stretch Device users and static stretching groups. The Rack® is another stretching device designed to work the ankle. An investigation by DePriest et al. (1999), using 14 male and 14 female swimmers, found it to be useful for increasing ankle plantar flexion.

Consumerism and Stretching Devices

In the "world of flexibility and stretching" inventors, marketers, coaches, and trainers and, of course, the public are always searching for the latest technological breakthrough. However, heed the warning "Let the buyer beware." Thomas and Quindry (1997) detailed 14 "red flags" culled from a review of the literature that should serve as warning signs to consumers. Several of these red flags are discussed and expanded as they relate to stretching machines.

- *Testimonials.* Testimonials and "before and after photos" lack substantiated evidenced for the efficacy of a product. The consumer should ask, for example, Was this martial arts expert already doing splits before using the device?

- *Money-Back Guarantees.* Are such clauses in the contract? Is the company reputable?

- *Cures or Miracles.* Claims that seem to be too good to be true should be held in doubt. Example: You will be able to perform splits in just 6 weeks!

- *Celebrity Endorsement.* Celebrities' and professional athletes' credentials are usually limited to personal experience and success in their profession. Furthermore, many celebrity endorsements in the area of stretching are made by those who have devoted years to mastering their flexibility. Often these celebrities are Olympic athletes or black belts in their respective martial arts.

- *Foreign Research.* References to research conducted in other countries (Russia, the former German Democratic Republic, or other former Eastern Bloc nations) must be considered carefully. Perhaps, these nations' athletes were successful because of a selection process that started with young children and a state-sponsored developmental training program that provided years of subsidized training with the best coaches and trainers in these nations.

- *Mass Media Marketing.* Here advertisers cite proven results from research. However, the research was never published in a peer-reviewed journal to verify its efficacy and safety.

- *Buzzwords.* Beware of buzzwords such as "secret," "miraculous," and "incredible."

- *Omission of Facts.* Advertisements may omit mention of any side effects or restrictions.

- *Highly Pedigreed.* Developers may claim they studied or worked at a prestigious institution or have a degree in a specific field. These claims can be exaggerated.

- *Express Mail.* Some companies will only ship through private mailing services to circumvent the federal (U.S.) restrictions on mail fraud.

Many products work; they are just unnecessary. You do not need to buy the machine; you can get the same results by just stretching.

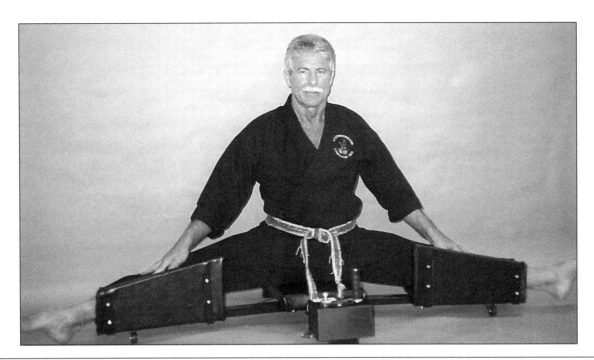

Figure 13.8   The Hurley Stretch Rack.
Courtesy of Carson Hurley.

The Rack System

The need for flexible groin and hamstrings muscles is essential in dance, gymnastics, and the martial arts. Various stretching machines have been invented to facilitate the performance of splits in all directions and high leg kicks. Many of these devices superficially appear to follow a similar "rack" design. However, some distinct differences exist. Because the rack system is the most popular and widely promoted device on the market, this design is analyzed in depth.

The frame of the rack can be constructed of steel, aluminum, or plastic. The quality and gauge of these materials will determine to a major extent the rack's durability. A pair of leg decks, which are often padded, are attached to the frame. Some racks have a seated back, whereas others do not. If the rack comes with a seated back, one should determine whether it can be adjusted while stretching and how many positions are available. Similar determinations should be made regarding the leg supports. Two accessories that come with some racks are the sidebar and the T-bar and handle, which assist the individual during the stretch. One of the most important components is the stretching mechanism, which may utilize a hand crank, worm drive, hydraulic system, or electric system. Each of these components has its advantages and disadvantages (e.g., simplicity, durability, possibility of leaking, or cost). An important safety component is a release mechanism to provide the user with a means to disengage the applied stretch to prevent possible injury. A measuring device permits the user to quantify the degree of stretch. Other factors to consider before purchasing a stretch device include the types of stretches permitted, the angle of stretch permitted, ease of use, safety, weight, and dimensions (see figure 13.8).

SUMMARY

Special stretching exercises and drills have been developed to achieve flexibility. Regardless of the method employed, overstretching may be produced in several ways, determined by the amount or intensity of stretch, the duration of the stretch, the frequency of movements performed in a given period, and the velocity or nature of the stretch. Techniques to increase ROM include static, ballistic, passive, active, PNF, muscle energy, strain-counterstrain, functional, mobilization, manipulation, traction, and nontraditional modalities. Additional research is necessary to identify the optimal method for a given person. Numerous disciplines and professions are involved in the development of the optimum ROM and stiffness. If history is any guide, most of them are dynamic fields open to new and innovative approaches. However, those innovations must always take into consideration those protocols that are the safest and most efficient.

14

Controversy Over Stretching and Controversial Stretches

Controversy surrounds the topic of stretching. Walsh (1985) recalled a statement attributed to Gordon Pirie, a British middle distance record holder of the 1950s: "Race horses don't stretch, so why should humans?" In a similar vein, Laughlin (2002a) writes:

> No cat I have ever seen stretches its hamstrings before sprinting away from the neighbor's dog—which some might see as justification for not stretching before an intense activity—but the difference is that cats are already perfectly flexible; their lifestyle (plenty of stretching and plenty of relaxing, too) encourages this.

Numerous articles have raised questions about the virtues and benefits of stretching and flexibility (Black and Stevens 2001; Davis 1988; Fixx 1983; Read 1989; Shrier 1999, 2000, 2001, 2002; Shrier and Gossal 2000; Wolf 1983). Some writers have even used this theme for humor; in a satirical essay, Frederick (1982) stated that the reason behind the increased interest in stretching is a highly skilled platoon of stretchers being training by the infamous Universal Church of Flexibility. These "stretchees" are charged with infiltrating the running community to spread the gospel of stretching and flexibility. In a more serious vein, orthopedic surgeon Richard H. Dominguez wrote that the public was being swept up by a "cult of flexibility" (Shyne 1982). Dominguez believed this trend began because naturally loose-jointed people would do stretching exercises and say, "Boy, this feels good." Consequently, many others would follow along. More recently, Tsatsouline (2001b) wrote: "Stretching in America is a cult. Every fitness-junkie guru preaches flexibility. They growl, they drool and they promise hell to the infidels who don't or won't stretch" (p. 13).

FLEXIBILITY CONTINUUM

Although flexibility is commonly assumed to reduce the incidence of injury, various authorities and researchers contend that flexibility training might actually increase the risk of injury! To understand this point, visualize flexibility on a continuum (Brody 1999; Surburg 1983). At one end is hypomobility, or decreased mobility. In the most extreme case, no flexibility or movement is possible, as in ankylosis (stiffness or fixation of a joint by disease, injury, or surgery). At the opposite end of the continuum is extreme flexibility or instability, that is, subluxation or dislocation. Brody (1999) challenges this concept. She maintains hypermobility should not be confused with instability because the latter is an excessive range of osteokinematic or arthrokinematic movement without protective muscular control. Somewhere between these two extremes lies the concept of relative flexibility and optimal level of flexibility that allows efficient execution of movement and diminishes the risk of certain types of injuries. The relationship between flexibility (ROM) and injury has been described as "U" shaped (Jones et al. 1993; Knapik et al. 1992). This relationship was discussed in chapter 2 and is further elaborated below.

Potential Disadvantages of Flexibility Training

One concern raised by several early writers (Bird 1979; Lichtor 1972; Lysens et al. 1991; Lysens et al. 1989; Nicholas 1970) is that increased joint laxity or looseness increases the likelihood of ligament injury, joint separation, and dislocation. Lichtor (1972) believed that individuals with loose joints do not have normal bodily control and coordination. Significantly, Lichtor did not define the term *loose joint* nor offer corroborative data. Nonetheless, he speculated such persons are not usually seen in professional sports, having been eliminated early by injury or poor performance. Barrack et al. (1983) investigated the relationship between joint laxity and proprioception in the knee. The study group consisted of members of a professional ballet company and a group of 12 healthy, active aged-matched control subjects. These investigators

Stretching in Humans and Animals

Perhaps, the most often cited stretching analogy by proponents of stretching is the cat. Cats are flexible and supple and often stretch after awakening. Therefore, based upon the observed action of cats, humans are encouraged to replicate its actions. However, is the stretching cat analogy valid? Obviously, no one knows what a cat feels or thinks. Therefore, assuming that a cat stretches because it knows stretching enhances its flexibility or because it feels good is presumptuous. A prudent course of action is to search out the relevant findings of scientific investigations related to this phenomenon.

Stretching and yawning upon awakening or after periods of inactivity are often, but not always, associated. Often, yawning is accompanied by stiffening of the extremities and trunk. What percent of the time cats yawn without stretching is unknown. Therefore, whether proponents of stretching include the action of yawning in their stretching analogy is pertinent. Yawning is an intriguing phenomenon. It is observed in humans, animals, birds, and possibly in reptiles under varied conditions (Argiolas-Antonio and Melis 1998). Currently, the physiological function of yawning is unknown, although numerous theories try to explain it (Argiolas-Antonio and Melis 1998; Askenasy 1989; Baenninger 1997; Barbizet 1958; Heusner 1946; Sato-Suzuki et al. 1998). Much evidence supports the view that yawning is an important mediator of behavioral arousal levels: maintenance or increase of arousal. This view is supported by a review of the endocrine, neuropeptide, neurotransmitter, and pharmacological mechanisms of yawning (Baenninger 1997).

If the cat stretching phenomena excludes yawning, what explains the stretching phenomena seen in cats? The answer again appears to be as a means of arousal. For example, Cerretelli and di Prampero (1987) reported,

"short isometric contractions as well as light rectangular isotonic loads elicit in humans a cardiac acceleration" and "the HR increase is the result of the suppression of cardiac vagal tone and not the consequence of increased sympathetic stimulation" (p. 322). Sandyk (1998), also supports the arousal hypothesis:

> The stretching-yawning syndrome elicited by ACTH [adrenocorticotropic hormone] is inhibited by treatment with cholinergic and dopaminergic antagonists (Ferrari et al. 1963; Yamada and Furukawa 1980; Ushijima et al. 1984) suggesting involvement of central cholinergic and dopaminergic neurons. Furthermore, electrophysiological studies using EEG recordings in cats have demonstrated that episodes of body stretching induced by ACTH are associated with cortical activation and additionally with shifts towards higher frequencies in hippocampal theta activity (Concu et al. 1974). Since the hippocampus is involved in arousal and attentional responses and in the regulation of sleep-wake mechanisms through a reciprocal interaction with the cortex (Green and Arduini 1954; Green 1964) and because the hippocampus contains a high density of cholinergic neurons and glucocorticoid receptors (Wood et al. 1978a, b; McEwen 1980; Gilad et al. 1985), it is believed that stretching behavior induced by ACTH reflects an arousal response involving activation of septohippocampal cholinergic neurons (Wood et al. 1978 a, b). (p. 108)

Thus, the stretching cat phenomenon does not appear to be a valid rationale for humans to stretch.

---

concluded that joint hypermobility may be a factor in decreased positional sense, which may produce hyperactive protective reflexes and thus increase the risk of acute or chronic injury. However, the investigators pointed out that an "unanswered question is whether clinical laxity and the implied associated decline in proprioception predisposes athletes to higher rates or certain types of injuries" (p. 135). Another argument against stretching is that tight-jointed individuals are better protected from severe injury because their characteristically bulky build limits the ROM of their joints. Similarly, some studies have suggested that in looser joints the stabilizing fibrous tissue that resists the impact is so low in quantity and

quality that the joints lose their parallelism (i.e., proper alignment) when they are hit, especially when the body or legs are fixed (Nicholas 1970) or during prolonged periods of weight bearing (Sutro 1947).

A vital question that must be addressed is whether joint looseness or flexibility training is potentially detrimental for some individuals. Numerous authorities are of the opinion that too much flexibility or ROM can be as dangerous as inadequate flexibility (Barrack et al. 1983; Bird 1979; Corbin and Noble 1980; Nicholas 1970). The literature also contains informal accounts in which international athletes report believing that they become less injury prone once they stop or diminish their stretching routines (Read 1989) or that they became more injury prone by participating in a stretching program (Fixx 1983; Walter et al. 1989). This issue is explored later in detail as it pertains to runners.

Excessive flexibility may destabilize joints (Balaftsalis 1982-1983; Corbin and Noble 1980; Nicholas 1970). For example, Klein (1961) contends that the deep squatting of weight lifters tends to weaken the knee ligaments and hence make the knee more vulnerable to injury. However, an investigation by Chandler (1989) demonstrated "no effect of squat training on knee stability" (p. 299). Their review of the literature also identified several works (Karpovich et al. 1970; Myers 1971; Ward 1970) indicating that the squat exercise does not cause a decrease in knee stability. Nonetheless, Nicholas (1970) reported, "independent of many other factors responsible for injury in football, an increased likelihood of ligamentous rupture of the knee occurred in loose-jointed football players" (p. 2239). However, Saal (1998) points out that "there was no clear separation between flexibility and laxity" (p. 86). Other researchers (Grana and Moretz 1978; Kalenak and Morehouse 1975; Moretz et al. 1982; Steele and White 1986) also found no correlation between hypermobility, ligamentous laxity, and the incidence or type of injury. Yet, another issue raised by Saal (1998) is that subsequent studies found a "wide variation in subjective assessment of joint laxity between different trained examiners" (p. 88). Expanding this thought, Lysens et al. (1991) point out "the lack of a clear definition of flexibility and the use of inadequate evaluation techniques" may be the main reason that no clear evidence supports the assumption that flexibility is associated with certain types of injury. Therefore, because so many other factors are involved, a correlation between flexibility and injury is almost impossible to establish. However, Knapik et al. (1992) found, at joints other than the hip and low-back region, a tendency for lower body injuries in those least flexible.

The ankle sprain is a common injury. Instability of the joint appears to be a problem in most patients. Lateral ankle instability possibly includes mechanical laxity and functional instability. Other factors could also include muscle weakness, joint proprioceptive disorder, or both. Many in vitro studies have demonstrated a significant role of joint flexibility in determining mechanical laxity of human cadaveric ankles after sectioning of the lateral ligaments. Liu et al. (2001) compared the differences in flexibility between ankles after the first sprains and ankles with repeated severe sprains and chronic symptoms. They reported, "a tendency was found that patients with multiple ankle sprains and chronic symptoms had a higher occurrence rate of mechanical laxity" (p. 243). The researchers suggested that their study "may also be interpreted that the ankles with mechanical laxity had a higher risk of re-injury and leading to chronic symptoms" (p. 237).

Another controversial issue is that joint hypermobility may predispose one to premature osteoarthritis. Beighton et al. (1999) present three possible explanations. First, "the particular collagen structure that contributes to hyperlaxity may be identical to that which leads to osteoarthritis" (p. 46). Second, the biomechanical factors associated with hypermobile joints assist in the "pathogenesis of the degenerative change" (p. 47). Third, research suggests, "that proprioception may be a causative link between hypermobility and osteoathritis" (p. 47). Additional research is required to evaluate the evidence that supports these hypotheses. However, Beighton et al. (1999) acknowledge, "Perhaps all three mechanisms contribute" (p. 47).

Conversely, studies have suggested that individuals participating in regular physical exercise may avoid osteoarthritis (Beighton et al. 1999; Bird 1979; Bird et al. 1980). Regular physical exercise may protect lax joints from osteoarthritis by stabilizing joints through increased muscular tone.

Summarizing the literature, the following statements can be made:

- Sufficient data are not presently available to conclusively determine whether exercises that stretch ligaments are detrimental to ligaments (Corbin and Noble 1980).

- "High muscle flexibility and joint mobility within the normal physiological range of motion seem to be no additional risk factors" (Lysens et al. 1991, p. 285).

- Restricting athletic participation based on ligamentous laxity testing is not warranted (Grana and Moretz 1978).

- Individuals with loose ligaments must increase strength through a strength-training program. The muscle-tendon unit is the first line of defense in protecting ligaments. Strengthening not only increases muscle but also probably protects the joint ligaments (Javurek 1982; Kalenak and Morehouse 1975; Moretz et al. 1982; Nicholas 1970).

- Conversely, although many authors recommend exercise for those with hypermobility, "few have any data on which to base that recommendation" (Russek 1999, p. 597).

- Individuals with less ROM or categorized as "tight" need to increase their flexibility through a flexibility-training program (Nicholas 1970).

Thus, three possible courses of action appear to be prudent based on empirical evidence. First, ROM should be reduced in joints where excessive flexibility is evident. Second, preventive and compensatory exercises should be incorporated into the training program to enhance the strength and stability of the joints (Arnheim and Prentice 2000; Corbin and Noble 1980; Javurek 1982; Kalenak and Morehouse 1975; Moretz et al. 1982). Third, a flexibility-training program is not indicated when the joint (or joints) in question is hypermobile or displays laxity (Corbin and Noble 1980).

Relationship Between Stretching or Warm-Up and Injuries

Several attempts have been made to statistically quantify the relationship of stretching or warm-up with the incidence of injury and pain in athletes. Kerner and D'Amico (1983) obtained data from 540 questionnaires. They found that "those runners who warmed up prior to running had a higher frequency of pain (87.7%) than those who did not (66%)" (p. 162). In addition, the comparison of warm-up time versus frequency of pain revealed a higher frequency of pain as warm-up time increased. In this study, stretching exercises were considered inclusively with warming up. Levine et al. (1987) found that although 92% of the subjects involved reported stretching their hamstrings, injury surveys revealed numerous hamstring strains. Consequently, they suggested their study "appears to cast doubt on the belief that stretching helps prevent injury" (p. 135).

Jacobs and Berson (1986) investigated injuries to runners in a 10-kilometer race. Of the 2,664 registrants for the National Championships, 550 were asked to complete a questionnaire, to which 451 runners responded. They found a positive correlation of injury to stretching. However, they caution, "it may be runners who are (already) injured stretch because of their injury" (p. 154). Stated another way, "because injured runners may be counseled to stretch before running, and because injured runners are at higher injury risk, it may appear that those who stretch are at greater risk for injury" (Brill and Macera 1995, p. 366). Furthermore, "no time frame was given for the questions on stretching and on other training techniques to assess if or how long runners used these techniques just prior to their injury" (Jacobs and Berson 1986). A related issue that could have implications for runners is proper stretching techniques (Brill and Macera 1995).

Walter et al. (1988) employed an 80-item questionnaire for 688 adult entrants in a 10-mile race in southern Ontario. The data revealed that the younger runners reported stretching more often and for longer periods than older runners. However, the percentage of male runners who experienced an injury during the preceding year was the same for both age groups (56.3%). In contrast, 53.1% of the women less than 30 years of age versus 62.5% of older runners experienced an injury during the preceding year. In evaluating these data, Walter et al. (1988) state:

Because stretching is considered an activity that might prevent running injuries, we might have expected a lower injury rate among the young runners. However, because other factors (e.g., differences in training habits, participation in other physical activities, constitutional factors) may have confounded some of the potential benefits of stretching, it would be presumptuous to question the effectiveness of stretching purely on the basis of our data. (pp. 112-113)

Walter et al. (1989) monitored 1,680 runners several times over a 12-month period. The data revealed that runners who say they never warm up had less risk for a new injury than those who do. In addition, runners who use stretching "sometimes" were determined to be apparently at a higher risk for new injury than those who usually or never use it. van Mechelen et al. (1993) initiated a 16-week injury intervention program for 421 male recreational runners that included warm-up, cool-down, stretching exercises, and health education information. "The intervention did not result in a reduction of running injury incidence expressed per hours of running exposure" (p. 718). As Jacobs and Berson (1986) succinctly point out, "Clearly, further research is needed to determine the risk and benefits of the various factors involved in running."

Macera et al. (1989) published a prospective study of 583 habitual runners (485 men and 98 women). The data revealed 54% of the men and 44% of the women stretched before running. The risk of injury or odds ratio (OR) was 1.1 for the men and 1.6 for the women. The strongest predictor of injury in the follow-up year was an initial report of running an average of 64 km (40 miles) or more per week and a 2.9 OR. These numbers indicated stretching was not a risk factor for running injuries among the participants evaluated.

Bixler and Jones (1992) tested the hypothesis that a 1.5-minute routine of warming up and a 1.5-minute stretching protocol after a halftime break for high school football players may reduce the incidence of third-quarter injuries. Fifty-five games by five Pennsylvania Mid-Penn Football Conference teams were played with 108 total injuries. The intervention teams sustained significantly fewer third-quarter sprains and strains per game than the nonintervention group, although no significant difference in total third-quarter injuries was noted. The investigators suggested "an association between post-halftime warm-up and stretching and reduced third-quarter sprain and strain injuries" (p. 131). Unfortunately, the study did not permit identifying whether the stretching or the warm-up was responsible for the improvement.

Bennell and Crossley (1996) evaluated the incidence, distribution, types and severity of musculoskeletal injuries sustained by track and field athletes spanning a 12-month period to identify risk factors for injury in this population. Out of 95 athletes, 72 sustained 130 injuries, giving an athlete incidence rate of 76%. Greater overall flexibility (among other factors identified) as measured by a combination of lumbar spine, hamstring, flexibility, calf muscle, and ankle measures were found associated with a greater likelihood of injury. Significantly, the investigators raised four pertinent points that must be considered when interpreting the data:

- Individual measurements were not related to injury occurrence.

- This research may indicate that a series of measurements are required to provide an adequate representation of one's flexibility profile.

- The relationship between past injuries and current flexibility is unclear.

- The greater flexibility observed in the injured athletes possibly reflects a greater amount of stretching in an attempt to prevent further injury in this group.

A retrospective study (Cross and Worrell 1999) of 195 Division III college football players analyzed the incidence of musculotendinous strains between 1994 and 1995. All variables were consistent between the two seasons except for the incorporation of a lower-extremity stretching program in the latter year. A statistical analysis of the data indicated "an association between the incorporation of a static stretching program and a decreased incidence of musculotendinous strains" (p. 13). The researchers were unable to report a cause and effect relationship because of confounding variables. Nonetheless, the researchers believed that the data supported "the incorporation of stretching programs as a means of preventing musculotendinous strains" (p. 13).

Pope et al. (1998) investigated the effects of ankle dorsiflexion and preexercise calf muscle stretching on the relative risk of five selected injuries in 1,093 male army recruits undertaking 12 weeks of intensive training. The study concluded that (1) "Restricted ankle dorsiflexion range confers an increased risk of lower limb injury, and particularly of ankle sprain, in Army recruits" (p. 171) and (2) "definitive evidence of an effect of stretching on injury risk was not found ($p = .76$), but the sample size may have been insufficient to detect such an effect" (p. 165).

Pope et al. (2000) published the results of a randomized trial of preexercise stretching for prevention of lower-limb injuries in 1,538 male army recruits. The 12-week training program included warm-up exercises and one 20-second static stretch for six major leg muscle groups. The investigation determined that "a typical muscle stretching protocol performed during preexercise warm-ups does not produce clinically meaningful reductions in risk of exercise-related injury in army recruits" (p. 271). Further elaborating on this point, they wrote,

Our best estimate of the effect of stretching is that it reduces all-injury risk by 5%, and we are able to rule out a 23% or greater reduction in injury risk with 95% certainty. When these results are expressed in absolute terms, the futility of stretching becomes apparent. Recruits stretched for 40 sessions over the course of training, and so, on average, each recruit would need to stretch for 3100 physical training sessions to prevent one injury. As it took 5 minutes to complete the stretches, an average of 260 hours of stretching would be required to prevent one injury (95% CI 50 hour to prevent one injury to 65 hour to produce one injury). Clearly, even the most optimistic effects consistent with our data are of dubious clinical significance. Most populations are at lower risk of injury than army recruits investigated in the present study, and so it is probable that the value of stretching is even less in those populations. (p. 275)

Several explanations were offered by the investigators to rationalize their findings. The muscle stretches employed in the study possibly were not sustained long enough to produce sufficient physiological changes in the musculotendinous unit to reduce the risk of injury. The age of the recruits was positively related to injury risk, with older recruits less likely to be injured. Perhaps army-style marching and running was new to most recruits, making them more susceptible to injury than habitual runners and walkers.

Contradictory results were found in an intervention study (Hartig and Henderson 1999) spanning 13 weeks of an infantry basic training course at Fort Benning, Georgia. The study employed a control group of 148 trainees and an intervention group of 150 trainees that added three hamstring stretching sessions to their already scheduled fitness program. The control group and intervention group had an incidence of lower-extremity overuse injury rate of 29.1% and 16.7%, respectively. The study demonstrated that the number of lower-extremity overuse injuries was significantly lower in infantry basic trainees with increased hamstring flexibility.

Yeung and Yeung (2001) performed a systematic search of the available evidence for randomized and quasirandomized studies that dealt with prevention of running injuries. Their analysis comprised five studies with 1,944 participants in intervention groups and 3,159 control subjects. The finding of their study was that "There is insufficient evidence to suggest whether stretching exercises are effective in preventing lower limb injuries" (p. 386).

Relationship Between Stretching Before Exercise and Muscle Injuries

Voluminous recommendations by coaches, experts, and pundits advise that stretching before exercise can reduce the risk of local muscle injury. Does clinical and basic science literature support this hypothesis? Shrier (1999, 2000, 2001), in a detailed review of the clinical and basic science literature found no supporting evidence. In fact, he identified five theoretical arguments why stretching before exercise would not prevent injury.

1. In animals, immobilization or heating induced increases in muscle compliance thereby causing tissues to rupture more easily.
2. Stretching before exercise should have no effect for activities in which excessive muscle length is not an issue (e.g., jogging).
3. Stretching would not affect muscle compliance during eccentric activity, when most strains are believed to occur.
4. Stretching can produce damage at the cytoskeletal level.
5. Stretching appears to mask muscle pain in humans.

Additional research is required to further substantiate the conclusions of Shrier (1999, 2000, 2001). However, a study by Krabak et al. (2001) appears to challenge the hypothesis that stretching appears to mask muscle pain in humans through a novel investigation utilizing anesthesia.

X-RATED EXERCISES

Stretching exercises and the development of flexibility should not be considered a panacea to enhance performance or reduce risk of injury in sport or allied disciplines. Virtually every exercise presents some degree of risk. The possibility of an injury depends on numerous variables, including the individual's state of training, age, previous injuries, structural abnormalities, fatigue, and improper technique.

The following sections investigate eight controversial exercises commonly cited in the literature as being potentially dangerous. Nonetheless, many of these stretches are considered an integral part of dance, gymnastics, martial arts, wrestling, and yoga training. These controversial stretches are (1) the hurdler's stretch, (2) the inverted hurdler's stretch, (3) the deep knee bend (squat or lunge), (4) the standing toe touch, (5) the arch and bridge, (6) the standing torso twist, (7) gravity inversion, and (8) the shoulderstand and the plow.

Hurdler's Stretch

The hurdler's stretch has been traditionally one of the most common exercises to stretch the hamstrings, along with the lower back muscles and related soft tissues (see figure 14.1). It was often recommended in texts written by athletic trainers, doctors of exercise physiology, physical therapists, and orthopedic physicians who deal with preventing or rehabilitating injuries (Alter 1996). The name of this stretch derives from its similarity to the position used by a track runner clearing a hurdle. This exercise is performed on the floor with the leg to be stretched straight forward (in hip flexion with the knee extended) and the opposite leg abducted, flexed, and internally rotated at the hip with knee completely flexed so that the heel is next to the buttocks. In yoga, the trianga mukhaikapada pashimottanasana corresponds to the hurdler's stretch.

Analysis of Risk Factors

Numerous authors have speculated that in the hurdler's stretch, the awkward knee position in the bent leg creates a stress point at the medial knee joint (Alter 1996, 1998; Anderson 2000; Beaulieu 1981; Cailliet and Gross 1987; Clippinger-Robertson 1988; Cornelius 1984; Lubell 1989; Ninos 1996b; Peters and Peters 1983; Tucker 1990; Tyne and Mitchell 1983). This problem is further compounded if the knee is externally rotated, allowing the rear foot to flare out to the side, because this position may result in overstretching of the medial collateral ligaments (Alter 1996, 1998; Anderson 2000). Consequently, this exercise is thought to promote medial knee instability. Cailliet and Gross (1987) cite three major problems associated with this exercise: (1) It stretches the knee ligaments, (2) it can result in twisting and side-slipping of the kneecap, and (3) it can crush the rear portion of the lateral meniscus. Yet, another disadvantage is that for most people who have tight hip flexor muscles, the position results in a slight sideways tilting of the pelvis and an improper stretch. When the position is correct, the body's weight is evenly distributed on both tuberosities of the ischium, and both iliac crests are level with the floor (Lasater 1983). The exercise may cause discomfort at the hip joint because "the leg that is tucked behind places the femur in a position of extreme rotation in the joint capsule" (Lubell 1989).

The lower back may also be susceptible to pain or injury when the hurdler's stretch (or the trianga mukhaikapada pashimottanasana) is incorrectly practiced. According to Lasater (1988a), this asana can cause problems for (1) structural or (2) functional reasons: (1) The lumbosacral part of the spine is handicapped because it lacks the same degree of support given by several strong ligaments to other regions of the spinal column. Hence, if the asana is practiced with a rounded spine, the already stressed ligaments can be overstretched, structurally weakening the lumbosacral area. (2) The asana can be complicated by functional factors such as a rounded back caused by the habit of sitting incorrectly in chairs. Therefore, Lasater (1988a) believes that practicing the asana incorrectly with excessive rounding of the lumbar spine can further aggravate the problem. However, not a single citation was found in the literature verifying any type of injury caused by performing this exercise.

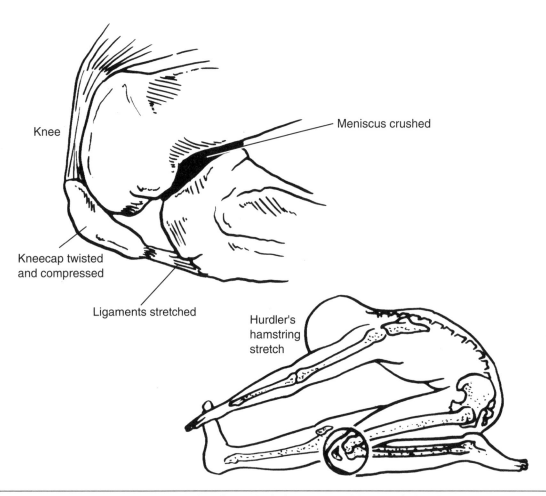

Figure 14.1   The hurdler's hamstring stretch will stretch the hamstring of the straight leg, but it can damage the bent knee by stretching the front knee ligaments, side-slipping the kneecap, and crushing the rear portion of the meniscus.

Reprinted, by permission, from R. Cailliet and L. Gross, 1987, *The rejuvenation strategy* (Garden City, NJ: Doubleday), 34.

Risk Reduction

The slight sideways tilting of the pelvis can be easily corrected by placing folded blankets or mats under the lower tuberosity until the pelvis becomes level. However, the problem with the knee remains. Here, the most prudent course is to either change the position of the knee or select an alternative stretch that accomplishes the same goal. The former can be achieved by pointing the foot of the flexed leg along the line of the lower leg, making the foot parallel to the thigh of the bent leg (Alter 1996, 1998; Anderson 2000).

Several solutions are available to reduce strain on the lower back. One solution is to perform the stretch from the hip joints with an elongated spine. Lasater (1988a) recommends placing the hands on the hip bones to feel the pelvis move forward as the trunk is elongated. If the hip bones do not move and the pelvis is held still, the spine becomes overly rounded, and the position is incorrect. A second alternative is to initiate the stretch sitting on a bench or table at approximately crotch level

(Alter 1996, Buckner and Khan 2002; Myers 1983). The nonstretched rear leg hangs freely over the edge, while the stretched leg is extended on the supporting surface. The trunk is lowered toward the thigh while keeping the upper back extended.

Another effective technique involves flexing the nonstretched rear leg so that the knee and thigh are brought close to the chest and the foot (rather than the shin) is placed flat on the floor. Then, during the forward stretch, the flexed leg is rotated outward, and the thigh is allowed to abduct. Thus, one is free to reach for the toes (Cailliet and Gross 1987). A more popularly cited variation (Anderson 2000; Beaulieu 1981; Cailliet 1988; Clippinger-Robertson 1988; Reid 1992; Tyne and Mitchell 1983) is to have the flexed leg fully abducted and rotated so that the outer side of the thigh and calf can rest on the floor, with the heel against the inner side of the opposite thigh. In yoga, the marichyasana and janu sirasana correspond to these two modified hurdler's stretches, respectively (Iyengar 1979).

Single-Leg or Double-Leg Inverted Hurdler's Stretch

The single-leg or double-leg inverted hurdler's stretch is used primarily for stretching the quadriceps muscles (see figure 14.2). However, it can also provide a powerful stretch for the anterior structures of the lower leg. In yoga, this exercise is known as the supta virasana, or reclining hero pose (Iyengar 1979; Lasater 1986). This exercise is quite effective in stretching the hip flexor. Its incorporation in a variety of programs has been recommended by American Academy of Orthopaedic Surgeons (1991), Ehrhart (1976), Lasater (1986), Reid (1992), Schuster (1988), Sing (1984), Smith (1977), and Weaver (1979). This stretch may drastically decrease the occurrence of debilitating episodes of periostitis (i.e., shin splints [O'Malley and Sprinkle 1986]). In addition, such quadriceps stretching may prevent Osgood-Schlatter disease, an avulsion of the tibial tuberosity in skeletally immature individuals by excessive pull of the patellar tendon (Kulund 1980). However, considerable contro- versy exists regarding its incorporation in a fitness or training program.

Analysis of Risk Factors

The inverted hurdler's stretch is postulated to place undue stress on the knee by opening the anterior portion of the articulation. Consequently, the exercise is believed to reduce joint stability by overstretching the ligaments, twisting and compressing the kneecap, and crushing the meniscus (Alter 1996, 1998; Anderson 2000; Cailliet and Gross 1987; Cornelius 1984). In addition, Lasater (1986) cautions that pregnant women should avoid prolonged backward bending after the fourth month to prevent a sudden drop in blood pressure caused by a compression of the inferior vena cava by the overlying fetus.

Risk Reduction

Two options are available for reducing the problems associated with the inverted hurdler's stretch. The first option is to incorporate alternative exercises that are easier and safer to execute. The second option is to learn how to

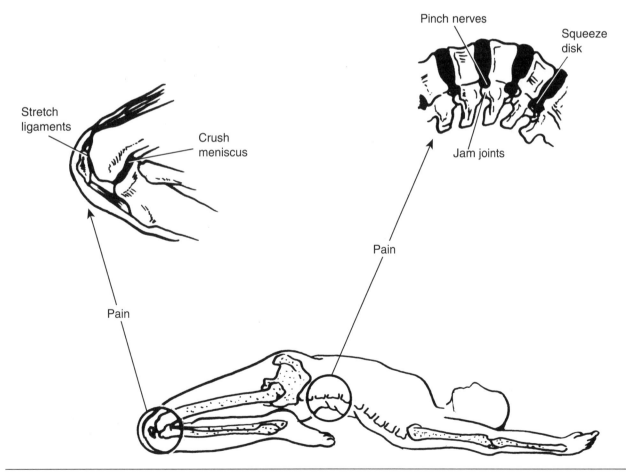

Figure 14.2 The single-leg or double-leg inverted hurdler's stretch. This exercise results in overstretching some tissues, crushing others, pinching nerves, and jamming joints.

Reprinted, by permission, from R. Cailliet and L. Gross, 1987, *The rejuvenation strategy* (Garden City, NJ: Doubleday), 37.

properly perform these stretches with detailed instruction from a competent instructor. The exercises should be mastered in a slow and sequential manner and with correct technique. The most commonly cited warning about technique is to avoid internally rotating the legs and flaring the feet out to the sides (Alter 1996, 1998; Anderson 1985, 2000; Lasater 1986; Luby and St. Onge 1986). Use of blankets, bolsters, mats, or props can further facilitate safely mastering this exercise (Lasater 1986; Luby and St. Onge 1986).

Deep Knee Bend

The deep knee bend (or lunge or squat) can enhance flexibility of the hamstrings, groin, calf, and Achilles tendon. It can also strengthen the muscles of the legs, especially the quadriceps. However, this exercise is potentially dangerous when performed incorrectly. The key factors responsible for injury are the velocity of the descent, the depth of the descent, and the positioning of the feet. The use of weights can potentially compound the risk of injury (see figure 14.3).

Analysis of Risk Factors

Problems develop with the deep knee bend when the bend is too deep and goes beyond the place where the muscles hold and control the body's weight. Beyond this point, the ligaments of the knees must bear the sudden and forceful weight (Alter 1983). According to Alter (1983) and Cailliet and Gross (1987), these exercises can strain the capsule and ligaments, compress the kneecaps, and crush the menisci. Several orthopedic surgeons (Fowler and Messieh 1987; Miller and Major 1994; Spindler and Benson 1994) point out that hyperflexion with a downward force on the anterior thigh is a common mechanism for posterior cruciate ligament (PCL) tear.

Squatting is a basic component of many disciplines and sports, including baseball, dance, gymnastics, handball, weightlifting, and wrestling. Hence, the avoidance of squatting is virtually impossible. However, squatting exercises should be avoided by laypeople, especially the middle-aged or elderly. The incorporation of squatting into a fitness or training program must always be evaluated on an individual basis.

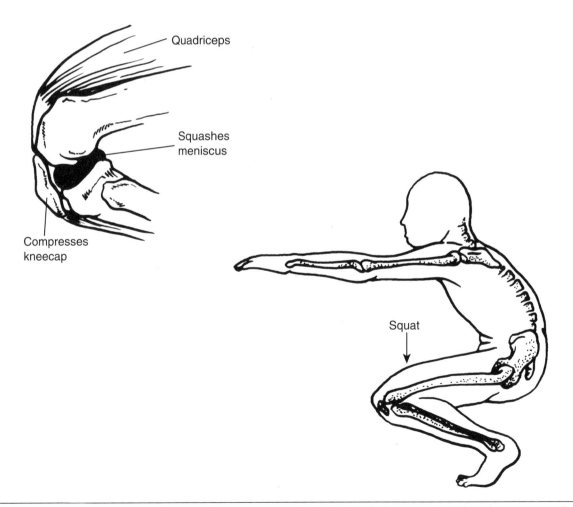

Figure 14.3 Deep knee bends endanger the ligaments of the knee and squash the meniscus. They also compress the kneecap. Partial knee bends, which strengthen the thigh muscles and strengthen the heel cords, are not dangerous.
Reprinted by permission, from R. Cailliet and L. Gross, 1987, *The rejuvenation strategy* (Garden City, NJ: Doubleday), 35.

Risk Reduction

One strategy to minimize the risk of injury when squatting is to reduce the movement velocity by slowly lowering the body with the control of the quadriceps, which can be done by holding on to something for support or squatting with the back against a wall (Anderson 1985; Benjamin 1978; Clippinger-Robertson 1988; Fisk and Rose 1977; Luby and St. Onge 1986). The second option is to reduce the depth of the descent by squatting to only a 90-degree angle at the knee (Clippinger-Robertson 1988). The knees should remain over the long axis of the foot (Anderson 1985; Benjamin 1978; Clippinger-Robertson 1988).

Standing Straight-Leg Toe Touch

The standing straight-leg toe touch is perhaps the most common stretching exercise. For many, it is the gold standard test of flexibility. Yet, it is perhaps one of the most controversial exercises. Yoga has three main variations of this exercise: The padahastasana is performed by bending forward and placing one's palms on the floor; the padangusthasana is performed by standing and catching the big toe in front of the body; and the uttanasana is performed by placing the hands on the floor well behind the feet while the upper torso rests on the thighs (see figure 14.4a-c). The purposes (both correct and incorrect) of these exercises include stretching the hamstrings, stretching the erector spinae (back extensor) muscles, stretching the spine, testing flexibility, and exercising the abdominal muscles. Exercising the abdominal muscles is the incorrect purpose.

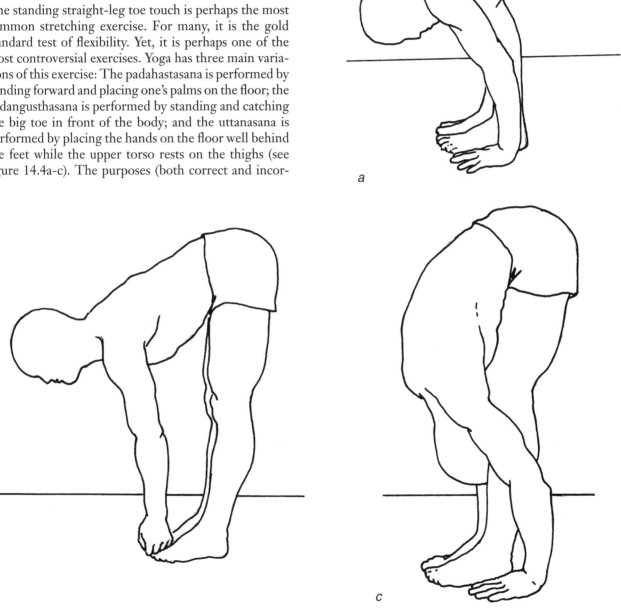

a

b

c

Figure 14.4 Variations of the standing straight-leg toe touch.
Reprinted from Alter 1990.

Analysis of Risk Factors

The standing straight-leg toe touch should be avoided, especially for people middle-aged or older who have a medical history of back problems (e.g., herniated disk). In addition, problems are most likely to occur in people with weak abdominal muscles or with tight hamstrings or low-back muscles (Falls and Humphrey 1989). Theoretically, the exercise is thought to put stress on the disks and posterior ligaments of the lower back and on the sciatic nerve (Alter 1996, 1998; Anderson 1985; Cailliet and Gross 1987; Dominguez, cited in Shyne 1982; Tessman 1980; Zacharkow 1984). The knees may be forced to hyperextend, resulting in permanent deformity, such as loose or "sway back" knees. The exercise is also thought to potentially damage the menisci (Cailliet and Gross 1987). Middle-aged and elderly participants may be at increased risk for loss of balance, resulting in falls and possible injuries (Daleiden 1990; Kauffman 1990). The higher the center of gravity and the narrower the base of support, the more unstable the position. This factor can also be compounded, especially in the elderly, by deficient postural control mechanisms (Daleiden 1990; Ochs et al. 1985), diseases (Daleiden 1990; Kauffman 1990), medication (Daleiden 1990; Tideiksaar 1986), and decreased strength (Kauffman 1990; Whipple et al. 1987).

The fully flexed posture while standing is also a potential occupational risk, especially among concrete reinforcement workers (rodmen) when tying reinforcement bar together (Rose et al. 2001). Consequently, the discussion that follows also has relevance for workers who assume this position for extended periods of time.

Upon reviewing the literature, one is struck by the question of what and whom to believe. Numerous experts present diametrically opposing views. Some contend that the standing straight-leg toe touch is dangerous and should not be practiced at all. Others provide cautions and warnings about its potential dangers or recommend using safer modifications. Still others recommend the exercise wholeheartedly or offer no precautions.

Among opponents who contend that the exercise is dangerous and should not be practiced are orthopedic professionals (Berland and Addison 1972; Dominguez and Gajda 1982; Seimon 1983; Williams 1977); doctors of physical medicine and rehabilitation (Cailliet and Gross 1987); a physical therapist (Zacharkow 1984), an athletic trainer (Tyne and Mitchell 1983), a professor of dance (Alter 1986), and a professor of physics (Tessman 1980). Equally impressive are the credentials of people who advocate the exercise, including orthopedic surgeons (Torg et al. 1987); medical doctors (Finneson 1980; Friedmann and Galton 1973; Grieve 1988; Kraus 1965, 1970; Wilkinson 1983), an osteopath (Stoddard 1979); and physical therapists (LaFreniere 1979; Van Wijmen 1986). Obviously, no consensus exists regarding the inherent risks and virtues of this exercise.

Risk Reduction

Several methods can minimize the risk when using a standing straight-leg toe touch in an exercise program. All things being equal, the greater the degree of flexibility and strength, the less the probability of an injury. Hence, only those individuals with adequate flexibility and strength should incorporate the exercise into their programs. However, in the real world things are seldom equal. Complicating factors include age, condition, injury, and vocation.

Working slowly and sequentially is one way to reduce the risk of injury. This strategy can include the use of various props or supporting devices. Eventually, by beginning with easier exercises and progressing to more difficult ones, many people should gradually develop the necessary flexibility and strength to successfully and safely master the standing straight-leg toe touch. Such a sequential program is described by Couch (1979), Carrico (1986), Luby and St. Onge (1986), and Grieve (1988).

Another method of reducing risk requires using correct technique. One school of thought advocates a flat back during the trunk-lowering phase (Couch 1979; Luby and St. Onge 1986). Lasater (1988b) describes the descending position as a gently arching curve and cautions against an overly rounded or overarched spine. Several explanations support keeping a relatively straight back. The most common explanation is that bending with a rounded back puts greater stress on the spine, sciatic nerve, and disks because the back muscles are not supporting the spine. Rather, the spine is primarily supported by the ligaments (Luby and St. Onge 1986). Another explanation is that "when the back is one unit, 'straight,' no one curve of the back is curving against its natural angle, so the discs and vertebrae are not forced out of alignment" (Couch 1979, p. 134).

In contrast, Siff (1992) advocates a natural or neutral position for the spine. In his opinion, "any major deviations from its natural curvatures will stress the spine unnecessarily" (p. 88). This, rationale is in part, based on the comments of Kapandji (1974). Kapandji points out "that the resistance of a curved column is *directly proportional to the square of its number of curvatures plus one . . .* Therefore, the vertebral column with its lumbar, *thoracic and cervical curvatures has resistance of 10, i.e., ten* times that of a straight column" (p. 20). Thus, Siff (1992) recommends, "the correct advice for spinal care is to maintain the neutral position of the spine" (p. 88).

A fourth approach is to slowly and smoothly lower the upper torso, as opposed to rapidly dropping the trunk. Ballistic types of movement should be avoided for two reasons. (1) By avoiding ballistic movement, the stretch reflex of the erector spinae muscles will not be initiated, thereby reducing the likelihood of back muscle contraction and the risk of opposing muscle tension and strain. (2) Ballistic stretching could generate large and uncontrollable amounts of angular momentum. The angular momentum may exceed the absorbing capacity of the soft tissues being stretched and may result in injury. The greater the amount of energy per unit of time a tissue must absorb, the greater is the stress and likelihood for injury. Hence, nonathletes, especially the middle-aged, the sedentary, and elderly, should generally avoid ballistic stretching.

Another technique of reducing strain during the descent is decreasing any load anterior to the vertebral body. The mechanics of the lumbar spine are such that any increased weight anterior to the vertebral column greatly increases the forces exerted on the lumbar spine. Holding the arms outstretched forward and lowering them horizontally to the floor increases the anterior load, whereas placing the hands on the hips or thighs during the descent will decrease the anterior load. Strain on the lower back can also be reduced by supporting the hands on the legs or thighs, a chair, a stack of books, or overhead straps or by supporting oneself on a counter with the elbows or outstretched arms (Alter 1986; Anderson 1985; Carrico 1986; Couch 1979; Knight and Davis 1984; Lasater 1988b; Luby and St. Onge 1986; White 1983). As one's strength and flexibility increase, one is gradually weaned off the support. Straddling the legs sideways can also reduce the strain. As flexibility and strength increase, the feet can be gradually placed closer together.

A final way to reduce strain on the hamstrings and lower back is to initiate the stretch from a squatting position. Flex the trunk forward to grasp the toes. Then slowly straighten the legs until a sensation of tightening or stretching is felt. At this point, the stretch should be maintained. This technique has been advocated by various authors (Alter 1986; Alter 1996, 1998; Hossler 1989; International Dance-Exercise Association n.d.; Luby and St. Onge 1986; Tyne and Mitchell 1983; Uram 1980).

Injuries can also occur during the trunk-ascending phase, most likely because of faulty reextension from the flexed position in which lordosis is regained before the pelvis is derotated (Cailliet 1988). Ideally, in reassuming the erect stance, the lumbar spine should act as an inflexible rod, and the back should be straight. With faulty reextension, the upper portion of the body rises too soon, so the lower back arches and the lordosis curve is forward of the center of gravity. This position places excessive stress on the lower back. As elaborated by Cailliet (1988), the supraspinous ligaments in full flexion and during reextension normally support the lumbar spine until the last 45°. (The reextension to the full upright posture is achieved mostly by pelvic derotation.) During the last 45° of extension, the erector spinae muscles straighten the spine. Hence, the lower back should regain its lordosis last. However, because of the short lever on which the erector spinae muscles act, this phase of reextension is inefficient, requiring a large amount of muscle tension to produce a small amount of movement. Furthermore,

when the erector spinae muscles fatigue, the task of maintaining and supporting the excessive load falls on the vertebral ligaments. Once these ligaments give way, the load falls on the joints, and subluxation of the joint results. The International Dance-Exercise Association (n.d.) prefers "rounding the upper torso up" rather than lifting up with a flat back. A similar position is offered by LaFreniere (1979).

Two additional variations can reduce the potential risks associated with the reextension phase. One variation involves bending the knees after the stretch has been maintained for the desired amount of time. Then, with the knees flexed, one can sit down on the floor. The other variation is to keep the knees flexed while the upper body rises until fully erect. This strategy has been described by several writers (Alter 1996, 1998; Nieman 1990; Peters and Peters 1983; Tyne and Mitchell 1983).

As a point of side interest, three additional studies deserve special consideration. First, Rose et al. (2001) found that in the vast majority of those tested in the flexed position, pain from the legs and not from the lower back limited the working ability. They suggested that "compression and shear forces on the vertebral discs are not sensed like muscle strain, and for non-muscle structures in the spine pain may not function as a warning signal." However, they point out "the fact that pain is sensed mainly from the legs does not necessarily imply that the legs have a higher risk of injury than the back" (p. 506). Because leg, hip, and back problems in occupations where fully flexed postures are common, further research in this area is warranted. Second, Jackson et al. (2001) examined the duration and pattern of recovery after 20 minutes of static lumbar flexion and found "full recovery of residual strain in the L4/L5 supraspinous ligament and multifidus activity was not obtained after 7 hours of rest" (p. 715). Based upon this research they inferred:

> That static flexion of the lumbar spine in occupational and sports activities is an extremely imposing function on its viscoelastic tissues because it is associated with severe tension-relaxation, residual strain, decrease in muscular stabilizing forces, and spasms. These implications of static lumbar flexion, even within the physiologic range and for relatively short periods, may expose the spine to potential disorders and require extremely long periods of rest before normal functions are reestablished. (p. 722)

This development raises a question: How do power lifters and weight lifters avoid injury when performing straight-leg deadlifts (morning exercises)? This exercise requires lifts (often with heavy loads) when the spine appears to be in full flexion. Cholewicki and McGill (1992) examined this very question in the third study using video fluoroscopy of the lumbar spine and movement in the sagittal plane. The research revealed that

"During their lifts, even though the subjects outwardly appeared to fully flex their spines, their spines were 2 to 3 degrees per lumbar joint from full flexion, thus explaining how they could lift magnificent loads without sustaining the type of injury that we suspected is linked with full flexion" (McGill 1998, p. 757). By chance, the investigators recorded an injury occurring. The lifter injured his back when "the L3-4 joint temporarily approached the calibrated full flexion angle and then exceeded it by 0.5 degrees while all other joints maintained their position" (p. 757).

This study and others (Cholewicki and McGill 1996) revealed that the spine appears to be most prone to failure because of *instability* when loading demands are low and the major muscles are not activated to high levels, or when very high loads are experienced. Elaborating on this point McGill (1998) writes, "Nonetheless, it appears that the chance of motor control error, which results in a short and temporary reduction in activation to one of the intersegmental muscles, would cause rotation of just a single joint to a point where passive or other tissues becomes irritated or possibly injured" (p. 757). The significance of this point should serve as a clear warning. Stretching even with low loads employing just one's own body weight, as when performing the straight-leg toe touch, requires concentration and vigilance in terms of technique.

Biomechanics

One method of analyzing the standing straight-leg forward toe touch is via myoelectric activity of the various muscle groups employed in the exercise. This evaluation could include the use of cinematography and electronic magnetoresistive movement sensors. A second way to analyze the exercise is by using mathematical models and mechanical analysis.

Myoelectric Activity During Back or Trunk Flexion.

Numerous electromyographic studies have investigated forward flexion and reextension of the trunk. Forward flexion is initiated (during the first few degrees of motion) by contraction of the abdominal muscles (Allen 1948; Floyd and Silver 1950) and then continued passively by gravity. As the upper trunk flexes forward, the hips shift backward, thus shifting the center of gravity behind the feet. Simultaneously, the pelvic girdle as a unit flexes on the femoral heads while the spinal column bends forward progressively from top to bottom, until the L5 vertebra flexes forward on the sacrum (Lee 1989). During the first portion of the flexion, strong myoelectric activity is found in the hip extensor muscles (gluteus maximus, gluteus medius, and hamstring muscles; [Okada 1970; Portnoy and Morin 1956]). This action stabilizes the pelvis and prevents motion at the hip joints, ensuring that all of the early motion occurs in the spine. As the spine bends forward, activity of the back muscles is increased

proportional to the angle of flexion and to the size of the load carried. The extent and rate at which the flexion proceeds is controlled by the eccentric contraction of the back muscles.

However, as the trunk flexion continues, myoelectric activity of the back muscles markedly decreases. Schultz et al. (1985) determined that EMG activity diminished at 40° flexion of the L1 vertebra. Eventually, at the *critical point* (CP) of forward flexion, the myoelectric activity in the back muscles ceases. Floyd and Silver (1950) called this phenomenon of a sudden decrease in activity of the erector spinae muscles *flexion relaxation* (flexion-relaxation response, or FRR). Older literature reported that the FRR phenomenon occurs between 40° and 70° of body flexion. However, more sophisticated research (Sihvonen 1997) determined back muscle activity ceased in lumbar flexion with a mean of 79°.

McGill and Kippers (1994) concluded that the "relaxation" of the lumbar muscles occurred only in an electrical sense because the lumbar muscles still generated substantial force elastically through passive stretching. Thus, they suggested that the term *flexion-relaxation* is inappropriate.

The critical point does not occur in all individuals or in all muscles. Schultz et al. (1985) cite Fick (1911) as the first to suggest that the erector spinae muscles need not be active in positions of full flexion. This observation has been confirmed by Allen (1948), Floyd and Silver (1951, 1955), Portnoy and Morin (1956), Pauly (1966), Schultz et al. (1985), Shirado et al. (1995), Tanii and Masuda (1985), and Wolf et al. (1991). Investigators have reported that some patients with low-back pain do not exhibit this phenomenon (Floyd and Silver 1951, 1955; Shirado et al. 1995; Sihvonen et al. 1991). In a study by Steventon and Ng (1995), the research implied "that either erector spinae activity is independent of speed in the slow to natural functional speed range or the flexion relaxation phenomenon is not related to changes in spinal ligamentous tension" (p. 239). However, a study by Sarti et al. (2001), found an increase in speed of movement "delayed the appearance of the electrical silence of the erector spinae muscles in the range of flexion" (p. E-416).

The effect of aging on the activity of the erector spinae during trunk flexion was investigated by Ng and Walter (1995). Their study comprised 22 normal females 20 to 25 years of age and 16 normal females 60 to 92 years of age. The investigation found the erector spinae "relaxed" at the critical position, which was 67% and 82% of full-trunk flexion for young and older subjects, respectively. Thus, "the CP in the older subjects occurred relatively later in the trunk flexion range than the young subjects" (p. 93).

No research has determined whether a difference exists in myoelectric activity between the flat-back and the rounded-back techniques. Hence, assuming that the same relaxation phenomenon occurs with both techniques, the argument that the rounded back creates greater stress on the spine is questionable because the back is supported primarily by the ligaments in both cases. This issue needs a detailed investigation to clarify the conflicting claims. A point of particular relevance to weight lifters who perform "morning exercises" (i.e., exercises using weights with the trunk in flexion) is that carrying weights during flexion causes the critical point to occur later in the range of vertebral flexion (Kippers and Parker 1984). It also increases the level of tension in the back muscles, increasing the risk of strain injury. Like the lower back muscles, the gluteus maximus relaxes as full flexion is approached. However, the hamstring muscles are significantly active from the onset and remain active throughout the trunk flexion.

The physiological basis of the critical point is unknown. Floyd and Silver (1951) hypothesized that "stretch receptors in the ligamenta flava and other ligaments are stimulated when these ligaments are stretched, and the afferent impulses from the stretch receptors cause reflex inhibition of the erectores spinae" (p. 134). Kippers and Parker (1984) have also suggested that this muscle relaxation may be the result of reflex inhibition initiated by proprioceptors in the lumbar joints and ligaments or in the muscle spindles.

A popular explanation for the FFR is that in the fully flexed position, the trunk flexion moment is resisted by structures other than muscles. That is, the passive resistance to stretching of the ligamentous tissues of the back substitutes for active muscle contractions in the flexed trunk position. Other structures that participate in creating this resistance are the thoracolumbar fascia and skin (Farfan 1973; Gracovetsky et al. 1977; Tesh et al. 1985). Because skin is farthest from the bending axis, it can contribute significantly to resisting the bending moment at even moderate stress levels. However, skin resistance is highly dependent on body build. As explained by Tesh et al. (1985), "loose and lax skin of an obese subject would not offer resistance, whereas the tighter skin of a lean subject would contribute considerably more to resisting forward flexion" (p. 186). Furthermore, dermal scar tissue is markedly less extensible than normal skin and can offer a higher resistance to forward bending. Altogether, normal skin can contribute up to 5% of the bending moment developed in full spinal flexion under body weight alone (Tesh et al. 1985).

The FFR has also been observed in the hamstrings and the cervical paraspinal muscles (McGorry et al. 2001; Meyer et al. 1993; Sihvonen 1997). However, they relax with different timing. For example, Sihvonen (1997) found hamstring EMG activity ceased when nearly full lumbar flexion 97° was reached. Beyond this point, "lumbar flexion and the last part of pelvic flexion happen without back muscle activity or hamstring bracing, respectively" (p. 486).

Although the FFR is thought to be reflexive in nature, it can be overridden by volitional or protective responses (Kaigle et al. 1998). The FRR may be absent or significantly impaired in cases of both acute and chronic low-back pain (Shirado et al. 1995; Sihvonen et al. 1991). Additional "research is needed to determine the extent to which detailed information of lumbar-pelvic rhythm can help when recognizing and differentiating back diseases clinically" (Sihvonen 1997, p. 489).

Myoelectric Activity During Back or Trunk Extension.

Extension of the trunk from the flexed to the upright position reverses the sequence of events observed when bending forward (Allen 1948; Donisch and Basmajian 1972; Floyd and Silver 1950, 1955; Morris et al. 1962; Okada 1970; Portnoy and Morin 1956). Segmental muscle recruitment progresses in the caudal-to-cephalad direction during trunk extension from full flexion in standing (McGorry et al. 2001). The gluteus maximus comes into action early and probably initiates hip extension together with the hamstrings (Okada 1970). Later, the posterior back muscles become active. The extensor muscle activity is greater while the trunk is being raised than while it is being lowered (Okada 1970) because concentric contractions require more active muscle tension than do eccentric contractions. Furthermore, lumbar lordosis increases myoelectric activity of the back muscles (Andersson et al. 1977; Okada 1970).

Mathematical Models and Mechanical Analysis of Trunk Flexion.

Estimation of stresses on various parts of the musculoskeletal system during dynamic activities requires a model that accounts for such factors as instantaneous positions and accelerations of the extremities, head, and trunk; changes in spinal geometry; and strength variations within different muscle groups (Pope et al. 1991). Macintosh et al. (1993) point out that flexion of the lumbar spine

> causes appreciable elongations of the lumbar back muscles and changes their orientation in relation to the lumbar spine. However, not all changes in orientation are in the same sense; some increase, others decrease. This discrepancy is because of the different orientation of different fascicles of the lumbar back muscles in the upright posture. (p. 889)

Nonetheless, a number of biomechanical models of spinal loading have been developed, based on the notion that the lumbar spine behaves like a set of small links with flexible articulations (disks) between them. With proper geometric and physiological data, the forces in each disk can be predicted.

The traditional mathematical model of the spine is a simple lever system (i.e., a cantilever model) in which a load carried in front of the body is balanced by the force generated by the spinal muscles. Aspden (1988) suggested that the spine instead should be considered as a series of linked rods that function like an arch. This model shows that spinal stresses are not as great as previously calculated.

Regardless of which model is used, the force, or moment, exerted on the spine when performing a standing straight-leg toe touch is proportional to the weight being moved and its distance from the axis of the body. The moment exerted on any lumbar vertebra is the product of the mass to be lifted and its horizontal distance from the vertebra. Consequently, a proportional increase in the compressive force on the low back is created by increasing the moment (National Institute for Occupational Safety and Health 1981). Moments can be magnified by increasing the weight or by increasing the horizontal distance of the weight from the body. This principle is utilized in exercise regimens, such as body building, power lifting, and weight lifting, in which weights are used to strengthen the back muscles (e.g., dead lifts and the morning exercise). Conversely, moments can be decreased by reducing the mass or by shortening its horizontal distance from the body. Most people should try to decrease the moment of force on the spine when exercising.

Adams and Hutton (1986) determined that when people adopt the static, fully flexed posture, the lumbar spine is flexed about 10° short of its elastic limit. This restriction in movement is probably caused by the protective action of the back muscles and lumbodorsal fascia. However, the margin of safety might be reduced or eliminated during rapid movements. Thus, most people performing a straight-leg toe touch should avoid ballistic stretching.

What posture or technique is optimal in performing a straight-leg toe touch? Assuming that the feet are placed together and parallel, and the knees are straight during trunk reextension, two back orientations are possible. Some authors recommend a *back-bowed-in* (BBI [i.e., in normal lordosis]), or a flat-back technique. Others recommend the *back-bowed-out* (BBO [i.e., curved in kyphosis]), or a slightly rounded position.

Delitto et al. (1987) performed an EMG analysis of lifting from the BBI and BBO positions. Erector spinae muscle activity during the initial period was greater in the BBI lift than in the BBO lift, and therefore the BBI position may provide optimal protection for the inert structures of the lumbar spine. This observation substantiates the finding of increased myoelectric activity with lordosis during extension (Andersson et al. 1977; Okada 1970).

Most information that may be extrapolated to the standing straight-leg toe touch was obtained from studies of weight lifting. Unfortunately, much of this research is concerned with lifting challenging weights (i.e., heavy to maximum resistance) from the classic squat-lift position

with the back nearly vertical. Comparing the extension phase of the standing toe touch with the squat-lift position, in which the trunk is already in extension and the pelvis in the rotated position, is difficult. Consequently, the forces acting on the pelvis and spine are not similar.

However, a biomechanical study by Gracovetsky et al. (1989) pertaining to the degree of lordosis during flexion-extension exercises may provide a solution to the dilemma of how flat the back should be during the exercise. The investigation indicated that the body naturally assumes the appropriate degree of lordosis or pelvic tilting. This model hypothesized that for every angle of forward flexion, a unique degree of lordosis will minimize and equalize the compressive stress within the spine. Because the connective tissues cannot contract by themselves, their degree of tension is a result of passive stretching and is thus controlled mainly by the geometric characteristics of the spine, in particular, the degree of lordosis (see figure 14.5a-c).

> Thus, when the moment to be balanced is highest (during the first phase of the return to the erect stance), it is advantageous to reduce the lordosis and support the load through ligamentous tension. When closer to the erect stance, the moment is lower, and the lordosis can be allowed to increase. (p. 415)

A mechanism that can protect the lower back during extension is isometric contraction of the abdominal muscles throughout the lift. This activity is thought to support the spine both by increasing the intraabdominal pressure and by tensing the thoracolumbar fascia through the attachments of the internal oblique and transverse abdominis muscles (Bartelink 1957; Bogduk 1984).

Reflexes

Another significant factor that influences the straight-leg toe touch while standing are two often neglected reflexes. One is the *positive support reaction* or extensor-thrust reflex. When pressure is exerted against the soles of the feet during standing, this reaction becomes operative and will stiffen the limbs and thus counter the desired objective (Guyton and Hall 1997). The pointine reticular nuclei of the vestibular nuclei excites the antigravity muscles of the body. In particular, they excite the muscles of the spinal column and the extensor muscles of the limbs. Functioning in association with the pointine reticular nuclei to excite the antigravity muscles are the vestibular nuclei. Consequently, toe-touching stretches in the standing and seated positions appear to be neuromuscularly different procedures (Siff and Verkhoshansky 1999). Another reflex discussed earlier is associated with eye positioning (see chapter 8). ROM can be increased by looking in the direction you desire to reach. For example, looking up will reduce lumbar flexion. In a similar manner, trunk rotation with the arms extended sideways is reduced by looking in the opposite direction the arms are positioned.

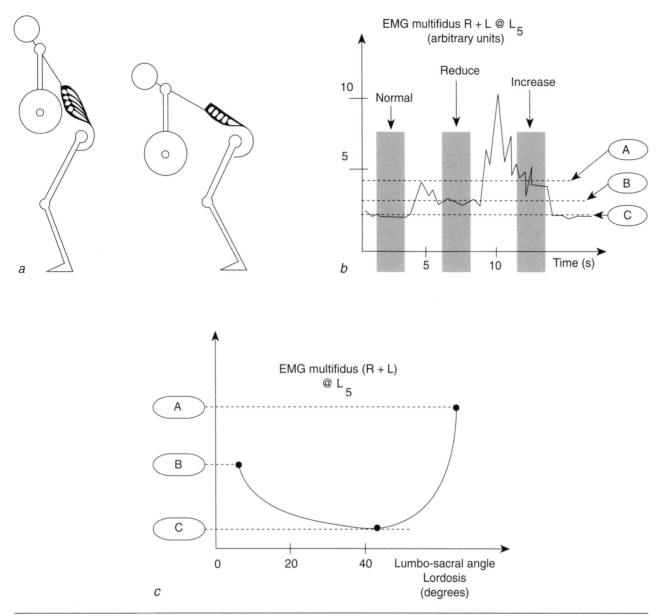

Figure 14.5 (*a*) Increased lordosis—ligaments slack. Decreased lordosis—ligaments tighten. (*b*) The integrated EMG activity is recorded bilaterally and superficial electrodes placed 2 cm to the right and left of the spinous process at L5. On this graph, the signal from right and left electrodes have been added. The levels corresponding to the most comfortable posture (normal) and reduced and increased lordosis are depicted by arrows. (*c*) Integrated EMG of multifidus showing relative activity vs. lumbosacral angle (lordosis). A = increased lordosis, B = decreased lordosis, C = normal.

Reprinted, by permission, from S. Gracovetsky, M. Kary, I. Pitchen, S. Levy, and R.B. Said, 1989, "The importance of pelvic tilt in reducing compressive stress in the spine during flexion-extension exercises," *Spine* 14(4), 415.

Rationale for the Standing Toe-Touch Exercise

What is the practical use of standing toe-touch exercise? How can it be justified? It is neither necessary nor recommended for the layperson, especially the middle-aged or elderly, because safer alternatives can stretch the same muscle groups. This exercise also is probably not necessary for many sports, but it may be considered essential in several sports. In some disciplines, this stretch position actually may be part of a compulsory or optional skill. In

3-meter and 10-meter diving, the deep flexed position is used in backward and forward multiple piked somersaults. Divers also use this position when pressing to a handstand on the edge of the platform. In gymnastics, this position can be seen in virtually every event

The risk of bending injury to the lumbar discs and ligaments depend on a variety of factors: the load, the loading rate, and loading history (Adams and Dolan 1996). Occupational risks among construction workers are high compared with those in other occupations. A review of literature by Rose et al. (2001) found the reported occupational accidents and diseases in Sweden for concrete reinforcement workers (rodmen) were 88.7/1000 employees in 1990, compared with a mean of 39.3/1000 for all occupations. "The fully flexed postures are very common among rodmen, and are dominant when tying reinforcement bars together" (p. 501). In other occupations, also (e.g., nursing and industrial assembly) a large amount of the working time is spent in fully flexed posture. Sustained lumbar flexion is also noted for occurring during two types of activity, typified by sitting and gardening (Adams and Dolan 1996). The question that needs to be resolved is whether stretching exercises such as the standing toe touch can reduce the risk of discomfort, fatigue, pain, or injury associated with activities or occupations in which much of the working time is spent in fully flexed postures.

Arch and Bridge

The arch and bridge (see figure 14.6) are two exercises primarily used to enhance the flexibility of the vertebral column and shoulders. They can also strengthen other parts of the body. The results depend on the variation of the arch or bridge performed and the method of achieving the final position. Many of these stretches are considered fundamental components of gymnastics, wrestling, and yoga.

Analysis of Risk Factors

Various types of arching and bridging exercises can range from potentially dangerous to life threatening. Flint (1964) criticized the common standing backbend exercise because, if the abdominal muscles are weak and a swayback condition exists, this exercise will exacerbate the condition. Cailliet and Gross (1987) believe that some arching is acceptable, but hyperarching is dangerous. Hyperextension of the low back can cause injury by excessively squeezing spinal disks, by jamming together the spinal joints, and by pinching the nerve fibers that emerge from the spinal foramina (openings) to form the sciatic nerve.

The concern of lumbar spine damage to gymnasts because of repetitive hyperlordosis and hyperextension (i.e., arching or bridging) has been addressed by several investigators (Fairbank et al. 1984; Goldstein et al. 1991; Jackson et al. 1976; Oseid et al. 1974; Sward et al. 1990). A result of such continuous insult to the vertebrae may be the development of spondylolysis or low-back pain. However, Tsai and Wredmark (1993) reported that former female elite gymnasts did not have more back problems than an age-matched control group.

Can relatively static skills such as the bridge or walkover cause spondylolysis, or is spondylolysis the result of chronic overloading during high-impact, weight-bearing activities (such as tumbling passes, vaulting, and dismounts from various apparatus) or of stresses imparted to the body during dynamic skills (such as giant swings on the horizontal bar, still rings, or uneven parallel bars)? A possible way to answer this question is to design a study that compares the vertebrae of three distinct groups that utilize hyperextension: artistic gymnasts, rhythmic gymnasts, and advanced practitioners of yoga.

Perhaps, the strongest criticism of this type of exercise was raised by Nagler (1973a, 1973b) and Hanus et al. (1977). In their medical opinion, the therapeutic value of these exercises for middle-aged people is not sufficient to justify the potential, although rare, risk of vertebral artery occlusion, which can result from forceful hyperextension of the cervical spine. The case of a 28-year-old female yoga enthusiast who performed the bridge was described by both Nagler (1973a) and Hanus et al. (1977). During the exercise, the woman reported a severe throbbing headache and later was unable to move without assistance. Five days later, a craniotomy was performed, and an ischemic infarct (stroke) with secondary hemorrhages was found in the left cerebellar hemisphere of the brain.

Risk Reduction

Before attempting a bridge, one should possess sufficient strength and suppleness to rise up and to support and maintain the position. Adequate suppleness in the hips, lower and upper torso, and shoulders are needed. Proper sequential learning through lead-up drills and exercises, using optimal technique, and the assistance of a knowledgeable spotter can substantially reduce the risk of injury. For the middle-aged and elderly, safer alternatives should be considered.

Rationale for the Arch and Bridge

For some disciplines, the bridge is merely a conditioning exercise. Yet, in other disciplines, including acrobatics, gymnastics, judo, and wrestling, the bridge or a variation thereof may be a required skill. For such disciplines, an arch or bridge exercise can be a part of a regular conditioning program, as long as proper precautions are employed to reduce the risk of injury.

Standing Torso Twist

The standing torso twist is used in many disciplines, including baseball, discus, golf, and the javelin throw. In the next section, risk factors of this exercise are discussed.

Analysis of Risk Factors

The potential danger associated with improperly executing the standing torso twist is that its momentum can exceed the absorbing capacity of the tissues being stretched (Alter 1996, 1998). In particular, failure to flex the knees can increase the risk of damage to their ligaments (Alter 1996, 1998; Anderson 1985). Other areas susceptible to injury include the muscles, ligaments, and additional soft tissues of the vertebral column.

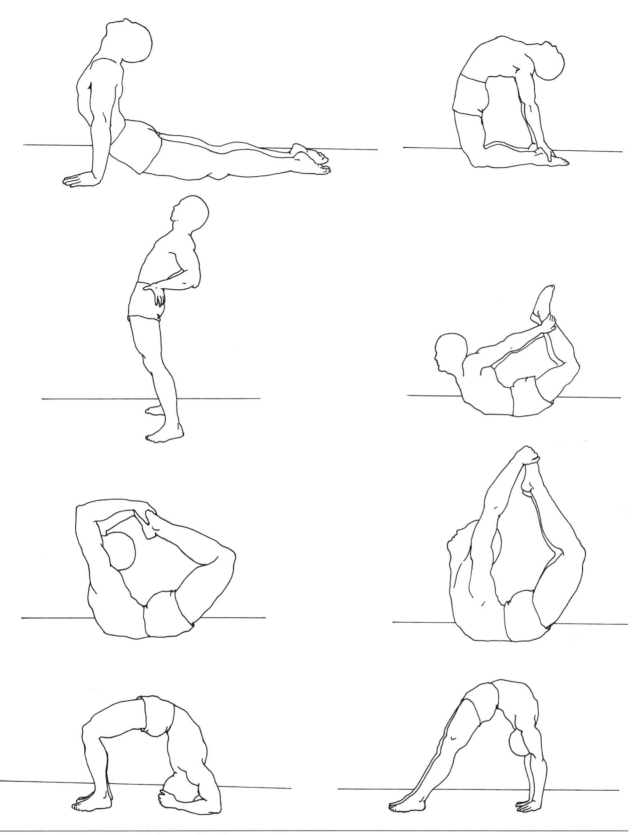

Figure 14.6   Variations of arching and bridging exercises.

Reprinted by permission, from M.J. Alter, 1990, *Sports stretch* (Champaign, IL: Human Kinetics), 108-110.

Risk Reduction

Risks associated with this exercise can be reduced by performing it with the hands on the hips (Rippe 1990). This position reduces the moment of inertia and consequently requires less muscle activity to rotate the torso and to brake the movement of the trunk. An alternative is to perform the stretch holding a broomstick across the back of the neck and shoulders while seated in a chair (Yessis 1986). Because the knees are not bearing weight, momentum and stress on the knees are reduced. If the exercise is performed standing, it should be executed with the knees slightly flexed.

Gravity Inversion

Gravity inversion exercises are traction techniques in which an individual is placed in an inverted position with gravity providing the tractive force. Gravity inversion devices can be classified into four major categories: (1) ankle boots that attach to a horizontal bar, (2) oscillating beds that allow moving from a horizontal to a completely inverted position by moving one's arms, (3) inversion chairs, and (4) inversion swings. These devices are popular in both medical and nonmedical settings.

Analysis of Risk Factors

Ploucher (1982) reported perhaps the first complication observed in two patients who participated in gravity inversion therapy. A 34-year-old woman and a 44-year-old man suffered periorbital petechiae (i.e., rupture of the blood vessels in the eye). Other researchers have expressed concern that inversion exercises may be potentially harmful, based on studies that show increases in pulse rate and blood pressure in the inverted position (Ballantyne et al. 1986; Heng et al. 1992; Klatz et al. 1983; Leboeuf et al. 1987) and even when moving from a seated to a supine position (Leonard et al. 1983). Increased intraocular pressure has also been reported during inversion (Friberg and Weinreb 1985; Klatz et al. 1983; Le Marr et al. 1984; Weinreb et al. 1984) and during movement from a seated to supine position (Galin et al. 1963; Krieglstein and Langham 1975). Another concern is the risk of potential retinal tear. Kobet (1985) reported a case of retinal tear without detachment that was presumed to be associated with hanging from gravity boots. Furthermore, the use of gravity inversion devices could be dangerous for anyone with glaucoma, hypertension, weakness in a blood vessel, or spinal instability and for anyone on anticoagulant drugs or aspirin therapy (Ballantyne et al. 1986; Friberg and Weinreb 1985; Klatz et al. 1983; Leboeuf et al. 1987; Ploucher 1982; Weinreb et al. 1984). Manufacturers also warn that inversion is contraindicated for those who are extremely obese, pregnant, have vulnerable areas of stress from recent surgery, hiatal hernia, ventral hernia, and history of space-occupying brain lesion, history of uncompensated congestive heart failure, carotid artery

sterosis, or osteopathia (e.g., cancer and tuberculosis of the bone).

Despite the preceding findings, proponents of gravity inversion argue that a person's blood pressure rises after any form of exercise. Perhaps of greater significance, de Vries and Cailliet (1985) and Cailliet (1985) believe that careful reinvestigations of previous findings have refuted many of the allegations against gravity inversion. Henry (1951), as quoted in de Vries and Cailliet (1985), stated:

> Protection against brain hemorrhage is given by the closed box of the skull. This protection is so effective that unprotected animals of human proportions can be exposed to 15 g without rupture of blood vessels, and no case of cerebral hemorrhage has yet been demonstrated following negative acceleration uncomplicated by asphyxia or trauma to the head. It is suggested that the danger of cerebral hemorrhage has been overestimated and that the risks of such accidental exposure of a human to 5 g are vanishingly small. (p. 127)

Consequently, the increases of arterial blood pressure should be of no clinical concern for individuals with a healthy cardiovascular system and without glaucoma.

Risk Reduction

As with all exercise programs, basic good health is a requirement for use of inversion devices. Prospective participants should seek medical advice before using these devices (Cailliet 1985; de Vries 1985; Jay and Rappaport 1983; Martin 1982). After medical clearance, competent supervision is required (de Vries 1985). Cailliet (1985) points out that those physicians who prescribe the use of gravity inversion need to specify its frequency, duration, indications or contraindications, and whether it is to be used passively or actively with an exercise program. Other factors that could reduce risk factors include the use of devices that are ergonomically well designed, well constructed, and well balanced (de Vries 1985).

Rationale for Gravity Inversion

Gravity inversion may relieve or prevent low-back pain via several mechanisms, including stretching of the paravertebral muscles, reduction of muscular spasm, decompression of the spinal segments, relief of nerve entrapment, and relief of neuromuscular tension (Kane et al. 1985; Nosse 1978; Vernon et al. 1985). The theoretical basis for the effectiveness of gravity inversion relates to the relaxation of peripheral neuromuscular tone. A vagotonic or parasympathetic influence on the cardiovascular system is also considered to cause reflex diminution of peripheral vascular resistance, leading to increased blood flow (Cailliet 1985; de Vries 1985; de Vries and Cailliet 1985). Cailliet (1985) reports that many patients who hang with their heads down or who meditate during headstand note this relaxation.

Proponents of inversion exercise claim it provides an important adjunct to military training by improving coordination and spatial orientation. Claims by manufacturers of inversion devices include relief of back ache, reduction of stress, combating fatigue, prevention of height loss, increased flexibility, combating body shape changes (middle-age spread) that come with age, and health maintenance (preventative fitness) (Teeter Hang Ups 2002).

Shoulderstand and Plow

The shoulderstand and the plow are the most controversial and potentially dangerous stretches for the cervical region. The shoulderstand is performed by lying supine and raising the legs and torso to a vertical inverted position, with weight borne by the back of the head, neck, and shoulders and the hands placed on the lower back for support (see figure 14.7 a-b). In yoga, this position, or asana, is the salamba sarvangasana, which means supporting or propping up the entire body (Iyengar 1979).

The plow is very similar, except that the feet are lowered downward over the head so that the toes rest on the floor. In yoga, this asana is known as halsana, meaning plow position (Iyengar 1979). A variety of plow positions can be performed with various degrees of difficulty and risk (see figure 14.7c-h).

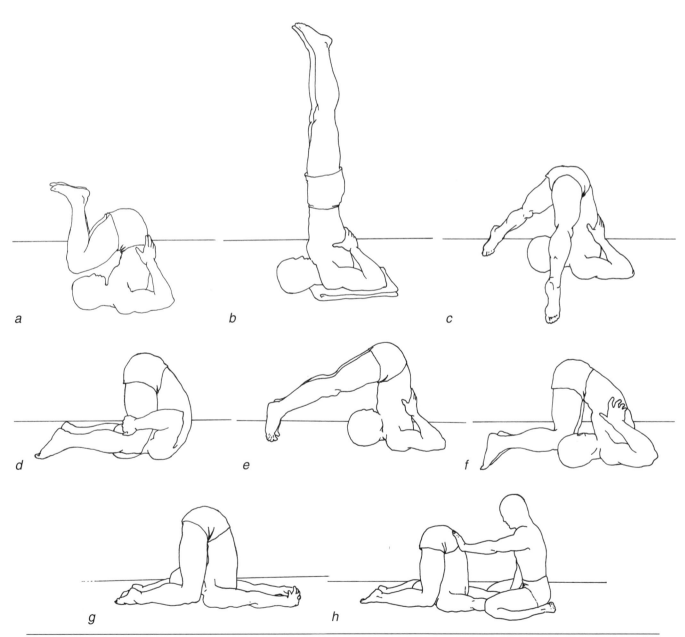

Figure 14.7 The shoulderstand *(a–b)* and the plow *(c–h)*, one of the most controversial stretches: intensified positions with a corresponding increased risk of injury.

Reprinted, by permission, from M.J. Alter, 1990, *Sports stretch* (Champaign, IL: Human Kinetics), 117-118, 128-130.

Analysis of Risk Factors

The shoulderstand and the plow are potentially detrimental for several reasons. The first problem with these exercises is the forward-head posture (Kisner and Colby 1996), which causes the body's weight to create a strong stretching force involving flexion of the upper thoracic region. This region frequently tends to be flexed from faulty posture. Hence, the exercise reinforces the faulty posture.

With age comes an almost universal tendency for a forward-head posture to develop (Paris 1990). This posture is thought to be a consequence of faulty postural habits and awareness, occupational and recreational activities, and genetics (Kauffman 1987; Paris 1990). Therefore, Paris (1990) believes that the forward-head posture should be discouraged, especially in middle-aged and elderly people. This condemnation includes such exercises as the shoulderstand and plow. Instead, exercise and therapeutic programs should emphasize trunk and neck extension.

A second point raised by Kisner and Colby (1996) is that the flexed, inverted position compresses the lungs and heart, decreasing their potential effectiveness by impairing both circulation and respiration. Luby and St. Onge (1986) contend that the plow position also compresses the blood vessels to the brain, upper spinal cord, and chest.

Alter (1983) hypothesizes that these exercises can potentially injure the bones of the cervical region in a gradual way. When the bones are irritated, in this case by bearing weight in a manner they are not meant to do, the body responds by sending calcium to the area. Consequently, the wear-and-tear type of arthritic calcium deposits can and do build up on the neck vertebrae. The literature does not substantiate this claim. However, this absence of evidence does not mean that this sequence of events is not plausible. A study to analyze X-rays taken of long-time practitioners of yoga may verify this hypothesis.

The most serious indictments of the shoulderstand and, more so, the plow deal with their potential risk to the vertebral joints. Numerous investigators (Beaulieu 1981; Berland and Addison 1972; Luby and St. Onge 1986; Shyne 1982; Tucker 1990; Tyne and Mitchell 1983) suggest that the plow creates a risk of tearing of the spinal ligaments, injury to the sciatic nerve, and a herniated disk. The more body weight that is supported by the upper vertebral column, the greater the risk. Additional force added by a partner could be disastrous.

Another risk factor is age. Children are generally more supple than adolescents, adults, and the elderly. However, this fact does not mean that the young are not susceptible to injury. The major problem confronting children during these exercises is a lack of discipline. Horseplay while one is in a compromised position could result in a permanent injury to the vertebral column.

Risk of injury increases with aging which results in a decreased ROM and a reduced margin of safety due to both quantitative and qualitative changes in the intervertebral disks. Among these changes are a decrease of water content in the nucleus pulposus, from 88% at birth to about 65% to 72% by age 75 years (Puschel 1930), an increase in the collagen content of the nucleus pulposus, and a decrease in the concentration of elastic fibers in the annulus, from 13% at the age of 26 years to about 8% at the age of 62 years. Consequently, aging presents a greater probability of muscular strain, ligamentous sprain, and disk damage, in addition to an increased likelihood of osteoporosis in women. The plow could thus be potentially risky because of the compression it places on the bones of affected people (Clippinger-Robertson, cited in Lubell 1989).

These stretches can be intensified by a number of variations (see figure 14.6). One method is to place the shins flat on the floor with the knees touching the shoulders. Another technique is to perform this modified position with a twist of the body. The greatest potential risk occurs when a partner accentuates the stretch.

Risk Reduction

The easiest way to reduce the risk of injury is to learn the exercise correctly in sequential stages. Adequate strength to support the body's weight and suppleness to withstand the tension of the stretch must be developed slowly As the level of fitness improves, the center of gravity can be permitted to move closer to the head, and the feet or shins can be allowed to rest on the floor. Cailliet and Gross (1987, p. 181) recommend an inverted bicycle modification of this exercise as part of a warm-up routine.

Rationale for Shoulderstand and Plow

The plow is considered basic and essential in certain sports and disciplines, such as track and field, wrestling, judo, and other martial arts (Alabin and Krivonosov 1987; Krejci and Koch 1979). Consequently, these exercises cannot always be avoided. However, they should not be practiced in a haphazard manner. Nor should they be part of most conditioning programs. Their practice must be slow, deliberate, and technically precise (Anderson 1978; Fitt 1988; Luby and St. Onge 1986; Peters and Peters 1983; Peterson and Renstrom 1986; Pollock and Wilmore 1990). Two physical therapists conclude, "We like the plow for its benefits, but one must recognize the restrictions of a critical area of the body caused by flexion of the cervical vertebrae. Care must be taken" (Peters and Peters 1983, p. 33). Luby and St. Onge (1986) concede:

> For the fitness of the average person, this exercise is too complicated. I don't feel one needs to accomplish it. [A well-designed routine can give] you a well-rounded program without the Plow. I recommend this exercise only for the advanced student and only [following specific directions]. (p. 123)

NO ABSOLUTE "NO-NOS"

Should these controversial stretches be incorporated into exercise programs? Opinion varies tremendously. Lubell (1989) sought the opinion of various experts, including Harold B. Falls, PhD, professor of biomedical science at Southwest Missouri State University, and James G. Garrick, MD, orthopedic surgeon and director of the Center for Sports Medicine at St. Francis Memorial Hospital in San Francisco, both editorial board members of *The Physician and Sportsmedicine*. Falls's response was, "There are no absolute no-no's . . . Everything depends on the individual. There are some exercises that some people can't do, and there are others that some people can do" (p. 191).

In a similar vein, Garrick said,

> Some exercises are discouraged because people look at the movements and say, "Folks shouldn't do that. That looks dangerous." But it's wrong to issue a blanket condemnation of an exercise. There are some people who can and should be doing that exercise . . . I think it is presumptuous for anyone to say you cannot do this or that. Under those conditions, up to one third of the exercises in the aerobic dance repertoire would be eliminated. (p. 191)

Another renowned expert, Mel Siff, PhD, researcher, author, and former editor of *Fitness and Sports Review International* presents another way to look at the controversy of supposedly dangerous exercises: "There is gener-ally no such thing as an unsafe stretch or exercise: only an unsafe way of executing any movement for a specific individual at a specific time" (Siff 1993b, p. 128).

SUMMARY

Flexibility exists on a continuum. At one end is immobility and at the opposite end is joint dislocation. Between these two extremes lies an optimum level of flexibility based on the needs of the individual. The literature is divided as to whether joint looseness and flexibility training are potentially detrimental. Empirical evidence indicates that stretching should be avoided in hypermobile joints and that instead a strength-training program should be initiated. For people who are physically able, common sense suggests participating in both flexibility and strength-training programs.

Stretching exercises are *not* risk free. However, certain exercises present a greater risk of injury. These exercises include the hurdler's stretch; the single-leg or double-leg inverted hurdler's stretch; deep knee bends, lunges, or squats (with or without weights); the standing straight-leg toe touch; the arch or bridge; the standing torso twist (with or without weights); inversion; and the shoulderstand or plow. Authorities disagree over the use of these and other exercises. The major argument for their use in athletics and other disciplines rests on the physical demands, technical requisites, and rules of the given discipline. If these exercises are to be incorporated in a training program, appropriate risk reduction strategies should be employed.

15

Stretching and Special Populations

People have always searched for the elixir of youth, a magic potion that will restore spent vigor or at least slow the relentless march of time (Shephard 1978). The evidence of the effectiveness of wellness and restorative programs for improving strength and endurance is extensive, but less abundant for ROM. This chapter investigates numerous topics pertaining to flexibility-training programs for geriatric, pregnant, and physically challenged populations.

FLEXIBILITY AND THE GERIATRIC POPULATION

Aging brings about a decrease in flexibility. Stretching exercises can improve flexibility, but the special health concerns of elderly people require precautions to avoid injury. In the following sections, we consider the effects of aging and their consequences for flexibility and stretching programs.

Defining the Elderly

When is a person old? Who are the elderly? In terms of chronological age, the elderly usually include individuals 65 years of age and older. Kramer and Schrier (1990) and May (1990) point out that subgroups of the elderly are commonly differentiated in the literature as the *young old* (age 65 to 74); the *old old*, *frail elderly*, or *aged* (age 75 and older); and the *oldest old* or *extremely old* (85 years of age and older). In contrast, the World Health Organization has adopted the following classification system:

Middle age: 45 to 59 years

Elderly: 60 to 74 years

Old: 75 to 90 years

Very old: over 90 years

Whatever classification system is used, the elderly constitute a group that is characterized by considerable variation in physiological, mental, and functional capacity.

Furthermore, dissimilarities among subgroups are often so pronounced that considering the elderly as a single group can be misleading (Kramer and Schrier 1990). These dissimilarities include genetic makeup, lifestyle, place of residence, and living arrangement.

Geriatric Demography

The numbers and proportions of older people are increasing in almost every country in the world. Furthermore, life expectancy will no doubt continue to increase. In the United States, people over 65 years of age represent the most rapidly growing population group, numbering over 36 million (see table 15.1). Society is faced with a growing segment of the population that has the greatest need for health services and the least capacity to respond to these services. Compounding matters, health-care reform legislation may limit the number of clinic visits (Henry et al. 1998). In addition, "many older adults are restricted to their homes by choice or circumstances and do not have access to formal exercise facilities. For this population, home-based exercise is a viable and important option for adopting a more active lifestyle" (Jette et al. 1998, p. 420). This need for health services and limited resources places extraordinary responsibilities on both the elderly themselves and on those who are responsible for wellness and restorative programs for the elderly.

Research Dealing With ROM in the Aged

ROM decreases with age in the cervical region (Ferlic 1962; Shephard et al. 1990), the shoulder (Allander et al. 1974; Bell and Hoshizaki 1981; Germain and Blair 1983; Shephard et al. 1990), the spine (Einkauf et al. 1986), the spines of women (Battié et al. 1987), the hip (Boone and Azen 1979), the ankle (Shephard et al. 1990; Vandervoort et al. 1992), and the wrist (Allander et al. 1974). Harris (1969b) reviewed two doctoral dissertation studies on flexibility in adults involving 510 men ranging in age

Table 15.1   Resident Populations by Sex and Age: 2005 to 2050*

Age (years)	2005			2010			2020	2030	2040	2050	Percent distribution			
	Total	Male	Female	Total	Male	Female					2005	2010	2020	2050
65-69	10,086	4,661	5,425	12,159	5,640	6,520	17,598	19,844	17,349	19,477	3.5	4.1	5.4	4.8
70-74	8,375	3,757	4,618	8,995	4,066	4,929	13,864	17,878	16,555	16,537	2.9	3.0	4.3	4.1
75-79	7,429	3,172	4,257	7,175	3,110	4,065	9,484	14,029	16,170	14,407	2.6	2.4	2.9	3.6
80-84	5,514	2,157	3,356	5,600	2,247	3,353	6,024	9,638	12,820	12,225	1.9	1.9	1.9	3.0
85-89	3,028	1,046	1,982	3,476	1,242	2,234	3,611	5,077	7,884	9,463	1.1	1.2	1.1	2.3
90-94	1,402	404	998	1,625	497	1,128	2,074	2,457	4,243	6,030	0.5	0.5	0.6	1.5
95-99	442	104	338	556	139	417	844	1,015	1,606	2,764	0.2	0.2	0.3	0.7
≥100	96	18	77	129	26	103	235	381	551	1,095	(Z)	(Z)	0.1	0.3
Total	36,372	15,319	21,051	39,715	16,967	22,749	53,734	70,319	77,178	81,998				
≥65	36,372	15,319	21,051	39,715	16,967	22,749	53,734	70,319	77,178	81,998	12.6	13.2	16.5	20.3
≥85	4,968	1,572	3,396	5,786	1,904	3,882	6,763	8,931	14,284	19,352	1.7	1.9	2.1	4.8
Total	41,338	16,890	24,448	45,501	18,870	26,631	60,497	79,249	91,461	101,351				

*Numbers in thousands.

Adapted from U.S. Census Bureau, National Population Projections—Summary Tables, January 13, 2000. www.census.gov/population/www/projections/natsum-T3.html.

from 18 to 71 years (Greey 1955) and 407 women ranging in age from 18 to 74 years (Jervey 1961) and found that flexibility decreased with age for most movements.

Research testing the effects of physical activity on the range of joint motion in the elderly has also increased. In a study by Frekany and Leslie (1975), 15 female volunteers, ranging from 71 to 90 years of age except for one volunteer who was 55 years of age, served as subjects for flexibility measurements. They exercised for one-half hour two times a week for approximately 7 months. The participants were also encouraged to exercise on their own as often as possible, preferably daily. A significant improvement in flexibility occurred in both the ankles and in the hamstrings and lower back. A 16-week study of men and women 60 to 83 years by Blumenthal et al. (1989) found a substantial (7% to 90%) increase of flexibility in a response to a program of either aerobic exercise or yoga plus flexibility exercises. Hopkins et al. (1990) studied women 57 to 77 years of age involved in stretching, walking, and dance movements for 12 weeks. A 9% improvement of sit-and-reach scores was found relative to those of control subjects.

Morey et al. (1991) found that over a 2-year program of aerobic, strength, and flexibility exercises, 65-year-old to 74-year-old veterans showed an 11% gain in flexibility as assessed by the hamstrings. Rider and Daley (1991) carried out a 10-week treatment of specific flexibility exercises. The group receiving specific flexibility exercises showed a significant gain over control subjects that received more general forms of exercise. Brown and Holloszy (1991) had 65-year-old volunteers perform general unsupervised exercise for 3 months. Significant improvements occurred in forward bend, straight-leg raise, hip extension, and hip internal rotation, but not in ankle ROM.

Ronsky et al. (1995) studied 59 normal, healthy, and active subjects aged 60 to 79 years to assess the effects of various physical activities on gait and mobility characteristics. The researchers found (1) differences in ankle joint ROM and gait variables were based on gender, and (2) no distinct benefit with respect to ankle joint ROM or gait characteristics was provided with participation in higher-energy intensive physical activities in comparison to physical activities requiring low to moderate energy expenditures (p. 41). The investigators speculated "other factors which may be gender specific such as lower limb strength, habitual footwear, or the cumulative amount of exercise over a lifespan may play a more important role in affecting joint ROM" (p. 48).

Chapman et al. (1972) initiated a study to determine the effect of an exercise program on joint resistance (stiffness) of young and old men. The older group consisted of 20 volunteers from 63 to 88 years of age. Both groups showed improvement in joint mobility after training. Gutman et al. (1977) compared the effects of a Feldenkrais exercise program (i.e., slow therapeutic movement)

with a conventional exercise program. Improvements in rotational flexibility occurred in both groups. However, the test design presented problems (Munns 1981).

Munns (1981) employed a 12-week exercise and dance program designed to work on the specific parts of the body to be measured. Twenty subjects over 65 years of age participated in a program that met three times a week for 1 hour each session. At the end of the program, the range of joint motion of the elderly subjects was significantly improved.

An investigation to determine the effectiveness of PNF flexibility techniques (see chapter 13) for improving hip-joint flexibility in older females and to determine whether local cold application could enhance the effectiveness of these techniques was carried out by Rosenberg et al. (1985). Thirty-one healthy subjects, ages 55 to 84 years, participated in the study, which concluded that PNF flexibility maneuvers enhance hip flexibility in older females to a greater degree than do traditional static stretching techniques and that local cold application had no significant effect on flexibility.

Raab et al. (1988) investigated the ability of weighted and nonweighted exercises to increase flexibility in 46 women aged 65 to 89 years. The subjects participated in an organized exercise program for 1 hour, 3 days a week, for 25 weeks. Similar flexibility increases were achieved through exercise with or without weights for shoulder flexion, ankle plantar flexion, and cervical rotation. Misner et al. (1992) had a group of 12 women volunteers participate in a 5-year study. The women participated in comprehensive ROM exercises plus water exercises. ROM increased significantly in all joints except the shoulder. Hong et al. (2000) investigated the beneficial effects of Tai chi chuan (TCC) on 28 male TCC practitioners with an average age of 67.5 years and 13.2 years of TCC experience. Compared with 30 sedentary men aged 66.2 serving as a control group, the TCC practitioners had better trunk and hamstring flexibility than their sedentary counterparts. This study confirmed the findings of Lan et al. (1996) that TCC improved hip-joint flexibility as measured by the stand and reach test scores. Feland et al. (2001) demonstrated that elderly subjects ranging from 65 to 97 years of age improved their ROM by stretching four times with a 10-second rest between stretches. However, for ROM gains to be maintained, stretching must be continued. All of these studies provide sufficient evidence that both general programs of physical activity and specific ROM exercises can enhance flexibility in old and very old subjects (Shephard 1997).

Rationale for Stretching for the Elderly

Properly designed and conducted physical activity programs can increase the range of joint motion of subjects of all ages. Everyday functional pursuits (activities of daily living, or ADLs) such as bathing and dressing may be limited by a lack of flexibility in major joints. For example, a person may have difficulty reaching something in the cupboard, combing the back of the head, tucking in shirts, or even putting on shoes and socks (May 1990). Stiffness in the back or neck could make turning and looking backward when backing up a car difficult or impossible, increasing the risk of an accident. Programs to increase flexibility can improve everyday functioning and enhance one's ability to meet the demands of everyday living. Thus, an improvement in the quality of life can result (American College of Sports Medicine 2000; Blumenthal and Gullette 2001; Galloway and Jokl 2000; Warburton et al. 2001a, 2001b).

A second commonly stated rationale for exercising and stretching is to reduce the likelihood of sprains and muscle tears (American College of Sports Medicine 2000; Galloway and Jokl 2000). Of particular importance is the potential for preventing or relieving low-back pain by maintaining abdominal strength and low-back flexibility through exercise (Pardini 1984). Although authorities offer numerous testimonials, no documented proof supports this contention. Nonetheless, the Centers for Disease Control and Prevention and the American College of Sports Medicine recommend that people maintain or improve their flexibility to avoid muscle sprains and tears (Pate et al. 1995).

Exercise programs for seniors often focus on flexibility, balance and light aerobics. Although such programs are commendable, they may in fact be short sighted. For example, Barrett and Smerdely (2002) suggested a progressive resistance-training program produced greater strength, balance and gait improvements than a nonspecific flexibility exercise group. This study implies the importance of including a relatively high-intensity

---

Age and Flexibility

Aerobic demand of walking and running is adversely affected by advancing age and by lower extremity orthopedic pathologies. Similarly, musculoskeletal flexibility also tends to decline with old age and joint pathologies. Thus, increased aerobic demand and reduced flexibility in these special populations are probably related. For example, flexibility declines could result in a modified gait pattern (e.g., shorter stride length) that is less economical or in increased muscular effort to produce the same gait pattern because of increased resistance to motion near extremes of the ROM. Unfortunately, little data are available that considers the potential link between flexibility and economy either for special populations, such as the aged and diseased, or for healthy young adults (Martin and Morgan 1992, p. 469).

---

training in exercise programs for older adults to ensure a well-rounded outcome.

Potential Risks Associated With Stretching in the Elderly

A stretching exercise program presents risks for the geriatric population, in particular, the susceptibility to a fall. Numerous factors influence the degree of risk exposure to the elderly whether they are active or inactive. The following sections analyze these risk variables, with special attention to the risk of falling. Significantly, the literature reveals that, "an estimated 25% to 35% of adults aged 65 years and older fall each year" (Boulgarides et al. 2003, p. 329).

Reduced Soft-Tissue Extensibility

The application of inappropriate stretching techniques can be potentially hazardous. Three other conditions prevalent in the geriatric population require special consideration: extensibility, osteoporosis, and arthritis. Ligaments, tendons, and muscles in the elderly are less elastic and pliable. Generally, this change is caused by decreased water content (i.e., dehydration), increased crystalline orientation, calcification, and the replacement of elastic fibers with collagenous fibers (see chapters 4 and 5). Consequently, these less extensible tissues are potentially subject to an injury such as a sprain or strain.

Osteoporosis and Arthritis

If an elderly person has been bedridden or immobilized or is in an advanced state of deconditioning, *osteoporosis* may be present. Osteoporosis is associated with the loss of bone density or mass. Hence, it is sometimes called the bone-robbing disease. This disease is eight times more common in women than in men. Furthermore, it affects primarily small-boned white and Asian women. Because black women tend to have greater bone mass than white or Asian women, they are less likely to experience the disorder. Special care must be employed to prevent overzealous stretching that may induce a fracture in people affected with osteoporosis (Kisner and Colby 2002).

Arthritis occurs in two different forms: osteoarthritis and rheumatoid arthritis. Osteoarthritis is a chronic degenerative disorder that primarily affects the articular cartilage of weight-bearing joints. Treatment for this condition depends on the joints afflicted and the degree of impairment. General treatment goals include decreasing pain, reducing stiffness, and preventing deformities. A program of passive, nonstressful ROM exercises is helpful. However, too much exercise or inappropriate, stressful exercise may aggravate symptoms (Wigley 1984).

Rheumatoid arthritis (RA) is a chronic joint (and systemic) disease, characterized by inflammation of the synovial membrane. The nature of stretching that is prescribed or allowed depends on the degree of inflammation and pain. The rule of thumb is that no strengthening or stretching exercise should cause severe pain at the time the exercise is performed, later pain lasting more than 2 hours, or increased joint inflammation or excessive pain on the day after the exercise regimen.

Reduced Strength

The decline in muscle strength that accompanies aging is often a result of reduced activity, rendering the individual progressively weaker. However, precise strength values vary because they depend on many factors. This decrease is caused in part by a reduction in the number of muscle fibers and nerve cells (Herbison and Graziani 1995). More important is the loss of contractile proteins within the muscle cell. Together these factors result in *atrophy*, or loss of muscle mass.

Muscular strength must be an important consideration in designing a stretching program for the elderly. Many elderly people may lack sufficient muscular strength to support themselves in an erect stance for a prolonged period, resulting in fatigue and a potential fall. A logical adaptation is to do mobility exercises on the floor, because of less chance of a fall. However, many programs for seniors rely on chairs for safe positioning, because many elderly people may lack sufficient strength to rise up from the floor (Rikkers 1986).

Balance, Proprioception, and Vision Changes

Balance is an important component in some stretching exercises, most notably those that are performed standing. Sensory impairments involving visual, auditory, vestibular, and proprioceptive modalities may affect balance. Progressive degeneration of the proprioceptors caused by aging can severely impair knowledge of one's position in space. This determination is further compromised by a reduction in peripheral vestibular excitability. Eventually, these changes in postural stability are manifested as an increase in body sway.

With increasing age, the visual contribution to equilibrium becomes the predominant method for assessing body position (Kulkarni et al. 1999). Eventually, it too can become compromised by such ailments as cataracts, glaucoma, and retinopathy. Collectively, these and other problems associated with aging can lead to misinterpretation of visual/spatial information (Kulkarni et al. 1999). Consequently, the risk of falling becomes greater.

Medication and Alcohol

Prescribed medications are ubiquitous among the elderly (Ray and Griffin 1990), and numerous sources have associated them with an increased risk of falls (Chapron and Besdine 1987; MacDonald 1985; Stewart 1987). The National Center for Health Statistics, cited by Ray and Griffin (1990), reported in June 1987 that in the United States, more than 80% of women and 70% of men 65 years of age and older who live outside nursing homes receive one or more prescription medications at any given time. In nursing homes, the prevalence of medication use is even higher. A consistent finding in the studies cited by MacDonald and MacDonald (1977) and by MacDonald (1985) was an increase in fall frequency among people taking more than one medication. Medications that are especially apt to predispose a person to falls include those that induce somnolence (hypnotics), postural hypotension (diuretics, nitrates, antihypertensive agents, and tricyclic antidepressants), and confusion (cimetidine and digitalis [Wieman and Calkins 1986]). Further compounding matters, Stewart (1987) points out that very few drugs have precise and narrow ranges of pharmacological effects; rather, many drugs have multiple pharmacological actions. For example, thorazine, a drug commonly used by nursing home patients, is associated with sedation, decreased blood pressure, decreased motor activity, lowered convulsive threshold, changed EEG patterns, adrenergic blockade, cholinergic blockade, and altered endocrine function. Many drugs can alter functions that may impact the elderly patient's ability to perform stretching exercises and may increase the risk of such exercise programs. Alcohol use also causes instability and falls (Kulkarni et al. 1999).

Noncompliance

Noncompliance is another potential risk factor for the elderly. Noncompliance may have a variety of causes (e.g., loss of intelligence, decreased ability to remember, or lack of a sense of time). Noncompliance with an exercise program could endanger the well-being of an elderly person.

Reduction Risk Strategies for Stretching Exercise Programs for the Elderly

With an elderly population, to err on the side of caution because of their risk of injury is always prudent. A variety of strategies can be implemented to reduce the risk of injury when stretching during an exercise class. In the following sections, several of these strategies are discussed.

Medical Prescreening

Ideally, the instructor should know of any exercise contraindications for the participants taking the class and whether any of the participants have any special needs (e.g., auditory or visual impairments). By being aware of participants' physical limitations, the instructor can plan accordingly. Medical screening is important because of legal considerations.

Environment and Facilities

The environment in which the activities are to be performed should be inspected for safety. The area should be large enough to accommodate all participants, with no obstructions or obstacles that the participants could kick, hit, or trip over. If the exercises are to be performed in a chair, it should be sturdy yet comfortable. If the exercises are to be practiced on the floor, a nonslip surface should be used. The carpeting or mat should be well padded to reduce potential discomfort and to cushion landings. Lighting and ventilation should be adequate.

Communication and Instruction

Communication is a major component in instruction. Many elderly people have impaired auditory or visual capabilities. Therefore, the following basic guidelines should be implemented when instructing the older client:

- Eliminate all distracting background noise.
- Face the person to whom you are speaking.
- Talk slowly and clearly.
- Provide concise and simple directions.
- Demonstrate the desired exercise or position. (If the participants are to mimic your movements while facing you, they will use the opposite arm or leg.)
- Use effective kinesthetic cues.
- Provide time for the elderly to process and internalize the instructions.
- Continually monitor the participants' feedback.

Use a Low Center of Gravity

A safety strategy employed in some class settings is lowering the center of gravity of the elderly participants to maximize their stability. This modification is achieved by having the participants perform their exercises sitting on a chair or resting on the floor. However, many senior programs do not include floor exercise, because many older people have real fears about lowering themselves to the floor and getting stuck there. They may not know how to get up safely, and the kneeling position may be uncomfortable for people with arthritis or prior injuries (Rikkers 1986).

Exercise Protocol

Before exercising, the participants should be adequately warmed up. The routine should be paced to the ability of the participants. As a general rule, ballistic movements should be avoided because they are potentially more injurious than other types of stretches. Participants should be instructed to breathe naturally and not hold their breath. The best form of exercise involves the entire body and is, above all, fun.

FLEXIBILITY AND PREGNANCY

What guidelines for exercise and stretching should women follow during pregnancy and the postpartum period? The American College of Obstetricians and Gynecologists (ACOG) has addressed this question (American College of Obstetricians and Gynecologists 1985, 1994). At the opening of their guidelines, ACOG (1985) cautions women to use common sense and discretion before adopting any exercise program:

> The number and type of exercise programs available now to pregnant and postpartum women have increased dramatically. Some of these programs were designed by nonprofessionals who lack the scientific background to appreciate potential problems and to take steps to minimize their occurrence. A recent review of several exercise programs being marketed to pregnant and postpartum patients revealed medical content that was often inappropriate, inaccurate, or incomplete.
>
> Exercise standards for pregnant women, one of the major subgroups in the general population, have not been set. At present, recommendations for pregnant and postpartum patients are based largely on intuition and "common sense." Little research has been done on the effects of exercise during pregnancy and the postpartum period, and ethical considerations make it almost impossible to define limits of safety. (p. 1)

Risk Reduction During Pregnancy

Perhaps the most prudent and important way to reduce risk during pregnancy is for "all pregnant women [to] obtain an obstetrical and medical examination early in gestation and before engaging in exercise programs" (Mittelmark et al. 1991, p. 301). Concurrent with the examination, the physician should provide specific advice to the patient regarding exercise. Mittelmark et al. (1991) state that patients should be educated to recognize and be alert to various symptoms that signal when to stop exercising and contact the physician:

> (a) pain of any kind; (b) uterine contractions (at 15-min intervals or more frequent); (c) vaginal bleeding, leaking amniotic fluid; (d) dizziness, faintness; (e) shortness of breath; (f) palpitations, tachycardia; (g) persistent nausea and vomiting; (h) back pain; (i) pubic or hip pain; (j) difficulty in walking; (k) generalized edema; (l) numbness in any part of the body; (m) visual disturbances; and (n) decreased fetal activity. (p. 301)

Factors That Increase the Risk of Injury During Pregnancy

The factors that increase the risk of injury during stretching for pregnant women are biomechanical, uteral, or hormonal. The biomechanical factors deal with forces and torques specific to the pregnant body. The influence of hormones renders parts of the body more susceptible to injury.

Biomechanical Factors

One important biomechanical factor that pregnant women contemplating exercise should consider is that total body mass increases. This weight increase is a product of the growing fetus and the mother's retention of fluids, development of fatty tissues, and enlarging breasts. A woman's center of gravity changes during the later stages of pregnancy because of the increased weight anterior to the body, altering stability and affecting the mechanical loading on the body. In particular, greater effort is required of the lower-back muscles to prevent the body from falling forward and downward. Therefore, pregnant women should avoid stretching exercises that exacerbate overloading of the back muscles. To improve stability, stretching exercises can be performed while sitting on the ground or on a chair.

Uteral Factors

Howard et al. (1953) made the first report of "supine hypotension" in late pregnancy. The hypotension occurred in patients assuming the supine position. As pregnancy progresses, the aorta and inferior vena cava may be compressed by the weight and size of the uterus. This condition can result in an obstruction of venous return and compromise cardiac output. Three to 7 minutes are generally required for the symptoms of significant hypotension to become evident: shortness of breath, dizziness, nausea, and tachycardia. In addition, supine hypotension can have important maternal hemodynamic consequences and, because of decreased uterine perfusion, may result in fetal hypoxia and bradycardia. Therefore, exercising in the supine position should be avoided (American College of Obstetricians and Gynecologists [ACOG] 1994; Arujo 1997; Requejo et al. 2002; Strauhal 1999).

Hormonal Factors

The loosening of the connective tissues because of the hormones estrogen, progesterone, and relaxin may compromise joint stability. This change, in combination with the changes in mechanical loading, may produce serious consequences for the pregnant woman, including increased strain on the sacroiliac and hip joints and, more rarely, separation of the symphysis pubis (ACOG 1985; McNitt-Gray 1991). Therefore, ballistic movements and deep flexion or extension of joints should be avoided, and stretches should not be taken to the point of maximum resistance (ACOG 1985). ACOG (1994) points out that, theoretically, hormonal influences may result in generalized increases in joint laxity, thus predisposing the pregnant woman to mechanical trauma or sprains. This hypothesis has been substantiated by objective data only in the metacarpophalangeal joints by Calguneri et al. (1982).

Developing an Exercise Program During Pregnancy

According to ACOG (1985), "The safety of the mother and infant is the primary concern in any exercise program prescribed in conjunction with pregnancy" (p. 1). Therefore, ACOG (1985) is of the opinion that "the goal of exercise during pregnancy and the postpartum period should be to maintain the highest level of fitness consistent with the maximum safety" (p. 1). No two women are alike. Some women are able to tolerate more strenuous exercise than others. Obviously, the guidelines for laywomen will differ from those for highly trained or professional athletes (Mittelmark et al. 1991). For either group, exercise programs should be tailored to meet the individual needs of the patient.

Stretching and Yoga for Pregnant Women

Stretching and yoga exercises are often recommended during and after pregnancy in books and magazines for the general public. Rationales offered by proponents are that such exercises facilitate relaxation and maintain muscle tone and flexibility (Baddeley and Green 1992). A popular belief is that various stretching and yoga exercises will improve the quality of the labor by loosening the pelvic area and helping prepare the pregnant woman for birth (Tobias and Stewart 1985). Exercise is also said to help relieve backache and other minor discomforts (Tobias and Stewart 1985). However, ACOG (1994) points out that "no level of exercise during pregnancy has been conclusively demonstrated to be beneficial in improving perinatal outcome" (p. 4).

FLEXIBILITY AND PEOPLE WITH PHYSICAL DISABILITIES

Another population that deserves recognition are people who have impairments and disabilities. An *impairment* is any disturbance or interference with normal structure and function of the body, such as loss of an anatomic part, blindness, deafness, cerebral palsy, or spinal cord injury. In contrast, *disability* is the loss or reduction of ability to carry out one's role as dictated by culture or family. Thus, impairments may predispose one to disability.

The importance of understanding the requirements and nature of the physically challenged cannot be overemphasized. ROM limitations can have an impact on functional performance. Laskowski (1994) details wheelchair road racers' specific needs that directly relate to flexibility and stretching. Many such athletes have dominance of one muscle group over another, which can result in imbalances of strength and ROM, disrupting the proper "kinetic chain" essential for optimal performance. Specifically, wheelchair road racers may be more susceptible to potential shoulder problems because of a relatively tight anterior capsule. Furthermore:

> Suboptimal flexibility can hinder maximal positioning and predispose the individual to complications such as pressure sores. As an example, the aerodynamic position of most current wheel road racers requires excellent flexibility in the hip, knee, and ankle groups. Performance can suffer and skin can be at risk if adaptive equipment and user interfaces are not optimal. (p. 222)

Varieties of pathologies cause disabilities or impairment. Each of these entities may present difficulties in a specific activity or sport. Nonetheless, many disabled or impaired individuals can participate in some type of stretching program. However, the exercises must conform to the limitations and needs of the individual. For many people with disabilities, stretching aids such as balls, ropes, sticks, and wands may be helpful. Besides being effective in enhancing ROM, such aids can also add creativity, enjoyment, and play to stretching. For those unable to stretch to increase flexibility (e.g., those with spastic cerebral palsy), the use of physical activity such as play-based therapy has been successful in enhancing ROM (Yaggie and Armstrong 2002).

SUMMARY

Flexibility generally decreases with age. Nevertheless, flexibility can be maintained and improved among most elderly people. However, exercising, and stretching in particular, can present a risk for the geriatric population. Preventive strategies should be employed in exercise programs to reduce the risk of injury to elderly people. Pregnant women are also cautioned to employ common sense and discretion before adopting any exercise program. The most important way to reduce risk is to obtain obstetrical and medical examinations throughout and after the pregnancy. To date, no scientific evidence exists that exercise results in shorter labors, easier labors, fewer complications, or benefit to the baby. People with physical disabilities can also benefit from a stretching program. However, the exercises must conform to the limitations and needs of the individual.

UNIT

ANATOMICAL (OR REGIONAL) ASPECTS OF FLEXIBILITY

Anatomy and Flexibility of the Lower Extremity and Pelvic Girdle

The lower extremity and pelvic girdle consists of the foot, ankle, leg, knee joint, thigh, gluteal region, iliac region, and hip joint. In general, the lower limb supports weight, provides a means of movement, and maintains balance. This chapter discusses this anatomical area's structure, function, limits on ROM, potential for injury, and preferred method of stretching. Furthermore, the chapter describes the flexibility of each region of the lower extremity, beginning with the toes and progressing toward the trunk. See *Sport Stretch* (Alter 1998) for a detailed description of stretching exercises covering the lower extremity and pelvic girdle.

THE FOOT AND TOES

The foot has three major anatomical parts: the hindfoot, consisting of the calcaneus and talus; the midfoot, comprising the navicular, cuboid, and three cuneiform bones; and the forefoot, formed by the metatarsals and phalanges. The foot contains 26 bones (seven tarsals, five metatarsals, and 14 phalanges) and four layers of interwoven and overlapping fascia, muscles, tendons, and ligaments. The foot is similar in structure to the hand but with adaptation to weight bearing, shock absorption, and propulsion.

The foot is an elastic, arched structure. The *plantar vault* is an architectural feature that unites all the elements of the foot—joints, ligaments, and muscles—into a single system. It acts as a shock absorber that is essential for the flexibility of the foot. However, the curvature and orientation of the vault depend on a delicate balance of muscles (Kapandji 1987). For example, the unusually high arch in *pes cavus* (claw feet) can result from contractures of the plantar aponeurosis or from the use of shoes with soles that are too rigid (Cailliet 1977, 1996; Kapandji 1987). Cailliet (1996) recommends exercises for this condition that stretch the toe extensors and distal toe flexors. *Pes planus* (flat feet) is the absence of the longitudinal arch. Pes planus is usually congenital but may be caused by muscle paralysis.

Significance of a Flexible Foot and Ankle

A supple foot and ankle absorb energy efficiently, resulting in less chance of injury. For individuals involved in ballet, flexibility in this region is a must, as explained by Hamilton (1978d):

Flexibility is needed in the instep or midfoot so that the foot in the pointe position becomes the projection of the axis of the tibia (shinbone). This position requires a total of ninety degrees of plantar flexion (combining motion at the ankle and instep), and actually, a few degrees more if the downward movement is going to compensate for the recurvatum most dancers have at the knee (see figure 16.1). If this motion is not present, the dancer will not be "all the way up" on pointe or demi-pointe. There is a tremendous difference between being all the way up and almost all the way up in terms of the extra energy required to maintain the pointe position. The result is chronic overstrain of the Achilles and other tendons. (p. 85)

Limits on Foot ROM

The ROMs in the foot depend on a variety of things: bony structure, joint articulations, fascia, ligaments, musculature, and tendon support. Like other parts of the body, the foot can become more flexible if its tissues are stretched. However, the foot is usually neglected because developing flexibility in it requires diligence and hard practice.

Interphalangeal and Metatarsophalangeal Joints of the Toes

The interphalangeal (IP) joints are located between the segments of the toes. Each toe has two IP joints, except

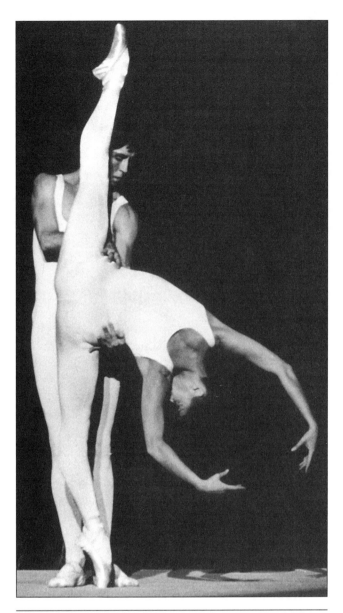

Figure 16.1 In a pas de deux, Soviet ballerina Galina Shlyapina demonstrates her perfect natural facility for pointe work and turnout.

Reprinted from Warren 1989. Photo by Juri Barikin.

for the big toe, which has only one IP joint. The metatarsophalangeal (MTP) joints are located where the toes attach to the foot; each toe has one MTP joint. Flexion of the IP and MTP joints involves bending the toes toward the sole of the foot. Flexion at these joints ranges from 0° to 90° at the IP joints and from 0° to 35° at the MTP joints (Kapandji 1987). Flexion is produced by both the intrinsic (i.e., muscles that have both origin and insertion within the foot) and the extrinsic (i.e., muscles that have their origin outside of the foot) phalangeal flexors. Factors that limit ROM in the toes are flexor muscle contractile insufficiency, passive tension of the extensor muscle tendons of the toes, and contact of the soft parts of the phalanges.

Extension of the IP and MTP joints involves drawing the phalanges away from the sole of the foot. Extension of the phalanges ranges from approximately 0° to 80°. This movement is primarily produced by the extrinsic extensors of the foot. Factors limiting ROM are contractile insufficiency and tension of the plantar and collateral ligaments of the toe joints. Extension may also be limited by tight plantar fascia or plantar fascitis (i.e., inflammation of the plantar fascia). Planter fascitis may cause severe pain when one runs on the balls of the feet.

The plantar metatarsal arch and plantar fascia can be stretched by using either one's own weight or hand. However, the literature is divided over the application of such stretching. Alter (1989-1990) believes that stretching the metatarsal arch and plantar fascia is detrimental or contraindicated. In contrast, a number of sources recommends stretching (American Academy of Orthopaedic Surgeons 1991, 2001; Baxter and Davis 1995; Bowman 2000; Brody 1995; Cramer and McQueen 1990; DiRaimondo 1991; Frey and Feder 1999; Graham 1987; Kraeger 1993; Linz et al. 2001; McPoil and McGarvey 1995; Scala 2001). Additional research is necessary to validate either of these claims.

THE ANKLE JOINT

The *talocrural*, or ankle, joint is a hinge joint formed by the tibia and fibula (bones of the lower leg) and talus (bone of the foot). The relationship among these three bones is maintained by a fibrous capsule, ligaments, and musculotendinous structures. The medial collateral ligament, or *deltoid ligament*, of the ankle has four components: the posterior tibiotalar, the tibiocalcaneal, the tibionavicular, and the anterior tibiotalar. The *lateral collateral ligament* comprises three bands: the anterior talofibular, the posterior talofibular, and the calcaneofibular. Because the bony stability is greater laterally than medially (because of the difference in length of the fibula and tibia), and because the deltoid ligament is stronger than the lateral collateral ligament, the joint is predisposed toward inversion (turning in). Most ankle ligament injuries are common inversion sprains, involving tearing structures on the lateral side. "Many findings from the literature support the view of a close interaction between the geometry of the ligaments and the shapes of the articular surfaces in guiding and stabilizing motion at the ankle joint" (Leardini et al. 2000, p. 602).

Effects of Excessive Talocrural Stress

The bone structure of an ankle and foot can be modified by excessive stress. For instance, dancers who begin training before age 12 years exhibit architectural changes in the tarsal bones that allow increased mobility and plantar flexion of the forefoot (Ende and

Wickstrom 1982; Nikolic and Zimmermann 1968). However, excessive stress can also result in decreased ROM. The formation of spurs on the anterior and posterior lips of the talus limit the range of dorsiflexion and plantar flexion, respectively (Brodelius 1961; Ende and Wickstrom 1982; Hamilton 1978c, 1978d; Howse 1972), which can result in asymmetrical pliés for dancers (Ende and Wickstrom 1982; Schneider et al. 1974). Excessive stress can cause osteophytes (small bone spurs) on the tibia impinging on the superior dorsal neck (in front of the ankle), limiting dorsiflexion of the talus. Ankle motion can also be limited by the presence of an extra bone behind the ankle, called an *os trigonum* (Brodelius 1961; Ende and Wickstrom 1982; Hamilton 1978b; Howse 1972).

Limits on Talocrural ROM

The ROMs of the ankle depend on its bony structure, joint articulation, fascia, geometry of the ligaments, musculature, and tendon support. The tissues of the joint can be stretched and its flexibility enhanced, as seen particularly in ballet dancers.

Eversion, or Pronation

Eversion, or pronation, of the ankle, is turning the sole of the foot so that it tends to move outward and face laterally. Pronation also includes abduction and dorsiflexion of the midfoot (Greene and Heckman 1994, p. 124). Eversion is produced primarily by the peroneus longus and peroneus brevis muscles and ranges from approximately 0° to 20°. The factors limiting eversion are evertor contractile insufficiency, passive tension of the deltoid ligaments, passive tension of the tibialis anterior and tibialis posterior muscles, tightness of the medial aspect of the joint capsule, and contact of the tarsal bones with the fibula laterally.

Inversion, or Supination

Inversion, or supination, of the ankle is turning the sole of the foot so that it tends to move or face medially. Supination also includes adduction and plantar flexion of the midfoot (Greene and Keckman 1994, p. 124). Inversion is produced by invertor muscles, primarily the tibialis anterior and tibialis posterior, and is assisted by the flexor digitorum longus, flexor hallucis longus, and medial head of the gastrocnemius. Inversion of the ankle ranges from approximately 0° to 45°.

The factors limiting the ROM are invertor contractile insufficiency, passive tension of ligaments (including the interosseous talocalcaneal ligament, the other tarsal interosseous ligaments, and the calcaneofibular ligament), passive tension of the evertor muscles (peroneus longus and peroneus brevis), tightness of the lateral aspect of the joint capsule, and contact of the tarsal bones with the tibia medially.

The Ankle and Flexibility

The Relationship Between Ankle and Calf ROM

Ankle ROM is inversely related to rear-foot pronation and internal tibia rotation. Consequently, tight calf (gastrocnemius) muscles are associated with greater amounts of rear foot pronation and lower-leg internal rotation. In excess, these two factors can contribute to foot, lower-leg, and knee problems (Brandon 2003).

The Relationship Between Ankle Sprains and Calf Muscles

Lysens et al. (1984) found a clear relation between tightness of the calf muscles and ankle sprains. They suggested that tightness of the calf muscles could be responsible for ground contact of the feet in a supinated position. In theory, this condition could result in a higher risk of an ankle sprain. This finding may explain how stretching of the calf muscles prevents ankle sprains (Lysens et al. 1991).

The Relationship Between Ankle Injuries and Hamstrings

Achilles tendon and plantar fascia injuries can result from tight hamstrings, which can limit extension and exaggerate flexion of the knee during running. This overflexion at the knee can increase dorsiflexion at the ankle during the landing phase of the running stride. Consequently, the increased flexion at the ankle creates an increased stress on the Achilles tendon, which in turn increases risk of injury. The increased stress on the Achilles pulls on the heel bone (calcaneus) and plantar fascia. Collectively, these actions magnify stress on the plantar fascia and can lead to plantar fasciitis (Anderson 2003b).

Plantar Flexion

Plantar flexion of the ankle is moving the top of the foot away from the front of the shin (i.e., physiological extension of the foot). Plantar flexion is produced by plantar flexor muscles, primarily the gastrocnemius and soleus, and is assisted by the tibialis posterior, peroneus longus, peroneus brevis, flexor hallucis longus, flexor digitorum longus, and plantaris. Ankle plantar flexion ranges from approximately 0° to 50°. Factors limiting ROM are plantar flexor contractile insufficiency, passive tension of the anterior talofibular and the anterior tibiotalar ligaments, passive tension of the dorsiflexor muscles, tightness of the dorsal aspect of the joint capsule, and bone contact of the posterior portion of the talus with the tibia.

Dorsiflexion

Dorsiflexion of the ankle is moving the top of the foot upward and toward the front of the shin (i.e., physiological flexion of the foot). Ankle dorsiflexion is produced primarily by the tibialis anterior and is assisted by the extensor digitorum longus, extensor hallucis longus, and peroneus tertius. Dorsiflexion ranges from approximately 0° to 20°. Factors limiting ROM are dorsiflexor contractile insufficiency, passive tension of the plantar flexors (especially the gastrocnemius and soleus, but also the tibialis posterior, flexor hallucis longus, flexor digitorum longus, peroneus longus, and peroneus brevis muscles), passive tension of the Achilles tendon, tension of the deltoid and calcaneofibular ligaments, tightness of the posterior aspect of the joint capsule, and bone contact of the talus with the anterior margin of the tibial surface.

Dorsiflexion range is greater with the knee flexed than with it extended because of the influence of a two-joint muscle, the gastrocnemius, which crosses both the ankle and knee joints. When the knee is flexed, the gastrocnemius is slack at the knee, allowing it to stretch more at the ankle. However, when the knee is extended, the gastrocnemius is stretched at the knee, allowing it to stretch less at the ankle (passive insufficiency).

Talocrural Injury Prevention

The ankle and foot are susceptible to many injuries, including fascial and ligamentous sprains, muscle strains, tendinitis (inflammation of a tendon or its connective tissue sheath), and stress (incomplete or partial) fractures. Risk of these injuries can be reduced by proper conditioning, adequate warm-up and stretching, utilization of proper technique, wearing appropriate shoes, avoiding hard surfaces, resting when fatigued, and avoiding overuse.

THE LOWER LEG

The *crus*, or lower leg, is the segment of the lower limb between the knee and ankle. It is analogous to the forearm of the upper limb. The lower leg is made up of the tibia, or shinbone, and its smaller companion, the fibula. The two bones are connected together by the interosseous membrane and surrounded by muscles that are susceptible to injury if not adequately stretched before activation. These muscles are all enclosed by a tough connective tissue sheath, the *crural fascia*.

The Posterior Calf Muscles

The *calf* comprises the posterior muscles of the lower leg, including three superficial muscles, the gastrocnemius, soleus, and plantaris, plus four deep muscles, the popliteus, flexor hallucis longus, flexor digitorum longus, and

tibialis posterior. The gastrocnemius muscle can flex the knee, but the primary function of the superficial muscles is plantar flexion of the ankle. The primary function of the deep muscles is flexion of the toes and inversion of the foot.

The gastrocnemius, the most superficial calf muscle, comprises two portions, or heads, and forms the greater bulk of the calf. The soleus is a broad, flat muscle situated immediately deep, or anteriorly, to the gastrocnemius. Together, they form a muscular mass called the *triceps surae*. The triceps surae contributes 90% of the total plantar flexion force of the posterior muscles. The tendons of the gastrocnemius and soleus form the tendo calcaneus, or Achilles tendon.

The tendo calcaneus is the largest and strongest tendon in the body. Its distal end is attached to the posterior surface of the calcaneus. The strength of the tendon approximates 1.24×10^8 N/m² (18,000 psi). Despite the tendon's tremendous strength, it is not invulnerable to injury.

Injuries to the Posterior Calf Muscles and Achilles Tendon

Cold muscles, inadequate warm-up, overuse, fatigue, improper technique, working on a hard surface, or stepping unexpectedly in a hole can cause pulls or strains of the calf. A pull of the calf has been dubiously named *tennis leg*, a misnomer because it often occurs in activities other than tennis. However, surgical exploration has demonstrated that tennis leg is caused by a tear of the musculotendinous junction of one of the heads of the gastrocnemius muscle; that is, where the gastrocnemius attaches to the Achilles tendon (Arner and Lindholm 1958; Feit and Berenter 1993; Irvin et al. 1998; Miller 1977).

The most common injury to the Achilles tendon is tendinitis, mainly caused by overuse. Treatment of tendinitis includes rest, ice, mild anti-inflammatory medicines, and appropriate medical assistance. The most catastrophic injury to a tendon is rupture. Rupture can be compared with the giving way of an old, frayed rope, because tendon fibers are coiled like rope. "Rupture of the Achilles tendon appears to have a multifactorial pathogenesis, with mechanical, degenerative, and ischaemic factors all contributing" (Ahmed et al. 1998, p. 595). Significantly, "the Achilles tendon has a poor blood supply throughout its length, as determined by the small number of blood vessels per cross-sectional area. Consequently, it is suggested that the poor vascularity may prevent adequate tissue repair following trauma, leading to further weakening of the tendon" (Ahmed et al. 1998, p. 591). Treatment of rupture consists of either prolonged immobilization in a cast or surgical repair. Prevention should include enhancing both the tendon's flexibility and strength.

Stretching the Posterior Calf Muscles and Achilles Tendon

The method used to stretch the lower leg's posterior muscles and tendons is virtually identical to the mechanism that often causes injury. To stretch these muscles, the feet are slowly dorsiflexed from a neutral position with the knee joint in flexion and then in extension. Injury is caused by a rapid or ballistic dorsiflexion (Feit and Berenter 1993). Safe, slow stretching prevents injury. Proper stretching of these muscles can be achieved by sitting upright on the floor, kneeling, or standing (see exercises 19 to 44 in *Sport Stretch*). In a modified hurdler's stretch position, the stretch is initiated when one pulls up on the toes toward the body (see exercise 9a, page 285). If the toes cannot be reached, a towel may be used (see exercise 9b, page 285). Another commonly employed stretch is to stand about 1 m (3 ft) from a wall and lean forward while keeping the heels down. One or both legs simultaneously may be stretched in a variety of ways (see exercises 23, 24, and 31 in *Sport Stretch*).

The Anterior and Lateral Lower-Leg Muscles

The lower leg has four anterior muscles (on the front of the shin). The tibialis anterior is anterolateral to the tibia and is the major dorsiflexor of the ankle joint and invertor of the foot. The extensor hallucis longus, the extensor digitorum longus, and the peroneus tertius assist in dorsiflexion, and the former two muscles also extend the toes.

Another set of lower-leg muscles, the peroneal group, is situated on the lateral side of the lower leg. The group consists of the peroneus longus and the peroneus brevis muscles. Both muscles assist in plantar flexion of the feet, but their primary function is to evert the feet.

Injuries to the Anterior and Lateral Lower-Leg Muscles

Pretibial periostitis, or shinsplints, is one of the most common injuries to the anterior and lateral regions of the leg. Fick et al. (1992) claim the term that better defines the injury is *medial tibial stress syndrome*. This catchall syndrome is thought to be most often a microscopic tearing of the attachments of the muscles from the tibia, resulting in tenderness or a dull pain. The etiology of shinsplints has been vaguely attributed to a number of causes, including practicing on hard surfaces, improper warm-up, poor technique, fallen foot arches, improper body balance from low-back strain, inherited tendency, insufficient conditioning, lack of flexibility, strength imbalance between the anterior and posterior calf muscles, fatigue, excessive eccentric muscle activity, and overuse (Michael and Holder 1985; Richie et

al. 1993; Thacker et al. 2002; Woods 2002). Shinsplints and stress fractures are suggested to be associated with ROM of ankle dorsiflexion. This belief is in part based on the assumption that the most common site of these injuries, the posteromedial tibia, borders the site of the medial soleus muscle origin (Pope et al. 1998; Michael and Holder 1985). However, Montgomery et al. (1989) measured the range of ankle dorsiflexion in 505 military trainees and reported no significant relationship between range of ankle dorsiflexion and risk of stress fracture. Another hypothesis is that the soleus muscle and its investing fascia are anatomically and biomechanically implicated, particularly when the heel is in a pronated position (Michael and Holder 1985).

Shinsplints can be treated with ice, warm soaks, whirlpool, gentle massage, stretching, taping, reduced activity, or rest, followed later by strengthening (Found et al. 1986; Woods 2002). A strategy to reduce pain is the use of nonsteroidal anti-inflammatory medications (Fick et al. 1992). O'Malley and Sprinkle (1986) and Woods (2002) claim that a deliberate and specialized series of stretching exercises to the anterior aspect of the legs before and after physical activity such as running or jogging can drastically reduce (or even eradicate) shinsplints. Several authors have suggested that stretching calf muscles will help reduce the possibility of shinsplints (Andrish et al. 1974; Ellis 1986; Flood and Nauert 1973). However, after a systematic review of the literature on prevention of shinsplints in sports, Thacker et al. (2002) concluded that "serious flaws in study design and implementation constrain the work in this field" (p. 32) and their review "yielded little objective evidence to support widespread use of any existing intervention to prevent [shinsplints]" (p. 32). Two specific reasons for differing opinions about shinsplints are (1) the definition of "shin" is confusing, varying from "the front part of the leg below the knee," to "the front edge of the tibia," to "the lower part of the leg," and (2) specific symptoms may vary by sport activity as different muscles and tendons are stressed.

Stretching the Anterior and Lateral Lower-Leg Muscles

The anterior lower-leg muscles can be stretched by slowly plantar flexing (see exercises 5 to 18 in *Sport Stretch*). A safe method is to apply a manual stretch by extending the ankle, with one leg crossed over the other while in a sitting position (see exercise 5, page 284). An easily employed method is to stand and lean against a wall with one foot turned under. Then, one's weight is shifted onto the top of the foot to develop the stretch. A method often cited in yoga texts and in numerous sports medicine sources is sitting on the shins with the toes facing back. However, this method must be used with caution because of the potential stress placed on the knees by their extreme flexion. Certain modifications can reduce the stress, such as sitting on a folded blanket placed on the calves or adjusting the separation between the buttocks and feet. With time, the blanket can be lowered until one is resting on the calves and heels. With increased proficiency, the body weight is gradually shifted backward. Maximum "isolation" of the tibialis anterior can be achieved from this sitting position by reaching behind, grasping the top portion of the toes (especially the big toe), and pulling them toward the buttocks (see exercise 4, page 284). Once again, go slowly and use caution.

The easiest and safest method to stretch the lateral lower-leg muscles is to apply a manual stretch by slowly plantar flexing and inverting the ankle, with one leg crossed over the other while in a sitting position (see exercise 5, page 284). A second method is to assume a modified hurdler's stretch position, reach down and grasp the outer portion of your foot (or use a towel if the foot cannot be reached), and slowly turn the outside of the foot medially (see exercise 11 in *Sport Stretch*). Last, standing on the soles of the feet on an inclined board at a 45° angle is another very simple method to stretch the lateral lower-leg muscles (see exercise 15 in *Sport Stretch*).

THE KNEE JOINT

The *genual*, or knee, joint is the largest joint in the body. It is formed by the articulation of three bones: the femur (thigh bone), tibia, and fibula. The knee is an example of a modified hinge joint. The patella (kneecap) glides in front of the femur. Because the bony arrangement of the knee joint is architecturally weak, compensation must be provided by the firm support of muscles and the joint's nine ligaments.

The knee moves almost exclusively in flexion and extension. Medial and lateral rotations of the tibia are possible only to a slight degree when the knee is flexed.

Knee Flexion

Flexion of the knee involves bringing the heel up to the back of the thigh. Flexion can be carried to about 120° with the hip joint extended, to about 135° with the hip joint flexed and to about 160° when a passive force, such as sitting on the heels, is introduced. During active movement of the unweighted leg, knee flexion is performed by two sets of biarticular muscles: the hamstrings and the gastrocnemius. ROM is limited by flexor muscle contractile insufficiency, passive tension of the quadriceps extensor muscles and their tendon, passive tension in the anterior parts of the capsule, passive tension of the posterior cruciate ligament (with moderate flexion) and both cruciate ligaments (in extreme passive flexion), and contact of the heel and posterior portion of the lower leg with the posterior portion of the thigh and buttocks. Stretches that enhance flexion of the knee are discussed in the section dealing with the anterior femoral muscles.

Knee Extension

Extension of the knee is the return movement from flexion. Extension beyond 0° has been referred to as *genu recurvatum* or swayback knee. However, the American Academy of Orthopaedic Surgeons (Greene and Heckman 1994) has adopted the term *hyperextension*, which is caused by ligamentous and capsular instability or bony deformity. It is one indication of the presence of the hypermobility syndrome (Beighton et al. 1973; Carter and Wilkinson 1964; Grahame and Jenkins 1972). Wynne-Davies (1971), in a study of 3,000 Edinburgh children, found that 15% of the 3-year-old children could extend their knee beyond 10°. However, this degree of extension was observed in less than 1% of children at 6 years of age. In two large studies of healthy adult males, the average knee extension was –2° ± 3°. Adults normally have a slight degree of flexion at the knee joint when standing (Greene and Heckman 1994). If hyperextension is present, stretching exercises that further extend the knee should be avoided. Even in nonhypermobile knees, one must be careful not to lock or press back the knee joint when stretching. Instead, bend the knee slightly, and bring it back to a straight, but strong, position. Then raise the kneecaps up toward the thigh (Follan 1981).

The powerful quadriceps muscle group, consisting of the rectus femoris, vastus lateralis, vastus medialis, and vastus intermedialis, produces extension of the knee. Factors limiting ROM are quadriceps contractile insufficiency, passive tension in the hamstring and gastrocnemius muscles, tension of the cruciate ligaments or of the tibial and fibular collateral ligaments, and tightness of the posterior aspect of the capsule. Any abnormal locking of the knee in flexion may also restrict extension and may be caused by a mechanical internal derangement, such as a loose body or torn meniscus. The knee is a sliding or gliding mechanism. Any foreign object that is interposed between two surfaces will block motion. Stretches for the knee's extensors are discussed in the section dealing with the posterior femoral muscles.

The Mechanical and Structural Disadvantages of the Muscles at the Knee Joint

One of the potentially detrimental aspects of the knee joint is that it is partially controlled by "two-joint," or biarticulate, muscles. This arrangement makes the hamstring muscle group susceptible to strain. The hamstrings, which flex the knee as well as extend the hip, and the rectus femoris, which extends the knee and flexes the hip, are examples of biarticulate muscles (Clanton and Coupe 1998; Fujiwara and Basmajian 1975; Jones 1970; Markee et al. 1955; Morgan-Jones et al. 2000). Trouble develops when both muscle groups are simultaneously moved to their extremes. The resulting tension on the muscles and tendons may become so great as to cause an injury. This action rarely occurs in normal daily activity. However, it is common in many sports and artistic disciplines. For example, the hamstrings are severely challenged when a hurdler's leading leg undergoes simultaneous hip flexion and nearly complete knee extension, when a cheerleader or dancer performs high leg kicks, or when a high jumper uses the straddle technique. Further exacerbating the risk is that the muscles are probably being loaded eccentrically. Compounding matters even more, the hamstring muscles have a relatively high proportion of type II fibers (Garrett et al. 1984), and these fibers are more susceptible to strains (Garrett et al. 1984). Stretching exercises for the knee's flexors are discussed in the section dealing with the posterior femoral muscles.

THE UPPER LEG

The *thigh* is the segment of the leg between the hip and knee. This limb segment contains a single bone, the femur. The femur is the longest and strongest bone in the body, and it is surrounded by the femoral muscles.

The Posterior Femoral Muscles

The posterior portion of the thigh consists of three muscles: the biceps femoris, the semitendinosus, and the semimembranosus (see figure 16.2). In lay terminology, these muscles are known as the *hamstrings*. This word evolved from the Anglo-Saxon *hamm*, meaning "back of the thigh." The biceps femoris is posterior and lateral in the thigh and is so named because it has two heads. The semitendinosus is located posterior and medial in the thigh and is named for the remarkable length of its tendon. The muscle is literally half tendon. The semimembranosus lies on the posteromedial aspect of the thigh. It is named for the flattened membranous form of its upper attachment.

The major functions of the hamstrings are to produce both flexion of the knee joint and extension of the hip joint. In flexion at the hip and in leaning forward, they resist gravity. When the knee is semiflexed, the biceps femoris can act as a lateral rotator and the other hamstrings act as medial rotators of the lower leg. When the hip joint is extended, the biceps femoris also laterally rotates the thigh while the other hamstrings act as medial rotators.

The balance of muscle strength between the quadriceps (anterior thigh muscles) and hamstrings is crucial to injury prevention. The hamstrings-to-quadriceps torque ratio varies among selected populations. Parker et al. (1983) found that high school football players had a ratio between 47% and 65%. Davies et al. (1981) reported

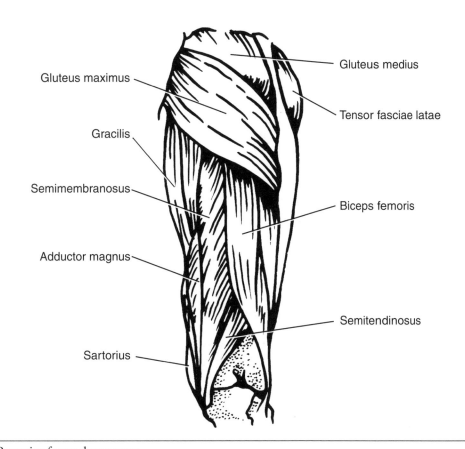

Figure 16.2 Posterior femoral extensors.

Reprinted, by permission, from J.E. Donnelly, 1982, *Living anatomy* (Champaign, IL: Human Kinetics), 139.

ratios between 51% and 64.9% for professional football players. Research on healthy soccer players indicated an average between 67% and 82%, depending on the speed of the contraction (Stafford and Grana 1984). Gilliam et al. (1979) calculated ratios in the range of 40% to 70% for children between the ages of 7 and 13 years. Siff and Verkhoshansky (1999, pp. 233-234) have criticized the concept of optimal ratio of quadriceps to hamstring strength as meaningless. They make the following arguments:

- Russian scientists have found that this ratio depends on the specific type of sport.

- The ratio changes not only with joint angle but also with velocity of measurement.

- Another confounding factor is the influence of the angle of nearby joints on the torque produced by given muscles about the joint in question.

Causes and Mechanisms of Injury to the Posterior Femoral Muscles

The hamstring strain, or "pulled hamstring," is caused by a violent stretch or rapid contraction of the hamstring muscle group, causing rupture within the musculotendinous unit. The injury is time consuming to treat, easily aggravated, psychologically devastating, and almost literally a "pain in the butt." A hamstring strain may occur in the muscle's belly or near the ends of the tendons. Therefore, the strain may occur just below the hip or posteriorly at midthigh level. An activity not usually thought to be associated with a hamstring injury is water skiing. However, this injury commonly occurs among waterskiers (Morgan-Jones et al. 2000). Sallay et al. (1996) have described a common mechanism of injury as improper body position resulting in forced, severe hip flexion while the knee was maintained in extension. This condition occurs when a skier attempts to get up on one or two skies from a submerged position (see figure 16.3). Athletes involved in kicking, punting, hurdling, and sprinting are often at higher risk. Strain is most likely to occur at the latter part of the swing phase as the hamstrings contract in an eccentric manner to decelerate the kicking leg.

Speculations have persisted about predisposing factors that might cause the hamstring muscle group to become strained. A strength imbalance between the hamstrings and quadriceps is one such factor (Burkett 1970; Yamamoto 1993). Currently, researchers are inclined toward the idea that a decrease from the normal 50% to 70% hamstring-to-quadriceps muscle strength ratio predisposes one to such hamstring injuries (Arnheim and Prentice 2000; Clanton and Coupe 1998; Gilliam et al. 1979; Liemohn 1978; Parker et al. 1983; Rankin and Thompson 1983; Sutton 1984). However, Bozeman et al. (1986) suggests that a criterion of 75% of the quadriceps strength be adopted because during parts of some movements, such as running, both the hamstrings and quadriceps contract at

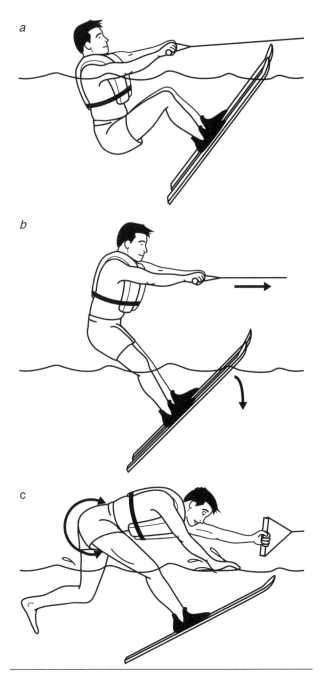

Figure 16.3 (*a*) Proper crouch position at the beginning of takeoff. (*b*) The novice skier tends to straighten the knees prematurely, causing the ski tips to submerge. (*c*) The continued forward momentum pulls the skier forward causing extreme flexion at the hip.

Reprinted from Sallay, Friedman, Coogan, and Garrett 1996.

the same time (Burkett 1975). Thus, opposing forces are in action. If one of these forces is greater than the other and resistance is maintained, something must give—usually the hamstring muscles, which are weaker than the quadriceps. Yet another important variable is that muscle strength and fatigue under stretch conditions affect the energy a muscle can absorb before failure (Garrett 1993; Garrett et al. 1987). Mair et al. (1996) investigated a rabbit muscle strained to failure "after" being fatigued. Mimicking a stretch to muscle failure, a decrease in energy absorption of 42% was seen in the first 70% of the length change. This point is where most muscle injuries occur. The researchers found only a 6% difference in the last 30% of the stretch.

Burkett (1971) showed that a strength imbalance between the right and left hamstrings may also initiate an injury. A strength difference of 10% or more would likely result in strain to the weaker hamstring. Resistance training could help to maintain these critical strength balances. Clinical studies on the benefits of weight training for hamstring strains have been conducted, but no data were presented regarding strength ratios (Gordon and Klein 1987). The actual ratios that constitute balance or imbalance have never been accurately defined (Grace 1985). In the opinion of Grace (1985), "what constitutes a significant discrepancy depends on the anatomical region, the sport, and the participant's size, age, and sex" (p. 80). Heiser et al. (1984) demonstrated a dramatic reduction in hamstring injuries in collegiate football participants with a specially designed prophylactic rehabilitation program that included correcting the hamstring-to-quadriceps ratio to 60%. However, Grace (1985) points out that "unfortunately the study was retrospective, without concurrent controls with a multifactorial rehabilitation program, therefore the actual relationship between imbalance and injury is unclear" (pp. 81-82).

Another explanation for the pulled hamstring is based on a neural mechanism (Burkett 1975). The injury could result from asymmetrical stimulation of the two nerves of the biceps femoris (the tibial nerve, which innervates the long head, and the common peroneal nerve, which innervates the short head) by the following mechanisms:

1. The stimulation to the short head is more intense than to the long head, causing an imbalance in the contraction phase.
2. The intensity of the stimulation does not change, but the timing of the stimulation to the two different heads is asynchronous.
3. Mechanisms 1 and 2 occur simultaneously.
4. The change from prime mover to stabilizer causes a lag in stimulation.

The presence of adverse neural tension has also been postulated as a factor in repetitive hamstring strain. An investigation of 14 male Rugby Union players who had a history of grade I repetitive hamstring strain revealed 57% with a positive slump test. These results suggested, "that adverse neural tension may result from or be a contributing factor in the etiology of repetitive hamstring strain" (Turl and George 1998, p. 16).

One of the most frequently cited causes of hamstring strain is lack of flexibility. Generally, the more flexible a person is, the less the chance of stretch injury. Conversely, the more inflexible a person is, the greater the likelihood of a pull. Limited muscle flexibility reduces the force absorption capability of the muscle (Garrett 1993; Wilson et al. 1991; Worrell and Perrin 1992; Worrell et al. 1994). Thus, greater flexibility may well reduce the incidence of muscle injury as a result of increased energy absorption decreasing the workload on muscles (Bennell et al. 1999a; Kirkendall et al. 2001). A lack of flexibility could also adversely affect the control of joint motion, thus predisposing one to injury (Garrett 1993). Klein and Roberts (1976) offered an explanation that pertains to runners: When the hip flexor muscles are tight and the pelvis tipped forward chronically in an altered posture, the hamstrings are in a state of overstretch because the origin of the attachment on the pelvis is lifted upward and the distance between the origin and insertion of the muscle is lengthened. This posture may account for early hamstring fatigue, one of the fundamental causes of hamstring injury.

Previous injury to the hamstring may also predispose one to injury (Arnheim and Prentice 2000; Drezner 2003; Garrett 1996; Kirkendall et al. 2001; Morgan-Jones et al. 2000). Worrell et al. (1991) reported that hamstring-injured subjects were significantly less flexible in both extremities compared with the noninjured group. Furthermore, they found hamstring symptoms and a high rate of reinjury were present in the hamstring-injured group. Therefore, Worrell and Perrin (1992) suggest, "it seems possible that the loss of hamstring flexibility is a possible sequalae to hamstring muscle strain" (p. 15).

Assuming a lack of flexibility is a cause of hamstring injury, the pertinent question is whether any tests screen for athletes at risk. The three most common tests for hamstring flexibility are the toe-touch test, the sit-and-reach test, and the straight-leg raise test. Bennell et al. (1999a) determined the toe-touch test is not a useful screening tool to identify Australian footballers at risk for hamstring strain.

The straight-leg raise test has numerous factors that may influence the results, among which are the pull of the gastrocnemius, the contralateral hamstrings, and the abdominal muscles (Mayhew et al. 1983). However, more significant is that the test is confounded by posterior rotation of the pelvis as the leg is raised (Bennell et al. 1999a; Bohannon 1982; Bohannon et al. 1985). Specifically, as the pelvis rotates posteriorly during hip flexion in the straight-leg raise test, the ischial tuberosity and the origin of the hamstring muscles moves in the same direction as the muscle insertion, so that little alteration occurs in muscle tension.

Another possible contributing factor to hamstring injury is the reduced ROM in the lumbar spine (Brukner and Khan 2002). During a variety of activities, the hips and lumbar spine form a related system of joints that move together in a coordinated manner. Consequently, an altered mobility of one of the component links in a multijoint system can produce compensatory movement in another that may lead to pathology, pain, and dysfunction. This condition has been demonstrated by Thurston (1985).

Beekman and Block (1975) have proposed a more complicated explanation for hamstring tightening that could potentially lead to a pulled hamstring. During gait, several determinants operate to smooth out the movement of the center of gravity, including the foot mechanism (eversion), the ankle mechanism (plantar flexion), and the knee mechanism (flexion). These systems are intimately related, so if one parameter is decreased, the others are increased. If a calcaneal varus (inversion) is present, the foot mechanism is inhibited. The knee is the only determinant that can effectively compensate for the effect of calcaneal varus at heel contact. Consequently, the knee mechanism must be more flexed when the foot contacts the ground, which means the hamstrings do not get properly stretched on each step. As a result, an acquired shortening takes place. This tightness could predispose one to a pulled hamstring. Another explanation is that during exercise, muscles swell and shorten. If the muscles are not flexible, they are more susceptible to strain during the next exercise period. Consequently, risk of injury is increased. Yet another variable is that the hamstring is a two-joint muscle group.

The hamstring muscle group fiber composition might have another intrinsic factor that predisposes one to injury: active force production by the muscle itself. The hamstrings contain a relatively higher proportion of type II fibers (Garrett et al. 1984). This fiber type is associated with a fast speed of contraction, high strength of contraction, and fatigability. In addition, the amount of active tension that a muscle can produce is proportional to fiber type content. With a faster speed of contraction or increased fatigue, athletes might be under greater risk of muscle strain.

Worrell et al. (1992) reviewed the literature concerning the relationship of hamstring muscle flexibility and hamstring muscle injury and found no standardized method of hamstring flexibility assessment. Several assessment methods included the sit-and-reach test, straight-leg raise test, and passive knee-extension test. Furthermore, assessment of hamstring muscle length can be confounded by many variables. Another important factor is the various types of flexibility: ballistic, static, passive, and active. Thus, additional research is clearly needed to ascertain the relationship of flexibility and injury.

Among other possible causes of pulled hamstrings are age, overuse, poor training methods and techniques, lack of endurance, fatigue, structural abnormalities (e.g., lumbar lordosis, leg length discrepancy, or flat feet), dyssynergic contraction, poor posture, electrolyte dehydration, mineral deficiency (e.g., magnesium deficiency), and prior injury (Clanton and Coupe 1998; Garrett 1996; Hennessy and Watson 1993; Kroll and Raya 1997; Langeland and Carangelo 2000; Morgan-Jones et al. 2000; Muckle 1982; Verrall et al. 2001; Worrell and Perrin 1992).

A review of the literature by Kroll and Raya (1997) and Sutton (1984) clearly substantiates that no single factor predisposes one to hamstring strain. Furthermore, because of the number of confounding variables, an accurate prediction of which individuals will suffer from hamstring strain is not yet possible with tests currently used. Therefore, more research is still needed. Nonetheless, one should incorporate lengthening and strengthening programs, as well as control the variables that are thought to predispose one to hamstring strains.

Stretching the Posterior Femoral Muscles

Stretching the hamstrings occurs with flexion of the hip and extension of the knee. This stretch is usually accomplished by lowering the upper torso toward the thighs while sitting or standing with one or both legs extended. Because of the significant interrelationship among the hamstrings, pelvis, and lower back, the lower-back muscles can also be stretched in this manner. Maintaining an anterior pelvic tilt and an extended upper torso when lowering toward the thighs is necessary. The ideal position forms a straight line from the sacrum to the back of the head. However, many untrained people round or slump the upper torso and tilt the pelvis backward rather than forward during the lowering phase. This position raises two significant questions. (1) Why does one naturally round the upper torso and tilt the pelvis posteriorly during the lowering and stretch phase? (2) Is the posture recommended by experts more effective than this more instinctive posture for increasing the stretch and facilitating an improvement in ROM?

Only one study (Sullivan et al. 1992) has partially investigated these questions. The head-to-knee position is commonly performed by flexing the cervical, thoracic, and lumbar spine in an attempt to bring the chin to the knee of the stretched leg or legs. This action could be natural or deliberate. Sullivan et al. (1992) postulate that in an anterior pelvic tilt position "the ischial tuberosity (hamstring origin) is placed superiorly and posteriorly, to a position farther from the proximal tibial and fibular hamstring insertions. Thus, greater tension would occur within the hamstring musculotendinous structure" (p. 1387). The investigators observed that patients immediately felt greater tension (and possibly pain) in the hamstring muscle group when stretching with the back in an extended position. Thus, the body may naturally attempt to compensate for the increased hamstring tension by assuming a back position that results in less musculotendinous tension. Such pelvic compensatory motion may occur because of the combined flexion patterns of the cervical, thoracic, and lumbar spine. This idea is based on Cailliet's (1988) concept of "lumbar pelvic rhythm." As the pelvis rotates posteriorly, the ischial tuberosity becomes displaced anteriorly and inferiorly and positions the hamstring's origin closer to its insertion.

The rounded-back position may be an attempt to "cheat" in getting the head to the knees. Slumping lets the spine avoid much of the angular or linear displacement when the chin is placed on the knees. That is, less ROM is needed. Hence, the cumulative flexions that occur throughout all the vertebrae can, in effect, create an illusion of a greater degree of hamstring flexibility.

The question remains as to which technique is more efficient in increasing muscle length. Sullivan et al. (1992), compared static stretching with the contract-relax-contract PNF technique. Their results suggested that, "the anterior pelvic tilt position was more important than the stretching method for increasing hamstring muscle flexibility" (p. 1383). This conclusion was based on the hypothesis that "this position allows for greater (passive) force within the musculotendinous unit that will increase hamstring muscle length more efficiently" (p. 1388).

The Medial Femoral Muscles: Adductors

The medial portion of the thigh consists of five muscles: the adductor brevis, adductor longus, adductor magnus, gracilis, and pectineus. These muscles are commonly known as the *groin* muscles, although the term is applied to the region that includes the upper part of the front of the thigh and the lower part of the abdomen. In medical terminology, the muscles of the medial femoral group are the *adductor* muscles. Their primary functions are to adduct, flex, and rotate the thigh. Furthermore, they serve to restrict abduction along with the ligaments of the hips.

Causes and Mechanisms of Adductor Injury

Like the hamstrings, the adductors are prone to strain. However adductor injuries are more difficult to manage than hamstring injuries because they are located in an area that is awkward both to treat and support (because of the proximity of the genitalia). Computed tomography, magnetic resonance imaging, and ultrasound have been widely adopted in establishing a correct diagnosis of injury (Thomeé and Karlsson 1995). The causes of groin strain are virtually the same as those of the pulled hamstring. In particular, the adductor muscles act as important stabilizers of the hip joint. Consequently, they are exposed to overloading and risk of injury if the stabilization of the hip joints is disturbed (Hölmich et al. 1999). Data indicate that between the years 1991 and 1997 the incidence of groin strain in the National Hockey League significantly increased. Injury is thought to occur in ice hockey because "in quick deceleration or acceleration or change of directions during a skating motion, the adductors are often under considerable tension during a strong contraction" (Emery et al. 1999, p. 155). According to Nicholas and Tyler (2002) and Emery et al. (1999), the exact incidence of adductor muscle strains in sport is unknown for two

reasons: (1) athletes play through minor groin pain and the injury goes unreported, and (2) misdiagnosis or overlapping diagnosis can skew the exact incidence.

With diligent and disciplined conditioning, the risk of groin strain can be reduced. Lengthening and strengthening programs and control of the variables that might predispose one to groin strains are necessary. Hölmich et al. (1999) demonstrated that a passive physical therapy program incorporated strategies such as transverse friction massage, stretching laser therapy, and transcutaneous electrical nerve stimulation (TENS) were ineffective in treating chronic groin strains. However, an 8-week to 12-week active strengthening program was effective. The program consisted of progressive resistive adduction and abduction exercises, wobble-board training, abdominal strengthening, and skating movements on a slide board. However, Morrissey (1999), cautioned that the study did not identify why the two programs caused different treatment effects and that a number of factors might explain the differences.

Stretching the Adductors

Adductors can be stretched abducting the hip, that is, by straddling the legs. This position can be performed while standing, sitting, kneeling, or lying, and the knees may be extended or flexed during the stretch (see exercises 82 to 118 in *Sport Stretch*). A method that deserves special attention is the straddle split in a standing position, in which one flexes at the hips and slowly straddles the legs as widely as possible. Biesterfeldt (1974) points out that this technique presents potential risks. Straddle splits apply direct sideways force on the knees. For people who are not fully mature, such forces can, if continued over time, cause permanent deformity, such as loose and knocked knees. Using a partner to apply pressure on the outside of the knees from behind must be totally avoided.

The Anterior Femoral Muscles: Quadriceps

The anterior portion of the thigh is made up of four quadriceps muscles: the sartorius muscle, the tensor fasciae latae, the gluteal aponeurosis, and the iliotibial band. The quadriceps are commonly called the *quads*. Each of the quadriceps is named for its respective position. Thus, the rectus femoris is located in front of the femur; the vastus lateralis is located on the lateral side of the femur; the vastus medialis is positioned on the medial side of the thigh; and the vastus intermedialis is situated between the femur and the rectus femoris. The name *sartorius* is derived from the Latin word for *tailor*, after the custom of tailors to sit cross-legged. All the quadriceps function to extend the knee. The rectus femoris also produces flexion of the hip. The sartorius flexes both the hip and the knee, and it rotates the hip laterally and the lower leg medially when the foot is off the ground. The tensor fasciae latae assist in flexion, abduction, and inward rotation of the hip.

Causes and Mechanisms of Quadriceps Injury

Injuries to the anterior thigh are common. Stiffness, soreness, and tenderness are associated with a number of possible causes, most common of which is direct trauma. The quadriceps may also spontaneously cramp. Such a cramp is popularly known as a charley horse. Other potential factors for quadriceps injury include insufficient warm-up and stretching, overtraining, and fatigue. A preventive approach to injury is both practical and prudent.

Stretching the Quadriceps

Three principal stretching methods for the quadriceps are (1) bringing the heel(s) to the buttocks without hip extension; (2) bringing the heel(s) to the buttocks with hip extension; and (3) hip extension with the legs relatively straight (see exercises 119 and 135 in *Sport Stretch*). Method 1 stretches predominantly the three vasti muscles. Method 2 stretches these muscles plus the rectus femoris (a maximal stretch of the rectus femoris can be achieved by a combination of hip extension and knee flexion). Method 3 stretches primarily the hip flexor muscles and the anterior hip-joint capsule and ligaments but also stretches the rectus femoris to some extent. For individuals with a medical history of knee problems, only method 3 should be used.

The reason method 2 results in a higher stretch sensation is based on anatomy. The rectus femorus muscle is a two-joint muscle. When the pelvis is tilted posteriorly (during extension of the hip) the origin and insertion of the rectus femoris is separated. Because of this tilt, method 2 also decreases the extension of the lumbar spine. Consequently, the rectus femoris and its connective tissues tighten up earlier when testing, which assures maximum stretch (Hamberg et al. 1993).

Two warnings should be heeded about three common quadriceps stretches. First, the quadriceps can be stretched by lying on the stomach and pulling one heel to the buttocks; standing upright and pulling one heel to the buttocks; and kneeling on both shins and leaning backwards. These stretches increase the risk of a meniscal injury (cartilage) injury. Therefore, care must be taken not to overcompress the cartilage or twist the legs (Alter 1996; Cailliet and Gross 1987; Ninos 1996a). Second, the hamstrings can easily cramp in a shortened position, tightening the hamstrings during these stretches must be avoided (Ninos 1996a).

Front Split

To perform a technically correct front split, both legs must be straight, the hips squared (facing directly forward, rather than twisted), and the buttocks flat on the floor. For aesthetic reasons, some people advocate a slight turnout of the rear hip. However, this rotation usually is carried to an extreme, primarily because of tight hip flexors or improper training.

To successfully master a front split, one must begin from a squared position and slowly lower into the split, while maintaining the correct alignment. This movement can be practiced from a modified kneeling position with both hands on the iliac crest. If maintaining balance is difficult, the split can be practiced between two chairs for support.

THE PELVIC REGION

The pelvic region can be divided into the iliac (anterior) and gluteal (posterior) regions. These regions are each discussed in the following sections.

The Iliac Region

The iliac region is so named because of its proximity to the ilium (anterior bone of the pelvis). This region contains three muscles: the psoas major, psoas minor, and iliacus (sometimes collectively referred to as the iliopsoas). The psoas major originates from the anterior surface and lower borders of the transverse processes of all the lumbar vertebrae and is attached to the lesser trochanter of the femur. It is the most important flexor of the hip. In front of the psoas major, within the abdomen, is the psoas minor, which is a weak flexor of the hip. The iliacus originates at the iliac fossa (inside the pelvis) and inserts into the lateral side of the tendon of the psoas major. This muscle assists in forward tilt of the pelvis, flexion of the hip joint, and outward rotation of the thigh.

Causes and Mechanisms of Iliac Region Injury

The muscles of the iliac region are susceptible to strain that can significantly impair movement. Without the full use of the iliopsoas, one is unable to maintain an upright posture easily or to move the thigh effectively. Potential factors for strain include insufficient warm-up and stretching, faulty technique, poor conditioning, overtraining, and fatigue.

Stretching the Iliac Region

To stretch the iliopsoas, the distance between their origin and insertion must be lengthened (Wirhed 1984). This lengthening can be achieved by kneeling on one knee (the opposite leg is flexed) with the top of the shinbone and instep resting on the floor. With one hand on the hip or buttocks, one should slowly extend the hip and push the front of the hip of the back leg toward the floor. An additional force can be applied by pushing on the buttocks or hip (see exercise 21, page 288). This stretch is an important lead up for those attempting to master a front split.

The Gluteal Region

The gluteal region is often referred to as the buttocks. This region contains nine muscles: three glutei and six smaller, more deeply situated muscles. The gluteus maximus, which is the largest and most superficial muscle in the region, is a hip extensor, and it assists in outward rotation at the hip. The gluteus minimus is the smallest and deepest of the glutei. The gluteus medius is intermediate muscle in both size and location. These two muscles abduct the hip joint and assist with inward and outward rotation of the thigh. The six smaller muscles—the piriformis, obturator externus, obturator internus, quadratus femoris, gemellus inferior, and gemellus superior—produce outward rotation at the hip.

Causes and Mechanisms of Gluteal Injury

Injuries to the gluteal region are common for a number of reasons, including overtraining and the use of poor technique. In addition, the gluteal region often experiences trauma, especially during falls. Like the adductor muscles, this area is awkward to treat and support.

Stretching the Gluteals

Stretching the gluteus maximus is usually accomplished by applying tension to the hip rotators. During stretching, the hip is flexed, adducted, and medially rotated. This stretch can be accomplished standing, sitting, or lying (see exercises 146 to 164 in *Sport Stretch*).

THE HIP JOINT

The coxal, or hip, joint is perhaps the most striking example of a ball-and-socket joint. It consists of the rounded femoral head, which articulates with the deep, cup-shaped fossa of the acetabulum (socket in pelvis). Because of the ball-and-socket arrangement, the hip is able to move through wide ROMs.

Factors Affecting Hip Stability and ROMs

Although the hip joint possesses considerable mobility, its chief function is to provide stability. Many factors contribute to the stability of the hip joint and determine its ultimate ROMs. These factors are discussed in the following sections.

The Acetabulum

The acetabulum is a somewhat hemispherical cavity that articulates with the femoral head. It is formed by the union of the three pelvic bones: the ilium, ischium, and pubis. When viewed anteriorly, it faces forward, downward, and laterally, a position that enhances stability for weight bearing.

Another structure that creates stability is the acetabular labrum, which is a fibrocartilaginous rim attached to the margin of the acetabulum that increases the depth of the joint and acts like a collar for the femoral head. It improves the fit between the two joining surfaces of the joint and keeps the femoral head firmly in place.

Shape of the Pelvis

The shape of the acetabulum is in part determined by the shape of the pelvis. The shape of the pelvis is determined by gender. The female pelvis differs from the male pelvis in ways that render it better adapted to pregnancy and childbearing. A woman's pelvis is shallower and shorter, the bones lighter and smoother, the coccyx more movable, and the subpubic arch angle more obtuse. It is also wider and almost cylindrical. Thus, the heads of the femur bones are more widely separated in women. Because the thighs curve toward the centerline of the body as they approach the knees, this outward flare at the hips brings the knees of a woman somewhat closer together than a man's. Broader hips give women a much greater potential ROM, such as the ability to do splits and high leg extensions more easily (Hamilton 1978b).

Angle of Femoral Inclination and Declination

The head and neck of the femur form angles of inclination and declination with the shaft of the femur. The *angle of inclination* is the neck-shaft angle in the frontal plane. At birth, newborns have angles of inclination of almost 150°. However, this angle decreases with age. By adulthood, the average angle is about 135° (see figure 16.4).

When the angle of inclination is larger than 135° in an adult, the resulting deformity is known as *coxa valga*. The range of abduction is increased. In extreme cases, it may reach a straight angle of 180°. With extreme coxa valga, no skeletal checks restrict ROMs, thus promoting dislocation (Kapandji 1987; Steindler 1977).

If the angle of inclination is less than 135°, the deformity is termed *coxa vara*. This more acute angulation results in a flaring or widening of the hips. With coxa vara, a restriction of the ability to abduct occurs because of impingement of the greater trochanter against the ilium. Inward rotation of the femur is also limited (Steindler 1977).

The *angle of declination* is the degree of forward angulation of the femur's head in relation to its shaft (see figure 16.4). In other words, it is the angle between the axis of the femoral neck and the frontal plane. This angle is normally rather high at birth (40°). However, with age, it decreases to about 12° to 15°. The angle of declination is also called the *angle of anteversion*. A decrease of this angle is *retroversion*.

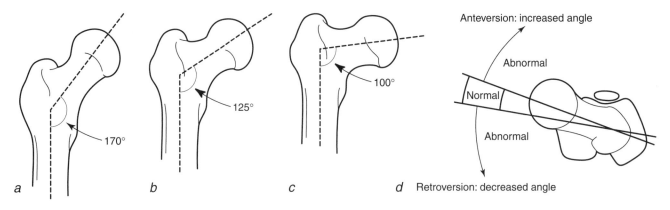

Figure 16.4 Femoral neck-shaft angles: *(a)* coxa valga causes increased femoral joint pressure, *(b)* normal position, *(c)* coxa vara produces increased stress on femoral neck, *(d)* relative position of the femoral neck and femora condyles.
Reprinted, by permission, from P.A. Houglum, 2001, *Therapeutic exercise for athletic injuries* (Champaign, IL: Human Kinetics), 349.

An increased angle of anteversion produces an increased internal torsion or medial rotation of the femur and leg, resulting in an in-toeing or a pigeon-toed gait. In contrast, retroversion produces an external torsion or lateral rotation of the femur and leg, resulting in an out-toeing or duck-toed gait. In ballet, this lateral rotation is referred to as *turnout*. Turnout allows one to increase hip abduction ROM. This technique is explained in greater detail later. Briefly, the skeletal conditions ideal for ballet (and for certain sports) are a long femoral neck with a small neck-shaft angle of inclination for maximum ROM, and retroversion for good, natural turnout. This combination is extremely rare (Hamilton 1978a).

Articular Capsule and Ligaments

Although the bony structure primarily determines the degree of motion of the hip, other factors also play a role. The most important of these factors are the articular capsule and the powerful ligamentous support apparatus. The heavy, fibrous articular capsule encloses the hip joint and the greater part of the femoral neck. Integrated into the capsule are the ligaments. At the hip, the principal ligaments are the iliofemoral, ischiofemoral, pubofemoral, and ligamentum teres. Their mechanism of checking joint motion is discussed later.

Muscular Reinforcement and Coordination

The stability of the hip joint is further enhanced by the muscles that run roughly parallel to the femoral neck. These muscles are the piriformis, obturator externus, gluteus medius, and gluteus minimus, and they help keep the femoral head in contact with the acetabulum.

An important factor in ROM is the role that the muscles play during active stretching, as opposed to the role of their tightness in passive stretch. For example, in active abduction of the legs, the limiting factor may be the lack of strength or coordination of the agonists (i.e., the abductor muscles) to create the movement.

Resistance of the antagonistic or opposing muscle group and its respective connective tissue sheaths are also a major factor in ROM. Thus, during abduction, the major limitation is tightness of the adductor muscles and their tissue sheaths.

Limits on Hip ROM

The six major movements of the hip (excluding circumduction) are flexion, extension, abduction, adduction, internal rotation, and external rotation.

Flexion

Hip *flexion* is a decrease in the angle between the thigh and abdomen. Flexion of the hip with the knee flexed ranges approximately from 0° to 120°, but with the knee extended, range is usually limited to about 90°. Tests for measuring hamstring muscle tightness include the passive toe-touch test, the passive unilateral straight-leg raise (SLR) test, and the active unilateral SLR test. The SLR test can also be used as a neurological test to assess adverse mechanical tension, lumbar nerve root compression, sciatic nerve normality, and intervertebral disk protrusion (Bohannon et al. 1985; Gajdosik and Lusin 1983; Göeken and Hof 1994; Hall et al. 1998; Urban 1981). However, Breig and Troup (1979) demonstrated that "If the SLR is to be a reliable and repeatable test, attention must be given to hip rotation as well as to the posture of the neck and trunk" (p. 249).

A number of instruments can be used to assess the SLR test (Hsieh et al. 1983; Lee and Munn 2000), including a simple universal goniometer, pendulum goniometer, electrogoniometer, and optical devices. Hunt et al. (2001) identified several problems associated with the reliability of the SLR test: consistency of instrument use, consistency of anatomic landmark technique, and identification of a consistent endpoint. Hunt et al. (2001) write: "Using the SLR test as an illustration, the AMA *Guides* [American Medical Association, 1993, *Guides to the Evaluation of Permanent Impairment*, 4th ed. Chicago, IL: American Medical Association, p. 127], for example, did not appear to give a definition of the SLR test or a description of the most appropriate endpoint to use for the test. Within the empirical SLR literature, at least seven different SLR endpoints have been used" (p. 2717).

Various factors may influence the results of the SLR test. Sutton (1979 cited by Oliver and Middleditch 1991) determined the SLR was influenced by hip adduction. Bohannon (1982) and Breig and Troup (1979) demonstrated that pelvic rotation could cast doubt on the findings of the SLR. In addition, Bohannon et al. (1985) found that posterior pelvic rotation began within 9° from the beginning of leg raising in the passive SLR test and that the angle of pelvic rotation increased in conjunction with the angle of leg raising. Their study found that 39% of the total supine passive SLR could be attributed to pelvic rotation. Further, in a study of the active SLR test, Mayhew et al. (1983) found that the degree of participation of the contralateral hamstrings and abdominal muscles might also contribute to potential variations.

Contraction of the erector spinae or gluteal muscles (Göeken and Hof 1994) might also restrict range of the SLR. In addition, pull of the gastrocnemius during dorsiflexion reduces ROM during the SLR (Boland and Adams 2000; Breig and Troup 1979). Hence, to minimize its pull, the ankle should be allowed to plantar flex slightly. Ankle plantar flexion with inversion can also influence the results (Butler and Gifford 1989). Alteration of the lumbar spine position (e.g., left SLR with lumbar spine lateral flexion to the right) is another influencing factor (Butler and Gifford 1989). Breig (1960) has demonstrated that the SLR is influenced by passive neck flexion. Furthermore, the amount of hip flexion in the SLR is decreased with various clinical problems, including lumbar spine disorders, muscle injuries, and hamstring contractures resulting from neurological disorders (Lee and Munn 2000).

Diurnal changes that occur throughout the day may also influence the reliability of the SLR test. Porter and Trailescu (1990) and Wing et al. (1992) found the straight-leg raise was decreased in the morning when measured clinically. Wing et al. (1992) suggest "that the morning restriction of straight leg raising may not be due to stiffness, but to an increase in tension on neural structures as a result of spine-to-spinal cord disproportion" (p. 765). Besides these physiological factors, another potential limiting factor in ROM between "stiff" and "flexible" subjects could be a different perception of the onset of pain. Thus, the restricted ROM could be a subjective variable (Göeken and Hof 1991) or an abnormal defense reaction for some populations (Göeken and Hof 1994).

Active flexion of the hip is produced primarily by the psoas major and iliacus and is assisted by the rectus femoris, sartorius, tensor fasciae latae, pectineus, adductor brevis, adductor longus, and adductor magnus. ROM is checked by hip flexor contractile insufficiency, contact of the thigh with the abdomen, and passive tension of the hamstring muscles. During flexion, all ligaments are relaxed and slack (figure 16.5). Thus, they provide no resistance. Active flexion of the hip is also impaired by peripartum pelvic girdle pain (Mens et al. 1999, 2002).

Extension

Hip *extension* is return from flexion to the anatomical, or neutral, position. Hyperextension begins when this movement continues beyond the neutral position. Active ROM is 10° of hip hyperextension with the knee flexed and 20° with the knee extended. Passive hyperextension attains 20° when one lunges forward and reaches 30° when the lower limb is forcibly pulled back (Kapandji 1987). To achieve a true test for the hip flexor muscles (which limit extension), one must lie with the back flat on a table with one leg flexed at the hip and knee and pulled to the chest, while the leg to be tested hangs over the table edge from the knee. If the thigh of the tested leg fails to touch the table while the back is flat, then tightness of the hip flexors is indicated (Kendall et al. 1971).

Primarily the gluteus maximus, semitendinosus, semimembranosus, and biceps femoris muscles produce active extension of the hip. ROM is limited by hip extensor contractile insufficiency, passive tension of the hip flexor muscles, locking of the spine that prevents anterior tilting of the pelvis, and tension in all the ligaments (see figure 16.5). These factors, for instance, make executing the rear leg portion of a front split with the hips squared difficult.

Abduction

Hip *abduction* is the lateral movement of the lower limb away from the midline of the body. It is produced primarily by the gluteus medius and gluteus minimus and is assisted by the tensor fasciae latae and the sartorius muscles. In one hip, abduction ranges from 0° to 45°. However, usually, abduction at one hip is automatically followed by a similar degree of abduction at the other hip. This opposite-hip motion becomes obvious after 30° of abduction in a standing position, when a lateral tilting of the pelvis away from the moving leg can be clearly seen. To produce 30° of apparent abduction in the moving leg, the pelvis tilts 15°, and the hip of the stationary leg abducts 15°. Thus, to produce 30° of apparent abduction, only 15° of hip abduction is required at each hip. Kapandji (1987) points out that as abduction continues, the vertebral column as a whole compensates for pelvic tilt by bending laterally toward the supporting side.

Hip abduction is limited by hip abductor contractile insufficiency, passive tension of the hip adductor muscles, passive tension of the pubofemoral and iliofemoral ligaments (see figure 16.5), and bone impact of the femoral neck on the acetabular rim. The vertebral column and pelvis can also serve as restraining factors in hip abduction, because the vertebral column is involved in movements of the hip, and any restrictions on the column

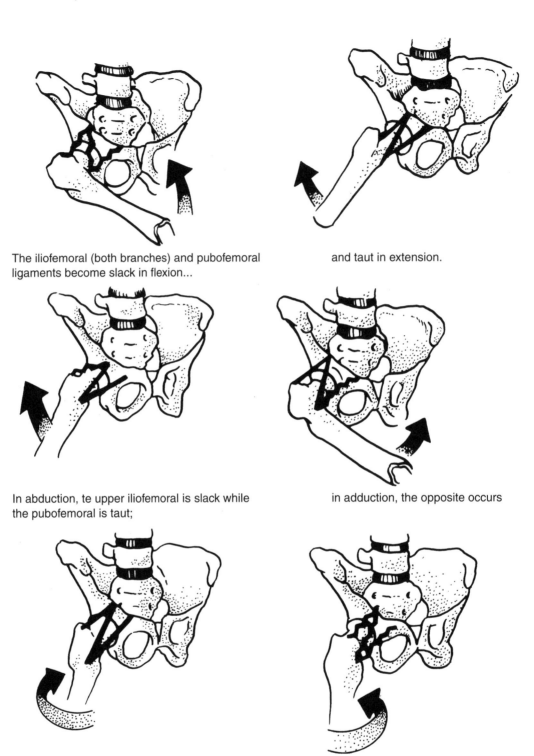

The iliofemoral (both branches) and pubofemoral ligaments become slack in flexion...

and taut in extension.

In abduction, te upper iliofemoral is slack while the pubofemoral is taut;

in adduction, the opposite occurs

The ligaments all become taut in lateral rotation...

and slack in medial rotation.

Figure 16.5 The iliofemoral and pubofemoral ligaments during various types of movement.
Reprinted from Calais-Germain 1993.

could in turn restrict compensatory actions required for pelvic tilting.

Can one maximize one's range of abduction? Yes! This skill can be performed in a static manner on the floor or actively in the air. In either case, when executed to 180°, pure abduction does not occur. After a certain point, hip movement is transferred to the pelvis and thereafter through the spine. The pelvis is tilted anteriorly while the vertebral column is hyperextended. Thus, the hip is put into a position of both abduction and flexion. This position reduces and minimizes the restraining action of the iliofemoral ligament because during hip flexion this ligament is relaxed (see figure 16.5).

Turnout can also enhance one's range of abduction. Turnout incorporates a lateral rotation of the hip joint, which results in a relaxing of the ischiofemoral ligament. However, all the anterior ligaments of the hip become taut, especially those bands running horizontally (i.e., the iliotrochanter band and pubofemoral ligament.) The second reason for the use of turnout is more significant, as explained by Chujoy and Manchester (1967):

> The principle of the turn-out is based on the anatomical structure of the hip joints. In normal positions the movements of the legs are limited by the structure of the joint between the pelvis and the hips. As the leg is drawn to the side, the hip (femoral)-neck meets the brim of the acetabulum and further movement is impossible. But, if the leg is turned out, the big (greater) trochanter recedes (moves posteriorly) and the brim of the acetabulum meets the flat side surface of the hip (femoral)-neck [Kushner et al. 1990; Watkins et al. 1989]. This turn-out allows the dancer to abduct the leg so that it forms an angle of ninety degrees or more with the other leg. The turn-out is not an aesthetic conception but an anatomical and technical necessity for the ballet dancer. It is the turn-out that makes the difference between a limited number of steps on one plane and the possibility of control of all dance movements in space. (p. 923)

Adduction

Hip *adduction* is movement of the lower limb toward the midline of the body. Adduction is produced primarily by the adductor longus, adductor brevis, and adductor magnus and is assisted by the pectineus and gracilis muscles. ROM is limited by adductor contractile insufficiency, passive tension of the abductors, tension of the iliotibial band, and contact with the opposite leg. When the thigh is flexed, the range increases from 0° to 60°. Here, motion is further restricted by tension of the abductor and hip lateral rotator muscles, tension of the iliofemoral ligament, and tension of the ligament of the femur's head.

Internal Rotation

Internal, or medial, rotation of the hip is inward rotation of the femur in the acetabulum toward the midline. Internal rotation is produced by the tensor fasciae latae, gluteus minimus, and gluteus medius. With the knee joint flexed, this movement ranges from approximately 0° to 45° and is somewhat less with the leg extended. Internal rotation is limited by contractile insufficiency, tension of the hip lateral rotators, and tension of the ischiofemoral ligament with the hip flexed and of the iliofemoral ligament when extended.

Mann et al. (1981) contend that stretching the hip by internal rotation can often eliminate knee pain associated with running. For instance, limited rotation of the hip, pelvis, or back can place more torque on the knee, leg, and ankle during running, especially during the foot-plant phase. Furthermore, if an external rotational deformity of the hip occurs, more torque is placed on the knee as speed is increased and the lower extremity attempts to rotate internally. Hence, the importance of stretching the external rotators. The external rotators can be stretched while one lies face down with the body extended and one knee flexed. A partner pulls the flexed leg away from the midline.

External Rotation

External, or lateral, rotation of the hip is outward rotation of the femur. External rotation is produced by the obturator muscles, gemelli, and quadratus femoris and is assisted by the piriformis, gluteus maximus, sartorius, and adductors. ROM is from approximately 0° to 45° with the knee joint flexed. The movement is limited by contractile insufficiency, passive tension of the hip medial rotators, and tension of the iliofemoral ligament. External rotation is seen in many yoga postures, such as the easy posture, perfect posture, and lotus posture, and in ballet when executing a turnout. When the hip is flexed, ROM for external rotation is greater because the iliofemoral ligament is slack (Calais-Germain 1993). Bauman et al. (1994) have suggested that loss of external rotation in the hip of ballet dancers may result from tight, highly developed external rotators, such as the glutei.

Because the turnout at the hip is determined mostly by the bony structure and by the surrounding hip-joint capsule and connective tissue, one may wonder to what extent this structure and flexibility can be affected by training. According to Hamilton (1978a), most medical literature indicates that spontaneous changes in anteversion occur most rapidly from birth to 8 years of age and that the process is mostly completed by 10 years of age. However, it is not completely finished until about 16 years of age. Later attempts to correct anteversion seem to have little effect. Rather, compensatory external rotation deformity is created in the tibia below the knee.

SUMMARY

The lower extremity and pelvic girdle is very complex. It is capable of numerous types of movement and through various ROMs. A host of factors can impede its optimal functioning. Through an understanding of the various structures and functions, optimal performance can be achieved most effectively and efficiently.

17

Anatomy and Flexibility of the Vertebral Column

The vertebral column (spine) is called the backbone, which describes its position in the body but not its structure and capabilities for movement. The vertebral column is not a single bone, but a stack of 33 bones that are flexibly connected, one above the other, and extending from the skull to the pelvis.

GROSS ANATOMY OF THE VERTEBRAL COLUMN

The vertebral column is made up of a series of irregular bones, many linked together by cartilage, disks, and ligaments. Twenty-four of the bones are movable. The vertebral column is generally grouped into five divisions as follows:

- Seven cervical vertebrae (neck)
- Twelve thoracic vertebrae (rib cage area)
- Five lumbar vertebrae (lower back)
- Five sacral vertebrae (base of the spine)
- Four coccygeal vertebrae (tailbone)

In the adult, the sacrum is a single bone that results from fusion of the five sacral vertebrae. Similarly, the coccyx is a single bone that results from fusion of the four coccygeal vertebrae. Therefore, a substantial amount of stability and virtually no mobility exists between the last nine vertebrae.

The vertebral column can be thought of as a massive transmitting and receiving tower supported by guy wires. The tower is the bony vertebral column, disks, and ligaments. The guy wires are the muscles that support the system and hold it erect. The base of the tower is the sacrum and pelvis, and the head is a transceiver. Another way to visualize the vertebral column is to imagine it as a flexible boom, like the mast of a sailboat.

In side view, the vertebral column has four distinct curves. At birth, an infant's spine has only one long curve.

This curve extends over its entire length and is convex posteriorly (C-shaped). However, once the infant starts to raise its head, the cervical curve develops. This anteriorly convex curve is the cervical lordosis. When the child begins to stand and walk, the lumbar curve develops in the lower back. This curve is also convex anteriorly and is the lumbar lordosis. In the adult, the thorax and sacrum retain their original posterior convexity.

Abnormal vertebral curves are present in some people. Deformities of flexion are called *kyphoses*. Kyphosis usually results from an exaggerated forward bend in the thoracic region. The deformity *lordosis*, results from excessive spinal hyperextension, most commonly seen only in the lumbar area. Lordosis is accompanied by a forward protrusion of the abdomen and a backward protrusion of the buttocks. Kendall and McCreary (1983) propose that individuals with "flat backs" (reduced lumbar curvature) while standing tend to have short hamstring muscles. The hypothesis is that the short hamstring muscles rotate the pelvis posteriorly, resulting in a concurrent reduction of lumbar lordosis. However, data from Li et al. (1996) did not support the assumption of Kendall and McCreary (1983). Furthermore, no other research finding has demonstrated correlation between postural alignment and muscle length. Flint (1963) found that "There is no significant relationship between lumbar lordosis and abdominal strength, back-extension strength, hip flexibility or hip-trunk flexibility" (p. 19). Toppenberg and Bullock (1986) found no relationship between pelvic tilt and lumbar curvature. However, longer abdominal muscles and shorter erector spinae muscles were associated with an increased lumbar curve. Heino et al. (1990) examined the relationships among hip extension ROM, standing pelvic tilt, standing lumbar lordosis, and abdominal muscle performance. No correlation was found among any of these variables. *Scoliosis* is an abnormal lateral deviation of the spine, seen in front or back view. Scoliosis is almost always primarily in the thoracic region.

FUNCTION OF THE VERTEBRAL COLUMN

The vertebral column has a number of different functions, the most important of which is protecting the spinal cord. The vertebral column also provides a firm support for the trunk and appendages. Thus, it is a supporting rod for maintaining the upright position of the body. The vertebral column also provides muscular attachments, serves as an anchor for the rib cage, acts as a shock absorber, and provides a combination of strength and flexibility that affords maximal protection and stability with minimal restriction of mobility.

THE VERTEBRAE

A typical vertebra is made up of the vertebral body (found anteriorly) and the vertebral arch (located posteriorly), which are actually several fused parts that, when dismantled, resemble a house (see figure 17.1). The foundation is the vertebral body, the largest part of the vertebra. It is located anteriorly, is cylindrical in shape, and is wider than it is tall. It is the weight-bearing part of the vertebra. The vertebral arch is composed of four smaller structures, two of which are the pedicles that form the supporting walls. The pedicles can withstand great forces placed on them. The other two parts of the

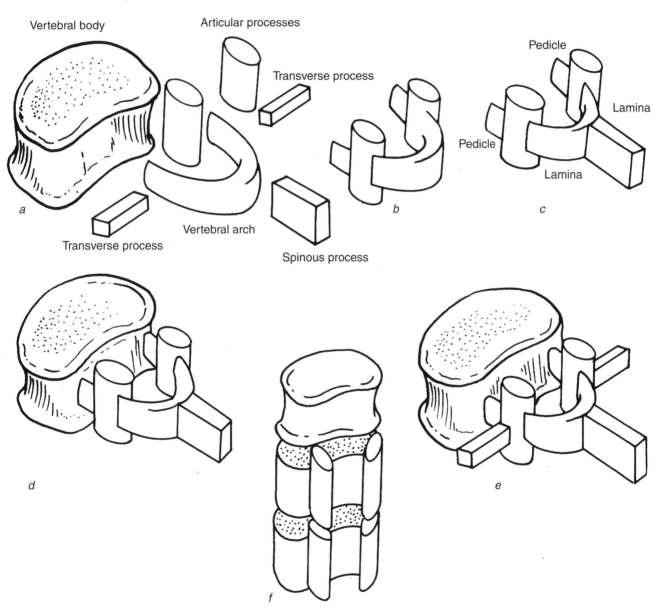

Figure 17.1   The vertebral segments.

Reprinted, by permission, from I.A. Kapandji, 1978, *The physiology of the joints: Vol. 3. The trunk and the vertebral column* (Edinburgh: Churchill Livingstone), 29.

vertebra are the laminae, which form the roof. Extending from the vertebral arch are three bony processes: two transverse processes and one spinous process. Protruding laterally from each pedicle-lamina junction are the right and left transverse processes. They may be thought of as the eaves or wings of the house. In the center is the midline spinous process, which protrudes posteriorly like a chimney on a roof. The spinous process is the most posterior part of the vertebra; its tip is seen when one bends forward.

The direction and degree of vertebral movement is determined by the orientation of the articular processes. In the thoracic region, the articular facets are nearly frontally oriented, with the superior and inferior facets facing posteriorly and anteriorly, respectively. This configuration permits rotation and lateral flexion. In the lumbar area, the articular facets are oriented in the sagittal plane. The superior facets face medially, and the inferior facets face laterally. This orientation allows flexion, extension, and lateral flexion.

THE INTERVERTEBRAL DISKS

Between the vertebral bodies are 23 intervertebral disks. The disks make up approximately 25% of the vertebral column. They function chiefly as hydraulic shock absorbers that permit compression and distortion, thus allowing motion between the vertebrae.

The thickness of the disks is extremely important, because the ROM in any region of the vertebral column depends in large part on the ratio between the height of the intervertebral disks and the height of the bony part of the column. Kapandji (1974) concisely describes the significance of disk thickness. Disk thickness varies with the region of the spine. The regions from thickest to thinnest are the lumbar (9 mm), thoracic (5 mm), and cervical (3 mm). However, more important than the absolute thickness is the ratio of the disk thickness to the height of the vertebral body. In fact, this ratio accounts for the mobility of the particular segment of the vertebral column because the greater the ratio, the greater the mobility. Thus, the cervical region is most mobile because its disk to body ratio is 2:5, or 40%. The lumbar region is slightly less mobile with a ratio of 1:3, or 33%. The thoracic region is the least mobile with a ratio of 1:5, or 20%.

An intervertebral disk consists of two parts: the nucleus pulposus and the annulus fibrosus. The liquid and elastic properties of the nucleus pulposus and annulus fibrosus, acting in combination, enable the disk to withstand great loads (see figure 17.2).

The Nucleus Pulposus

The nucleus pulposus is composed of an incompressible gellike protein polysaccharide encased in an elastic container. The nucleus pulposus is strongly hydrophilic. It can bind nine times its volume of water (the imbibing pressure of the nucleus pulposus has been found to reach 250 mmHg).

At birth, the water content of the nucleus pulposus is 88% (Puschel 1930). Like all fluids, it cannot be compressed in volume. Furthermore, because it exists in a closed container, it must conform to Pascal's law: "Any external force exerted on a unit of a confined liquid is transmitted undiminished to every unit of the interior of the containing vessel" (Cailliet 1981, p. 3). The container deforms in response to pressure. Thus, the nucleus pulposis acts as a hydraulic shock absorber.

When the spine is flexed, the disks become wedge shaped, becoming thinner anteriorly and thicker posteriorly. This deformation allows the vertebrae to come closer together anteriorly and to separate posteriorly, thereby increasing the flexion curve of the spine. Conversely, during spinal hyperextension, the disks become thinner posteriorly and thicker anteriorly. This deformation allows the vertebrae to come closer together posteriorly and to separate anteriorly, thereby increasing the extension curve of the spine.

As the nucleus pulposis ages, it loses its water-binding capacity. By age 70 years, the water content diminishes to 66%. The dehydration, which appears to be a natural process of aging, results from a decrease in the content of the protein polysaccharide and from the gradual replacement of the gelatinous material of the nucleus with fibrocartilage. Adams and Muir (1976) demonstrated that with advancing age, a change occurs even in the molecular size of the proteoglycans in the nucleus pulposus and annulus fibrosus and their specific content, which would be expected to affect the mechanical properties of the disk. Hence, fluid content decreases. After the second decade, the disk's vascular supply disappears. By the third decade, the disk receives its nutrition only by diffusion of lymph through the vertebral end plates. The consequence of the dehydration is extremely significant. It causes the loss of both spinal flexibility and height in the aged, as well as the impaired ability of the aged to regain elasticity in an injured disk (Cailliet 1988).

The nucleus pulposus receives primarily vertical forces from vertebral bodies and redistributes them radially in a horizontal plane. The surrounding annulus fibrosus then resists the created tension. To better understand this action, imagine the nucleus as a movable swivel (see figure 17.3). A summary of these actions is presented in table 17.1.

The Annulus Fibrosus

The annulus fibrosus consists of approximately 20 concentric layers of fibers (see figure 17.2), arranged so that the layers cross each other at oblique angles. This pattern allows controlled motion to occur. For example, when a shearing force is applied (i.e., a force that causes one layer of an object to slide over another layer), the oblique fibers in one direction will tighten, while the opposing fibers relax (see figure 17.4).

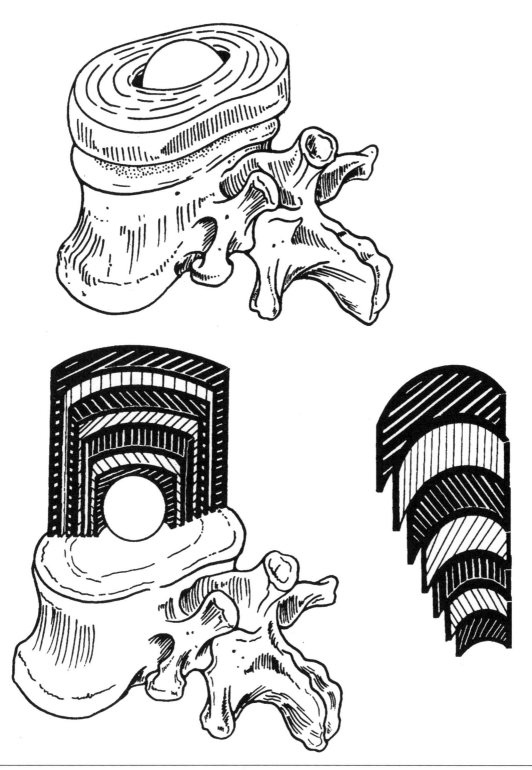

Figure 17.2 Structure of the intervertebral disk.

Reprinted, by permission, from I.A. Kapandji, 1978, *The physiology of the joints: Vol. 3. The trunk and the vertebral column* (Edinburgh: Churchill Livingstone), 29.

The annulus fibrosis receives the ultimate effects of most force transmitted from one vertebral body to another. This function may seem strange because the major loading of the disk is from vertical compression (weight bearing), but the annulus fibrosus is constructed to best resist shear. However, the nucleus pulposus trans-forms the vertical thrust into a radial or bulging force, which is restricted by the elastic and tensile strength of the fibers.

The annulus fibrosus loses much of its elasticity and resilience with age. In young and undamaged disks, the fibroelastic tissue of the annulus fibrosus is predominantly

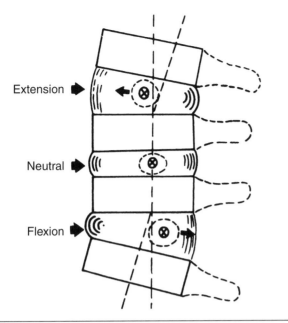

Figure 17.3 The fulcrum of movement in flexion and extension of the lumbar spine.

Reprinted, by permission, from J.W. Fisk and B.S. Rose, 1977, *A practical guide to management of the painful neck and back* (Springfield, IL: Charles C Thomas), 37.

elastic. However, with aging (or as a result of injury), a relative increase occurs in the percentage of fibrous elements. In the older annulus fibrosus, the highly elastic collagen fibrils are replaced by large fibrotic bands of collagen tissue devoid of mucoid material. The disk loses its elasticity and its hydraulic recoil mechanism and is therefore less able to return to its original shape after compression (Cailliet 1988; Panagiotacopulos et al. 1979; Walker 1981).

As a disk becomes more inelastic, it becomes more susceptible to injury and trauma. Each episode of trauma increases the possibility of extrusion of the nucleus pulposus into the tears of the annulus fibrosus. Thus, even a minor stress might tip the scales and result in major injury (Cailliet 1988). Furthermore, because of the reduced vascular supply and the inability of an injured disk to regain its elasticity with aging, herniated, ruptured, and bulging disks are found more often in the elderly than in the young (Cailliet 1988; Panagiotacopulos et al. 1979).

THE VERTEBRAL LIGAMENTS

Ligamentous structures and other connective tissues also contribute to the stability of the spine (see figure 17.5).

Table 17.1   Functions of the Nucleus Pulposus

Action	Flexion	Extension	Lateral flexion
The upper vertebrae will tilt:	Anteriorly	Posteriorly	Toward the side of flexion
Therefore, the disk will flatten:	Anteriorly	Posteriorly	Toward the side of flexion
Therefore, the disk will enlarge:	Posteriorly	Anteriorly	Toward the side opposite flexion
Therefore, the nucleus will be driven:	Posteriorly	Anteriorly	Toward the side opposite flexion

Reprinted, by permission, from M.J. Alter, 1988, *Science of stretching* (Champaign, IL: Human Kinetics), 130.

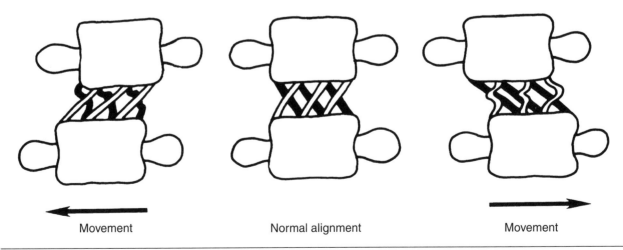

Movement   Normal alignment   Movement

Figure 17.4 The elastic fibers of the annulus fibrosus are in part responsible for the controlled motion of the vertebral column. When a horizontal force is applied to the vertebrae, the oblique fibers in one direction will tighten, while those in the other relax.

Reprinted, by permission, from M.J. Alter, 1988, *Science of stretching* (Champaign, IL: Human Kinetics), 130.

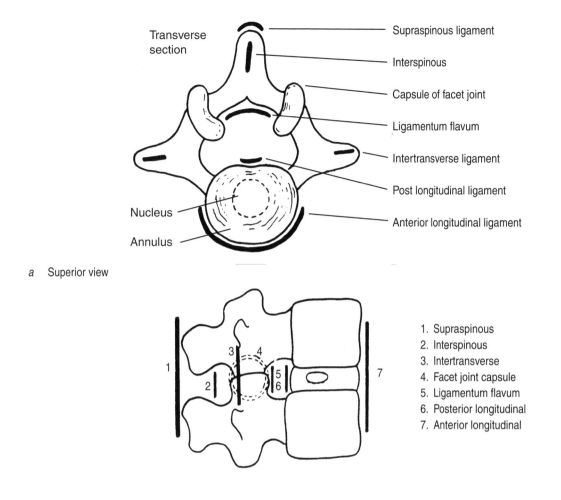

Figure 17.5   Restraining ligaments of the spine.

Reprinted, by permission, from J.W. Fisk and B.S. Rose, 1977, *A practical guide to management of the painful neck and back* (Springfield, IL: Charles C Thomas), 37.

They limit or modify movement occurring at a joint. For maximal stability, ligaments must be short, thick, and strong. However, for maximal ROM, ligaments must be long. Hence, long, thick, and strong ligaments are ideal but rarely occur.

How effectively a ligament checks excessive movement depends not only on its length and size but also on its location and distance from the axis of motion. The greatest strain falls on those ligaments and structures farthest away from the axis or fulcrum of movement. Conversely, those structures closest to the center of rotation are least able to check excessive movement.

Spinal Flexion and Extension

Because the greatest load falls on those ligaments farthest from the fulcrum of movement, the structures limiting flexion (in order of increasing contribution) are the posterior annulus fibrosus, the posterior longitudinal ligament, the ligamentum flavum, the facet joint posterior capsule,

the intertransverse ligaments, the interspinous ligaments, and the supraspinous ligament. The greatest stress falls on this last ligament. The erector spinae muscles of the lower back and the lower lumbodorsal fascia may also assist in restricting flexion. The lower lumbodorsal fascia is a dense sheath of connective tissue that encompasses the erector spinae muscles (Farfan 1973; Fisk and Rose 1977). Conversely, spinal hyperextension is limited by the anterior portion of the annulus fibrosus and the anterior longitudinal ligament, supplemented by the abdominal muscles and the fascia (the rectus sheaths).

Lateral Spinal Flexion

Lateral flexion is limited by all ligamentous structures lateral to the midline. Again, the greatest load falls on those structures farthest from the fulcrum of movement. Accordingly, the quadratus lumborum muscle (connecting the upper edge of the pelvis to the lower ribs), erector spinae muscles, abdominal oblique muscles, three layers of lumbodorsal fascia, and the facet capsular ligaments are most important, and the intertransverse ligaments are least important.

LIMITS ON RANGE OF MOTION OF THE THORACIC-LUMBAR REGION

The ROM between any two successive vertebrae is slight. However, the sum total of these movements is considerable when the vertebral column is considered as a whole. The ROMs of the various regions of the vertebral column depend on numerous factors. Following is a description of the thoracic and lumbar regions of the trunk and their ROMs in flexion, extension, and lateral flexion.

Trunk Flexion

Flexion of the trunk is bending or moving the chest towards the thighs. This movement is produced primarily by the rectus abdominis and assisted by the external and internal abdominal oblique muscles. Trunk flexion from a standing position is produced primarily by gravity and controlled by eccentric contraction of the spinal extensor muscles. The rectus abdominis performs trunk flexion against gravity, as when one bends from the supine position. ROM is limited by trunk flexor contractile insufficiency, tension of the spinal extensor muscles, passive tension of spinal posterior structures (the posterior annulus fibrosus, posterior longitudinal ligament, ligamenta flava, facet joint capsules, intertransverse ligaments, interspinous ligaments, and supraspinous ligaments), bony apposition of the lips of the vertebral bodies anteriorly with surfaces of adjacent vertebrae, stiffness of the ribs (see figure 17.6), compression of the ventral parts of the intervertebral fibrocartilaginous disk, and contact of the ribs with the abdomen. Flexion of the trunk occurs almost exclusively in the lumbar region, because of the unfavorable orientation of the articular facets in the thoracic region.

Standard methods of measuring joint motion are difficult to apply in the thoracic and lumbar spine (Greene and Heckman 1994). Alternative methods of measurement

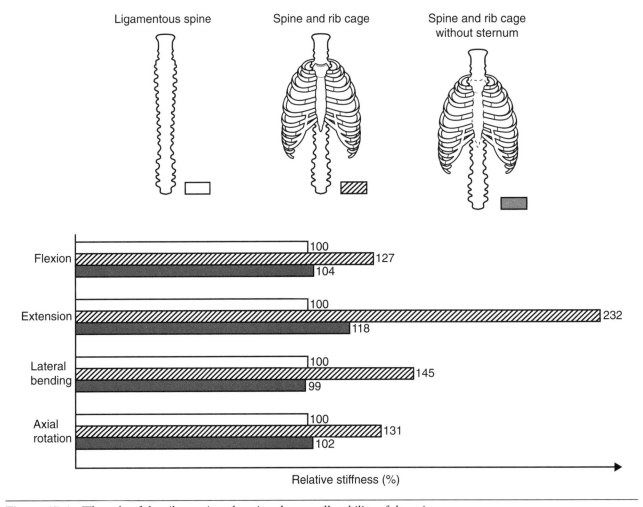

Figure 17.6 The role of the rib cage in enhancing the overall stability of the spine.

Adapted, by permission, from A.A. White and M.M. Panjabi, 1990, *Clinical biomechanics of the spine*, 2nd ed. (Philadelphia: Lippincott), 59.

have been devised and advocated but without agreement on which method is best. Standard methods of assessing thoracic and lumbar spine motion include visual estimation, skin distraction, goniometric measurements, and inclinometer techniques.

Trunk Extension

Extension of the trunk is returning from flexion to neutral, or erect, posture. Hyperextension of the trunk is bending dorsally. This movement is associated with an accentuation of the lumbar curvature and is produced by the erector spinae muscles of the lower back. ROM is restricted by extensor contractile insufficiency, tension of the anterior abdominal muscles, tension of the anterior spinal structures (annulus fibrosus and anterior longitudinal ligament), stiffness of the rib cage (see figure 17.6), and bony contact of adjacent spinous processes and of the caudal articular margins with the laminae.

Trunk Lateral Flexion

Lateral flexion of the trunk is a sideward inclination of the torso. This movement is produced by the external and internal abdominal oblique muscles and is assisted by the erector spinae muscles contracting unilaterally. ROM is limited by contractile insufficiency of these muscles, tension of the oblique abdominal muscles on the side opposite flexion, tension of spinal structures (the annulus fibrosus between the vertebrae, contralateral ligamenta flava, and intertransverse ligaments), interlocking of the articular facets on the side of the movement, and apposition of adjacent ribs (Huang et al. 2001).

INTERRELATIONSHIP OF STRETCHING THE LOWER BACK, PELVIS, AND HAMSTRINGS

One of the most commonly performed, least understood, and potentially dangerous flexibility exercises or tests is hip flexion with the knees extended. Although numerous variations exist, this exercise is often performed as a toe touch from one of four positions: standing, sitting, a modified hurdler's stretch, or supine (i.e., a straight-leg raise).

When stretching or testing for flexibility, one must be careful to distinguish between tight, normal, and stretched muscles. One must also make sure that only the desired muscle groups are stretched. Often, the true results of flexibility testing are masked or obscured (Kendall et al. 1971). For example, the fingertip-to-floor method is well known as an inaccurate parameter of lumbar ROM because "it neither differentiates movement of the hip from that of the lumbar spine nor does it take into consideration different arm lengths" (Ensink et al. 1996, p. 1341). In addition, it does not take into

consideration the influence of the hamstrings on hip flexibility. Therefore, some additional knowledge of the structures that are involved is necessary.

Most, if not all, of the forward flexion occurs in the lumbar spine. Specifically, 5% to 10% of flexion occurs between L1 and L4, 20% to 25% occurs between L4 and L5, and 60% to 75% occurs between L5 and S1 (see figure 17.7). Furthermore, most of the spinal flexion occurs by the time the trunk is inclined 45° forward. In actuality, total lumbar flexion is limited to the extent of reversing of the lordosis curve (Cailliet 1988). If a person bends forward to touch his or her fingers to the floor without bending at the knees or at the hips, more flexion is required than is attributed to the lumbar spine. Hence, if this lumbar curve reversal were the only flexion possible, one could not bend even half the distance to the floor. How is the additional flexion possible? Flexion also occurs at the hip joints.

Flexion at the hips is possible because of the mobility of the pelvic girdle. The hip is a ball and socket formed by the rounded heads of the femurs fitted into the cuplike acetabular sockets (see chapter 16). Consequently, the pelvis is capable of rotation around the fulcrum of the two lateral hip joints, like a seesaw or teeterboard (Cailliet 1988; Kapandji 1974). Therefore, during hip flexion, the anterior portion of the pelvis descends and the posterior

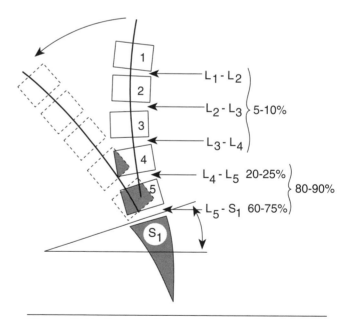

Figure 17.7 Segmental site and degree of lumbar flexion. The degree of flexion noted in the lumbar spine is indicated as a percentage of total spinal flexion. The major portion of flexion (75%) occurs at the lumbosacral joint; 15% to 20% of flexion occurs between L4 and L5; and the remaining 5% to 10% is distributed between L1 and L4. The diagram indicates the mere reversal past lordosis of total flexion of the lumbar curve.

Reprinted, by permission, from R. Cailliet, 1981, *Low back pain syndrome*, 3rd ed. (Philadelphia: F.A. Davis), 40.

aspect ascends. With reextension, the pelvis rotates back to its erect position (see figure 17.8).

Optimal and safe stretching requires a blend of adequate flexibility, strength, and mechanics. For example, when performing hip flexion with the knees extended, several factors may restrict ROM, the most common being tight low-back muscles and tight hamstring muscles. Obviously, with tight low-back muscles, lumbar flexion is restricted. However, with tight hamstrings, the pelvis is restricted

from rotating because the hamstrings are attached to the posterior portion of the knee and to the pelvis at the tuberosity of the ischium (Cailliet 1988). Other limiting factors include defects in the disks, ligaments, or bony structure; irregular curvature of the spine; impingement of the intervertebral joints (see figure 17.9); sciatic nerve irritation; and any muscle imbalance (Cailliet 1988).

When developing trunk flexibility, safety must always come first. For example, performing a standing straight-

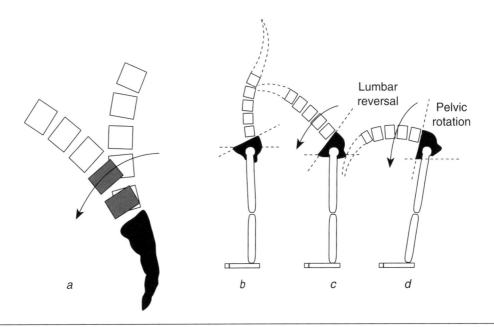

Figure 17.8 Lumbar pelvic rhythm. With pelvis fixed, flexion-extension of the lumbar spine occurs mostly between the lower segments L5 and S1.

Reprinted, by permission, from R. Cailliet, 1981, *Low back pain syndrome*, 3rd ed. (Philadelphia: F.A. Davis), 44.

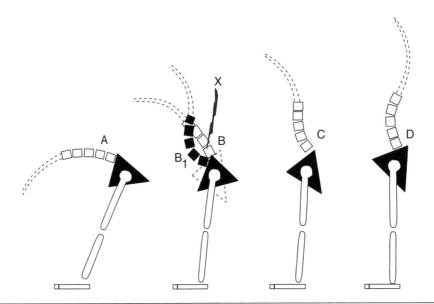

Figure 17.9 Mechanism of acute facet impingement. *(a–d)* The proper physiological resumption of the erect position from total flexion with reverse lumbar-pelvic rhythm. (B₁) Improper premature lordotic curve that cantilevers the lumbar spine anterior to the center of gravity. This position approximates the facets at X and, coupled with the eccentric leading of the spine, requires greater muscular contraction of the erector spinae group. Facet impingement can occur.

Reprinted, by permission, from R. Cailliet, 1981, *Low back pain syndrome*, 3rd ed. (Philadelphia: F.A. Davis), 64.

leg toe touch makes the body susceptible to injury and pain, especially when tight muscles in the lower back or hamstrings are overstretched (see figure 17.10) and especially with ballistic stretching. Faulty mechanics can also cause injury. The mechanics of the lumbar spine are such that any increased weight anterior to the vertebral column greatly increases the forces that are exerted on the lumbar spine. Consequently, during trunk flexion the resultant forces at the fulcrum, which is the lower lumbar segment, are very high. These forces are increased if the movement is performed with the arms horizontal to the floor. Placing the hands on the hips reduces the strain on the back (Segal 1983; White and Panjabi 1978).

Schultz et al. (1982) found that twisting and bending the trunk laterally did not load the spine more than bending forward. Lateral bending can load the spine moderately but not nearly as much as the forward flexion. The trunk cannot be laterally offset very much, so the moment imposed cannot become very large, and the lateral abdominal wall muscles act on the spine through a relatively large moment arm, so they need not contract strongly to counterbalance the offset weight moment (Schultz et al. 1982). Nonetheless, the possibility of injury still exists. Segal (1983) points out that in side bending, when one puts the opposite arm overhead, additional and unnecessary stretch is placed on the lower-back muscles on the same side as the extended arm. The risk of injury is further compounded if the lateral rotation is combined with excessive rotation and flexion or excessive rotation and extension (Garu 1986). Performing this exercise in a ballistic manner makes the potential for injury even greater.

Low-back injury or pain can be caused by faulty reextension from the flexed position, in which the lumbar lordosis is regained before the pelvis is derotated (Cailliet 1988). When one reassumes the erect stance, the lumbar spine should be kept straight and fully extended (Cailliet 1988). With faulty reextension, the upper portion of the body rises early, so that the lower back arches and the lordosis curve is in front of the center of gravity (see figure 17.11). Consequently, this position places an excessive stress on the lower back. Pelvic derotation should occur before lordosis is regained when reextending; the erector spinae muscles should straighten the spine and the lower back should regain its lordosis during the last 45° of extension. However, because of the short lever arm to which the erector spinae muscles are attached, this portion of reextension is inefficient and can potentially strain these muscles. When the erector spinae muscles fatigue, the task of maintaining and supporting the excessive load falls on the vertebral ligaments. The lumbar spine is normally supported by the supraspinous ligament when in full flexion until the last 45° of extension (Cailliet 1988) (see figure 17.12).

The erector spinae are not active during full-trunk flexion. Thus, a significant load is applied to the ligaments during trunk flexion, creating the possibility of a sprain or tear of the ligaments. If the ligaments give way, the load falls on the joints, and subluxation of the joints may occur.

A toe touch from a sitting position or modified hurdler's stretch also requires caution, especially when

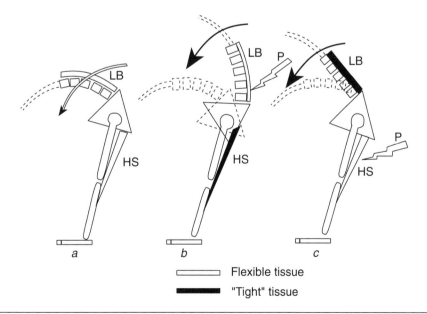

Figure 17.10   Mechanism of stretch pain in the tight hamstring and the tight low-back syndromes. (*a*) Normal flexibility with unrestricted lumbar-pelvic rhythm. (*b*) Tight hamstrings (HS) restricting pelvic rotation and thereby causing excessive stretch of low back (LB), resulting in pain (P). (*c*) Tight low back (LB) performing an incomplete lumbar reversal and thus, by placing excessive stretch on the hamstrings (HS), causing pain (P) in both the hamstrings and the low back as well as a disrupted lumbar-pelvic rhythm.

Reprinted, by permission, from R. Cailliet, 1981, *Low back pain syndrome*, 3rd ed. (Philadelphia: F.A. Davis), 65.

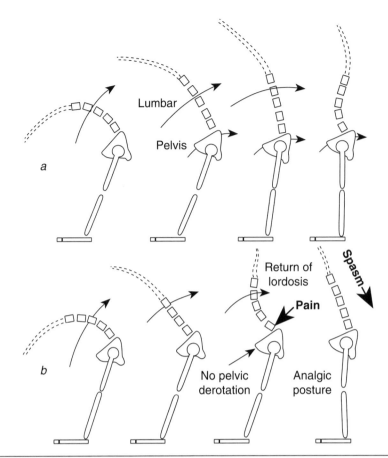

Figure 17.11 Proper versus improper flexion and reextension. *(a)* Proper simultaneous resumption of the lumbar lordosis with pelvic rotation. *(b)* Regaining of pelvic lordosis with no pelvic derotation, causing painful lordotic posture with the upper part of the body held ahead of the center of gravity.

Reprinted, by permission, from R. Cailliet, 1981, *Low back pain syndrome*, 3rd ed. (Philadelphia: F.A. Davis), 132.

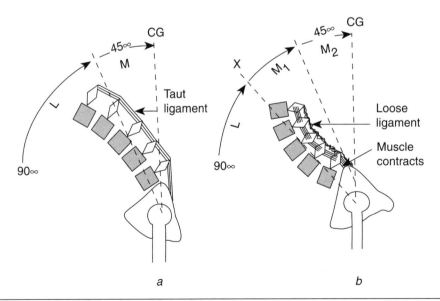

Figure 17.12 Faulty reextension of the lumbar spine. *(a)* Correct reextension. Until the last 45°, the lumbar spine (L) is supported by supraspinous ligaments requiring no muscular effort. Muscles normally become active in the last 45° (M) when the carrying angle is close to the center of gravity (CG). *(b)* Premature lumbar lordosis with pelvis not adequately derotated causes the erector muscles (M_1) to contract before having reached the last 45°. The ligaments loosen, and the muscles take the brunt and contract inefficiently and forcefully, resulting in pain.

Reprinted, by permission, from R. Cailliet, 1981, *Low back pain syndrome*, 3rd ed. (Philadelphia: F.A. Davis), 133.

stretching with a partner. Injury often occurs when a partner unknowingly applies a little too much stretch. Anticipation and communication can prevent such accidents.

THE CERVICAL VERTEBRAE

The neck's skeletal framework is made up of seven cervical vertebrae. The best known are the first and second vertebrae below the head, the atlas and axis, respectively. These vertebrae have a unique structure. The atlas, which directly supports the head, forms a bony ring. The axis has a small, upward bony projection that forms a peglike pivot. The atlas rotates around this pivot when the head is turned from side to side. Thus, this structure determines much of the direction and extent of head motion.

MOVEMENTS OF THE CERVICAL REGION

The cervical region is capable of flexion, extension, lateral flexion, and rotation. This region is most mobile and has the most unencumbered ROM of all the vertebrae because the disks are thickest in relation to the height of the vertebral body. The ratio of disk to body is 2:5, or 40% (Kapandji 1974). Furthermore, because the width of the vertebral body is greater than its height or depth, a greater capacity exists for flexion and extension than for lateral bending.

The major determinants of the direction and extent of motion is the shape of the vertebral bodies and the contours and orientations of the intervertebral articulations. The ligaments, fascia, and capsules also provide constraints to motion. When their elastic limits are reached, the tension halts motion. Following is a brief description of the factors that limit ROM in the cervical region.

Cervical Flexion

Cervical flexion is moving the head forward to the chest. Typically, when the body is vertical, neck flexion is produced by gravity. However, when the body is supine, the head is lifted against gravity. The primary muscle involved in flexion is the sternocleidomastoid (SCM), assisted by the scalenes, rectus capitis anterior, longus capitis, and cervicis. Flexion of the neck is limited by SCM contractile insufficiency, tension of posterior spinal structures (the posterior longitudinal ligament, ligamenta flava, interspinal ligaments, and supraspinal ligament), tension of the posterior muscles and fascia of the neck, the apposition of the anterior lips of the vertebral bodies with the surfaces of the adjacent vertebrae, compression of the anterior portion of the intervertebral fibrocartilage, and the chin coming to rest on the chest. Cervical flexion always moves the lumbar cord in a cephalad (head) direction (Lew et al. 1994).

The most controversial and potentially dangerous stretch for the cervical region is the plow (see chapter 14). In brief, the authorities and experts are divided on the issue. For individuals involved in gymnastics, judo, wrestling, and yoga, this stretch may be essential in their discipline. However, for most laypeople and athletes, safer alternatives should be used.

Effective stretching of the extensors of the cervical region to increase flexion requires anchoring and stabilization of the scapula and shoulder girdle. This position can be easily achieved lying flat on the floor (see exercise 231 in *Sport Stretch*). The key to the stretch is pulling the head off the floor and drawing the chin to the chest while keeping the shoulder blades flat on the floor. If the shoulder blades lift off the floor, most of the stretch is lost. Another effective demonstration of the importance of stabilizing the scapula and shoulder girdle is standing upright while holding a pair of dumbbells or a barbell. With the shoulders depressed by the weight, looking down and slowly bending the head toward the chest as if nodding stretches the upper back and cervical region.

Cervical Extension

Cervical extension is returning the head from the flexed (on the chest) position to the upright position. Drawing the head backward beyond the upright position is *cervical hyperextension*. This movement is produced by several posterior neck muscles (upper trapezius, semispinalis cervicis and capitis, splenius cervicis and capitis, rectus capitis posterior major and minor, obliquus capitis superior and inferior, and interspinales). ROM is limited by extensor contractile insufficiency, passive tension of the anterior longitudinal ligament, tension of the anterior neck muscles and fascia, bony approximation of the spinous processes, the locking of the posterior edges of the articular facet, and contact of the head on the muscle mass of the upper trunk. (An effective self-stretch using positioning and gravity is demonstrated in exercise 245 in *Sport Stretch*.)

Cervical Lateral Flexion

Cervical lateral flexion is tilting the head so that the left ear moves nearer the left shoulder or the right ear draws closer to the right shoulder. Lateral flexion of the neck is produced by many muscles (the SCM, scalenes, splenius cervicis and capitis, semispinalis cervicis and capitis, rectus capitis lateralis, rectus capitis posterior major and minor, obliquus capitis superior and inferior, intertransversarii, and longus cervicis and capitis) acting unilaterally. ROM is restricted by the contractile insufficiency of these muscles, passive tension of the intertransverse ligaments, tension of the neck muscles and fascia on the side opposing flexion, and impingement of the articular processes. Table 17.2 summarizes factors limiting lumbar, thoracic, and cervical movements.

Effective stretching of the lateral portion of the cervical area also necessitates anchoring the shoulder girdle, which can be accomplished by sitting in a chair and grasping a leg or the seat or by holding weights. The stretch is applied by pulling on the head with the hand opposite the side of the stretch or by self-positioning and the use of gravity. If the chair or weights is released, the shoulder on the stretched side will rise and the stretch is lost.

Cervical Rotation

Cervical rotation is turning the head and neck so that the face looks over one shoulder. Most rotation occurs at the atlantoaxial joint between vertebrae C1 and C2. Cervical rotation is produced by many muscles (on the opposite side by the SCM, semispinalis capitis and cervicis, and obliquus capitis superior; on the same side by the splenius capitis and cervicis, obliquus capitis inferior, rectus capitis posterior major, and rectus capitis lateralis). ROM is restricted by the contractile insufficiency of these muscles, passive tension of ligaments (particularly the

Table 17.2   Factors Limiting Lumbar, Thoracic, and Cervical Movement

Factor	Lumbar region	Thoracic region	Cervical region
Flexion			
Articular facet joint orientation	Sagittal plane (*no* contact/jamming occurs with flexion)	Frontal plane (contact/jamming *does* occur with flexion)	45° between frontal and horizontal planes (some sliding occurs with flexion)
Ratio of disk thickness to vertebral body thickness	Thick disks (allow considerable disk wedging prior to vertebral body contact anteriorly)	Thin disks (allow minimal disk wedging prior to vertebral body contact anteriorly)	Moderate ratio (allows moderate disk wedging prior to vertebral body contact anteriorly)
Rib cage	None	Contact of 12th rib with abdomen and incompressible sternum	None
Connective tissue tension	All posterior ligaments, facet joint posterior capsules	All posterior ligaments, facet joint posterior capsules	All posterior ligaments, facet joint posterior capsules
Muscle tension	Spinal extensor muscles (erector spinae and transversospinalis groups)	Spinal extensor muscles (erector spinae and transversospinalis groups)	Neck extensor muscles (erector spinae, transversospinalis, and suboccipital groups)
Extension			
Articular facet joint orientation	Sagittal plane (*no* contact/jamming occurs with hyperextension)	Frontal plane (contact/jamming *does* occur with hyperextension)	45° between frontal and horizontal plane (some sliding occurs with hyperextension)
Vertebral spinous process length	Short process, projects posteriorly (allows much hyperextension prior to impingement)	Long process, projects inferiorly, overlapping like roof shingles (no hyperextension is allowed)	Moderate length, projects nearly posteriorly (allowing moderate hyperextension prior to impingement)
Ratio of disk thickness to vertebral body thickness	Thick disks (allow considerable wedging prior to vertebral body contact posteriorly)	Thin disks (allow minimal wedging prior to vertebral body contact posteriorly)	Moderate ratio (allows moderate wedging prior to vertebral body contact posteriorly)
Rib cage	None	Attachment of ribs to inextensible sternum	None
Connective tissue tension	Anterior longitudinal ligament, facet joint anterior capsules	Anterior longitudinal ligament, facet joint anterior capsules	Anterior longitudinal ligament, facet joint anterior capsules
Muscle tension	Trunk flexor muscles (rectus abdominus)	Trunk flexor muscles (rectus abdominus)	Neck flexor muscles (many)

Factor	Lumbar region	Thoracic region	Cervical region
Lateral flexion (side-bending)			
Articular facet joint orientation	Sagittal plane (contact/jamming *does* occur with flexion)	Frontal plane (*no* contact/jamming occurs with flexion)	45° between frontal and horizontal planes (some sliding occurs with lateral flexion)
Ratio of disk thickness to vertebral body thickness	Thick disks (allow considerable wedging prior to vertebral body contact laterally)	Thin disks (allow minimal wedging prior to vertebral body contact laterally)	Moderate ratio (allows moderate wedging prior to vertebral body contact laterally)
Rib cage	None	Contact between adjacent ribs on shortened side of trunk	None
Connective tissue tension	Intertransverse ligaments, facet joint lateral capsules	Intertransverse ligaments, facet joint lateral capsules, and costovertebral ligaments	Intertransverse ligaments, facet joint lateral capsules
Muscle tension	Intertransversarii spinal extensor muscles, quadratus lumborum, abdominal obliques on lengthened side	Spinal extensor muscles, intercostal muscles on lengthened side	Neck lateral muscles (many) on lengthened side
Rotation			
Articular facet joint orientation	Sagittal plane (contact/jamming *does* occur with rotation)	Frontal plane (contact/jamming *does* occur with rotation)	45° between frontal and horizontal plane (*no* contact/jamming rotation)
Rib cage	None	Rib attachments to spine and sternum limit relative motion between adjacent ribs	None
Connective tissue tension	All spinal ligaments somewhat and facet joint capsules	All spinal ligaments somewhat and facet joint capsules	All spinal ligaments somewhat and facet joint capsules
Muscle tension	Back extensor oblique group/transversospinalis group (multifidi, semispinalis, rotatores)	Back extensor oblique group/transversospinalis group (multifidi, semispinalis, rotatores)	Neck rotator muscles (anteriorly: sternocleidomastoideus; posteriorly: splenius, obliquus capitis superior and inferior)

Reprinted by permission, from M.J. Alter, 1996, *Science of flexibility*, 2nd ed. (Champaign, IL: Human Kinetics), 276-277.

atlas ligaments between C2 and the skull), tension of the opposing neck muscles, and impingement of the articular processes. Table 17.2 summarizes these factors.

SUMMARY

The vertebral column is made up of a series of separate bones, the vertebrae, linked together by cartilaginous disks and ligaments. These components form a structural and functional unit capable of performing many functions. Among several factors that determine ROM are the intervertebral disks, the height of the vertebrae, the orientation of the facets, the intervertebral ligaments, and the passive tension of various connective tissues. The optimal efficiency of the vertebral column may be impaired by aging, attrition, disease, and trauma. ROM of the vertebral column can be maintained or enhanced through purposeful stretching exercises.

CHAPTER 18

Anatomy and Flexibility of the Upper Extremity

The upper extremity consists of the shoulder girdle, shoulder joint, arm, elbow joint, forearm, wrist joint, and hand. It is described in terms of structure, function, limitation to ROM, and methodology of stretching.

THE SHOULDER GIRDLE AND ARM

Each shoulder girdle and shoulder-arm complex consists of a clavicle, humerus, and scapula bone, plus an attachment to the single midline sternum. In combination, these bony segments articulate at three major joints: the glenohumeral, sternoclavicular, and acromioclavicular joints. According to Kapandji (1982), the subdeltoid and the scapulothoracic joints should be included, although neither of these junctions are anatomical joints. Although many movements appear to occur in the glenohumeral joint, they often involve simultaneous movement at other adjacent joints. Without the assistance of these joints, movements of the upper limb would be seriously restricted.

Gross Anatomy of the Shoulder Girdle

The three major joints that provide motion in the shoulder girdle are the glenohumeral joint, the sternoclavicular joint, and the acromioclavicular joint. The scapulothoracic joint, although not a true joint, is very important in shoulder movement.

Glenohumeral Joint

The glenohumeral, or scapulohumeral, joint is a modified ball-and-socket joint consisting of the humeral head and the shallow glenoid fossa (i.e., cavity) of the scapula. This joint structure is one of the most mobile and least stable in the human body. The lack of stability is caused primarily by the joint's weak bony architecture. Support for the joint is provided by the large, enveloping musculature. A secondary line of support comes from the capsular-ligamentous complexes. These complexes include the glenoid labrum, the fibrous capsule, and the glenohumeral, coracohumeral, and transverse humeral ligaments.

Sternoclavicular Joint

The sternoclavicular (SC) joint is a synovial joint formed by the articulation of the medial end of the clavicle with the first rib and manubrium of the sternum. The sternoclavicular joint is the only bony attachment of the upper limb to the axial skeleton. The joint is afforded little stability by the bony arrangement but is strongly supported by its ligaments and the intervening disk.

Acromioclavicular Joint

The acromioclavicular (AC) joint between the acromial end of the clavicle and the medial margin of the acromion of the scapula obtains its primary stability from the ligamentous binding rather than from its bony architecture. Despite the ligamentous binding, the joint is generally weak and easily dislocated. It is also prone to degenerative changes and functional impairment.

Scapulothoracic Joint

The scapulothoracic joint is not a true joint, but instead rides on the scapula on the posterior surface of the thoracic cage—no articulation of bones occurs. The scapulothoracic joint is the most important joint of the shoulder-arm complex, although it cannot function without the scapulohumeral and subdeltoid joints, which are mechanically linked to it (Kapandji 1982).

Description of Shoulder Motion

Clavicular movements at the sternoclavicular and acromioclavicular joints are always associated with movements of the scapula, and movement of the humerus and clavicle usually accompanies scapula movements. The six scapular movements are elevation, depression, protraction, retraction, and upward and downward rotation. Similarly, movements of the upper arm at the glenohumeral joint are always associated with movements of the scapula and the previously mentioned shoulder joints. Glenohumeral joint movements are best described in relation to the humeral segment moving on the trunk. These arm movements include abduction, adduction, flexion, extension, internal rotation, external rotation, horizontal (transverse) abduction, and horizontal (transverse) adduction.

Arm Abduction

Abduction at the glenohumeral joint is the upward movement of the arm in the coronal (or frontal) plane from anatomical position, that is, raising the arm to the side (Greene and Heckman 1994). The range of abduction at the glenohumeral joint depends on the type of movement and rotation of the humerus. *Active* abduction is limited to about 90° because the greater tuberosity of the humerus impinges on the acromial process and the coracoacromial ligament. Active abduction is also limited by a lack of mechanical advantage of the deltoid muscle.

Passive abduction is limited to 120°. For the greater tuberosity to pass under the coracoacromial hood during arm abduction, simultaneous depression and external rotation of the humerus must occur. Thus, when the arm is raised overhead (180° abduction), only two-thirds (120°) of that movement actually occurs at the glenohumeral joint. However, if the humerus is maintained in internal rotation, it will not abduct beyond 60°, because of earlier impingement. This portion is the *true glenohumeral motion*, as opposed to the scapulothoracic motion (American Orthopaedic Association 1985). The remaining 60° abduction is achieved by upward rotation at the scapulothoracic joint.

The smooth, integrated movement of the humerus, the scapula, and the clavicle is the *scapulohumeral rhythm*. The intricate articulations of these bones result in coordinated shoulder motion. During the initial *setting phase* (i.e., 30°) of abduction, the motion is mainly glenohumeral, with the scapula making very little contribution. The scapula remains fixed, moves laterally or medially, or oscillates as it seeks stabilization. As abduction continues, the ratio of scapular to humeral motion remains about 1° of scapular motion for every 2° of humeral motion at low speeds (see figure 18.1). Thus, for every 15° of abduction of the humerus, 10° occurs at the glenohumeral joint, and 5° occurs from rotation of the scapula at the scapulothoracic joint. Consequently, if either of these articulations is fixed by injury or disease, the loss of motion is proportionate, with glenohumeral fixation causing twice as much restriction as scapulothoracic fixation (Turek 1984). However, ratios at high speed are not fixed and differ significantly from those at low speed. Specifically, "glenohumeral motion at high speed was more dominant at the beginning of abduction or adduction except in the setting phase

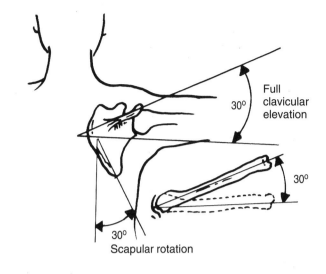

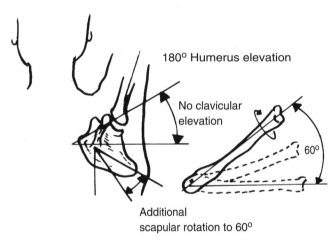

Figure 18.1 Scapular elevation resulting from clavicular rotation. The upper drawing shows the elevation of the clavicle without rotation to 30°. The remaining 30° of scapular rotation, which is imperative in full scapulohumeral range, occurs by rotation of the crank-shaped clavicle about its long axis.

Reprinted, by permission, from R. Cailliet, 1966, *Shoulder pain* (Philadelphia: F.A. Davis), 65.

and decreased according to the arm movement compared with that at low speed " (Sugamoto et al. 2002, p. 119). The muscles primarily responsible for the first phase of action are the deltoid and supraspinatus. ROM at the glenohumeral joint is limited by abductor contractile insufficiency, impingement of the shoulder as a result of the greater tuberosity hitting the superior margin of the glenoid or the acromion, passive tension of the shoulder adductor and internal rotator muscles, passive tension of the inferior portion of the shoulder joint capsule, and tension of the shoulder ligaments.

The claviculohumeral mechanism is another integral component of humerus abduction. During the first 90° of humerus abduction, the clavicle moves at the sternoclavicular joint, with the distal end elevating 4° for every 10° of abduction. Thus, at 90° of arm motion, the clavicle has elevated approximately 36° at the sternoclavicular joint. The motion at the acromioclavicular joint occurs both early (30°) and late (135° to 180°) in arm elevation. This motion consists of an upward swing of the scapula on the distal end of the clavicle. Without the cranklike action caused by the clavicle, full 180° abduction of the arm would be impossible (see figures 18.2 and 18.3).

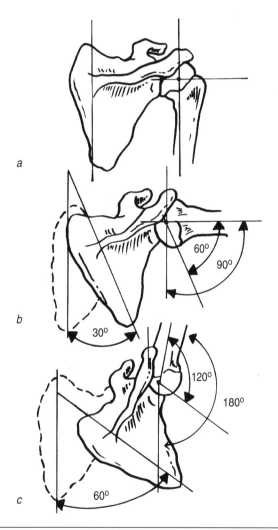

Figure 18.2 Scapulohumeral rhythm. *(a)* The scapula and the humerus at rest with the scapula relaxed and the arm dependent, both at 0°. Abduction of the arm is accomplished in a smooth, coordinated movement during which, for each 15° of the arm abduction, 10° of motion occurs at the glenohumeral joint and 5° occurs because of scapular rotation on the thorax. *(b)* The humerus (H) has abducted 90° in relationship to the erect body, but this movement has been accomplished by 30° rotation of the scapula and 60° abduction of the humerus at the glenohumeral joint, a ratio of 2:1. *(c)* Full elevation of the arm: 60° at the scapula and 120° at the glenohumeral joint.

Reprinted, by permission, from R. Cailliet, 1966, *Shoulder pain* (Philadelphia: F.A. Davis), 65.

The second phase of arm abduction ranges from 90° to 150°. This phase proceeds only with assistance of the shoulder girdle. The muscles responsible for this movement are the trapezius and serratus anterior. ROM is restricted by contractile insufficiency of the shoulder abductor, scapular upward rotator, and scapular elevating muscles; tension of the shoulder adductor, scapular depressor, and scapular downward rotator muscles (i.e., the latissimus dorsi and pectoralis major); and passive tension of the middle and inferior bands of the glenohumeral ligament. The third phase of arm abduction is from 150° to 180°. Attaining a vertical position of the arm may require movement of the vertebral column, which is accomplished by the exaggeration of the lumbar lordosis (Kapandji 1982). At the end of abduction, all the abductor muscles are in contraction. Limiting factors are the same as in the second phase.

Arm Adduction

Adduction of the glenohumeral joint is returning the humerus from the abducted position to its naturally hanging position (i.e., moving the arm toward the midline of the body) or beyond. Adduction is produced primarily by the pectoralis major and latissimus dorsi muscles. Movement is restricted when the humerus makes contact with the trunk.

Arm Flexion

Flexion, sometimes called *elevation* or *forward elevation*, is the upward motion of the arm toward the front of the body. Pure flexion at the glenohumeral joint ranges from 0° to 90°, and if modified, up to 180°. For purposes of analysis, the movement is divided into three phases. The first phase is the *setting phase* (Inman et al. 1944) and ranges from 0° to 60°. The muscles primarily responsible for this phase are the anterior fibers of the deltoid, the coracobrachialis, and the clavicular fibers of the pectoralis major. ROM is limited by their contractile insufficiency, tension of the coracohumeral ligament and inferior joint capsule, and tension of the teres minor, teres major, and infraspinatus muscles.

The second phase of arm flexion is from 60° to 120°. At this point, as in abduction, the scapulohumeral rhythm of the humerus and scapula comes into play. The ratio of motion in the scapulothoracic and glenohumeral joints is a constant 1° of scapular motion for each 2° of humeral motion. So for every 15° of humerus movement, the scapulothoracic movement is 5° and the glenohumeral movement is 10°. Again, as in abduction, when either of these articulations is fixed by injury or disease, the loss of motion is proportional, with glenohumeral fixation causing twice as much restriction as scapulothoracic fixation (Turek 1984). The muscles assisting during this phase are the trapezius and infraspinatus. Movement is restricted by contractile insufficiency, tension of the latissimus dorsi and serratus anterior, as well as anything that impedes the scapulohumeral rhythm.

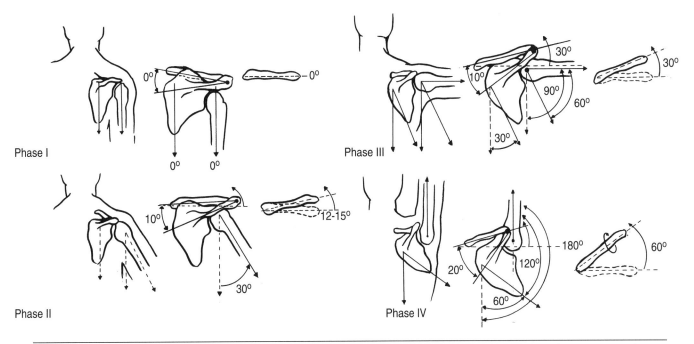

Phase I

Phase II

Phase III

Phase IV

Figure 18.3 Accessory movement of the scapulohumeral (SH) rhythm other than the glenohumeral movement. Phase I, the resting arm: 0° scapular rotation (S), 0° spinoclavicular angle (angle formed by the clavicle and the scapular spine, SCA), 0° movement at the sternoclavicular joint (SC), no elevation of the outer end of the clavicle (C), no abduction of the humerus (H). Phase II, humerus abducted 30°: outer end of the clavicle elevated 12° to 15° with no rotation of the clavicle; elevation occurs at the sternoclavicular joint; some movement occurs at the acromioclavicular joint as seen by increase of 10° of the spinoclavicular angle. Phase III, humerus (H) abducted to 90° (60° glenohumeral, 30° scapular): clavicle elevated to its final position, no rotation of clavicle as yet, all movement at the sternoclavicular joint, no change in the SCA. Phase IV, full overhead elevation (SH 180°, H 120°, S 60°): outer end of clavicle has not elevated further (at the sternoclavicular joint), but the SCA has increased 20°. Because of the clavicle's rotation and its cranklike form, the clavicle elevates an additional 30°. The humerus through this phase has rotated, but this has not influenced the above degrees of movement.

Reprinted, by permission, from R. Cailliet, 1966, *Shoulder pain* (Philadelphia: F.A. Davis), 65.

Flexion during the final phase is from 120° to 180°. When flexion is restricted at the glenohumeral and scapulothoracic joints, movement of the spinal column becomes necessary, which is accomplished by exaggeration of the lumbar lordosis (Kapandji 1982). The muscles responsible for movement and the factors limiting ROM are the same as in the previous two phases. For a complete 180° flexion, the humerus moves 120° at the glenohumeral joint, and the scapula moves upward and forward 60° at the scapulothoracic joint. The 60° of scapular motion would be impossible without the 40° and 20° elevation of the clavicle at the sternoclavicular and acromioclavicular joints, respectively.

Arm Extension

Extension of the glenohumeral joint is the return of the arm from the flexed or elevated position back to anatomical position (arm at the side). *Hyperextension* is the posterior motion of the humerus in the sagittal plane of the body (i.e., lifting the arm backward and behind the hip). Greene and Heckman (1994) of the American Academy of Orthopaedic Surgeons have not adopted this terminology, contending that hyperextension refers

only to atypical or asymmetrical motion, such as at the elbow or knee. Extension of the shoulder is sometimes called posterior elevation. Internal rotation is required for maximum posterior elevation, which ranges up to 60° (Browne et al. 1990). Posterior elevation occurs in the backswing during bowling. This movement is produced by the deltoid, latissimus dorsi, and teres major and is assisted by the teres minor and long head of the triceps. ROM is limited by contractile insufficiency, tension of the shoulder flexor muscles, tension of the coracohumeral ligament, and contact of the greater tubercle of the humerus with the acromion posteriorly.

Arm Internal, or Medial, Rotation

Internal, or *medial* (inward) *rotation*, of the glenohumeral joint may be measured by three different methods: rotation with the arm at the side, rotation with the arm in 90° of abduction, and rotation with the arm extended posteriorly. Greene and Heckman (1994) believe that the abdomen prevents accurate measurement of internal rotation with the arm at the side position. Internal rotation is produced by the scapularis, pectoralis major, latissimus dorsi, and teres major muscles and is assisted by the deltoid muscle. ROM is restricted by contractile insufficiency, tension of the superior portion of the capsular ligament, and tension of the external rotator muscles (i.e., infraspinatus and teres minor).

Arm External, or Lateral, Rotation

External, or *lateral* (outward), *rotation* of the glenohumeral joint is also measured by two methods. The first method is with the arms at the sides (neutral position), the elbow flexed at 90°, and the forearm parallel to the sagittal plane of the body. The second method is from a zero starting position with the arm abducted 90° while aligned with the plane of the scapula and the elbow flexed 90° with the forearm parallel to the floor. Kronberg et al. (1990) found that a larger angle of humeral head retroversion was consistent with an increased range of external rotation. The average angle of retroversion is 33° on the dominant side and 29° on the nondominant side. Hence, the dominant side is associated with an increased range of external rotation. An exaggerated torsion of the humerus might make the glenohumeral joint more vulnerable to instability or dislocation (Brewer et al. 1986; Debevoise et al. 1971). External rotation of the humerus is produced by the teres minor, supraspinatus, and infraspinatus. This movement is limited by contractile insufficiency, tension of the superior portion of the capsular and coracohumeral ligaments, and tension of the internal rotator muscles (i.e., subscapularis, pectoralis major, latissimus dorsi, and teres major).

Arm Horizontal Abduction

Horizontal abduction is moving the humerus laterally and backward with the humerus elevated to a horizontal position. Horizontal abduction ranges approximately from 0° to 30°. This motion is displayed during the cocking or setting phase of a forehand stroke with a tennis racquet. Horizontal abduction is produced by the posterior fibers of the deltoid, the infraspinatus, and the teres minor. ROM is limited by contractile insufficiency, passive tension of the anterior fibers of the capsule of the glenohumeral joint, and tension of the pectoralis major and anterior fibers of the deltoid muscles.

Arm Horizontal Adduction

Horizontal adduction is moving the humerus medially and forward with the humerus elevated to a horizontal position. Horizontal adduction ranges approximately from 0° to 130°. This movement is produced primarily by the pectoralis major and anterior fibers of the deltoid. It is seen in the follow-through of a swing of a baseball bat or a forward stroke in various racquet sports (e.g., racquetball, table tennis, tennis). ROM is limited by contractile insufficiency; tension of the glenohumeral's extensor muscles (i.e., latissimus dorsi, teres major, posterior fibers of the deltoid, and teres minor); and contact of the humerus with the trunk.

Descriptions of Movements at the Scapulothoracic Joint

The scapulothoracic joint is capable of several types of motion: scapular elevation, scapular depression, abduction of the scapula, adduction of the scapula, backward extension of the scapula, upward rotation of the scapula and downward rotation of the scapula.

Scapular Elevation

Elevation is upward movement of the scapula. The muscles involved are the upper trapezius, levator scapulae, and serratus anterior. Scapular elevation is restricted by contractile insufficiency, tension of the antagonistic muscles, tension of the costoclavicular ligament, and tension of the lower part of the capsule.

Scapular Depression

Depression is downward movement of the scapula. Passive depression is caused by gravity and the weight of the limb. Depression can be made active by pressing downward (or resting on the parallel bars). Simple depression, against no resistance, is produced by the pectoralis minor, subclavius, pectoralis major, and latissimus dorsi. ROM is limited by contractile insufficiency, tension of the antagonistic muscles, tension of the interclavicular and sternoclavicular ligaments, and the articular disks.

Scapular Abduction, Protraction

Scapular abduction, or *protraction*, is forward movement of the scapula, which is seen in all forward-pushing or thrusting movements. Protraction is produced by the serratus anterior, pectoralis minor, and levator spinae. ROM is restricted by contractile insufficiency, tension of the antagonistic muscles, tension of the anterior sternoclavicular ligament, and tension of the posterior lamina of the costoclavicular ligament.

Stretches to facilitate protraction are usually directed at the rhomboids. However, shrugging the anterior portion of the shoulders is not very effective, nor is swinging both arms through horizontal adduction. The most effective stretch for this muscle group requires a partner (see exercise 230 in *Sport Stretch*).

Scapular Adduction, or Retraction

Scapular adduction, or *retraction*, is backward movement of the scapula and is exemplified by pulling. It is produced by the trapezius and rhomboids and is assisted by the latissimus dorsi. ROM is limited by contractile insufficiency, tension of the antagonist muscles, tension of the posterior sternoclavicular ligament, and tension of the anterior lamina of the costoclavicular ligament.

Upward Scapular Rotation

Upward rotation of the scapula occurs as the arm is raised in abduction. The trapezius and the serratus anterior muscles produce this movement. ROM is restricted by contractile insufficiency or tension of the antagonistic muscles.

Downward Scapular Rotation

Downward rotation of the scapula occurs as the arm is lowered in adduction. This movement is produced by the latissimus dorsi, assisted by the pectoralis major and minor, rhomboids major and minor, and levator scapulae. ROM is restricted by contractile insufficiency or tension of the antagonistic muscles.

Shoulder Complex Injuries, Stretching, and Testing

Injuries to the shoulder girdle and shoulder-arm complex are common. Preventive actions include proper warm-up; proper exercise technique; building endurance, strength, and flexibility; and proper sleep posture.

Prolonged Stretching

A prolonged stretch occurs when an individual sleeps in a side-lying position with the lower shoulder pushing forward, causing the scapula to abduct and lift forward. This position stretches the lower trapezius muscle and possibly the rhomboid muscles. The top shoulder is susceptible to problematic stretching when the arm is heavy and the thorax is large, causing the arm to pull the scapula into the abducted, forward position. The humeral head in the glenoid also moves into a forward position (Sahrmann 2002, p. 20).

Flexibility should be developed in all directions and through the full ROM. However, when stretching or testing this region, one must carefully separate shoulder girdle motion from vertebral column motion. For example, to achieve a true stretch or to test glenohumeral flexion, one must position the body in hip flexion and lumbar spine flexion. Thus, lie with the lower back on the floor, both legs flexed, and the heels near the buttocks. Slowly raise the humerus. Once the lower back arches, the maximum range of flexion is determined. A partner may push down on the ribs to keep the back flat on the floor as glenohumeral flexion continues.

THE ELBOW JOINT AND FOREARM REGION

The elbow joint of the upper extremity is midway between the shoulder and wrist. The elbow is a relatively stable joint. However, an excessive force can cause a dislocation.

The elbow is primarily stabilized by its bony arrangement and ligaments.

Gross Anatomy of the Elbow

Three bones form the basic skeletal structure of the elbow: the humerus, radius, and ulna. The elbow is a hinge joint. It has three articulations but only two are mentioned here: the humeroulnar-radial joint, involved solely in flexion and extension in a sliding fashion, and the radioulnar joint, involved solely in pronation and supination.

Description of Elbow Movements

Four major movements occur at the elbow joint: flexion, extension, pronation, and supination.

Elbow Flexion

Flexion of the elbow is decreasing the angle between the humerus and forearm. The primary flexors of the elbow are the biceps brachii, brachialis, and brachioradialis, and the accessory flexors are the pronator teres, wrist and finger flexors, and radial wrist extensors (Turek 1984). The short head of the biceps brachii is a major supinator of the forearm. Flexion of the elbow ranges approximately from 0° to 150° when the flexors are hardened by contraction and up to 160° when the muscles are relaxed (Kapandji 1982). ROM is limited by contractile insufficiency, contact of the muscles of the upper arm on the forearm, impact of the head of the radius against the radial fossa and the coronoid process against the coronoid fossa, tension of the posterior capsular ligaments, and passive tension in the triceps.

Stretching of the elbow extensors facilitates motion in the flexion pattern. This stretch can be easily accomplished by leaning forward with the forearms resting on a table (see exercise 297 in *Sport Stretch*). Use of light dumbbells can increase both strength and stretch through a slow eccentric contraction. Most often, stretches of the elbow's extensors concentrate on the short head of the triceps and ignore the long head. Stretching the long head of the triceps requires flexing the elbow joint with the humerus in full flexion. This flexing can be accomplished by placing the elbow about head height against a wall and pulling down on the wrist using a towel (see exercise 299 in *Sport Stretch*) or by having a partner apply the stretch.

Elbow Extension

Extension of the elbow is returning from the flexed position or beyond the zero starting position (the elbow extremely straight). The primary extensors of the elbow are the triceps brachii and anconeus. ROM from the zero starting position varies from 0° to 10°. Extension beyond 10° is *hyperextension* (Greene and Heckman 1994). Hyperextension is one of the signs of hypermobility syndrome (Carter and Wilkinson 1964). Hyperextension is usually more common in women than in men. One explanation for the difference is the presence of a supratrochlear foramen, an aperture linking the coronoid and olecranon fossae of the humerus (Amis and Miller 1982). Two other explanations are the presence of a deep olecranon fossa or a small olecranon process (Hamill and Knutzen 1995). When hypermobility or joint laxity is present, stretching should not go beyond elbow extension. Cummings (1984) investigated whether extension of the elbow in normal female adults is limited primarily by muscle or by the ligaments and capsule and concluded, "elbow extension in the normal adult woman is limited primarily by muscle" (p. 170). ROM is limited by contractile insufficiency; impact of the olecranon process on the olecranon fossa; tension of the anterior, radial, and ulnar ligaments at the elbow; and tension of the flexor muscles (e.g., biceps brachii).

Stretching the flexors of the forearm facilitates extension of the elbow joint. The dilemma is how to stretch the biceps when the elbow joint is extended to 180°. One method is eccentrically contracting the flexors (see exercise 294 in *Sport Stretch*). However, the most effective technique is to stand with the back to a doorframe or pole with one hand grasping it. The arm must be internally rotated at the shoulder, the forearm extended, and the hand pronated with the thumb pointing down. While the thumb faces down, the biceps are turned upward (see exercise 295 in *Sport Stretch*). This stretch is essential for all athletes, especially those who use a throwing motion, because the throwing motion (especially of a curve ball) causes insult to the biceps tendon. During the throw of a curve ball, the elbow joint passes from flexion to extension while supinating the forearm. The biceps are the most important supinator of the forearm. Over the course of a season, the biceps receive thousands of insults. The importance of stretching the biceps cannot be overemphasized.

Description of Forearm Movements

The forearm has two main movements: pronation and supination.

Forearm Pronation

Pronation is turning the hand and forearm from the neutral, or thumb-up, position to the palm-down position. Pronation ranges approximately from 0° to 80° and is seen when topspin is applied in racquet sports. It is produced by the pronator teres and the pronator quadratus. ROM is restricted by contractile insufficiency; tension of the dorsal radioulnar, ulnar collateral, and dorsal radiocarpal ligaments; tension of the lowest fibers of the interosseous membrane; and the radius crossing and impacting against the ulna.

Forearm Supination

Supination is the outward rotation of the forearm from the neutral palm-down to the palm-up position. Supina-

tion ranges approximately from 0° to 90°. The primary supinators of the forearm are the biceps brachii, supinator, and brachioradialis. ROM is limited by contractile insufficiency, tension of the volar radioulnar ligament and ulnar collateral ligament of the wrist, tension of the oblique cord and lowest fibers of the interosseous membrane, and tension of the pronator muscles.

Injuries of the Elbow and Forearm

Injuries to the musculotendinous and ligament complex of the elbow have many causes, but the most common are activities that demand forceful and repetitive contractions of the forearm muscles, which produce strains. Strains are often experienced by tennis, racquetball, and baseball players. Inflammation of the lateral or medial epicondyle is called *epicondylitis*, or *tennis elbow*. The most effective exercise to prevent lateral epicondylitis is stretching the supinators of the elbow and forearm by grasping a broomstick, golf club, or tennis racquet in a dorsal grip (the back of the hand faces down and the thumb grasps under the handle [see exercise 306 in *Sport Stretch*]). This stretch is intensified by hanging from a chin-up bar with a dorsal grip (see exercise 307 in *Sport Stretch*).

A preventive approach is the most practical and prudent way to deal with elbow and forearm injuries. This approach includes proper warm-up, avoidance of excessive overloading or overuse, optimal technique, and exercises to develop flexibility, strength, and endurance.

THE WRIST JOINT

The *radiocarpal joint*, or wrist, is an ellipsoid joint formed by the articulation of the distal end of the radius and three of eight carpal bones in the hand. Ligaments bind the carpals closely and firmly together in two rows of four each. The first, or proximal, row comprises the scaphoid, lunate, triquetrum, and pisiform bones. The last carpal does not participate in the formation of the radiocarpal joint. The second, or distal, row comprises the trapezium, trapezoid, capitate, and hamate bones.

Stability of the Wrist Joint

The wrist is a very stable joint. It is stabilized primarily by the ligaments of the joint and the numerous muscle tendons that pass over it and secondarily by the bony arrangement. The major ligaments of the wrist are the palmar radiocarpal, palmar ulnocarpal, dorsal radiocarpal, radial collateral, and ulnar collateral.

Description of Wrist Movements

The wrist joint allows several active movements, including flexion, extension, abduction, adduction, and circumduction. All but the last are discussed in the following sections.

Wrist Flexion

Wrist *flexion* involves drawing the palm toward the forearm and ranges approximately from 0° to 90°. It is greatest when the hand is in the neutral position (i.e., neither abducted nor adducted). The chief flexors of the wrist are the flexor carpi radialis, flexor carpi ulnaris, and palmaris longus.

Flexion is limited by contractile insufficiency, tension of the wrist extensor muscles (i.e., extensor carpi radialis longus, extensor carpi radialis brevis, and extensor carpi ulnaris), and tension of the dorsal radiocarpal ligament. Flexion is minimal when the wrist is in pronation (Kapandji 1982). Movement is also diminished when the fingers are flexed, because of the increased tension of the extensor muscles. Flexion can be facilitated by stretching the wrist extensors (see exercises 304 to 307 in *Sport Stretch*).

Wrist Extension

Wrist *extension* occurs when the palm is moved away from the forearm. This movement ranges approximately from 0° to 85°. Extension is greatest when the hand is in the neutral position. The main extensors of the wrist are the extensor carpi radialis longus, extensor carpi radialis brevis, and extensor carpi ulnaris. ROM is restricted by contractile insufficiency, tension of the wrist flexor muscles (i.e., flexor carpi radialis, flexor carpi ulnaris, and palmaris longus), and tension of the palmar radiocarpal ligament. Extension is minimal during pronation (Kapandji 1982). Stretching the wrist flexors enhances wrist extension. This enhancement can be achieved by a number of stretches (see exercises 306 to 311 in *Sport Stretch*).

Wrist Abduction, or Radial Deviation

Radial deviation of the wrist is flexion of the hand toward the side of the forearm where the radius bone resides (the side of the thumb). Most movement occurs at the midcarpal joint, ranging approximately from 0° to 20°. Radial deviation is less than ulnar deviation because of the buttressing effect of the radial styloid process as the carpus becomes mechanically blocked (Greene and Heckman 1994; Volz et al. 1980). The range of radial deviation is generally minimal when the wrist is fully flexed or extended because of the tension developed in the carpal ligaments (Kapandji 1982). Radial deviation is produced by the flexor carpi radialis, in conjunction with the extensor carpi radialis longus, extensor carpi radialis brevis, abductor carpi radialis longus, and extensor pollicis brevis. ROM is limited by contractile insufficiency, tension of the antagonistic muscles, and, at extreme limits, the radial and ulnar collateral radiocarpal ligaments.

Wrist Adduction, or Ulnar Deviation

Ulnar deviation of the wrist is flexion of the hand toward the side of the forearm where the ulna bone resides (the side of the little finger). Ulnar deviation has a range two to three times larger than that of radial deviation: approximately from 0° to 30°. The greater range of ulnar deviation may be associated with the shortness of the styloid process of the ulna (Williams et al. 1995). Ulnar deviation is produced by the flexor carpi ulnaris in conjunction with the extensor carpi ulnaris. ROM is restricted by contractile insufficiency, tension of the antagonistic muscles, and impingement of the wrist.

SUMMARY

The upper extremity consists of the shoulder girdle, shoulder joint, arm, elbow joint, forearm, wrist, and hand. Many types of movements take place in the upper extremity and through various ROMs. Often these movements involve simultaneous actions at other adjacent joints. Without the assistance of the appropriate joints and muscles, efficient movement would be impossible. Causes of reduced efficiency of the upper extremity include aging, lack of use, disease, and trauma. However, optimal upper-extremity efficiency can be maintained or enhanced through purposeful warm-up, stretching, strengthening, and endurance exercises.

UNIT

5

SPECIFIC DISCIPLINES

CHAPTER

19

Functional Aspects of Stretching and Flexibility

Numerous factors go into creating optimal performance, including endurance, power, strength, and mental toughness. In addition to these attributes, flexibility is generally recognized as a crucial factor in skilled movement (Garhammer 1989a). Consequently, flexibility plays a significant role in determining the outcome of various performances or competitions. Flexibility enhances and optimizes the learning, practice, and performance of skilled movement. Therefore, some skills may be enhanced more effectively by purposefully increasing or decreasing the ROM around certain joints until the apparent optimal flexibility is reached (Hebbelinck 1988).

AESTHETIC ASPECT OF SKILLS

Aesthetically, flexibility is definitely a requirement for skilled movement. However, the effects of increased flexibility on artistic and sports performance may range from obvious to subtle. For instance, the need for excellent flexibility in such disciplines as ballet, diving, figure skating, and gymnastics is obvious. These disciplines have an aesthetic component, and optimal flexibility obviously enhances performance because it is part of the scoring system (Stone and Kroll 1991). Flexibility allows the individual to create an appearance of ease, smoothness of movement, graceful coordination, self-control, and total freedom. Flexibility also helps the individual to perform more skillfully and with greater self-assurance, elegance, and amplitude. The concept of amplitude is further elaborated by George (1980):

> Essentially, amplitude refers to the "range" through which a body moves and can be subdivided into two basic types. The first type, "external amplitude," is used to describe the range through which the *total* body unit moves relative to the ground and/or apparatus . . . However, the "hidden component" that allows the gymnast to take full advantage of technique is her own internal power . . .

The second type of amplitude, "internal amplitude," focuses upon range of motion *within* the joints of the body. More specifically, it refers to the range through which one or more of the individual body segments move relative to each other . . . Just as power is the hidden component underlying external amplitude, joint range of motion or *flexibility* is the key factor for obtaining maximum internal amplitude. (pp. 7-9)

Thus, without suppleness, a highly skilled performance would be impossible in many disciplines. The difference between an average and an outstanding performance may simply be a matter of flexibility.

BIOMECHANICAL ASPECT OF SKILLS: ROM

Biomechanics is the application of mechanical laws to living structures. It examines the forces that act on a body and the effects of these forces. For example, in tennis, an increased ROM allows one to apply forces over greater distances and longer periods of time. Similarly, in gymnastics, an increase in distance through which force can be applied improves the potential for a more vigorous and effective forward headkip (George 1980). Greater range can increase velocities, energies, and momenta involved in physical performance (Ciullo and Zarins 1983). Many skills depend on a close interaction between internal and external amplitude (George 1980).

Flexibility may be needed in lengthening contractions that immediately precede active muscle contraction. An increased ROM can permit a greater stretch on the involved muscles. Those muscles can produce even greater forces because a prestretched muscle can exert more force than a nonstretched muscle. Prestretched muscles function with greater efficiency because elastic energy is stored in the muscle tissue during stretching and recovered during the subsequent shortening (Asmussen and Bonde-Petersen 1974; Boscoe et al. 1982; Cavagna et al. 1968; Cavagna et al. 1965; Ciullo and Zarins 1983; Grieve 1970; Komi and Boscoe 1978). Ciullo and Zarins (1983) compared this phenomenon with cocking an air rifle. However, Hill (1961) found that when relaxation of the muscle is allowed to occur between the stretching and shortening phases, the preloaded condition provides no advantage, and the stored elastic energy is dissipated as heat. Komi (1984) showed that a delay of 0.9 seconds between eccentric and concentric contractions eliminated the increase in performance expected from elastic recoil. Thus, timing is an all-important component of this use of flexibility.

Biomechanical Aspects: Compliance and Stiffness

Compliance refers to a material easily elongated by low levels of force. In contrast, stiffness is a measure of a material's elasticity or property to resist deformation from a force and quickly return to its normal shape. The mechanical measure of a material's elasticity is stiffness. Therefore, compliance is inversely related to stiffness. A relationship exists between musculotendinous compliance, stiffness, and performance in various sports and activities. This section reviews the relationship.

Joint Tissues and Flexibility

The current emphasis on flexibility neglects the equally important mechanical qualities of the tissues composing the joints, in particular their stiffness and damping ratio. In other words, these tissues must offer each joint an effective balance between mobility and stability under a wide range of operating conditions. For instance, a joint whose tissues have low stiffness (or can be stretched easily) but a low damping ratio (or poorly absorbs tensile shocks) is especially susceptible to overload injuries.

Therefore, in analyzing flexibility, one has to consider the separate and the interrelated effects of the ROM of the joints and the mechanical properties of the tissues they comprise (Siff and Verkhoshansky 1999, p. 174).

Strength, Power, and Jumping Performance

Van Bevern (1979), cited by Kroll et al. (1997), demonstrated a decrease in strength after a long-term stretching program in subjects with varying initial hamstring length. Davies et al. (1992), cited by Young and Elliott (2001), found that static stretching significantly reduces leg strength. Similarly, Öberg (1993) cited an example in which a group of handball players were tested for strength

in the thigh muscles, jump performance, and flexibility before and after a set of stretching exercises. The results showed decreased torque in eccentric contractions and in jump performance. Rosenbaum and Hennig (1995) investigated the acute effects of stretching and warm-up exercises on the Achilles tendon of 50 male athletes. "The stretching treatment had a generally impairing effect on active force production, which may have been caused by mechanical changes such as increased tendon slack" (p. 489).

Walshe et al. (1996) postulated that a complex relationship between musculotendinous stiffness and performance appeared to be "dependent on the type of muscular contraction involved" and "the way force is developed within the muscle" (p. 338). The researchers discussed the idea that "musculotendinous stiffness was significantly related to both concentric and isometric performance such that the stiffer subjects were able to develop force more rapidly" (p. 338).

Kokkonen et al. (1998) investigated whether acutely stretching the hip, thigh, and calf muscles after five different static stretching activities alters the performance of a 1-repetition maximum lift (RM). Stretches were performed three times with and without assistance. Each stretch was held 15 seconds and followed by a 15-second recovery time between repetitions. The static stretching group had a decline of 7.3% and 8.1%, respectively, for 1 RM of knee flexion and 1 RM for knee extension., Fowles et al. (2000b) monitored the time course of plantar flexor strength deficit after 30 minutes of maximum, passive stretching. A 20% decrease in force was produced 5 minutes after stretching. This decrease was also accompanied by a significant 13% decrease in activation as measured by the interpolated twitch technique and a nonsignificant 15% decrease in EMG activity. Furthermore, voluntary strength decreased for up to an hour.

In an investigation by Behm et al. (2001), 12 subjects performed a 5-minute warm-up on a cycle ergometer, followed by 5 sets of static and passive stretches. Each stretch was held for 45 seconds and followed by a 15-second relaxation period. After stretching, a significant 12% decrement occurred in maximal voluntary contraction force with no significant changes in the control group. Nelson et al. (2001) also found a deleterious impact of stretching activities on maximal torque production (decrease in a muscle's capacity to generate force). The study suggested "that the inhibitory relationship between acute stretching and force production is velocity-specific, with the greatest decrements seen at slower movement velocities" (p. 246).

Jumping performance is negatively impacted by stretching. Ten males and 10 females warmed up for 3 minutes on a lifecycle followed by three 15-second static stretches of the hamstrings, quadriceps, and calf muscles. Three maximal-effort vertical jumps were performed, with the mean score used for statistical analysis. The effect of stretching was not uniform among the participants, with 55% showing a decrease in peak vertical velocity (7.5%) after stretch and 45% showing no change or an increase in peak vertical velocity (2.4%) after stretching. Young and Elliott (2001) found "that static stretching produced a significant decrement in drop jump performance and a significant decrease in nonconcentric explosive muscle performance" (p. 278). McNeal and Sands (2001) found an 8.2% loss in jumps in 14 female gymnasts as a result of static stretching for 30 seconds. They pointed out that "This reduction in performance could mean the difference between landing safely and under-rotating a tumbling skill." Similarly, Church et al. (2001) demonstrated a decreased vertical jump performance for a PNF treatment group. Young and Behm (2003, p. 26) also found two minutes of static stretching "appeared to elicit a negative influence on concentric and SSC explosive force measures and jumping performance." In contrast, Hunter and Marshall (2002) concluded, "Stretching (flexibility training) appeared to offer no added benefits to drop jump height and had no effect on drop jump technique" (p. 486). Further research is necessary to ascertain the mechanism of acute decreases in jump height from stretching.

Rationales for Decreased and Increased Performance

Investigators have postulated several explanations for the decrease in strength and power after stretching. Some researchers suggest that a portion of the stretch-induced force can be attributed to changes in viscoelastic properties of the muscle, altering its compliance (Kokkonen et al. 1998; Nelson et al. 2001; Young and Elliott 2001). Wilson et al. (1994) suggested that a more compliant system could result in a loss of force production by the contractile component because of altered intramuscular length and velocity conditions. At a given magnitude of contraction, a compliant musculotendinous unit goes through a period of rapid and virtually unloaded shortening, which continues until the elastic components are altered sufficiently to transmit the generated force to the bone. An alternate explanation is that a transient increase in muscle length caused by stretching might negatively impact the excitatory stretch reflex originating from the muscle spindles (Fowles et al. 2000b). However, muscle spindles recover immediately after stretch (Guissard et al. 1988).

Negative acute effect of static stretching might be related to "an inhibitory neural mechanism" (Young and Elliott 2001, p. 278). However, several researchers challenge the explanation of motor-unit inhibition via proprioceptors (e.g., Golgi tendon organs and low-threshold pain receptors) (Nelson et al. 2001). This explanation is questionable because autogenic inhibition is limited to the duration of the stretching maneuver (Guissard et al. 1988). Further research is required to identify whether the poststretch deficit in strength is related to a change in neural or mechanical status.

Several investigators have postulated reasons for improved performance. Wilson et al. (1994) proposed that a stiffer musculotendinous unit may facilitate some performances by improving the force production capabilities of the contractile component because of a combination of improved length and rate of shortening, and additionally by enhancing initial force transmission. Another explanation is provided by Walshe and Wilson (1997):

> A stiffer MTU with relatively less tendinous extension would transfer most of an imposed length change to the contractile element. In turn, this would effectively increase the afferent response via greater spindle distortion, resulting in higher levels of excitatory reflex feedback. This could facilitate stretch-shortening cycle performance, either by direct myogenic potentiation or by altering extrinsic stiffness. (p. 119)

Relationship of Flexibility and Stiffness to Aerobic Performance

Another related biomechanical result of stretching and flexibility is enhanced economy of energy utilization. Successful performance in many aerobic activities such as walking, running, and swimming are determined by the optimum use (expenditure) of energy stores within the body. Genetic factors play a role in poorly developed oxygen transport systems and in their efficiency. Improvements in gait economy were evinced by a reduction of the metabolic cost in young, asymptomatic males after a single bout of static stretching and PNF stretching (Godges et al. 1989). They attributed the improvement in running economy to factors such as improved balance and coordination, greater pelvic symmetry, and reduced resistance to limb motion resulting from the stretching program. However, studies by Gleim et al. (1990), Craib et al. (1996), and Jones (2002) contradicted these findings. Contrary to what might be initially expected, athletes with a decreased ROM (misleadingly described by several researchers as being "stiffer") tend to have a lower VO_2 at submaximal running speeds. For example, Gleim et al. (1990) found that subjects with greater flexibility (ROM) used 10% more energy to accomplish the same speed than the subject with less ROM. Similarly, Craib et al. (1996) suggested that "inflexibility in hip and calf regions of the musculoskeletal system is associated with improved running economy in sub-elite male distance runners" (p. 743). The primary finding by Jones (2002) was "that lower limb and trunk flexibility (as assessed by the sit-and-reach test) is negatively related to running economy in international standard male distance runners" (p. 41). In other words, the least flexible runners are also the most economical. Craib et al. (1996) suggested that a decrease in flexibility in the trunk and hips might improve running economy by "stabilizing the pelvic region of the body at the time of foot impact with the ground, thereby reducing the need for excessive and metabolically expensive stabilizing muscular activity" (p. 742).

Potential reasons for the enhanced economy might also relate to stiffness (not ROM) of musculotendinous structures. Jones (2002) stated that "it is possible that stiffer musculotendinous structures reduce the aerobic demand of submaximal running by facilitating a greater elastic energy return during the shortening phase of the stretch-shortening cycle" (p. 40). Additional research must quantify the optimum amount of stiffness and ROM within specific disciplines.

Stiffness in the lower extremity is a vital factor in athletic performance in various sports and activities. Leg stiffness has a positive influence on the amount of stored energy and its utilization during the positive (concentric) phase of jumping. Furthermore, an optimal leg stiffness value to maximize the mechanical power during the positive phase of drop jumps has been determined (Arampatzis et al. 2001). Maximization of mechanical power apparently is not achieved by a maximum activation, but rather by an optimum activation of the leg muscles during the preactivation phase.

ADDITIONAL IMPEDIMENTS

An adequate amount of flexibility (ROM) is also essential to ensure that performance is not compromised. For example, strength training may be impaired if the muscle group cannot work its full ROM. Excessive muscle activity may be required, leading to premature fatigue (Hutson 2001). Inadequate flexibility (ROM) in one part of the body may impact other parts of the body. Thus, if motion is limited at one location, "substitution and faulty movement patterns occur" (Brody 1999, p. 100). These actions can impede performance and cause injury.

JOGGING, RUNNING, AND SPRINTING

The objective in competitive and recreational jogging, running, or sprinting is to cover a given distance in the shortest time. This speed is a product of two interdependent factors: *length* and *frequency* of stride. To improve speed, a runner must increase one or both of these variables without causing the other to be reduced by a comparable (or, worse yet, a more than comparable) amount (Hay 1993). Maximum running efficiency occurs only when length and frequency of stride are in optimal proportions. These factors depend on the weight, build, strength, coordination, and flexibility of the runner (Dyson 1986).

Increasing the Length of Stride

One explanation of how flexibility reduces running times is that an increase in the body's mobility and joint range results in a greater length of stride, leading to better performance. The length of stride is most conveniently measured from the front of the toe print to the front of the succeeding toe print (Slocum and James 1968). One stretching machine manufacturer has referred to this greater length of stride as the "geometry of winning." Following is an example from their brochure analyzing a 100-yard dash (TRECO 1987):

> If a runner has a 96 inch stride it would mean 37.5 strides would be required to run the dash (discounting the shorter starting strides). If this were done in 10 seconds then each stride would have averaged .266 seconds. With no more than a 2 inch increase the 96 inch stride becomes 98 inches. This means that 36.74 strides are now needed to run the 100 yards. If each stride still takes .266 seconds then the 10 second 100 yard dash time will drop to 9.8 seconds. A person running a 9.8 second 100 yard dash will finish nearly 6 feet in front of a 10.0 second runner.

Another example of the "geometry of winning" is illustrated in table 19.1 (Dintiman and Ward 1988). On a purely biomechanical level, an increased flexibility in the lower limbs should result in an increased stride length. With all other factors remaining constant, running time should be lowered.

However, stride length is thought to depend on the speed, angle, and height of projection of a runner's center of gravity (Carr 1997; Steben and Bell 1978), acceleration of the thigh angle (i.e., the angle between the thighs at

Table 19.1   Stride-Length Increase and Its Effect on 40-Yard Dash Time With a Flying Start

	Stride length	Stride rate	Feet per sec	Approximate 40-yd-dash time
Original speed	6 ft ×	4.0 steps per sec	= 24	5.0 sec
New speed	6 ft 6 in. ×	4.0 steps per sec	= 26	4.6 sec

Reprinted, by permission, from G. Dintiman and R. Ward, 1988, *Sport speed* (Champaign, IL: Human Kinetics), 149.

the moment of first surface contact) (Kunz and Kaufmann 1980), hip-joint mobility and lower-extremity flexibility (Carr 1997; Dintiman and Ward 1988), and the power of the runner's legs (Carr 1997; Dintiman and Ward 1988; Dyson 1986; Ecker 1971; Robison et al. 1974). The more powerful the leg drive, the greater the thrust against the ground with each step and the longer the stride. The increase in stride length that results from this forward projection of the body is believed to be the best method for achieving an increase in stride length because it does not interfere with the mechanical efficiency of the runner's motion. At each footstrike, the support leg is underneath the runner's center of gravity (Steben and Bell 1978). Attempting to increase stride length by "stretching out" causes overstriding (the support leg being forward of the center of gravity at footstrike), which, in turn, causes braking on each step, a decrease in stride frequency, and a slower time (Ecker 1971; Robison 1974).

Because the beneficial increase in stride length is a result of foot-ground interaction, the importance of stride frequency becomes apparent: Too slow a cadence causes a loss in efficiency of movement, whereas too great a stride length decreases the number of strides possible in a given distance, thus reducing momentum. When humans increase their stride frequency at a given running speed, the most important adjustment to the body's spring system is stiffening leg spring. Thus, "between the lowest and highest possible stride frequencies, the stiffness of the leg spring more than doubles" (Farley and Gonzalez 1996, pp. 185-186).

Another factor that can influence the stride length is the degree of *crossover*, which may be related to flexibility. Crossover is a measure of how far a runner's legs cross over the midline of the body while running (figure 19.1). This phenomenon is also referred to as *asymmetrical leg action*. Prichard (cited by Cailliet 1991 in Brant 1987; Neff 1987) postulated that these crossover inches can add a substantial extra distance to long-distance races. For example, a typical marathoner takes about 1,000 strides per mile (620 strides per km) or 26,000 strides per race. If the degree of crossover is reduced by 2 inches (5 cm) per stride, the reduction in distance run is 4,333 feet (1,320 m).

What causes runner crossover? One possibility is poor technique. However, Prichard (cited by Brant 1987) believes that crossover can result from any one or combination of three factors: leg length differences, inflexibility of the adductor muscles on the insides of the legs, and *upper body torque* (i.e., tightness in the upper torso). Upper body torque is most often the result of inflexibility of the shoulders, which in turn results from tightness in the chest muscles. For example, as a runner's right arm goes back, it pulls the left arm across the body. Consequently, the right leg crosses over to the left in a compensating movement. This crossover is referred to as *asymmetrical arm action* (Hinrichs 1990, 1992). Enhanc-

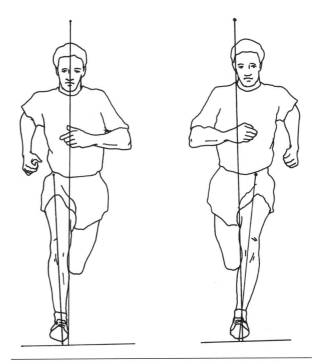

Figure 19.1 Excessive upper body torque, which pulls the legs across the midline of the body, is a frequent cause of running injury.

Reprinted from Prichard (1984).

ing the flexibility and reducing the stiffness of the upper torso will decrease upper body torque and increase performance. Another postulated detriment of excessive arm movement across the trunk is injury to the knees and lower limbs (Brant 1987; Cailliet 1991; Prichard 1984; Volkov and Milner 1990). Additional research on the subject is needed before any conclusions can be drawn about the actual causes of the asymmetries and whether the runner's performance is helped or hindered by them (Hinrichs 1990, 1992).

Increasing the Range of Force Application

A second means by which flexibility can reduce running times is by increasing the runner's velocity. Velocity is increased by increasing the distance or range over which a muscle force is applied. Tolsma (1985) identified the posterior and anterior muscles of the lower leg (ankle plantar flexors and dorsiflexors, respectively), the anterior thigh muscles (quadriceps), and the posterior buttock muscles (gluteals) as muscle groups whose enhanced flexibility will increase the range over which a force can be applied. Following is an analysis based on the work of McFarlane (1987), Slocum and James (1968), and Tolsma (1985).

The Ankle Plantar Flexors

The support phase of running is divided into three distinct periods: *footstrike*, *midsupport*, and *takeoff*. Footstrike begins when the foot first contacts the ground and continues through the brief moment that the foot becomes firmly planted. Midsupport starts once the foot is fixed and continues until the heel rises from the ground. Takeoff commences when the heel rises and continues until the toes leave the running surface. During the midsupport phase, the knee is flexed 30° to 40° as the heel remains on the ground. This position places the posterior muscles of the lower leg in an elongated position. However, if the runner has very short calf muscles, the heel lifts off the ground prematurely. Consequently, the force applied to the ground by contraction of the calf muscles is through a shorter ROM (see figure 19.2). The result is a decrease of force. Accordingly, in a warm-up stretching program the calf should be stretched with the knee somewhat bent to simulate the leg position in running, during which these muscles are stretched.

The Ankle Dorsiflexors

During the later stages of takeoff, the propulsive action of the calf is very important, and the farther the foot can be plantar flexed, the longer this driving force can be sustained. Hence, the importance of stretching the anterior portions of the lower leg, ankle, and foot. The difference between the ranges of force application of a flexible and inflexible ankle is shown in figure 19.2.

The Quadriceps

Flexibility in the quadriceps can also significantly affect running efficiency. During takeoff, the hip joint goes through extension. Consequently, the hip flexors (e.g., rectus femoris, iliacus, and psoas muscles) are stretched. With enhanced flexibility, the hip flexors allow a longer application of force to the ground. Once again, the result is the facilitation of force. Schache et al. (2000) reported that static hip extension flexibility measured using the modified Thomas test did not appear to be reflective of peak hip extension ROM at a submaximal running speed.

The Gluteals

The gluteal muscles can also potentially maximize running efficiency. Their function is extension of the hip joint. During the *forward swing* period of running, the thigh begins to move forward and stops when the hip reaches maximum flexion. At this point (i.e., when the knee is brought toward the chest) these muscles are stretched. Theoretically, the higher the knees can be efficiently raised, the greater the range through which a runner can subsequently apply the forces of hip extension. (Raising the knee too high results in reduced efficiency and slower running time.)

Reduced Muscular Resistance

Stretching and flexibility reduces the muscular and passive forces that resist motion (de Vries 1963; Tolsma 1985). Hubley-Kozey and Stanish (1990) describe this phenomenon as running without excessive soft-tissue resistance, whereas McFarlane (1987) refers to it as running with lower internal-muscle resistance. A muscle passively stretched

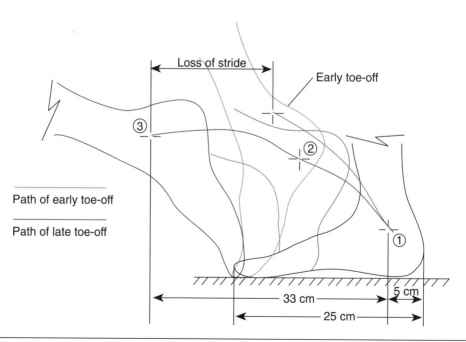

Figure 19.2 Effect of early and late takeoff on stride length. Early takeoff caused by decreased ankle flexibility results in a shorter stride and more vertical displacement of the center of mass, creating a less efficient running style than later takeoff, which enhances stride length and lessens vertical displacement.

Reprinted, by permission, from D. Martin and P. Coe, 1997, *Better training for distance runners, 2nd ed.* (Champaign, IL: Human Kinetics), 27.

opposes stretch by a force that increases slowly at first and more rapidly with increased elongation. The longer or more flexible the muscle, the later in the movement this resistance is encountered (Tolsma 1985). Consequently, the resultant force in the muscle being opposed (agonist) is higher without any additional expenditure of energy and promotes greater local endurance (Kulakov 1989; Tolsma 1985). Findings in the literature regarding stretching and decreasing passive tension are contradictory. For example, Toft et al. (1989), using the contract-relax stretching technique, found that ankle dorsiflexion passive tension can be decreased in subjects irrespective of their flexibility through stretching. In contrast, Muir et al. (1999) found that static calf-stretching exercises did not produce a significant reduction in the resistive torque during ankle dorsiflexion. Perhaps, the discrepancies reflected different stretching techniques. However, another possibility is that the reduction in passive resistance found by Toft et al. (1989) resulted directly from the stretching exercises or from the preconditioning of the connective tissues during the testing protocol (Muir et al. 1999).

How Much Flexibility Is Necessary for Running?

Some degree of flexibility is necessary for optimal running efficiency. However, three basic questions must be asked. (1) How much flexibility is actually required for optimal running? (2) Does stretching soft tissues to an extreme ROM provide any benefit? (3) Do runners need enough flexibility to perform splits? Runners routinely attempt almost contortionistic stretches before a big race. This behavior has been criticized by several leading experts (Dominguez, cited by Shyne 1982; Fixx 1983; Frederick 1982; Wolf 1983).

Unfortunately, little information is available for assessing the average ROMs required in different athletic activities (Hubley-Kozey and Stanish 1990). Nonetheless, a careful biomechanical analysis of various angles that the legs pass through while running may help to establish a minimal requirement for certain joints. Distance runners require a much smaller ROM than do dancers or gymnasts. In a normal running stride, when the hip is flexed, the knee is also flexed. Hence, a long hamstring position is never reached. Consequently, a runner does not need extreme flexibility in the hamstrings (Tolsma 1985). A runner needs an ROM that permits running without excessive soft-tissue resistance (de Vries 1963; Hubley-Kozey and Stanish 1990; Martin and Coe 1997). Once again, the question of the specific amount flexibility necessary is raised. Prichard (cited by Brant 1987) suggests that recreational runners should have a *stride angle* of at least 90° and competitive runners at least 100° (figure 19.3). The stride angle is the composite of the angle of flexion of the front leg and the angle of extension of the back leg. Additional research is needed in this area to substantiate the foregoing estimates.

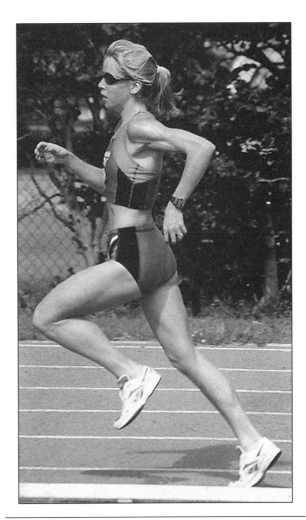

Figure 19.3 A runner's stride angle should equal 90°— 100° would be even better.

Reprinted from Martin and Coe (1997).

SWIMMING AND WATER POLO

The objective in competitive swimming and in some recreational swimming is to cover a given distance in the shortest time. Average swimming speed is a product of two factors: the average stroke length and the average stroke frequency (Hay 1993). The two forces that govern stroke length are the *propulsive force*, which drives the swimmer through the water and is produced by the swimmer's movements, and the *resistive force*, which the water exerts on the swimmer in opposition to the swimmer's motion (Hay 1993). The following sections analyze how flexibility in five specific areas of the body influences swimming.

Increasing the Range of Force Application

Flexibility can reduce swimming times by increasing the swimmer's velocity. This improvement is accomplished by increasing the distance or range through which the force is applied. Lewin (1979) has identified five major parts of the body that deserve special attention in developing flexibility to enhance swimming: the ankles, hips, spinal column, shoulders, and knees.

The Ankles

Swimming the front crawl, back crawl, and butterfly requires good plantar flexion of the ankles. The best swimmers use an up-and-down (flexion and extension) motion known as the flutter kick (Hay 1993; Hull 2002). In the downbeat, the top of the extended foot produces propulsion as hip flexion moves the leg downward. During the upbeat, the sole of the foot applies thrust force as the leg moves from a flexed to an extended position. Cureton (1930) concluded that the upbeat was more effective than the downbeat for propulsion.

Because the application of backward force depends on foot position, flexible ankles are necessary for an efficient flutter kick (Bunn 1972; Counsilman 1968, 1977; Hull 1990-1991, 2002; Lewin 1979). Robertson (1960) found significant relationships between ankle flexibility and propulsive force. Thus, to improve this type of flexibility, the anterior muscles of the lower leg (i.e., dorsiflexors of the ankles and toes) must be stretched. Swimmers have more flexibility than nonswimmers in the ankle (Bloomfield and Blanksby 1971; Hull 2002; Oppliger et al. 1986).

The importance of dorsiflexing the feet toward the shins is also significant in swimming. This movement is particularly relevant in the breaststroke (Bunn 1972; Counsilman 1968; Hay 1993; Lewin 1979; Rodeo 1984). The most efficient leg action in the breaststroke is the *whip kick* (Hay 1993). Two explanations have been proposed as to why dorsiflexion enhances the breaststroke. (1) During the catch phase, the knees are flexed more than 90° with the feet above the buttocks, close to each other, and the ankles are everted. The soles of the feet face backward and upward, and the feet are turned so that the toes point laterally (Rodeo 1984). When the feet start to spread, ankle dorsiflexion begins. This position presents a large surface to "catch" and push the water backward through the downsweep of the kick (Counsilman 1968; Gaughran 1972; Rodeo 1984). Thus, if the swimmer performs this action and the feet remain pointed backward during the power phase, the kick is less effective (Gaughran 1972). (2) Lewin (1979) contends that the greater the amplitude of flexion of the foot, the faster the athlete can get a grip on the water in the transition between the recovery phase (pulling up the legs) and the power phase (extending the legs). Nimz et al. (1988) found that no outstanding flexibility is necessary for swimming the whip kick.

The Hip Joint

The four Olympic competitive strokes utilize some degree of hip flexion and extension, with the breaststroke incorporating the most motion. Hip abduction and adduction are associated with the breaststroke. Lewin

(1979) believes that, despite the fact that the full movement amplitude is not used once the swimmer develops an optimal swimming technique, high movement amplitudes in executing straddle movements (abduction) are important for the breaststroker.

The Spinal Column

The literature often discusses the subject of swimming flexibility exclusively in terms of the ankle and shoulder joints. Flexibility in the vertebral column is also essential for optimal performance. A high level of trunk hyperextension is essential for backstrokers (Bloomfield et al. 1994). A high level of hyperextension enables backstrokers to enter their body into the "hole" opened by the hands and head at the start of the race and thereby reduce drag. A flexible back is also necessary for optimal performance of the breaststroke. As explained by Engesvik (1993), swimmers with very flexible backs look rather like ducks because their shoulders are high above the surface and their hands may recover over the surface. They appear to "hump" over the water. This technique causes less resistance than underwater recovery and improves speed. Lewin (1979) also addresses the importance of spinal flexibility:

> The significance of flexibility of the spinal column is often underestimated in developing an optimum swimming technique. And yet it is an important factor, for it is a necessary condition for adapting the trunk to the changing conditions during a movement cycle in such a manner as to minimize the body's drag in the water and thereby raising the efficiency of the swimming movements. The flexibility (suppleness) of the spinal column in all planes should be developed and improved; flexibility of the spinal column in the sagittal plane is particularly important for the breast and dolphin swimmer, while for the crawl swimmer and backstroker flexibility in the frontal plane is important. It is also essential for being able to twist the body (turning the shoulder line and the hip line in opposite directions around the central body axis). Special attention should be paid to improving the flexibility of the cervical section of the spinal column, because the greater the flexibility of this part of the spinal column, the less detrimental the influences of the movement of the head during breathing on the posture and movement of the trunk and the extremities. (p. 121)

The Shoulder Joint

Good flexibility in the shoulder joint is critical for all swimming strokes. In the front crawl, limited shoulder flexibility results in the swimmer recovering the arm with a low elbow. This technique is both incorrect and inefficient (Bloomfield et al. 1985; Counsilman 1968; Hay 1993; Lewin 1979). As described by Counsilman (1968), to recover the arms and clear them over the water rather than drag them in the water, the inflexible swimmer must roll the body and make a flatter and wider sweep of the arms during the recovery than does a more flexible swimmer. This poor technique produces a greater reaction or lateral thrust of the legs and initiates an unwanted rotation about the anteroposterior axis that tends to move the body out of alignment in a lateral direction (Hay 1993). Consequently, swimmers with tight shoulders must frequently adopt a two-beat crossover kick to keep the legs in alignment (Counsilman 1968). Swimmers with a higher arm recovery seem to have fewer shoulder problems (Greipp 1986).

The butterfly stroke requires shoulder flexibility (Counsilman 1968; Johnson et al. 1987; Rodeo 1985a, 1985b). As the arms leave the water, the palms of the hands face almost directly upward (Counsilman 1968). The arms are backward in extension and internal rotation. This position decreases the mobility of the shoulder joint (Counsilman 1968). Hence, as soon as the hands leave the water, the swimmer must rotate the arms outward and swing them forward and around. The hands should enter the water at a point only slightly outside the shoulder line, but if the swimmer lacks adequate shoulder flexibility, the shoulder rotation and hand placement in the water is inefficient. According to Souza (1994), "it is essential that at hand entry the hand enter the water slightly outside of shoulder width to maintain neutral shoulder position allowing movement in mainly the coronal plane" (p. 114).

Shoulder flexibility is vital in the backstroke crawl. The swimmer's arm, with the elbow straight, most efficiently enters the water in line with and directly over the shoulder (Counsilman 1968) or above and slightly to the side of the shoulder at almost full reach (Hay 1993). Thus, the recovery arm should move in essentially a straight line in the vertical plane (Counsilman 1968, 1977). However, the tighter the shoulder, the farther out of line the arm enters the water and the less efficient the stroke. Deviation sideward from this plane because of limited shoulder flexibility will result in a sideward displacement of the hips and legs. Consequently, the resistance or drag that the swimmer creates will increase (Counsilman 1977).

The Knees

The significance of knee flexibility is probably the most underestimated in developing swimming technique. However, flexible knee joints in concert with flexible hip joints is particularly significant in the breaststroke. According to Lewin (1979), "the ability to move one's lower legs as far out sideways as possible (abduction) is essential, because this determines the arc of the thrust planes during the power phase of the leg movement" (p. 120).

Reduced Muscular Resistance

Stretching and developing flexibility are thought to reduce the muscular and passive forces that resist motion in swimming. See the earlier section on reduced muscular resistance (page 262).

How Much Flexibility Is Needed for Swimming?

More often than not, swimmers are too flexible rather than insufficiently flexible (Falkel 1988). Several stretching exercises are now recognized as "detrimental, either worsening underlying pathology or initiating a problem" (Litchfield et al. 1995, p. 53). Marino (1984) cites Douglas (1980) who states that swimming coaches and swimmers appear to be determined to destroy the anterior capsule of the shoulder joint by performing damaging passive shoulder stretching exercises. Hence, Marino (1984) addresses the need for coaches and swimmers to distinguish between *muscle flexibility* and *capsular laxity*. "Perverse stretching maneuvers such as horizontal abduction of the humerus to the point where the elbows cross behind the back do not promote muscular flexibility, and they do not maintain adequate range of motion" (p. 223). Furthermore, this behavior may actually lead to an increased likelihood of anterior dislocation (Dominguez 1980; Litchfield et al. 1995). Another exercise criticized by Litchfield et al. is "stretching the painful shoulder in the overhead position in forward flexion is probably unwise, due to the exacerbation of an impingement process" (p. 53). Hence, the swimmer not only should know how much flexibility is needed but also which stretches are good or bad.

Water polo players are also at risk for shoulder pain because of the repetitive nature of swimming combined with throwing (Elliott 1993). In very flexible water polo players, the repeated forced lateral rotation causes the anterior capsule to become lax, resulting in instability. In turn, overzealous stretching can exasperate this laxity. Excessive stretching can also predispose the player to dislocation. According to Rollins et al. (1985) shoulder dislocation is frequent among water polo players. The mechanism of injury is the striking of the arm by an opposing player with forced abduction, extension, and lateral rotation. For flexible water polo players, strengthening the shoulder girdle complex must override the need to stretch.

Pain is common among competitive swimmers. Weldon and Richardson (2001) found prevalence rates of shoulder pain in swimmers ranging from 3% to 80%. A review of literature revealed average yardage for midseason swimmers is 8,000 to 20,000 yards per day (Beach et al. 1992). Counsilman (1968) proposed a 4:1 ratio of running to swimming, in which 4 miles of running are exertionally equivalent to 1 mile of swimming. Therefore, the average swimming yardage would be equivalent to running more than 32,000 to

80,000 yards per day—or more than 45 miles per day (Beach et al. 1992; Johnson et al. 1987). Furthermore, the average collegiate swimmer is estimated to perform more than 1 million strokes annually (Kammen et al. 1999; McMaster et al. 1989; Rockwood and Matsen 1998).

Consequently, repetition or overuse is a major factor in the development of pain. Several components, including training errors, improper technique, performance level, strength imbalance, and increased shoulder ROM have been suggested as etiologic factors that contribute to overuse shoulder problems (Bak and Magnusson 1997). One simplified model proposes that reduced stability leads to subluxation of the glenohumeral joint, which, when combined with repetition, leads to inflammation and pain (Weldon and Richardson 2001). The pertinent question is whether a correlation exists between flexibility and shoulder pain. Some authors (Greipp 1985; Johnson et al. 1987; Johnson et al. 2003; Richardson et al. 1980) have suggested that a lack of shoulder flexibility in swimmers contributes to shoulder injury. On the other hand, Dominguez (1980), Falkel (1988), Johnson et al. (2003) and McMaster (1986) have discussed the potential influence of hyperflexibility and overstretching in swimmers and the role it may play in developing shoulder problems.

Data on the relationship between shoulder ROM and pain are conflicting. For example, Bak and Magnusson (1997) reported changes in shoulder ROM seem unrelated to the occurrence of shoulder pain. In contrast, Greipp (1985) found a strong correlation between lack of flexibility and incidence of swimmer's shoulder. A study of 28 competitive swimmers between 15 and 21 years of age found that "flexibility data showed an extremely low, nonsignificant correlation to shoulder pain" (Beach et al. 1992, p. 267). No correlation was found between flexibility and pain in elite water polo players (Elliott 1993).

Zemek and Magee (1996) have demonstrated a direct relationship between the amount of increased shoulder laxity and level of success in swimmers. However, increased shoulder ROM can reduce stability of the glenohumeral joint and predispose a swimmer to injury. In addition, a shoulder with capsuloligamentous laxity can decrease the force produced by the muscles of the rotator cuff (Weldon and Richardson 2001) and thereby impair performance.

How much flexibility does a swimmer need? A conservative response is that a swimmer needs ROM that will permit swimming without excessive soft-tissue resistance and that will facilitate optimal technique. Once again, to cite Hubley-Kozey and Stanish (1990, p. 22), "there is little information available for assessing the average ranges of motion required by different athletic activities." Therefore, "physicians and therapists (and coaches) must rely on their experience and knowledge of a particular sport and the available literature when suggesting how much an athlete should stretch."

THROWING AND PROJECTING

One skill that begins in early childhood is throwing. According to Bunn (1972), throwing is second only to running as the most common element in sport. Lindner (1971) has suggested that throwing motions in various disciplines share a common trait of lateral deviation of the upper part of the body from the throwing arm, which must be considered a natural movement. Atwater (1979) corroborated the hypothesis that the throwing angle between the arm and the trunk in projecting a football, javelin, tennis racquet, or baseball are essentially the same. Furthermore, Atwater (1979) reported similarity in the nearly completed extension of the forearm and the elbow joint at release or impact as evidence of a commonality of joint and segment actions in sport skills employing the overarm pattern. However, Anderson (1979) pointed out that slight to moderate spatial-temporal differences between various sport skills require adjustments within the general overarm pattern.

Flexibility is a vital factor for throwing. An increase in ROM permits one to exert muscle forces over greater distances and longer periods of time. Consequently, this ability can increase velocities, energies, and momenta associated with physical performance (Ciullo and Zarins 1983; Northrip et al. 1983). If flexibility is high, then antagonist muscle activity may be reduced, which would also lead to high limb velocity (Kraemer et al. 1995). In short, an increased ROM permits a greater prestretch on the involved muscles and thus allows them to produce even greater forces.

Upper-Extremity Flexibility Needs

Studies among athletes who use repetitive throwing movement patterns show that they are potentially subject to changes in shoulder strength, ROM, and physical deformation, depending on the quantity and quality of overload. Among baseball players, significantly increased external rotation is found between the dominant and nondominant shoulders. In contrast, significantly decreased internal rotational ROMs are found in the dominant and nondominant shoulders (Baltaci et al. 2001; Bigliani et al. 1997; Brown et al. 1998; Cook et al. 1987; Magnusson et al. 1994; Werner et al. 1993). During the cocking phase of pitching, maximal external rotation has been reported to be between 160° and 185° (Dillman et al. 1993; Feltner and Dapena 1986; Fleisig et al. 1995; Pappas et al. 1985). The mechanism of external rotation is "the inertial lag of the forearm and hand as the more proximal segments rotate forward" (Feltner and Dapena 1986, p. 254). The changes in ROM are an adaptive response to the unique repetitive stresses placed on the glenohumeral joint and its surrounding structures during the throwing motion. Sandstead (1968) found that throwing velocity was significantly related ($r = .77$) to the range of external shoulder rotation in college varsity baseball players. According to

Tullos and King (1973), this increase in external rotation improves the efficiency of the internal rotator muscles and thus allows the ball to be delivered with greater velocity (see figure 19.4).

Atwater (1979) points out:

> Since several anterior shoulder injuries seem to be associated with the position of *maximum* shoulder lateral rotation and since there is a strong positive relationship between throwing velocity and range of shoulder lateral rotation, those pitchers who rely on the delivery of fastballs or those youngsters who practice for hours to increase the speed or distance of their throw, may be most susceptible to anterior shoulder injuries. (p. 73)

An increase in shoulder external rotation and a decrease in shoulder internal rotation, particularly on the dominant side, have also been reported in javelin throwers (Herrington 1998) and tennis players (Chandler et al. 1990; Chinn et al. 1974; Ellenbecker et al. 1996). However, a longitudinal study by Roetert et al. (2000) found external rotation of ROM did not significantly change in nationally ranked junior tennis players tested

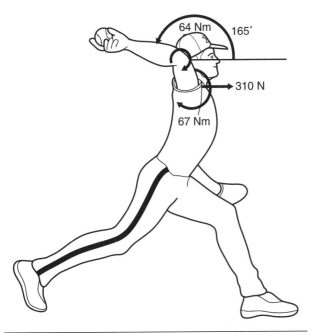

Figure 19.4 External rotation of a pitcher. Shortly before maximum external rotation was achieved, the first critical instant occurred; at this instant, the arm was externally rotated 165°, and the elbow was flexed 95°. Among the loads generated at this time were 67 N-m of internal rotation torque and 310 N of anterior force at the shoulder, and 64 N-m of varus torque at the elbow.

Reprinted, by permission, from G.S. Fleisig, J.R. Andrews, C.J. Dillman, and R.F. Escamilla, 1995, "Kinetics of baseball pitching with implications about injury mechanisms," *American Journal of Sports Medicine* 23(2), 238.

between the ages of 14 and 17 years. In contrast, internal rotation of the dominant arms revealed a significant increase between ages 14 and 15 years and between ages 14 and 16 years, with a slight decrease at age 17 years. Similar to Sandstead (1968), Cohen et al. (1994) found a correlation between both strength and flexibility and serve velocity. Investigations of elite volleyball athletes by Wang and Cochrane (2000) and Wang et al. (2000) found that active ROM of internal rotation on the dominant side was smaller than on the nondominant side, whereas external rotation was not statistically different between the two sides.

Adaptation of the shoulder is a lengthening of the posterior shoulder musculature and capsular structures by the tennis serve or overhead smash (Zarins et al. 1985). This adaptation occurs because the shoulder is stretched to the extremes of external rotation and abduction during the backswing phase of a serve (Chinn et al. 1974; Nirschl 1973). This critical part of the serve is the *back-scratch* position (Nirschl 1973) in reference to its appearance. The increased range of external glenohumeral rotation possibly allows the muscles producing the arm acceleration to internally rotate the humerus through a wider range for a longer time, thereby imparting added momentum to the ball (Michaud 1990). Cohen et al. (1994) demonstrated that numerous flexibility measures, including dominant wrist flexion and dominant shoulder forward flexion, are related to tennis serve velocity.

Over the years, repeated insults and microtrauma may produce fibrotic changes in the capsule and ligaments of the posterior shoulder, where the traction stresses of follow-through are concentrated. Consequently, these fibrotic changes may maintain the overall stability of the joint structure by decreasing capsular distensibility in the posterior portions. Concomitantly, this fibrosis reduces full range of internal rotation in tennis players (Chandler et al. 1990; Chinn et al. 1974). Athletes who use overhead arm movements often show significant tightness of the posterior capsule and deltoid, which can contribute to anterior subluxation symptoms (Harryman et al. 1990). Consequently, "in these athletes, a stretching program emphasizing cross-body adduction and internal rotation is instituted" (Dahm and Lajam 2002, p. 7).

However, Aberdeem and Joensen (1986) discovered a significant difference in range of rotation values at the shoulder joint when comparisons between right and left sides were made in 73 normal right-handed subjects, and this difference was related to handedness. In right-handed people, the range of right external rotation is normally greater than the range of left external rotation, and the range of left internal rotation is normally greater than right internal rotation.

Adaptation from prolonged unilateral training can cause permanent asymmetrical physiological changes in the upper extremity (Magnusson et al. 1994; Renstrom and Roux 1988). The most common shoulder changes are *hypertrophy* (increased muscle mass and size of the humeral bone) and *depression* (low carrying angle of the scapula). Because scapular depression is common among tennis players, it has been dubbed *tennis shoulder*. According to Priest (1989), two possible mechanisms cause tennis shoulder. (1) The muscles that elevate the shoulder, the joint capsule, the ligaments, and the tendons are recurrently stretched during the serve and overhand smash. Repeated elongation of structures beyond their usual lengths increases laxity in the overloaded shoulder, eventually causing the shoulder to droop (Priest 1989; Priest and Nagel 1976). (2) The greater weight of the playing extremity that has hypertrophied draws the shoulder downward (Priest 1989). Numerous photographs in the literature illustrate this feature (King et al.1969; Priest et al. 1977; Priest and Nagel 1976). In extreme cases scoliosis (lateral curvature of the spine) can develop (Priest 1989; Renstrom and Roux 1988).

Sport-specific upper-extremity strain, mostly unilateral, can also lead to adaptations of bone. Pieper (1998) documented an increased humerus retrotorsional angle in handball professionals' throwing arm. The increased humeral retrotorsion "allows for more rotation of the shoulder joint before the humeral head is constrained by the anterior capsule and the glenohumeral ligaments. It therefore enables the handball player to extend the cocking phase and thus further accelerate the throw" (p. 252). Furthermore, increased retrotorsion will "lead to an earlier restraint of the humeral head by the posterior capsule and thus limit internal rotation." Therefore, the increase in humeral retrotorsion could be "interpreted as a protective mechanism for the anterior capsulolabral complex" (p. 253).

Pappas et al. (1985) states the reason the freedom of movement in all positions of a pitcher's shoulder is necessary to ensure a fluid delivery:

> Every movement pattern of the arm has an expected relative contribution of the glenohumeral and scapulothoracic components. A deterioration of any of the structures that control a component leads to the loss of flexibility. From pitching, the shoulder complex is susceptible to loss of flexibility from two sources, musculotendinous tightness and reactive fibrous tissue formation in the anterior and posterior capsule. Therefore, the shoulder tightness frequently seen in pitchers occurs from either or both the muscular and capsular structures.
>
> When assessing loss of flexibility in a pitcher's shoulder, particular attention needs to be given to the specifics of a movement, not the movement as a whole. Loss of flexibility in one component results in a compensatory increase in the other component so that the movement can be achieved. In the process of compensation, the usual synchrony of muscle action is interrupted and patterns of movements are established which lead to various pathologic problems, e.g., loss of flexibility. (p. 227)

The relationship between decreased internal rotation and risk of injury, along with its impact on performance of tennis players, has been subject to discussion (Chandler et al. 1990; Kibler et al. 1996; Marx et al. 2001; Roetert et al. 2000). One possible result of decreased internal rotation of the shoulder may create an athlete "who is susceptible to injury and less able to withstand the extrinsic demands of the sport" (Kibler et al. 1996, p. 284). Reviews of the literature by Ellenbecker et al. (1996) and Roetert et al. (2000) revealed that decreases in internal rotation affect normal joint arthrokinematics and can subject the joint to abnormal forces and translations, leading to injury. Ellenbecker and Roetert (2002) examined the effects of a 4-month season on glenohumeral joint internal and external ROM of 11 elite female collegiate tennis players. The study found no significant changes in ROM. The 4-month study was most likely not long enough for significant ROM alterations to occur. Another part of the body susceptible to injury is the lower back. Low-back pain is a common complaint among elite tennis players. However, the relative contribution of the flexibility of each muscle group is not known and may vary among individuals (Chandler et al. 1990).

Additional research analyzing the interrelationship between ROM and injury and performance is needed. A sample of topics for future study has been provided by Kibler et al. (1996):

- Can these deficits be modified and, if so, what is the most efficient method of modification?

- If these deficits are modified, what is the relationship to performance and risk of injury?

- Do these deficits continue to decline in a linear direction, or does a curvilinear pattern occur with an absolute maximum?

- Were these deficits compounded by variables such as the amount of weight training, other conditioning practices, or previous childhood activities?

Lower Extremity Flexibility Needs

If shoulder ROM is vital to throwing performance, what about the need for ROM in the lower extremity? Tippett (1986) investigated lower extremity ROM between the stance leg and kick leg in 16 college baseball pitchers and found ROM of ankle plantar flexion, hip internal rotation, and hip extension to be greater in the stance leg than in the kick leg. Conversely, the kick leg had greater active hip flexion than the stance leg did. The biomechanical explanation of the interrelationship between the lower extremity's ROM and the stage of pitching follows.

- Internal rotation of the stance leg is facilitated during the *gathering stage*. This rotation allows the trunk to coil on the fixed stance leg to "load" for an efficient transfer of momentum from the leg to the hip, the hip rotators, the torso, and finally the arm.

- The hip flexion of the kick leg corresponds to the flexion of the knee forward and across the body. This movement provides significant momentum to produce significant rotational force on the fixed stance.

- During the *drive stage*, proper alignment of the kick leg originates with knee extension, hip abduction, and external rotation. As the pitcher strides toward the plate, the stance leg provides power via hip extension. During this stage, the stance leg displays an increase in hip extension and ankle plantar flexion. "Theoretically, the greater motion can allow for a greater ability for corresponding muscles to generate force" (p. 13).

What flexibility regimen should be followed by athletes who use throwing motions? Tennis players obviously would benefit from a level of shoulder joint mobility that permits the desired racquet movement during a serve (Bloomfield et al. 1985). Prudent athletes who use high-velocity throws (e.g., pitchers) must exercise their shoulders for flexibility to allow the ROM needed in cocking, without producing excessive joint laxity or instability (Boscardin et al. 1989). A purposeful exercise program for the nonthrowing extremity should be employed to prevent asymmetrical development of the shoulders and arms (Priest 1989). Failure to develop either sufficient flexibility or strength might result in decreased performance and an increased likelihood of injury.

WRESTLING

The importance of flexibility to wrestling performance is mainly theoretical. Empirical evidence indicates that adequate flexibility is necessary for many offensive and defensive movements (Evans et al. 1993). For instance, flexibility in the hips and legs permits a wrestler to lower the center of gravity in the defensive position (Sharratt 1984). Consequently, the greater ROM of the hip allows more techniques from a defensive position (Song and Garvie 1976). "This can be a chain in thought, that is, this increase in confidence while in the defensive position will allow the wrestler to attack freely and not become pre-occupied by fear of making a mistake and ending up on the bottom only to be pinned" (p. 15). Also, "flexibility enables the wrestler to 'deform' enough to avoid tissue tearing as well as to slip out of positions that would otherwise be disabling" (Kreighbaum and Barthels 1985, p. 297). For example, the shoulder girdle is often used as a point of attack, particularly when both wrestlers are on

the ground. Hence, wrestlers with tight shoulders must go with the move put on them or suffer injury (Sharratt 1984) (see figure 19.5). The greater the active flexibility, the better a wrestler is able to wrap the body, arms, and legs around the opponent (Kreighbaum and Barthels 1985). A study by Song and Garvie (1980) of 44 wrestlers training at the Canadian Olympic Training Center reported no significant relationship between flexibility and the different weight classes.

The need for flexibility is also recognized in sumo wrestling. Because sumo wrestling requires considerable speed and agility, stretching is a major component of their training regimen.

WEIGHT LIFTING, POWER LIFTING, AND BODYBUILDING

Weight lifting, power lifting, and bodybuilding are three disciplines that utilize weight training. Olympic weight lifting has two compulsory lifts: the overhead snatch and the clean-and-jerk. Power lifting is competitive lifting of maximum weights in one repetition (1 RM). These lifts include the bench press, the squat, and the dead lift. Bodybuilding is concerned with the development of muscular hypertrophy and definition, body symmetry, and the reduction of body fat (Garhammer 1989b).

Resistance, or weight, training is also utilized to strengthen the areas of the body directly involved in performing skills required in other sports or activities. Such training is valuable for the enhancement of recreational and competitive performance.

Much remains to be researched on the interrelationship of flexibility and weight training. Theoretically, however, along with reducing the risk of injury, stretching and the development of flexibility are thought to improve the performance of the weight lifter by facilitating the use of optimal technique and enhancing muscular hypertrophy and strength.

Facilitating the Use of Optimal Technique

Flexibility, or mobility, in the joints is an important component of physical preparation in weight training. Good flexibility helps in executing the technical elements necessary to establish stable and steady lifting techniques of the classic exercises (Dvorkin 1986). For instance, without the requisite flexibility, a lifter cannot successfully execute the catch and receiving positions during the snatch lift.

The snatch lift requires full shoulder flexibility for external rotation so that a lifter can bail out by *rotating out* if the weight gets behind him or her. Rotating out means that a lifter completely rotates the shoulders from behind the back, getting the weight away from the body so it will not cause injury if dropped (Burgener 1991; Dvorkin

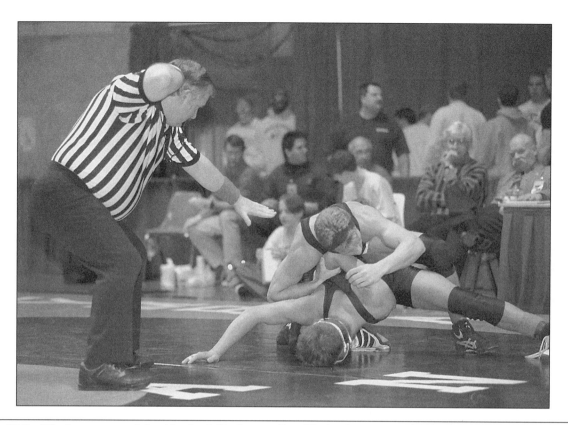

Figure 19.5   The importance of shoulder flexibility in wrestling. Notice the extreme shoulder hyperextension being forced on the man on the bottom by the man above him.

Reprinted, by permission, from M. Mysnyk, B. Davis, and B. Simpson, 1994, *Winning wrestling moves* (Champaign, IL: Human Kinetics), 151.

1986; Kulund et al. 1978). To achieve this specific flexibility, shoulder dislocation exercises with a broomstick are commonly recommended (Kulund et al. 1978; Vorobiev 1987; see exercise 284 in *Sport Stretch*).

Lifters also need flexibility in the spinal column and elbow joints. Although no substantiating data was presented, Vorobiev (1987) states that high indices of flexibility in the spinal column correlate with high achievement in the snatch lift. A significant (extreme) decrease in mobility in the spinal column makes getting under the barbell (literally) and fixing the barbell (catching the barbell in a controlled position with the back fairly upright and the bar overhead) in the snatch lift more difficult. Insufficient flexibility in the elbow joint is postulated to result in poor "locking" (elbow extension).

Other areas of the body that require flexibility in weight lifters are the quadriceps, the adductors, and the Achilles tendon, which are all stretched during the squat position of the snatch and clean-and-jerk lifts. In the opinion of Webster (1986),

> The need for flexibility in the Achilles and ankles is not well-known and needs greater attention. Tight Achilles and ankles result in the heel raising from the floor, reducing the size of the base and making the lift less stable. Furthermore, the

ability to steeply incline the shins forward, well in advance of the toes, gives a much better position by reducing the tilt of the pelvis, which in turn reduces the lumbar curve. (p. 91)

Hence, a certain degree of flexibility is required for optimal performance (see figure 19.6).

Female lifters have been suggested to be more flexible than male lifters and thus are able to master weight-lifting techniques more readily than men (Giel 1988).

Enhancing Muscular Hypertrophy, Strength, and Bodybuilding Performance

Zulak (1991) contends that stretching a muscle, and specifically its fascia, facilitates muscular hypertrophy by reduction of a hypothesized inhibiting factor that somehow slows muscle growth (i.e., tight fascia does not provide room in which muscle can grow). John Parrillo, a nutritionist and bodybuilding expert, believes that stretching a muscle is not only important but also absolutely essential for bodybuilders to develop "maximum muscle size, shape and separation" (Zulak 1991, p. 108). Parrillo contends that stretching the fascia is

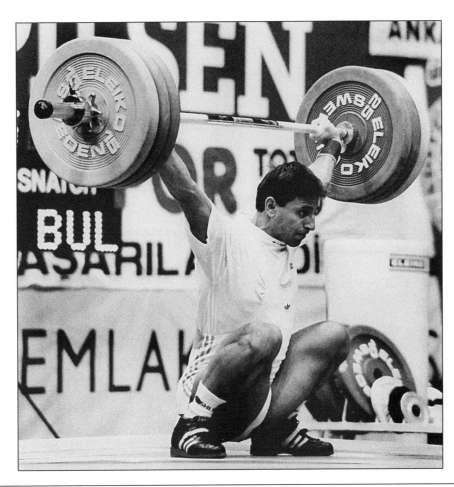

Figure 19.6   The importance of flexibility in weight lifting. Notice the flexibility of the ankles, knees, groin, shoulders, elbows, and wrists. Yoto Yotev of Bulgaria (155 kg) performs the snatch at the 1994 World Championships in Istanbul.

Photo by Bruce Klemens.

the key to success because "thickened, toughened fascia limits muscle growth and gives a bodybuilder's development a flat appearance" (Zulak 1991, p. 107). Additional stretching gives the muscle underneath the fascia greater room in which to grow. According to Parrillo, the fascia should be stretched when the muscles are fully pumped up (full of blood) and after every set.

Parrillo has proposed several other reasons why stretching is advantageous for bodybuilders. Stretching can increase one's strength on a neurological level by as much as 15% to 20%. This improvement is theoretically made possible by raising the GTOs' threshold (see chapter 6). Consequently, one is capable of handling heavier weights and more repetitions. Stretching helps to "recharge" the muscles by enhancing the removal of lactic acid that hinders muscular contraction. The loosening effect of stretching helps the bodybuilder breathe better during the workout, increasing the oxygen utilization for improved energy levels. Stretching may cause muscle fibers to split and increase in numbers (i.e., hyperplasia). Stretching gives the body a more graceful appearance—essential when posing in a routine. Clearly,

clinical testing under controlled conditions is necessary to substantiate these claims.

Flexibility training properly performed has several benefits for bodybuilders.

- It allows the bodybuilder to perform the choreographed poses.
- It allows the bodybuilder to display muscle groups that otherwise would be impossible to see.
- It allows the bodybuilder to perform with greater ease and economy of motion.
- It allows the bodybuilder to coordinate the movements of the trunk, head, hips, and limbs in a harmonious manner.
- It allows the body builder to execute well-coordinated movements in an aesthetically appealing manner.
- It allows the bodybuilder to flow through routines that are enjoyable to watch.
- It allows the bodybuilder to win (or place higher) in a competition.

Weider (1995) contends that many "bodybuilders attempt to mask their muscle tightness by performing twisting poses instead of remedying the condition by enhancing flexibility" (p. 136).

Relationship Between Tension and Muscular Hypertrophy

Tension is one of the many important factors involved in the regulation of skeletal muscle size and hypertrophy (Vandenburgh 1987). Other factors include force, strain, damage and repair, metabolic stress, and hormonal influences (Fowles et al. 2000a). Studies on developing embryos show that passive stretch plays an important role in muscular development. Stretch has been implicated in such processes as early muscle growth and development (Ashmore 1982; Barnett et al. 1980; Holly et al. 1980), denervation hypertrophy (Goldspink et al. 1974), dystrophic muscle (Ashmore 1982; Day et al. 1984; Frankeny et al. 1983), neurogenic atrophy (Pachter and Eberstein 1985), and compensatory hypertrophy (Gutmann et al. 1971; Schiaffino 1974; Schiaffino and Hanzlíková 1970; Thomsen and Luco 1944). Although mechanical stretching of skeletal muscle has been known to increase its metabolic rate for more than 80 years, the mechanism involved is still unknown (Vandenburgh and Kaufman 1979). Passive stretching increases DNA and RNA concentrations in chickens (Ashmore 1982; Barnett et al. 1980; Carson and Booth 1998) and rats (Loughna and Morgan 1999), oxidative enzyme activity in chicken muscle (Frankeny et al. 1983; Holly et al. 1980), and proteolytic enzyme activities in chicken muscles (Day et al.1984). Although these studies are interesting, they dealt only with animals. Consequently, the relevance of these studies to humans has been questioned (Alter 1996; Kadi 2000; Lowe and Alway 2002).

Because both forceful contraction and passive stretch result in an increase in muscle tension, does the increase in tension per se, independent of whether it is produced by active contraction or passive stretch, create the stimulus for protein synthesis and muscle enlargement? Fowles et al. (2000a) employed an isolated bout of maximal tolerated passive stretch for 27 minutes on the soleus muscle of human volunteers. The study determined that an acute bout of maximum passive stretch of the calf muscle is not a sufficient stimulus to elevate the fractional muscle protein synthetic rate. Thus, because the duration of the stretch (27 minutes) greatly exceeded the total time (1 to 2 minutes) that a muscle might be subject to a stretch in a typical resistance-training session, "it is reasonable to conclude that passive stretch per se is not a major contributor to the elevation in FSR observed following weightlifting" (p. 178).

Using an animal model in lieu of human stretching exercises for studying muscle hypertrophy or elongation

offers two primary advantages. (1) The investigator has tight experimental control of the subjects. (2) After the experiment, animals can be sacrificed, and muscles and other soft tissues can be removed.

The chief disadvantage of using animal models is the extent to which the results can be generalized to humans (Lowe and Alway 2002). Thus, the applicability of the foregoing animal research to humans is only speculative. Additional clinical research is needed to substantiate the practical implications of these findings.

RIB CAGE FLEXIBILITY, PERFORMANCE, AND RESPIRATION

The tissues of the *thoracic cage* have elastic recoil or its reciprocal, *compliance*. The elements responsible for elastic recoil and compliance include the diameter and shape of the chest; the height of the individual; the mass of the musculature; the amount of body fat and abdominal fluid; and the integrity of the skeletal system, muscular system, lung tissue, and connective tissue. In individuals with large, heavy, bony frames and heavy musculature, the increased mass of the upper torso muscles cause increased stiffness of the relaxed chest wall. Consequently, a greater muscle force is needed to expand the chest. Similarly, a woman with large breasts or an obese person must exert additional force to lift the added weight with each respiration. Posture also influences compliance of the chest cage. In individuals with hunched and rounded shoulders or a head-down posture, the weight of the shoulder girdle pulls down on the chest girdle. Thus, tight and inflexible intercostal or pectoral muscles decrease chest compliance and increase the burden of respiration.

Can modifying the chest compliance enhance athletic performance? A flexible and mobile chest enhances athletic, exercise, and vocational performance. As described by Bowen (1934), "With a mobile chest the muscles can more easily move the amount of air needed in quiet breathing and the subject does not so soon reach his limit in exercise that demands great increase of respiration" (p. 249).

A study of the relationship between chest girth and vital capacity was undertaken by Louttit and Halford (1930). Data from 100 boys with an average age of 15.7 years showed little or no relation between chest girth or expansion and vital chest capacity in normal boys. Barry et al. (1987) investigated the relationship between lung function and thoracic mobility in 51 normal subjects with ages ranging from 17 to 27 years. Statistically significant relationships (r = .27 to .42; $p < .05$) existed between the lung function and chest expansion variables. However, they conflicted with the findings of Louttit and Halford (1930). Neither lateral flexion of the trunk nor thoracic rotation were significantly related to lung function.

Grassino et al. (1978) demonstrated that restriction of the chest wall compartments is associated with a compensatory increase in the displacement of the abdomen to maintain a given tidal volume. Hussain et al. (1985) expanded this study and investigated whether the compensatory mechanisms influenced high-intensity cycling performance. Their investigation determined that restricted movements of the rib cage decreased tidal volume, decreased inspiratory and expiratory time, decreased diaphragmatic contractility, increased abdominal muscle recruitment in expiration, and altered the pattern of breathing in normal subjects. Perhaps of greater significance was a reduced exercise time (decreased endurance) in high-intensity exercise.

Compliance of the chest wall has rarely been modified as a controlled variable in investigations of such problems as asthma, emphysema, adult respiratory distress syndrome (ARDS), and general aging. Instead, a general mention is made about the use of stretching and mobilization for treating these conditions (Cassidy and Schwiep 1989; Neu and Dinnel 1957; Warren 1968; Watts 1968). A review of the literature located only one study dealing with stretch gymnastics training in asthmatic children (Kanamaru et al. 1990). This study found that some patients were able to relieve their dyspneic sensation (i.e., difficult or labored respiration) solely by increasing chest flexibility.

This research is potentially significant for people who have a deformity of the rib cage or respiratory illness, for healthy people, and for athletes. The question of whether exercises that increase chest expansion and upper torso flexibility improve function in these three populations should be examined in a clinical setting. To establish the existence of a causal link between chest expansion and lung function, chest expansion must be deliberately manipulated as an independent variable (Barry et al. 1987).

SPRINGBOARD AND PLATFORM DIVING

Both men's and women's springboard (1 or 3 meter) and platform diving (10 meter) are recognized by the Federation Internationale De Natation (FINA), the worldwide swimming sports governing organization. *Fina Diving Rules (D) New Rules 2001-2002* recognizes six groups of dives (forward, backward, reverse, inward, twisting, and armstand) and four basic midair body positions (straight, pike, tuck, and free).

Judging

Section D8 of FINA's diving rules pertains to judging and describes the technical requisites for the four body positions. Points are deducted from a diver's performance

for a variety of reasons. Several examples directly related to flexibility are grace, body position, pointed toes, and entry into the water. Without adequate flexibility, divers cannot fulfill the technical requisites of each dive. Therefore, without the highest level of flexibilities, the aesthetic positions needed to gain high marks in the various maneuvers cannot be obtained (Blomfield et al. 1994; Tovin and Neyer 2001) nor can the skill be executed.

Biomechanics

Two other reasons flexibility is required in diving relates to biomechanics. (1) The rate of rotation (angular velocity) of a somersaulting diver can be increased by making the body more compact or decreased by making it less compact. (2) When the body is in a tight compact tuck position, its resistance to rotation is at its lowest, and its angular velocity is at its greatest (about four times as great) (see figure 19.7).

A tighter tuck and faster rotation offers two advantages. (1) The diver has additional time to establish visual contact and "spot" the water. (2) The diver has additional time to kick out (open) before entering the pool.

Failure to attain the deep tucked position could be caused by a lack of flexibility.

Anatomical Considerations

Several parts of the body deserve special attention in developing flexibility to enhance diving ability: the neck

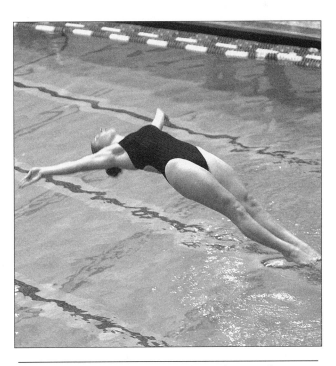

Figure 19.7 Flexibility is critical for achieving the proper biomechanics in diving.

and shoulder girdle, the lats and upper torso, the lower back and hamstrings, and the ankles.

Neck and Shoulder Girdle

Divers must develop a supple neck (cervical flexion) and shoulder girdle to facilitate the compact pike and tucked positions. Besides increasing the rotation, this added dimension enhances the aesthetic quality of the dive.

Chest, Lats, and Upper Back

Flexibility in the chest, lats, and upper back is necessary to maintain a straight armstand (handstand) position. In addition, adequate flexibility is required to execute a streamlined and vertical angle of entry into the water. The bodyline must be stretched and tight. The technical requisites state that "the arms shall be stretched beyond the head and in line with the body." However, this technique can only be performed with the necessary suppleness.

The most spectacular and ultimate entry into the pool is a *rip entry*, a head-first entry with a very low splash. Divers use the palms of their hands to create a "hole" in the water for their body to "rip" through. The more streamlined the body, the less surface area contacting the water and the greater the rip. A perfect rip entry leaves only foam, no splash. Failure to attain a streamlined entry into the water can be caused by inadequate flexibility. The lack of flexibility required by divers is a predisposing factor to shoulder injury (Carter 2001).

Hamstrings and Lower Back

The hamstrings and lower back of divers require extreme flexibility to execute the deep pike seen in many multiple-somersault dives. The deep pike increases the angular momentum and enhances the aesthetics of the dive. Hamstring and lower back flexibility is also required to perform a straight leg press to a handstand.

Ankles: Technique and Force

All divers must have a high level of ankle extension (plantar flexion). Pointed ankles and toes add to the aesthetics of the dive and assist the entry into the pool. The last thing the judges see and the final impression of the dive are the diver's ankles and toes. Thus, they are the final exclamation mark.

GOLF

According to the Bestcourses.com (2002), the United States has more than 26.7 million golfers age 12 years and over. Japan has 17 million golfers (Japan Information Network 2002 [www.jinjapan.org]), and the United Kingdom has another 4 million (Ask.com). A multitude of interacting factors determine success or failure in golf. One of these factors can be flexibility.

The full golf swing (see figure 19.8) is one of the most complex movements in sports. It necessitates strict coordination, balance, timing, strength, and flexibility. The swing is most often used when teeing off or hitting long shots from the fairway. The primary goal of the golfer is to drive the ball a desired distance and place it in the ideal position on the golf course. Each phase of the swing places unique demands on the golfer's body and results in specific numbers and types of injuries. For purposes of analysis, the swing is broken down into five major phases.

Addressing the Ball

Addressing the ball (see figure 19.8a) is taking the correct grip and proper stance in preparation to making a stroke. During this phase, the golfer typically flexes the knees. The slightly flexed knees enable the golfer to (1) lower the center of gravity, which, in turn, increases the balance by placing the center of gravity closer to the base, (2) produce greater torso rotation, (3) stretch the leg extensor muscles , (4) flatten the swing arc, and (5) gradually absorb the force during the follow-through (Maddalozzo 1987). According to Carranza (2002), subtle knee flexion works in two ways: (1) it allows the lower body to comfortably coil or rotate during the back swing and down swing, and (2) it keeps the lower body out of the way so as to allow the arms and hands to hang freely from the shoulders. Pedersen (2003) points out that flexed knees (1) allow body to make a relaxed, comfortable first swing and (2) encourage a more synchronized swing from the ground up. Flexing the knees while maintaining the feet flat on the ground requires flexibility in the gastrocnemius-soleus complex and Achilles tendon.

During the address, the golfer also flexes forward from the pelvis to the midthoracic spine with the back fairly straight, but not rigid. The flexion at the hip facilitates proper alignment and extension that follows. This action requires flexibility in the lower back.

The Takeaway (Backswing)

The backswing is bringing the club in a backward motion from the ground until it stops over the head (see figure 19.8b). The backswing establishes a perfectly balanced, powerful position at the top of the swing (Maddalozzo 1987). The arc of the backswing should be natural and simultaneously around the body and upward. This action can be likened to compressing a coil, which is the body. During the backswing, the shoulders rotate away from the target as the golfer pivots around the vertebral column. At the same time, the hips should barely move. McTeigue et al. (1994) found "on the backswing, the upper body rotates first to initiate the takeaway, and it rotates faster than the hips" (p. 55). A 90° (shoulder turn) turn is optimum so the golfer's back is directly facing the target. This movement requires the golfer to rotate his or her cervical spine a minimum of 70° to the left to maintain good head position, hence the importance of good spinal flexibility.

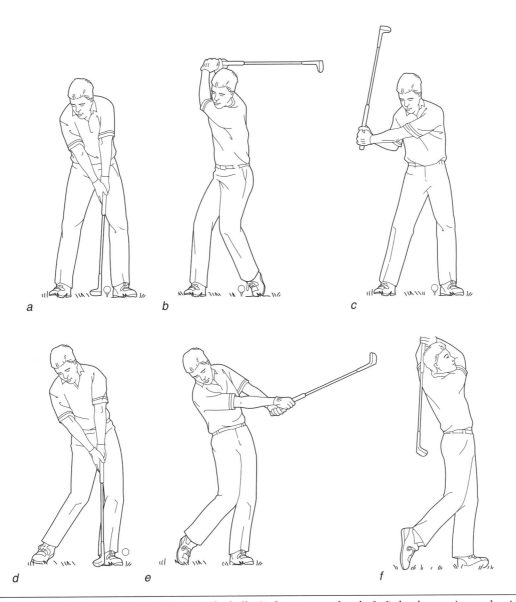

Figure 19.8   Phases of a golf drive: *(a)* addressing the ball, *(b)* the stop overhead, *(b-d)* the downswing and point of impact, and *(d-f)* the follow-through.

Reprinted by permission, from G. Carr, 1997, *Mechanics of sport* (Champaign, IL: Human Kinetics), 136-137.

During the backswing, the right-handed golfer hyper-adducts the left thumb and then radially deviates the left wrist. This action is referred to as *cocking* (i.e., to bend the wrists backwards in the back swing). Cocking naturally permits bringing the shoulders through a 90° arc and the hips through a 45° arc. At the top of the backswing, the right wrist further dorsiflexes. Not cocking the hands reduces power and distance. Repeated stress during the backswing may cause tendonitis of the wrist and epicondylitis. Other areas of stress to the golfer's body include the left hip and right shoulder (McCarroll 1986).

At the top of the backswing, the shaft of the golf club is approximately horizontal. Professional players achieve a higher backswing position than amateurs. This position is the classic and idealized position seen in many photo-graphs. However, a golfer should avoid going farther than this horizontal point because of the potential sacrifice of control. The high shaft position (horizontal) provides several advantages if properly utilized:

- The increased ROM allows the golfer to apply forces over greater distances and longer periods of time.

- The greater range allows the golfer increased velocities, energies, and momenta.

- The increased ROM permits the golfer a greater stretch on the involved muscles. As a result, those muscles can produce even greater forces because a prestretched muscle can exert more force than a nonstretched muscle.

The need for flexibility in the hip rotators during a backswing is concisely described by Ninos (2001):

> During the back swing of a right-handed golfer, tightness in the right hip external rotators and left hip internal rotators can affect range of motion. As the trunk is rotating to the right, the right hip will internally rotate while the left hip will externally rotate. Tightness in the opposite muscle groups will inhibit the hips' ability to accomplish these needed motions. (p. 26)

McCarroll et al. (1982) found 21% of all injuries occur during the backswing. In 75 injuries the most common during the takeaway were to the back (28), wrist (25), elbow, neck, and knee (9), hand (7), and shoulder (6).

The Downswing

The downswing is the motion of swinging a club from the top of the swing to the point of impact (see figure 19.8b-d). The change in direction should be a continuous motion (kinetic sequence) with a continuing acceleration. McTeigue et al. (1994) found that the hips initiated the change in direction with professional players during the downswing. Furthermore, they found that professional players have faster rotation, contributing to greater clubhead speed. During this phase, the body uncoils and turns in the direction of the swing. Jones (1999), found that 16 recreational golfers participating in an 8-week training study employing PNF stretching strategies had a significant increase in clubhead speed. During the downswing, the golfer also transfers weight from the right side to the left side and releases the wrist from radial to ulnar deviation (Murray and Cooney 1996). McLaughlin and Best (1994) substantiate that delaying adduction of the wrist (i.e., keeping the wrists in a cocked position) to the last possible moment produces the most effective golf swing. Releasing the wrists at the beginning of the downswing is referred to as *casting* and is generally associated with *coming over the top*. This action dissipates power and prohibits hitting the ball crisply.

Hosea et al. (1990), Lindsay and Horton (2002), and Sugaya et al. (1999) have identified the downswing, rather than the backswing, as the part of the swing where most stress and injuries occur. Flexibility in the shoulders, vertebral column, and hips is vital for an optimum downswing. Thus, golfers should warm-up properly before playing, as well as engage in regular stretching exercises, to improve maximum available trunk ROM (Geisler 2001; Lindsay and Horton 2002; Sugaya et al. 1999).

Ball Strike

McCarroll (1986) divides ball strike (see figure 19.8d) into preimpact and impact phases: "As the player starts to hit the ball the right wrist is in maximum dorsiflexion; the left thumb is hyperabducted; the left ulnar nerve, right elbow, and forearm muscles are under tension; and the left hip is rotated" (p. 10). Then, "at impact, the left wrist moves from a position of radial deviation through neutral to slight ulnar deviation, while the right wrist moves from a dorsiflexed, radially deviated position to a more neutral position with slight ulnar deviation" (Murray and Cooney 1996, p. 86). Impact coincides with compression at the wrist. At this moment, a substantial transfer of force from the clubhead to the hands and wrists occurs. Then, beyond impact, "the left forearm supinates and the right forearm pronates creating the 'roll-over' action of the hands" (Murray and Cooney). Thus, the right hand begins to climb over the left (Maddalozzo 1987).

Murray and Cooney (1996) state, "The range of motion required of the wrist in the golf swing exceeds the functional range of motion requirements of the wrist. Perhaps, it is the catapulting function of the left wrist at impact, as well as the increased range of motion of both wrists, which make the wrists of the golfer vulnerable to injury" (p. 86).

More injuries occur during the impact phase of the swing than any other time (McCarroll 1986). Because the clubhead accelerates from zero to over 100 miles per hour, a tremendous potential for injury exists. In particular, the compression of impact with an object other than the ball, such as when the golfer makes a divot (hits the ground), may injure the wrist and elbow. Other upper-extremity injuries that can occur during this phase include carpal fractures, carpal tunnel syndrome, tibial collateral ligament stress, and tendinitis.

Recovery, or Follow-Through

The final phase of the full swing is the follow-through (see Figure 19.8 d-f). It commences with the termination at impact. During this phase, the rolling over action of the hands continues. The wrists are fully released through ulnar deviation and back into radial deviation. The shoulder too, is subject to stress. The left shoulder raises and flexes forward, and the left elbow begins to flex. In contrast, the right shoulder rotates internally as it crosses the body. Right shoulder pain caused by stretching the long thoracic nerve is also possible (Schultz and Leonard 1992). The lumbar and cervical spinal areas rotate and hyperextend, and the hip continues to rotate. These movements are facilitated by the clubhead speed, with its resultant centrifugal force exerting an outward pull on the arms, body, and legs.

At the finish of the swing, the hips have turned along with the shoulders, so the golfer faces the intended target. Also, the head turns to accommodate the full finish of the swing and to see the shot result. During this phase the golfer passes through the classic reverse "C" position. Although this position is essential to playing better golf, it can cause injury to the back if the reverse "C" position is exaggerated. Hosea and Gatt (1996) reported that peak forces and torques at the L-3/L-4 level of the lumbar spine occur during the forward swing and follow-through, confirming many golfers' subjective reports of pain just after impact. Morgan et al. (1997) hypothesize that lateral bending and axial rotation velocities in combination contribute to lumbar degeneration and injury. They have termed this effect the *crunch factor*. A study (McCarroll et al. 1982) of injuries associated professional golfers found 106 injuries occurring during the follow-through. The injuries were located in the back (43), shoulders (18), ribs (12), knees (10), wrist (9), neck (6), elbow (4), and hand (4).

The hip region must not be overlooked. During the follow-through, a substantial amount of torque is also applied at the hip. However, the hips do not share equally in these stress reactions, because a much greater force passes through the left hip joint of a right-handed player. This fact becomes significant when considering hip replacement and postoperative recommendations (Stover et al. 1976). Furthermore, during follow-through, the right hip externally rotates while the left hip internally rotates. "These motions can be affected by tightness in the right internal rotators and left external rotators" (Nimos 2001, pp. 26-27). Hence, once again, the importance in maintaining an optimum ROM via a flexibility-training program. Further elaborating on this point, Geisler (2001) writes:

> The follow-through phase requires sufficient flexibility of both upper quarters and hips to reach the full finish position. Limitations in hip internal or external rotation or the shoulders will not allow the golfer to fully follow through and thus not allow sufficient time to safely decelerate the swing. Lumbar extension is also required to swing through the ball and finish in a high, balanced position. When physical limitations such as these are not addressed, increased stresses and compensatory actions inevitably can become a consistent component of the golf swing. (p. 215)

Golfers must be cognizant that just one tight link can compromise the efficiency of the entire chain. Thus, stretching can help prepare the body for the proper sequencing of the swing. On the other hand, golfers must also warm up before stretching and initially stretch slowly. All golfers must recognize that stretching programs are compulsory not only to reduce the risk of injury but also to enhance performance. However, stretching should also be accompanied by incorporating a program of strengthening, muscular endurance, and cardiovascular exercises.

BALLET AND OTHER FORMS OF DANCE

Theatrical dance includes classical ballet and modern dance; each is distinct in its origin, form, and fundamental physical demands (Wiesler et al. 1996, p. 754). Those who attain the apex and pinnacle of their specialty are the product of a rigorous and unforgiving selection process. Hardaker et al. (1984) described this selection process as a "Darwinism of dance." Various factors contribute to the weeding out process: body shape and weight, femoral anteversion, genu valgum or varum, leg length, rigid pes planus, pes cavus, coordination, rhythm, musicality, strength, power, endurance, and flexibility (Gelabert 1989; Huwyler 1989; Kushner et al. 1990; Stone et al. 2001). Whether "successful" dancers are a result of nurture (training) or nature (genetic predisposition) remains to be resolved. Studies of ballet students and professional dancers, both male and female, report superior flexibility when compared with control subjects (Chatfield et al. 1990; Grahame and Jenkins 1972; Klemp and Learmonth 1984; Klemp et al. 1984; Micheli et al. 1984). The one area of exception is a decrease in hip internal rotation compared with nondancers (DiTullio et al. 1989).

Anatomical Considerations

Dancers are renowned for their extreme flexibility in virtually every part of their bodies. However, two parts of the body deserve special attention in developing flexibility to enhance performance: the ankles and hips.

The Ankle

Female dancers, especially ballet dancers when dancing *en pointe*, have greater needs for ankle flexibility, specifically plantar flexion. Weisler et al. (1996) found that female ballet dancers have a decreased ankle ROM in eversion and inversion compared with modern dancers. This finding is predictable because ballet dancers have very little need to use their feet in these two positions. Khan et al. (2000) found that elite dancers 16 to 18 years of age who enter full-time ballet training do not augment their ankle dorsiflexion to any appreciable degree.

Quirk (1994) suggested that ankle ROM may be related to future ankle injuries. However, Weisler et al. (1996) "found little evidence to support the hypothesis that abnormalities in ankle range of motion serve as predictors for subsequent injury" (p. 757).

The Hip

The ideal 180° (90° per leg) external rotation demanded of professional ballet dancers is usually achieved with 60° to 70° of external rotation from above the knee and 20° to 30° from below the knee (Hardaker et al. 1984) (see figure 19.9). Turnout is often forced at the knees and feet by those who cannot perform sufficient hip lateral rotation. This attempted compensation places increased external torsional stress on the knees and can produce medial knee strain and patellar subluxation. The most common method of forcing the turnout is *screwing the knee*. This movement is accomplished by performing a demi-plié (half knee bend), allowing a 180° position of

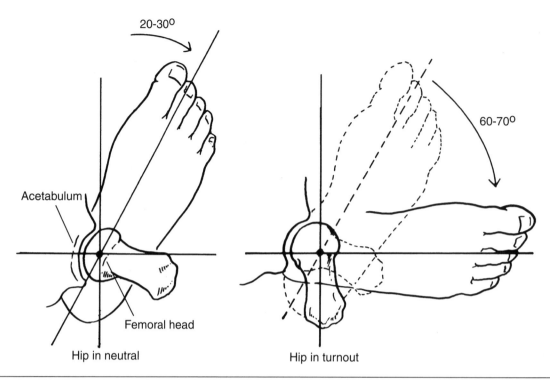

Figure 19.9 The dancer's hip turnout. In ideal circumstances, the 90° of desired turnout is achieved by a combination of external rotation at the hip, knee, and ankle joints. Theoretically, the majority of external rotation (60° to 70°) occurs at the hip with the remaining 20° to 30° occurring from the combined outward inclination of the foot, ankle, and knee joints.

Reprinted, by permission, from W.T. Hardaker, L. Erickson, and M. Myers, 1984, The pathogenesis of dance injury. In *The dancer as athlete*, edited by C.G. Shell (Champaign, IL: Human Kinetics), 12-13.

the feet, then straightening the knees without moving the feet (Ende and Wickstrom 1982; Hald 1992; Stone et al. 2001; Teitz 1982). The effect is similar when a football player firmly plants a cleated shoe in the ground and then rotates the leg (Miller et al. 1975). Forcing the feet into 180° of turnout places stress on the medial aspect of the ankles and feet, potentially leading to pronated feet and flattening of the plantar arches.

Because the turnout at the hip is determined mostly by the bony structure and by the surrounding hip-joint capsule and connective tissue, one may wonder to what extent this structure and flexibility can be affected by training. According to the consensus of medical literature, spontaneous changes in anteversion occur most rapidly from birth to age 8 years, and the process is nearly finished by age 10 years. However, it is not completely finished until about age 16 years. Later attempts to correct anteversion seem to have little effect. Rather, compensatory external rotation deformity is created in the tibia below the knee. Khan et al. (2000) conducted a 12-month study of 28 female and 20 male elite first-year and second-year professional ballet dancers aged 16 to 18 years to see if they could improve hip ROM. Among both sexes, the first-year students significantly increased their left hip external rotation greater than the second-year students.

The investigators suggested the difference might be the result of a training effect during the first year that reached a plateau in the second year. Nonetheless, they cautioned that not all 16-year-old to 18-year-old dancers have the capacity to improve their external rotation.

Bauman et al. (1994) found that dancers who had excellent turnout also had lower than average femoral neck angles. Consequently, "it appears that the soft tissues, rather than the skeleton, must allow for increased external rotation and turnout at the hip" (p. 61). G.W. Warren (1989), further addressing this issue, succinctly states:

> Very few human bodies possess the capacity for perfect turn out. Students should remember that they are trying to achieve more than the ability simply to turn their legs outward. Their goal must be to develop the muscular strength to *control* and *maintain* their own maximum degree of turn-out *at all times* while they are dancing. (p. 11)

Another consequence of the emphasis on abduction flexibility may cause limited adduction ROM secondary to tightness of the iliotibial band. In turn, this imbalance may further contribute to pain in the anterior hip, lateral hip, or lateral knee (Reid et al. 1987; Hald 1992).

Stretching Cessation and Its Effect on Flexibility

In a study (Koutedakis et al. 1999) of 17 professional ballerinas (mean age 27.2 years), volunteers examined the effects of a 6-week summer break on selected physiological parameters, including flexibility. Compared with prebreak data, the 6-weeks of holiday was followed by a 15% overall increase in three flexibility tests. The findings were in contrast with the current literature, according to which, deconditioning occurs when formal exercise ceases. Elaborating on their findings, Koutedakis et al. (1999) write:

> The present findings also contradict the dancers' general perception of rest, especially on parameters such as muscle flexibility and joint mobility. Traditionally, professional dancers start their season with many hours of "stretch" exercises in an attempt to regain the supposedly lost, or reduced, muscle flexibility and joint mobility. Clearly, our data do not support such practices, since flexibility levels were higher at the end of the rest period than at the beginning. (p. 382)

Additional research is necessary for an understanding of the mechanisms associated with this finding.

MUSICIANS

According to the Gallup Organization, more than 62 million amateur musicians aged 5 years and older live in the United States. Six in 10 American households include someone who has experience playing a musical instrument; in half of these households, one or more people currently play (Gallup Organization 2000, p. 2). Multitudes of factors, often interacting, determine success or failure in the field of music. One factor may be flexibility. The following sections analyze two broad categories of music performance potentially impacted by flexibility: vocal and selected instrumental.

Vocal

The body is a singer's instrument. A singer has no external pedals and no special wood to deepen and enrich her tone. Her work centers on making changes inside her body—not just changes that lead to better voicing but changes that lead to artistic singing. Her sense of rhythm, pacing, emotion, phrasing, and drama—all the nuances of a beautiful sung work—start and stop inside her body. (Caldwell and Wall 2001, p. 7)

"Singing is a sensory-motor phenomenon that requires particular balanced physical skills" (Bunch 1997, p. 7). One important factor that can affect a singer's performance is flexibility. The major reasons flexibility is important fall under the categories of physiological parameters, psychological parameters, and aesthetics.

Physiology

Any study of the physiology of vocal production reveals the complexity of the various anatomical parts and the intricate coordination needed for these parts to produce sound. Furthermore, singing is intimately connected to breathing. Breathing, in turn, is dependent upon the mechanics of the upper trunk, in particular, the ribs, thoracic spine, and intercostal muscles. The ribs must move freely for the lungs to work optimally. When the rib cage cannot properly expand, the vacuum created in the lungs brings in less air. Tightness in the ribs, which is actually tightness in the intercostals that connect the ribs, may have many causes (Nelson and Blades-Zeller, 2002, p. 89), but the focus here is on tight intercostal muscles.

During inhalation, the short external intercostal muscles contract and expand the rib cage and increase the anterior-posterior (AP) diameter of the chest. Simultaneously, the sternum moves forward and upward, also expanding the AP dimensions. In contrast, during forced exhalation, the internal intercostals contract and pull the ribs closer together, as well as down and in. This action decreases the size of the thoracic cavity. Therefore, optimum lung capacity requires a flexible rib cage.

> The significance of a flexible body must not be underestimated. Tension in muscles of the shoulder and chest affects the singer's estimation of how much air is needed or is available for use. A false sense of fullness can be produced which misleads the singer into believing that he has an adequate supply, and only when he begins to sing does he realize that little air was taken in and therefore very little breath is available. (Bunch 1997, p. 53)

Another aspect of singing is chest-wall vibrations (Sundberg 1983). According to Sundberg, "it seems likely that the sensations of chest vibrations can serve as a useful nonauditory and hence room-independent signal for the voluntary control of phonation" (p. 329). Assuming then, that a tight chest can impact sensations of chest-wall vibrations, stretching hypothetically may beneficially influence this useful internal feedback signal. However, a controlled study is necessary to substantiate this theory.

Physiologically, the benefits of stretching for singers are thought to be similar to warm-up for athletes. Anecdotal claims extolling positive psychological advantages are found throughout musical literature (Jerome 1988;

Paull and Harrison 1997). Several significant benefits are thought to include improved relaxation, facilitated unwinding and decompression, and providing a mental period of transition from preperformance to performance.

Additional anecdotal and theoretical (Bruser 1997, pp. 30-32; Sirbaugh 1995; Sundberg 1983; *Teaching Music* 2001) benefits of stretching include

- facilitating unwinding and decompression,
- relieving the stress of daily situations,
- releasing tense muscles and preparing them for work,
- preparing the body's muscles for their major task,
- loosening up the spine and freeing the spinal cord and its attaching sensory and motor nerves, which, in turn, increases sensitivity to sounds and sensations,
- while fully breathing, making the space inside the body more fluid so the organs can expand and move more freely,
- facilitating musical vibrations that can then move more easily through the organs, bringing the singer into a more complete engagement with the music while singing and, thus, creating a more full-bodied tone, and
- facilitating greater expressive ability.

Another vital component in a performance is the aesthetic appeal. An artist can sing every note technically correct and with incredible energy. However, if the visual presentation appears lacking because of a "constricted" or "tight" appearance, the actual qualitative aspect of the performance may suffer. Hearing a recording of a singer is one thing; actually seeing the singer on stage is another. A singer needs to be able to perform with a flexible and expressive body that actively supports the changing needs of the performance (Caldwell and Wall 2001, p. 7).

Instrumental

Musicians endowed with flexibility in those areas of the body related to their chosen instrument may have a predisposition to excel because with many musical instruments, manual dexterity is essential for optimum performance (Beighton et al. 1999). The relationship between flexibility and instrumentalists is reviewed in this section. Two major groups of instrumentalists that are examined are string players and keyboard players.

String Instrumentalists

Among the better known and most numerous string instruments are the violin, viola, cello, double bass, and guitar. Each instrument has its own distinct technical requisites and physical demands. Two pertinent questions that relate to string instrumentalists are the relationship between flexibility and successful careers and the relationship between flexibility and injury.

The ability to span the fingerboard is one of the requisites for successful performance. Instrumentalists might be assumed to have above average ROM in their upper extremity. Niccolo Paganini (1782-1840), a virtuoso violinist is a frequently cited example of a musician widely suspected having suffered from Marfan's syndrome (Beighton et al. 1999; Brandfonbrener 2000; Schoenfeld 1978; Wolf 2001). This syndrome is associated with joint laxity. However, this diagnosis is questionable, because no evidence supports, and considerable evidence discounts, his having a diffuse connective tissue disorder (Brandfonbrener 2000, p. 72). Mantel (1995, p. 44), writing on cello techniques, emphasizes the need for extensibility of the body to facilitate both physical performance and aesthetic impression.

A study by Kloeppel (2000, p. 23) of cellists, guitarists, and a control group found all groups showed more "spreadability" of the fingers on the left hand than on the right hand. The reason for this difference is not known. Other findings were that only negligible changes of the finger span occur because of the influence of playing the cello or the guitar, and a significantly greater difference existed in favor of the left-hand span between the index and small fingers only in cellists and in none of the guitarists. The increased span can possibly be attributed to practice.

Hypermobility of the thumb and wrist (including the fingers) can be an asset in playing instruments such as the flute, violin, and piano (Larsson et al. 1993). However, hypermobility of joints providing support, such as the spine, and to some extent the knee, can be a liability during long periods of practice and performance. A study (Kihira et al. 1995) of wrist motion of right-handed violinists found that the right wrist used a wider ROM in both flexion/extension and radioulnar deviation than did the left wrist in playing several pieces of music.

Compared with professional instrumentalists, dedicated amateurs share "many epidemiologic, etiologic, and diagnostic parameters" (Dawson 2001, p. 152). Approximately 5% to 7% of the general population has a condition known as *benign laxity* (Biro 1983, p. 701), meaning they have moderately hyperextensible joints in the absence of any other associated connective tissue defects. Nonetheless, Brandfonbrener (1990, 1997) found that more than 20% of instrumentalists with hand and arm pain are hyperextensible. Consequently, Brandfonbrener (2001) believes that "excessive laxity of certain joints of the hand and fingers may increase the potential for a variety of overuse injuries and painful syndromes" (p. 24). Dawson (1995) has raised concern about extrapolating the relationship between hypermobile instrumentalists and pain. In 16 patients, "overuse" diagnoses were made, thus relegating the hypermobile condition to that of an associated or coexisting diagnosis.

In general, musicians with hypermobility of specific joints report definite symptoms more often than those who do not have hypermobility of the same joints (Larsson et al. 1993). Two explanations (Brandfonbrener 1997, 2000) have been offered to explain the association between hyperlaxity and musicians' pain: (1) Joints with a supranormal ROM presumably are subject to increased mechanical wear and tear and potentially to ligamentous strain and sprains. (2) The inability to stabilize a finger on a given string or key increases muscle tension when stability is not provided by the ligaments.

Brandfonbrener (1990) recommends that methods be developed to compensate for preexistent laxity and to provide protection from damage caused by the unstable joints.

Another possible cause of injury to musicians' wrists can be a restricted flexibility (hypomobility) in the upper extremity. Because the wrist joint is just one part of a kinematic chain, restricted flexibility may result in an additional compensatory strain on the wrist (Schuppert and Wagner 1996).

Anecdotal and empirical testimony advocates a wide range of strategies to reduce the risk and severity of injury and improve performance. Among these strategies are avoiding overuse, avoiding misuses, maintaining proper posture, warming up, applying self-massage, taking stretch breaks, employing two short rehearsals rather than one long, intense session, never playing through pain, getting sufficient rest and sleep, reducing stress, and visiting a health-care provider when in doubt (Arskey 2001; Davies 2002; Frederickson 2002; Medoff 1999; *Teaching Music* 2001).

Keyboard Instrumentalists

Keyboard instrumentalists play principally the piano, fortepiano (literally, "soft-loud", because it responded to the weight of the player's touch), harpsichord, clavichord, organ, and synthesizer. This section is primarily devoted to the piano.

The piano was invented by Bartolomeo Cristofori in Italy around 1709. Over the years, significant alterations to the instrument have included the size of both its keys and its keyboard. Today, the standard piano has an 88-note keyboard that spans 48 inches, substantially larger than the keyboard played on and written for by musicians such as Bach and Beethoven. Two pertinent questions are examined. (1) What is the relationship between finger spreadability (flexibility) or hand size of pianists and successful careers? (2) What is the relationship between flexibility of pianists and injury?

Sarcastically, Donison (1998) recalls two great, related secrets in the world of piano playing: The instrument is much easier to play with larger hands, and the instrument

is impossible to play with smaller hands. Donison points out that the female is on average 15% smaller than males. Consequently, the standard keyboard is too large for most women. In search of improved spreadability, some musicians have utilized several strengthening and stretching devices for the hand (Kloeppel 2000). Perhaps the most celebrated example was the nineteenth century composer and pianist Robert Schumann. He purportedly invented a machine to stretch his fingers and improve his technique. The result was a finger paralysis that ended his playing career (Chissell 1967; von Wasielewski 1975). Sams (1971), however, contends that Schumann's hand injury was caused by either mercury poisoning or syphilis.

What then, does the research indicate regarding ROM and playing piano? Wagner (1988) found a greater passive movability in pianists than in the general population. However, piano playing employs active flexibility, not passive flexibility. Furthermore, to date, no studies demonstrate the long-term exercise/fingering protocol to detect any resulting changes in spreadability. However, Kloeppel believes "If one takes into consideration that the increase of spreadability and finger length takes place, if at all, in the range of a few or even 1 millimeter, the possibility for influencing the predispositioned conditions seems very remote" (p. 30).

Wagner (1974, p. 26) cites Trendelenburg (1923) and Ortmann (1962) in stating that the degree of finger flexibility may be a limiting factor in performance or difficulties of technique. In the opinion of Ortmann (1962), the limit to the ROM, whether it is stiffness or looseness, is caused by the bones and the soft parts surrounding the joints. Wagner (1974) has demonstrated that "passive finger flexibility varies to an extraordinarily high degree: Spreading and hyperextension showed coefficients of variation between 23% and 47%" (p. 259). Wagner (1974) found a small decrease in flexibility during the middle period of life. Does this decrease have any functional significance on the slight decrease of finger dexterity? "For some professions, especially the musician whom depends on a constant level of fine motor abilities far beyond the 50th year, this problem has great practical importance" (Piperek 1971, cited by Wagner 1974, p. 275).

Currently, "no study has examined the link between range of motion at the piano and the possible development of injury" (Wristen 2000, p. 63). However, many proposed causes have been postulated as having the potential to contribute to injury development (Wristen 2000, pp. 56-62). Further study is required to verify these hypotheses.

The advantages of stretching and warm-up for piano players are analogous to those previously mentioned.

- Stretching facilitates unwinding and decompression.

- Stretching relieves the stress of daily situations.
- Stretching releases tense muscles, preparing them for work.
- Stretching preparing the body's muscles for their major task.
- Stretching loosens up the spine and frees the spinal cord and its attaching sensory and motor nerves, which in turn, increases sensitivity to sounds and sensations (Bruser 1997; Norris 1993; Roskell 1998; Sirbaugh 1995; *Teaching Music* 2001).

Stretching can possibly facilitate greater expressive ability of the pianist. In turn, greater expressiveness can enhance the aesthetic appeal of performance. For example, if a pianist appears "constricted" or "tight," the actual qualitative aspect of the performance may suffer. Krugman (1995) described the posture of several master pianists who performed at Carnegie Hall. The following selected comments relate to posture and flexibility.

- Pianists whose trunk, head, and hips are relatively less mobile as they play seem to produce unnecessary effort in their hands, wrists, and arms, especially when reaching for very high or very low notes or in passages that require crossing of the arms.
- Pianists whose trunk, head, and hips are freely mobile as they play seem to move their hands, wrists, and arms with greater ease and economy of motion and less effort.
- The pianists who seem the most at ease at the piano are those who coordinate the movements of the trunk, head, hips, and limbs in a harmonious manner. Such easy, well-coordinated movement is a pleasure to watch (Krugman 1995).

A pianist's flexibility can and does impact the quality of performance.

Percussionists

Percussion instruments were probably the first musical instruments developed by humans. Percussion instruments have no strings or mouthpieces. Instead, they are struck by hand or hit, banged, or tapped with an implement such as a drumstick. Percussion instruments are classified as those with definite pitch, such as the timpani, piano, harp and xylophone, and those with indefinite pitch, such as the bass drum, triangle and woodblock. Some of the other percussion instruments include the marimba, cymbals, glockenspiels, timpanis, wooden chickitas, maracas, castanets, sonajero, tambourine, bells, and gong.

Percussionists share a commonality with all other musicians: they can benefit by stretching and enhancing their ROM. Stretching is thought to enhance performance, reduce the risk of injury, and improve the general wellness of the percussionist. Journals devoted to this discipline regularly publish articles detailing the benefits of stretching and how to do it properly (Haley 2000; Mikula 1998; Workman 1999, 2002).

SUMMARY

Numerous factors go into creating optimal performance, and flexibility is generally recognized as one of these crucial factors. Flexibility enhances and optimizes the learning, practice, and performance of such skills as dance and music. Because ROM is specific to many disciplines, some skills may be enhanced more effectively by purposefully increasing or decreasing the ROM around certain joints until the apparent optimal flexibility is reached. Stretching may enhance muscular hypertrophy and improve respiratory function for people with respiratory disorders. These and other claims need to be investigated to substantiate any practical implications.

Stretching Exercises

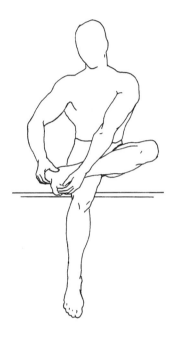

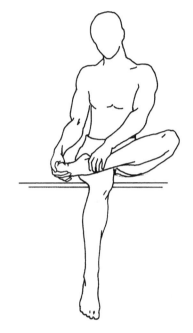

1—Plantar Arch

1. Sit upright in a chair or on the floor with one leg crossed over the opposite knee.
2. Grasp your ankle with one hand.
3. Grasp the underside of your toes and ball of the foot with your other hand.
4. Inhale, and pull your toes toward your shin (extension of the toes).
5. Hold the stretch and relax.
6. You should feel the stretch in the sole of the raised foot.

2—Anterior Aspect of the Toes

1. Sit upright in a chair or on the floor with one leg crossed over the opposite knee.
2. Grasp your ankle and heel with one hand.
3. Grasp the top portion of your foot and toes with your other hand.
4. Inhale, and slowly pull the bottom of your toes toward the ball of your foot (flexion).
5. Hold the stretch and relax.
6. You should feel the stretch on the top of the foot and toes.

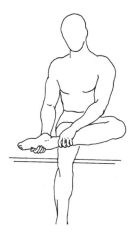

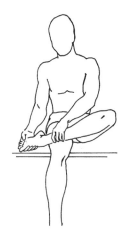

3—Anterior Portion of the Ankle and Lower Leg

1. Sit upright in a chair or on the floor with one leg crossed over the opposite knee.
2. Grasp your leg above your ankle with one hand.
3. Grasp the top portion of your foot with your other hand.
4. Inhale, and slowly pull the sole of your foot toward your body (plantar flexion).
5. Hold the stretch and relax.
6. You should feel the stretch in the instep and top of the ankle.

5—Anterior and Lateral Aspect of the Ankle and Lower Leg

1. Sit upright in a chair or on the floor with one leg crossed over the opposite knee.
2. Grasp your ankle and heel with one hand.
3. Grasp the top outside portion of your foot with the other hand.
4. Inhale, and slowly invert your ankle (turn it upward).
5. Hold the stretch and relax.
6. You should feel the stretch in the anterior and lateral aspect of the ankle and lower leg.

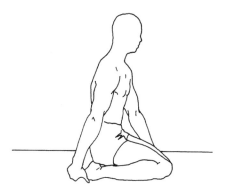

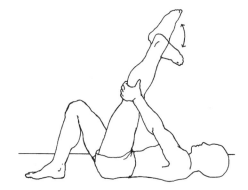

4—Anterior Portion of the Ankle and Lower Leg

1. Kneel with your toes pointing backward. If this position is uncomfortable, place a blanket under your shins.
2. Exhale, and slowly sit on the top of your heels (if you can).
3. Reach around, grasp the top portion of your toes, and pull them toward your head.
4. Hold the stretch and relax.
5. You should feel the stretch along the shin. The muscle primarily targeted is the tibialis anterior. *Note:* This stretch is used to prevent shinsplints. However, make sure your hips sit on top of the heels and *not* between the feet. (The latter position is called W sitting and is bad for the knees.) This stretch should be avoided by people with a history of knee problems.

6—Achilles Tendon and Posterior Lower Leg

1. Lie on your back with the legs extended.
2. Flex one leg and slide the foot toward the buttocks.
3. Raise the opposite leg toward your face and grasp behind the knee.
4. Inhale, and slowly dorsiflex the foot toward your face.
5. Hold the stretch and relax.
6. You should feel the stretch in the Achilles tendon. *Note:* If you have back problems, after the stretch you should flex the extended leg and slowly lower it to the floor.

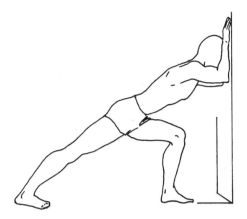

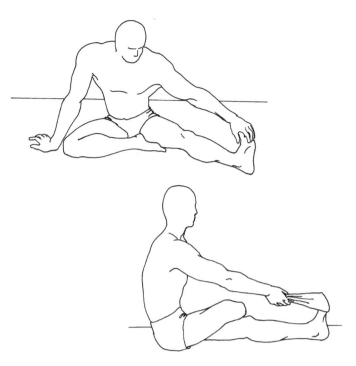

7—Gastrocnemius and Achilles Tendon

1. Stand upright slightly more than arm's length from a wall.
2. Bend one leg forward and keep the opposite leg straight.
3. Lean against the wall without losing the straight line of your head, neck, spine, pelvis, rear leg, and ankle.
4. Keep the heel of your rear foot down, sole flat on the floor, and foot pointing straight forward.
5. Exhale, bend your arms, lean toward the wall, and shift your weight forward.
6. Exhale, and flex your forward knee toward the wall.
7. Hold the stretch and relax.
8. You should feel the stretch in the calf and Achilles tendon. *Note:* To stretch the soleus, flex the rear leg at the knee.

9—Back of the Knee

1. Sit upright on the floor with the legs straight.
2. Keep one leg straight and bend the opposite leg in until its heel touches the groin of the extended leg.
3. Exhale, lean forward, and grasp your foot.
4. Exhale, keep your leg straight, and pull your foot back toward your trunk.
5. Hold the stretch and relax. *Note:* If you cannot reach your foot, use a folded towel. To intensify the stretch, cross the bent leg and rest the heel on the opposite knee, and then apply the stretch.

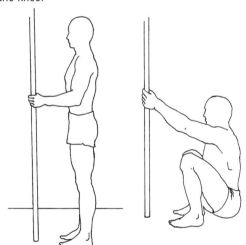

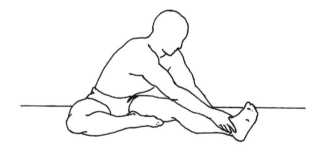

8—Quadriceps

1. Stand upright, with your feet parallel and about 30 cm (1 ft) apart, holding a pole.
2. Exhale, lean backward slightly, keeping your heels flat on the floor and knees behind your toes, and squat as low as you can.
3. Hold the stretch and relax.
4. You should feel the stretch in the quadriceps.
5. Inhale and return to the starting position. *Note:* This stretch may also be felt in the adductors (i.e., groin) and Achilles tendon of those who are tight in these areas.

10—Hamstrings

1. Sit upright on the floor with both legs straight.
2. Flex one knee and slide the heel until it touches the inner side of the opposite thigh.
3. Lower the outer side of the thigh and calf of the bent leg onto the floor.
4. Exhale, and while keeping the extended leg straight, bend at the hip and lower your extended upper torso from the hips onto the extended thigh.
5. Hold the stretch and relax.
6. You should feel the stretch in the hamstrings.

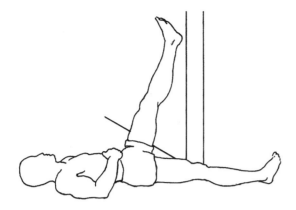

11—Hamstrings

1. Lie flat on your back in a doorway.
2. Position your hips slightly in front of the doorframe.
3. Raise one leg and rest it against the doorframe, while keeping this knee extended and your bottom leg flat on the floor. To increase the stretch, slide the buttocks closer to the doorframe or lift the leg away from the doorframe.
4. Hold the stretch and relax.
5. You should feel the stretch in the hamstrings. *Note:* To intensify the stretch, use a folded towel wrapped around the foot of the raised leg. By pulling on the towel, the leg can be pulled away from the doorframe and closer to your chest.

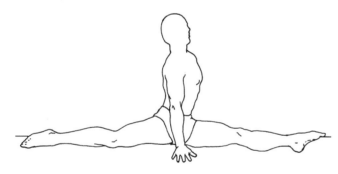

12—Hamstrings

1. Kneel on the floor with both legs together and your hands at your sides.
2. Lift up one knee and place your foot slightly in front for support.
3. Exhale, bend at the waist, lower your upper torso down onto the front thigh, and place your hands slightly in front of the front foot for support.
4. Exhale, slowly slide your front foot forward, straighten both legs and straighten back into an upright position as you extend into the split position.
5. Hold the stretch and relax.
6. You should feel the stretch in the hamstrings. *Note:* A split is one of the more advanced stretches for the hamstrings. To perform a technically correct split, both legs must be straight, the hips squared (facing front, not twisted sideways), and the buttocks flat on the floor. For aesthetic reasons, some people advocate a slight

turnout of the rear hip. However, due to tight hip flexors or improper training, this turnout can be too extreme. To increase the stretch one can extend the upper torso and lower the chest onto the forward thigh, or perform the split with the forward leg placed on top of a folded blanket. This latter method should be avoided by the vast majority of even advanced athletes since it can possibly strain the posterior knee.

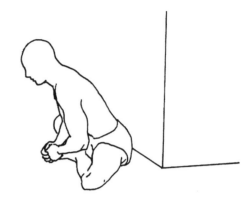

13—Adductors

1. Sit upright on the floor with your buttocks against a wall, your legs flexed and straddled, and heels touching each other.
2. Grasp your feet or ankles and pull them as close to your groin as possible.
3. Exhale, lean forward from the hips without bending your back, and attempt to lower your chest to the floor.
4. Hold the stretch and relax.
5. You should feel the stretch in the groin (adductors). *Note:* A common error is rounding the back.

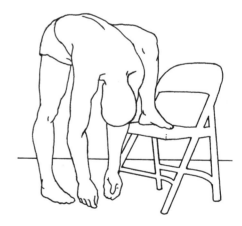

14—Adductors

1. Stand upright with one leg raised and the foot resting on the seat of a chair.
2. Exhale, bend at the hip, and lower your hands toward the floor.
3. Hold the stretch and relax.
4. You should feel the stretch in the groin (adductors).
5. Inhale while raising your upper torso to return to the upright position.

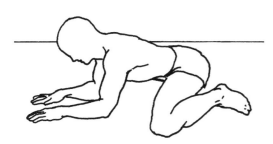

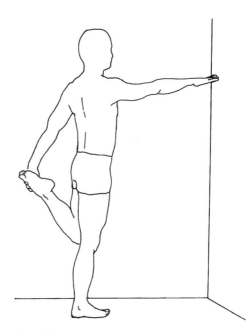

15—Adductors

1. Kneel on all fours with your toes pointing out to the sides.
2. Bend your arms and rest your elbows on the floor.
3. Exhale, slowly straddle (spread) your knees, and attempt to lower your chest to the floor.
4. Hold the stretch and relax.
5. You should feel the stretch in the groin (adductors). *Caution:* This stretch is one of the most intense exercises for the adductors—it's extremely deceptive.

17—Quadriceps

1. Stand upright with one hand against a surface for balance and support.
2. Flex one knee and raise your heel to your buttocks.
3. Slightly flex the supporting leg.
4. Exhale, reach behind, and grasp your raised foot with one hand.
5. Inhale, and pull your heel toward your buttocks *without* overcompressing the knee.
6. Hold the stretch and relax.
7. You should feel the stretch in the quadriceps.

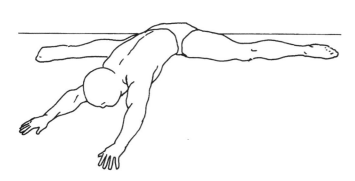

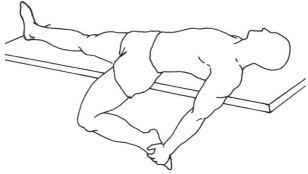

16—Adductors

1. Sit upright with your legs straddled and straight.
2. Exhale, and slowly lower your chest and belly onto the floor while keeping your back flat.
3. Hold the stretch and relax.
4. You should feel the stretch in the groin (adductors). *Note:* Ideally, your legs should form a straight line when executing a straddle split. People with greater flexibility can roll the hips forward and backward.

18—Quadriceps

1. Lie on your back at the edge of a table with one side near the edge.
2. Exhale, slowly lower the outside leg off the table at the hip, and grasp the ankle or foot with the outside hand.
3. Inhale, and slowly pull your heel toward your buttocks.
4. Hold the stretch and relax.
5. You should feel the stretch in the middle to upper thigh. *Note:* This exercise can be an intense stretch. To protect your lower back, lift up your head and contract the abdominal muscles.

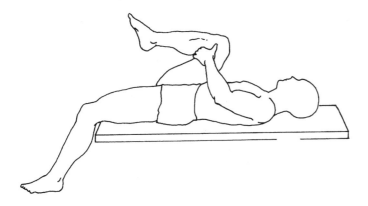

19—Hip Flexors

1. Lie on a table, flat on your back, with both legs hanging over the edge at the knees.
2. Inhale, flex one hip, and raise the knee toward your chest.
3. Interlock your hands behind the raised knee.
4. Inhale and bring your knee to your chest as you keep the opposite leg hanging over the edge.
5. Hold the stretch and relax.
6. You should feel the stretch in the upper thigh.

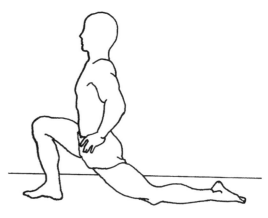

21—Hip Flexors

1. Stand upright with the legs straddled (spread sideways) about 60 cm (2 ft) apart.
2. Flex one knee, lower your body, and place the opposite knee on the floor.
3. Roll the back foot under so that the top of the instep rests on the floor.
4. Place your hands on your hips (some people may prefer placing one hand on the forward knee and one hand on the buttocks) and keep the front knee bent at a 90° angle as much as possible.
5. Exhale, and slowly push the front of the hip of the back leg toward the floor.
6. Hold the stretch and relax.
7. You should feel the stretch in the upper thigh.

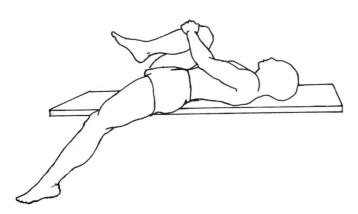

20—Hip Flexors

1. Lie on a table near the side, flat on your back.
2. Allow the outside leg to hang over the side of the table at the hip.
3. Inhale, flex the opposite knee, grasp it with your hands, and bring it to your chest.
4. Inhale and compress your thigh to your chest.
5. Hold the stretch and relax.
6. You should feel the stretch in the upper thigh.

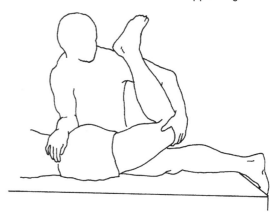

22—Hip Flexors

1. Lie face down with your body extended and one knee flexed.
2. Your partner is positioned at your side, standing or resting on one knee, with one hand under your knee (on front of thigh) and the other slightly above or on the side of the buttocks.
3. Contract your gluteals (buttock muscles) as you allow your partner to anchor down the belly to the table or floor with one hand and gently lift your leg higher with the opposite hand.
4. Hold the stretch position and relax.
5. You should feel this stretch in the upper thigh. *Note:* This exercise creates an intense stretch and must be used with extreme caution.

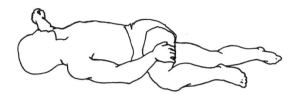

23—Lateral Buttocks and Hip

1. Lie flat on your back with your legs extended.
2. Flex one knee and raise it to your chest.
3. Grasp your knee or thigh with the opposite hand.
4. Exhale, and pull your knee sideways across your body to the floor, while keeping your elbows, head, and shoulders flat on the floor.
5. Hold the stretch and relax.
6. You should feel the stretch in the lateral buttocks and hip.

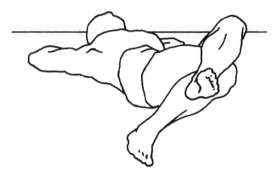

24—Buttocks and Hip

1. Lie flat on your back, knees flexed, and your hands interlocked underneath your head.
2. Lift your left leg over your right leg and hook your leg.
3. Exhale, and use your left leg to force the inside of your right leg to the floor, while keeping your elbows, head, and shoulders flat on the floor.
4. Hold the stretch and relax.
5. You should feel the stretch in the buttocks and hip.

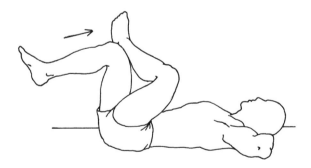

25—Buttocks and Hip

1. Lie flat on your back with your left leg crossed over your right knee.
2. Inhale, flex your right knee, lifting your right foot off the floor, and let it push your left foot toward your face, while keeping your head, shoulders, and back flat on the floor.
3. Hold the stretch and relax.
4. You should feel the stretch in the buttocks and hip.

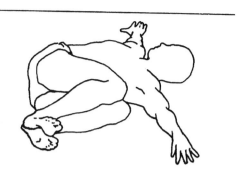

26—Buttocks, Hips, and Trunk

1. Lie flat on your back, with your knees flexed and arms out to the sides.
2. Exhale, and slowly lower both legs to the floor on the same side, while keeping your elbows, head, and shoulders flat on the floor.
3. Hold the stretch and relax.
4. You should feel the stretch in your buttocks, hip, and lower trunk.

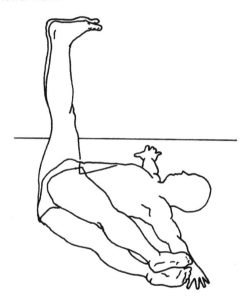

27—Buttocks, Hip, and Trunk

1. Lie flat on your back, your legs raised and straight, and your arms out to the sides.
2. Exhale, and slowly lower both legs to the floor on the same side, while keeping your elbows, head, and shoulders flat on the floor.
3. Hold the stretch and relax.
4. You should feel the stretch in the buttocks, hip, and lower trunk.

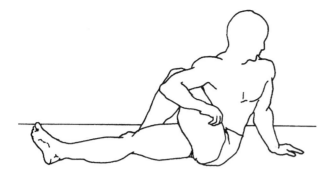

28—Buttocks and Hip

1. Sit upright on the floor, with the hands behind your hips for support and your legs extended.
2. Flex your left leg, cross your left foot over your right leg, and slide your heel toward your buttocks.
3. Reach over your left leg with your right arm, and place your right elbow on the outside of your left knee.
4. Exhale, and look over your left shoulder while turning your trunk and pushing back on your knee with your right elbow.
5. Hold the stretch and relax.
6. You should feel the stretch in the buttocks and hip.

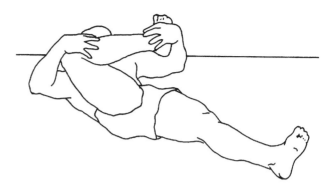

30—Buttocks and Hip

1. Lie on the floor with your body extended.
2. Flex one leg and slide the heel toward your buttocks.
3. Grasp your knee with the same-side hand and your ankle with the opposite hand.
4. Inhale, and slowly pull your foot to the opposite shoulder, while keeping your head, shoulders, and back flat on the floor.
5. Hold the stretch and relax.
6. You should feel the stretch in the buttocks and hip.

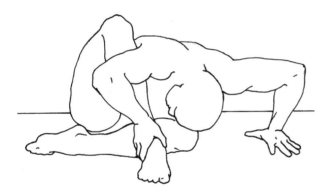

29—Buttocks, Hip, and Trunk

1. Sit upright on the floor with the outside of your left leg resting on the floor in front of you, with your knee flexed and your foot pointing to your right.
2. Cross your right leg over your left leg and place the foot flat on the floor.
3. Exhale, round your upper torso, and bend forward.
4. Hold the stretch and relax.
5. You should feel the stretch in the buttocks, hip, and trunk.

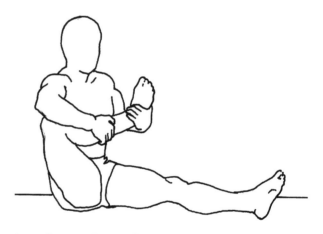

31—Buttocks and Hip

1. Sit upright on the floor with your back flat against a wall.
2. Flex one leg and slide your heel toward your buttocks.
3. Hold your knee with the same-side elbow and grasp your ankle with the opposite hand.
4. Inhale, and slowly pull your foot to the opposite shoulder.
5. Hold the stretch and relax.

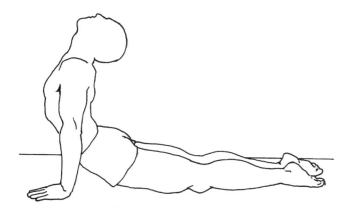

32—Abdomen and Hip Flexors

1. Lie face down on the floor with your body extended.
2. Place your palms on the floor by your hips with your fingers pointing forward.
3. Exhale, press down on the floor, raise your head and trunk, and arch your back while contracting the gluteals to prevent excessive compression on the lower back.
4. Hold the stretch and relax.
5. You should feel the stretch in the abdomen and upper thighs.

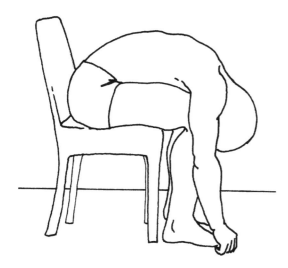

33—Lower Back

1. Sit upright in a chair with your legs separated slightly.
2. Exhale, extend your upper torso, bend at the hip, and slowly lower your stomach between your thighs.
3. Hold the stretch and relax.
4. You should feel the stretch in your lower back.

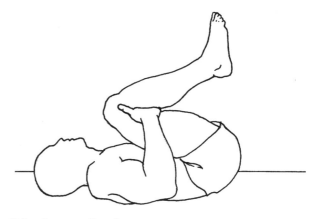

34—Lower Back

1. Lie flat on your back with your body extended.
2. Flex your knees and slide your feet toward your buttocks.
3. Grasp behind your thighs to prevent hyperflexion of the knees.
4. Inhale, pull your knees toward your chest and shoulders, and elevate your hips off the floor.
5. Hold the stretch and relax.
6. You should feel the stretch in your lower back.
7. Exhale and reextend your legs slowly one at a time to prevent possible pain or spasm.

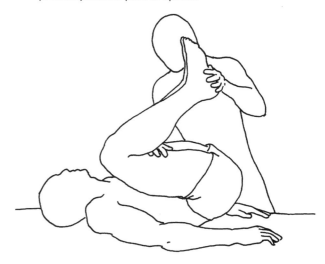

35—Lower Back

1. Lie flat on your back with your body extended.
2. Flex your knees and slide your feet toward your buttocks.
3. Your partner is positioned to your side, with one hand under your hamstrings and the other grasping your heels.
4. Exhale as you allow your partner to bring your thighs closer to your chest, lifting your buttocks and lower back from the floor.
5. Hold the stretch and relax.
6. You should feel the stretch in the lower back.

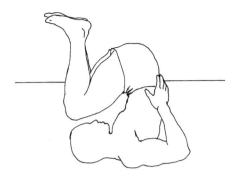

36—Lower Back

1. Lie flat on your back with your arms at your sides, palms down.
2. Inhale, push down on the floor with your palms, and raise your legs up in a squat position so the knees almost rest on your forehead.
3. Support the weight of your hips with your hands.
4. Hold the stretch and relax.
5. You should feel the stretch in your lower back. *Caution:* Use this controversial stretch with care. Avoid excessive flexion of the neck.

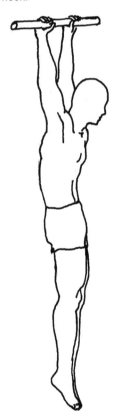

37—Lateral Trunk

1. Hang from a chin-up bar with your arms straight, hands almost touching, and your body slightly flexed in a C shape (convex toward the front).
2. Exhale, place your chin on your chest, and sink in your shoulders.
3. Hold the stretch and relax.
4. You should feel the stretch in the lateral trunk and upper back.

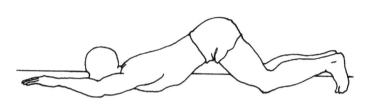

38—Upper Back

1. Kneel on all fours.
2. Extend your arms forward and lower your chest toward the floor.
3. Inhale, extend your shoulders, and press down on the floor with your arms to produce an arch in your back.
4. Hold the stretch and relax.
5. You should feel the stretch in your upper back.

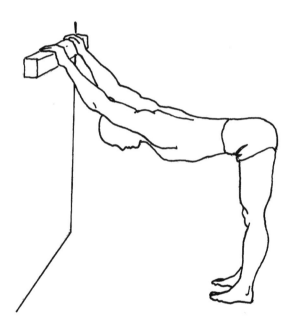

39—Upper Back

1. Stand upright, feet together, about 1 m (3 ft) from a support surface that is approximately waist to shoulder height, and your arms overhead.
2. Exhale, keep your arms and legs straight, flex at the waist, flatten your back, and grasp the supporting surface with both hands.
3. Exhale and press down on the supporting surface to produce an arch in your back.
4. Hold the stretch and relax.
5. You should feel the stretch in your upper back.

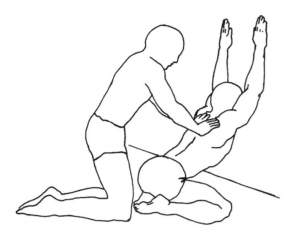

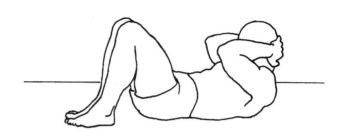

40—Upper Back

1. Sit upright, knees straddled, facing a wall about an arm's length away.
2. Raise your arms with your elbows straight, lean forward, and place your palms against the wall shoulder-width apart with your fingers pointing upward.
3. Exhale, raise your arms, press down against the wall, open your chest, and produce an arch in your back.
4. Your partner is positioned directly behind with his or her hands placed on the upper portion of your shoulder blades.
5. Exhale, as you allow your partner to gently push down and away from your head. Communicate with your partner and use great care.
6. Hold the stretch and relax.
7. You should feel the stretch in your upper back.

42—Posterior Neck

1. Lie flat on the floor with both knees flexed.
2. Interlock your hands on the back of your head near the occiputs.
3. Exhale and pull your head off the floor and onto your chest while keeping your shoulder blades flat on the floor.
4. Hold the stretch and relax.
5. You should feel the stretch in the upper back and posterior neck.

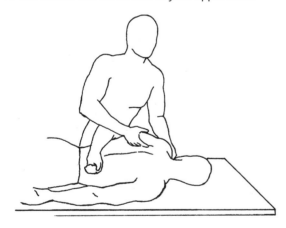

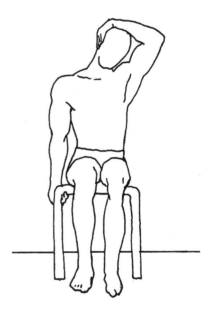

41—Serratus Anterior and Rhomboids

1. Lie flat on your chest, head turned to the left, with your left elbow flexed and forearm resting on the lower back.
2. Your partner is positioned to your side with his or her left hand grasping the top front portion of your shoulder.
3. Exhale, as you allow your partner to lift up your front shoulder to expose the scapula (shoulder blade).
4. The partner places his or her right hand under your scapula and gently lifts it upward.
5. Hold the stretch and relax.
6. You should feel the stretch in the rhomboids.

43—Lateral Neck

1. Sit or stand upright.
2. Place your left hand on the upper right side of your head.
3. Exhale, and slowly pull the left side of your head onto your left shoulder (lateral flexion).
4. Hold the stretch and relax.
5. You should feel the stretch in the lateral side of the neck.

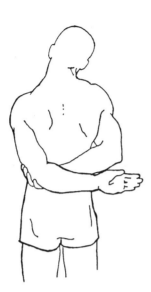

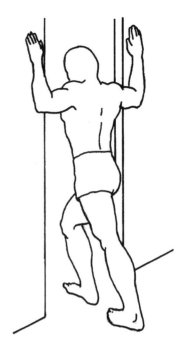

44—Lateral Neck

1. Sit or stand upright with your left arm flexed behind your back.
2. Grasp the elbow from behind with the opposite hand and pull your elbow across the midline of your back to keep the left shoulder stabilized.
3. Exhale and lower your right ear to the right shoulder.
4. Hold the stretch and relax.
5. You should feel the stretch in the lateral side of the neck.

46—Pectorals

1. Stand upright facing a corner or open doorway.
2. Raise your elbows to shoulder height at your sides, bend your elbows so that your forearms point straight up, and place your palms against the walls or doorframe to stretch the sternal section of the pectoralis muscles on both sides.
3. Exhale and lean your entire body forward.
4. Hold the stretch and relax.
5. You should feel the stretch in your upper chest (pectorals).

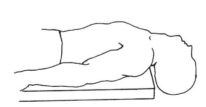

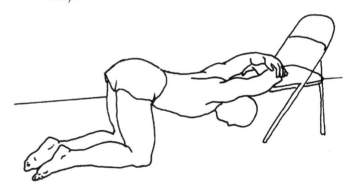

45—Anterior Neck

1. Lie flat on a table with your head hanging over the edge.
2. Hold the stretch and relax.
3. You should feel the stretch in the anterior part of the neck.

47—Pectorals

1. Kneel on the floor facing a barre or chair.
2. Interlock your forearms above your head and bend forward to rest them on top of the barre or chair, with your head dropping beneath the supporting surface.
3. Exhale and let your head and chest sink to the floor.
4. Hold the stretch and relax.
5. You should feel the stretch in your upper chest (pectorals).

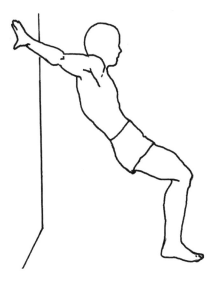

48—Anterior Shoulder

1. Stand upright, your hands behind you at about shoulder height resting on a wall and your fingers pointing upward.
2. Exhale and flex your legs to lower your shoulders.
3. Hold the stretch and relax.
4. You should feel the stretch in the anterior shoulder.

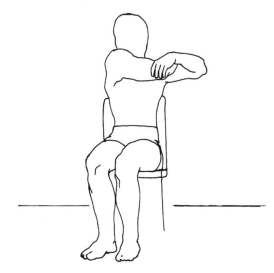

49—Lateral Shoulder

1. Sit or stand upright with one arm raised to shoulder height.
2. Flex your arm across to the opposite shoulder.
3. Grasp your raised elbow with the opposite hand.
4. Inhale and pull your elbow toward your back.
5. Hold the stretch and relax.
6. You should feel the stretch in the lateral shoulder.

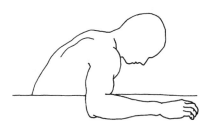

50—Shoulder Internal Rotators

1. Sit upright with your side next to a table.
2. Rest your forearm along the table edge with your elbow flexed.
3. Exhale, bend forward from the waist, and lower your head and shoulder to table level.
4. Hold the stretch and relax.
5. You should feel the stretch in the upper and medial shoulder.

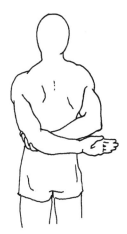

51—Shoulder Abductors

1. Sit or stand upright with one arm flexed behind your back.
2. Grasp the elbow (or wrist if unable to reach elbow) from behind with the opposite hand.
3. Inhale and pull your elbow across the midline of your back.
4. Hold the stretch and relax.
5. You should feel the stretch in the posterior part of the shoulder.

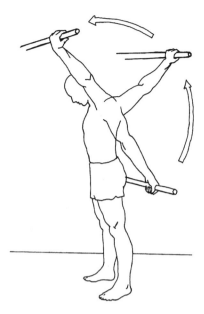

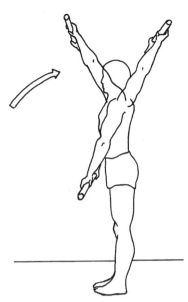

52—Shoulder Internal and External Rotators

1. Stand upright, feet straddled, and grasp a pole or towel with both hands behind your hips with a wide, reverse grip (your palms facing forward and thumbs on the outside).
2. Inhale and slowly raise your arms overhead, keeping both straight and symmetrical, with no twisting to the side as your arms rotate forward in the shoulder joint and end in an L grip (the palms of the hands face up and the thumbs under the pole).
3. Inhale, then reverse the direction.
4. You should feel this stretch in the shoulders (especially the posterior region).

53—Shoulder Internal and External Rotators

1. Stand upright, feet straddled, and grasp a pole or towel in front of your hips with a wide overgrip (palm facing down).
2. Inhale and slowly raise your arms overhead, keeping them both straight, symmetrical, and with no twisting to the side as they rotate in the shoulder joint and end up behind your head.
3. Inhale, then reverse the direction.
4. You should feel this stretch in the shoulders (especially the anterior region).

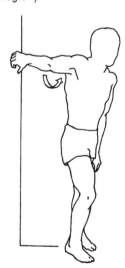

54—Biceps Brachii

1. Stand upright with your back to a doorframe.
2. Rest one hand against the doorframe with your arm internally rotated at the shoulder, forearm extended, and your hand pronated with your thumb pointing down.
3. Exhale and attempt to roll your biceps so they face upward.
4. Hold the stretch and relax.
5. You should feel this stretch in the biceps brachii.

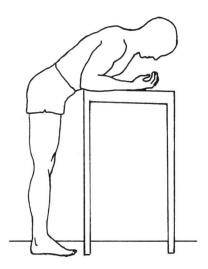

55—Triceps Brachii

1. Stand upright with your forearms resting on a table with the palms facing up.
2. Exhale, bend forward, and bring your shoulders to your wrists.
3. Hold the stretch and relax.
4. You should feel the stretch in the triceps brachii.

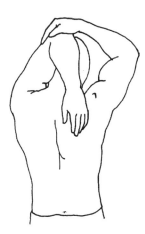

56—Triceps Brachii

1. Sit or stand upright with one arm flexed, raised overhead with elbow next to your ear, and your hand resting on your opposite shoulder blade.
2. Grasp your elbow with the opposite hand.
3. Inhale and pull your elbow behind your head.
4. Hold the stretch and relax.
5. You should feel the stretch in the triceps brachii.

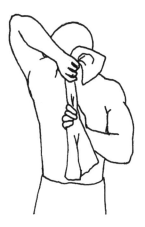

57—Triceps Brachii

1. Sit or stand upright with one arm behind your lower back, placed as far up on your back as possible.
2. Lift your other arm overhead, while holding a folded blanket or towel, and flex your elbow.
3. Grasp the blanket or towel with your lower hand.
4. Inhale as you slowly pull your hands together.
5. Hold the stretch and relax.
6. You should feel the stretch in the triceps brachii.

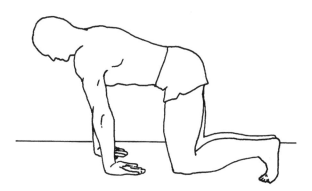

58—Brachioradialis

1. Kneel on all fours, flex your wrists, and place the tops (dorsa) of your hands against the floor, with fingers pointing toward your knees.
2. Exhale and lean against the floor.
3. Hold the stretch and relax.
4. You should feel the stretch in the brachioradialis.

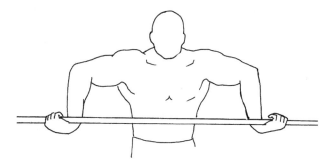

59—Brachioradialis

1. Hold a pole in front of you in an L grip (the palms of the hands face up and the thumbs on the outside).
2. Exhale and flex your elbows.
3. Hold the stretch and relax.
4. You should feel the stretch in the brachioradialis.

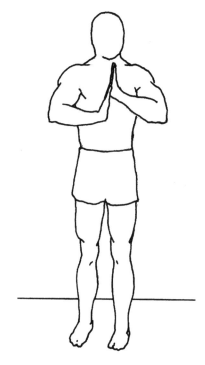

60—Forearm Flexors

1. Sit or stand upright on the floor with your wrists hyper-extended (bent backwards).
2. Place the heel of one hand against the palmar surface of the fingers of your other hand.
3. Exhale and press the heel of your hand against your fingers.
4. Hold the stretch and relax.
5. You should feel the stretch in the forearm flexors.

References

Aarskog, D., K.F. Stoa, and T. Thorsen.1966. Urinary oestrogen excretion in newborn infants with congenital dysplasia of the hip joint. *Acta Pædiatrica Scandinavica* 55(4), 394-397.

Aberdeen, D.L., and E. Joensen. 1986. A study of the relevance of handedness to the range of rotation at the glenohumeral joint. *European Journal of Chiropractic* 34(2), 67-87.

Abraham, W.M. 1977. Factors in delayed muscle soreness. *Medicine and Science in Sports* 9(1), 11-20.

Abraham, W.M. 1979. Exercise-induced muscular soreness. *The Physician and Sportsmedicine* 7(10), 57-60.

Abrahams, M. 1967. Mechanical behaviour of tendon *in vitro*: A preliminary report. *Medical & Biological Engineering & Computing* 5(5), 433-443.

Abramson, D., S.M. Roberts, and P.D. Wilson. 1934. Relaxation of the pelvic joint in pregnancy. *Surgery, Gynecology, and Obstetrics* 58(3), 595-613.

ACOG. *See* American College of Obstetricians and Gynecologists.

Adair, S.M., and C. Hecht. 1993. Association of generalized joint hypermobility with history, signs, and symptoms of temporomandibular joint dysfunction in children. *Pediatric Dentistry* 15(5), 323-326.

Adams, M.A., and P. Dolan. 1996. Time-dependent changes in the lumbar spine's resistance to bending. *Clinical Biomechanics* 11(14), 194-200.

Adams, M.A., P. Dolan, and W.C. Hutton. 1987. Diurnal variations in the stresses on the lumbar spine. *Spine* 12(2), 130-137.

Adams, M.A., and W.C. Hutton. 1986. Has the lumbar spine a margin of safety in forward bending? *Clinical Biomechanics* 1(1), 3-6.

Adams, P., and H. Muir. 1976. Qualitative changes with age of proteoglycans of human lumbar discs. *Annals of the Rheumatic Diseases* 35(4), 289-296.

Adler, S.S., D. Beckers, and M. Buck. 2000. *PNF in practice: An illustrated guide.* 2nd ed. New York: Springer-Verlag.

Agre, J.C., D.C. Casal, A.S. Leon, C. McNally, T.L. Baxter, and R.C. Serfass. 1988. Professional ice hockey players: Physiologic, anthropometric, and musculoskeletal characteristics. *Archives of Physical Medicine and Rehabilitation* 69(3), 188-192.

Agre, J.C., L.E. Pierce, D.M. Raab, M. McAdams, and E.L. Smith. 1988. Light resistance and stretching exercise in elderly women: Effect upon stretch. *Archives of Physical Medicine and Rehabilitation* 69(4), 273-276.

Ahmed, I.M., M. Lagopoulos, P. McConnell, R.W. Soames, and G.K. Sefton. 1998. Blood supply of the Achilles tendon. *Journal of Orthopaedic Research* 16(5), 591-596.

Ahtikoski, A.M., S.O.A. Koskinen, P. Virtanen, V. Kovanen, and T.E.S. Takala. 2001. Regulation of synthesis of fibrillar collagens in rat skeletal muscle during immobilization in shortened and lengthened positions. *Acta Physiologica Scandinavica* 172(2), 131-140.

Akagawa, M., and K. Suyama. 2000. Mechanism of formation of elastin crosslinks. *Connective Tissue Research* 41(2), 131-141.

Akeson, W.H., D. Amiel, and D. LaViolette. 1967. The connective tissue response to immobility: A study of the chondroitin 4- and 6-sulfate and dermatan sulfate changes in periarticular connective tissue of control and immobilized knees of dogs. *Clinical Orthopaedics and Related Research* 51, 183-197.

Akeson, W.H., D. Amiel, G.L. Mechanic, S. Woo, F.L. Harwood, and M.L. Hammer. 1977. Collagen crosslinking alteration in joint contractures: Changes in reducible crosslinks in periarticular connective tissue collagen after nine weeks of immobilization. *Connective Tissue Research* 5(1), 15-20.

Akeson, W.H., D. Amiel, and S. Woo. 1980. Immobility effects on synovial joints: The pathomechanics of joint contracture. *Biorheology* 17(1/2), 95-110.

Akster, H.A., H.L.M. Granzier, and B. Focant. 1989. Differences in I band structure, sarcomere extensibility, and electrophoresis of titin between two muscle fiber types of the perch (*Perca fluviatilis* L.). *Journal of Ultrastructure and Molecular Structure Research* 102(2), 109-121.

Alabin, V.G., and M.P. Krivonosov. 1987. Excerpts from training aids and specialized exercises in track and field. *Soviet Sports Review* 22(2), 73-75.

Albert, H., M. Godskesen, J.G. Westergaard, T. Chard, and L. Gunn. 1997. Circulating levels of relaxin are normal in pregnant women with pelvic pain. *European Journal of Obstetrics & Gynecology and Reproductive Biology* 74(1), 19-22.

Alexander, M.J.L. 1991. A comparison of physiological characteristics of elite and subelite rhythmic gymnasts. *Journal of Human Movement Studies* 20(2), 49-69.

Alexander, R.M. 1975. *Biomechanics.* London: Chapman and Hall.

Alexander, R.M. 1988. *Elastic mechanisms in animal movement.* Cambridge: Cambridge University Press.

Allander, E., O. Bjoörnsson, O. Olafsson, N. Sigfússon, and J. Thorsteinsson. 1974. Normal range of joint movements in shoulder, hip, wrist and thumb with special reference to side: A comparison between two populations. *International Journal of Epidemiology* 3(3), 253-261.

Allen, C.E.L. 1948. Muscle action potentials used in the study of dynamic anatomy. *British Journal of Physical Medicine* 11, 66-73.

Allen, D.G. 2001. Eccentric muscle damage: Mechanisms of early reduction of force. *Acta Physiologica Scandinavica* 171(3), 311-319.

Almeida-Silveira, M-I., C. Pérot, and F. Goubel. 1996. Neuromuscular adaptations in rats trained by muscle stretch-shortening. *European Journal of Applied Physiology* 72(3), 261-266.

Almekinders, L.C. 1993. Anti-inflammatory treatment of muscular injuries in sports. *Sports Medicine* 15(3), 139-145.

Alnaqeeb, M.A., N.S. Al Zaid, and G. Goldspink. 1984. Connective tissue changes and physical properties of developing and aging skeletal muscle. *Journal of Anatomy* 139(4), 677-689.

Al-Rawi, Z.S., A.J. Al-Aszawi, and T. Al-Chalabi. 1985. Joint mobility among university students in Iraq. *British Journal of Rheumatology* 24(4), 326-331.

Alter, J. 1983. *Surviving exercise.* Boston: Houghton Mifflin.

Alter, J. 1986. *Strength & strengthen.* Boston: Houghton Mifflin.

Alter, J. 1989-1990. Book review. *Kinesiology and Medicine in Dance* 12(1), 41-43.

Alter, M. 1996. *Science of flexibility.* 2nd ed. Champaign, IL: Human Kinetics.

Alter, M. 1998. *Sport stretch.* 2nd ed. Champaign, IL: Human Kinetics.

Alvarez, R., I.A.F. Stokes, D.E. Asprinio, S. Trevino, and T. Braun. 1988. Dimensional changes of the feet in pregnancy. *Journal of Bone and Joint Surgery* 70(2), 271-274.

American Academy of Orthopaedic Surgeons. 1991. *Athletic training and sports medicine.* 2nd ed. Rosemont, IL: Author.

American Academy of Orthopaedic Surgeons. 2001. *Essentials of musculoskeletal care.* 2nd ed, ed. W.B. Greene 487-490. Rosemont, IL: Author.

American Alliance for Health, Physical Education, and Recreation. 1968. *School safety policies with emphasis on physical education, athletics, and recreation.* Washington, DC: Author.

American Chiropractic Association. 1991. *Chiropractic: State of the art 1991-1992.* Arlington, VA. Author.

American College of Obstetricians and Gynecologists [ACOG]. 1985. *Exercise during pregnancy and the postnatal period. ACOG home exercise programs.* Washington, DC. Author.

American College of Obstetricians and Gynecologists [ACOG]. 1994. *Exercise during pregnancy and the postpartum period* (ACOG Technical Bulletin, No. 189). Washington, DC: Author.

American College of Sports Medicine. 2000. *ACSM's guidelines for exercise testing and prescription*. 6th ed. Philadelphia: Lippincott Williams & Wilkins.

American College of Sports Medicine Position Stand. 1998. The recommended quantity and quality of exercise for developing and maintaining cardiorespiratory and muscular fitness, and flexibility in healthy Adults. *Medicine and Science in Sports and Exercise* 30(6), 975-991.

The American contortionist. 1882. *Lancet* 1, 618.

American Medical Association. 1993. *Guidelines to the evaluation of permanent impairment*. 4th ed. Chicago: Author.

American Orthopaedic Association. 1985. *Manual of orthopaedic surgery*. Chicago: Author.

Amis, A.A., and J.H. Miller. 1982. The elbow. *Clinics in Rheumatic Disease* 8(3), 571-593.

Amnesty International 2001. *2001 Annual report*. [Online]. Available: www.amnesty.org/ailib/aireport/index.html [December 1, 2001].

Anderson, B. 1978. The perfect pre-run stretching routine. *Runners World* 13(5), 56-61.

Anderson, B. 2000. *Stretching*. New revised ed. Bolinas, CA: Shelter.

Anderson, B. 1985. Stretch: A key to body awareness. *Shape* 4(3), 37-42.

Anderson, M.B. 1979. Comparison of muscle patterning in the overarm throw and tennis serve. *Research Quarterly* 50(4), 541-553.

Anderson, O. 2003a. Okay, but does stretching really lower the risk of injury? Here's what science says. *Peak Performance*. [Online]. Available: www.pponline.uk/encyc/0852.htm. [October 31, 2003].

Anderson, O. 2003b. Running foot injuries—Describing plantar fasciitis is easy: It's simply an inflammation of the fascia on the bottom of the foot. Getting rid of plantar fasciitis is hard. *Peak Performance*. [Online]. Available: www.pponline.uk/encyc/0180.htm [October 31, 2003].

Andersson, G.B.J., T.N. Herberts, and R. Örtengren. 1977. Quantitative electromyographic studies of back muscle activity related to posture and loading. *Orthopaedic Clinics of North America* 8(1), 85-86.

Andren, L., and N.E. Borglin. 1961. Disturbed urinary excretion pattern of oestrogens in newborns with congenital dislocation of the hip. I. The excretion of oestrogen during the first few days of life. *Acta Endocrinologica* 37(3), 423-433.

Andrish, J.T., J.A. Bergfeld, and J. Walheim. 1974. A prospective study on the management of shinsplints. *Journal of Bone and Joint Surgery* 56A(8), 1697-1700.

Ansell, B.A. 1972. Hypermobility of joints. In *Modern trends in orthopaedics*, ed. A.G. Apley, 25-39. New York: Appleton-Century-Crofts.

AOSSM [American Orthopaedic Society for Sports Medicine] Research Committee 1998. Hyperbaric oxygen therapy in sports. *American Journal of Sports Medicine* 26(4), 489-490.

Apostolopoulos, N. 2001. Performance flexibility. In *High-performance sports conditioning*, ed. B. Foran, 49-61. Champaign, IL: Human Kinetics.

Araujo, D. 1997. Expecting questions about exercise and pregnancy. *The Physician and Sportsmedicine* 25(4), 85-93.

Arampatzis, A., G.-P., Brüggemann, and G.M. Klapsing. 2001. Leg stiffness and mechanical energetic processes during jumping on a sprung surface. *Medicine and Science in Sports and Exercise* 33(6), 923-931.

Argiolas-Antonio, A., and M.R. Melis. 1998. The neuropharmacology of yawning. *European Journal of Pharmacology* 343(1), 1-16.

Armstrong, C.G., P. O'Connor, and D.L. Gardner. 1992. Mechanical basis of connective tissue disease. In *Pathological basis of the connective tissue diseases*, ed. D.L. Gardner, 261-281. Philadelphia: Lea & Febiger.

Armstrong, R.B. 1984. Mechanisms of exercise-induced delayed onset muscle soreness: A brief review. *Medicine and Science in Sports and Exercise* 16(6), 529-538.

Armstrong, R.B., R.W., Ogilvie, and J.A. Schwane. 1983. Eccentric exercise-induced injury to rat skeletal muscle. *Journal of Applied Physiology* 54(1), 80-93.

Armstrong, R.B., G.L. Warren, and J.R. Warren. 1991. Mechanisms of exercise-induced muscle fibre injury. *Sports Medicine* 12(3), 184-207.

Arner, O., and A. Lindholm. 1958. What is tennis leg? *Acta Chirurgica Scandinavica* 116(1), 73-77.

Arnheim, D.D., and W.E. Prentice. 2000. *Principles of athletic training*. 10th ed. Boston: McGraw-Hill.

Arskey, M. 2001. Daily bow vitamins: Build relaxed, flexible muscles thirteen ways. *American String Teacher* 51(4), 43-45.

Ashmen, K.J., C.B. Swanik, and S.M. Lephart. 1996. Strength and flexibility characteristics of athletes with chronic low-back pain. *Journal of Sport Rehabilitation* 5(4), 275-286.

Ashmore, C.R. 1982. Stretch-induced growth in chicken wing muscles: Effects on hereditary muscular dystrophy. *American Journal of Physiology* 242 (Cell Physiology 11), C178-C183.

Askenasy, J.J.M. 1989. Is yawning an arousal defense reflex? *Journal of Psychology* 123(6), 609-621.

Asmussen, E. 1953. Positive and negative work. *Acta Physiologica Scandinavica* 28(4), 364-382.

Asmussen, E. 1956. Observations on experimental muscle soreness. *Acta Rheumatologica Scandinavica* 2,109-116.

Asmussen, E., and F. Bonde-Petersen. 1974. Storage of elastic energy in skeletal muscles in man. *Acta Physiologica Scandinavica* 91(3), 385-392.

Asterita, M.F. 1985. *The physiology of stress*, New York: Human Science Press.

Aspden, R.M. 1988. A new mathematical model of the spine and its relationship to spinal loading in the workplace. *Applied Ergonomics* 19(4), 319-323.

Aten, D.W., and K.T. Knight. 1978. Therapeutic exercise in athletic training: Principles and overview. *Athletic Training* 13(3), 123-126.

Athenstaedt, H. 1970. Permanent longitudinal electric polarization and pyroelectric behaviour of collagenous structures and nervous tissue in man and other vertebrates. *Nature* 228(5274), 830-834.

Atwater, A.A. 1979. Biomechanics of overarm throwing movements and of throwing injuries. *Exercise and Sport Sciences Reviews* 7, 43-85.

Aura, O., and P.V. Komi. 1986. Mechanical efficiency of pure positive and pure negative work with special reference to the work intensity. *International Journal of Sports Medicine* 7(1), 44-49.

Avela, J., H. Kyröläinen, and P.V. Komi. 1999. Altered reflex sensitivity after repeated and prolonged passive muscle stretching. *Journal of Applied Physiology* 86(4), 1283-1291.

Axelson, H.W., and K.-E. Hagbarth. 2001. Human motor control consequences of thixotropic changes in muscular short-range stiffness. *Journal of Physiology (London)* 535(1), 279-288.

Baatsen, P.H., W.K. Trombitás, and G.H. Pollack. 1988. Thick filaments of striated muscle are laterally interconnected. *Journal of Ultrastructure and Molecular Structure Research* 98(3), 267-280.

Bachrach, R.M. 1987. Injuries to dancer's spine. In *Dance medicine*, eds. A.J. Ryan, R.E. Stephens, 243-266. Chicago: Pluribus Press.

Baddeley, S., and S. Green. 1992. Physical education and the pregnant woman: The way forward. *Midwives Chronicle & Nursing Notes* 105(1253), 144-145.

Badtke, G., F. Bittmann, and D. Lazik, D. 1993. Changes in the vertebral column in the course of the day. *International Journal of Sports Medicine* 14(3), 159.

Baenninger, R. 1997. On yawning and its functions. *Psychonomic Bulletin & Review* 4(2), 198-207.

Bak, K., and S.P. Magnusson. 1997. Shoulder strength and range of motion in symptomatic and pain-free elite swimmers. *American Journal of Sports Medicine* 25(4), 454-459.

Baker, M.M. 1998. Anterior cruciate ligament injuries in the female athletes. *Journal of Women's Health* 7(3), 343-349.

Balaftsalis, H. 1982-1983. Knee joint laxity contributing to footballers' injuries. *Physiotherapy in Sport* 5(3), 26-27.

Baldissera, F., H. Hultborn, and M. Illert. 1981. Integration in spinal neuronal systems. In *Handbook of physiology. Sec. 1. The nervous system*. (Vol. 2, Part 1, 509-595). Bethesda, MD: American Physiological Society.

Ballantyne, B.T., M.D. Reser, G.W. Lorenz, and G.L. Smidt. 1986. The effects of inversion traction on spinal column configuration, heart rate, blood pressure, and perceived discomfort. *Journal of Orthopaedic and Sports Physical Therapy* 7(5), 254-260.

Balnave, C.D., D.F. Davey, and D.G. Allen. 1997. Distribution of sarcomere length and intracellular calcium in mouse skeletal muscle following stretch-induced injury. *Journal of Physiology* 502(Pt. 3), 649-659

Baltaci, G., R. Johnson, and H. Kohl. 2001. Shoulder range of motion characteristics in collegiate baseball players. *Journal of Sports Medicine and Physical Fitness* 41(2), 236-242.

Bandy, W.D., and J.M. Irion. 1994. The effect of time on static stretch on the flexibility of the hamstring muscles. *Physical Therapy* 74(9), 845-850.

Bandy, W.D. 2001. Stretching activities for increasing muscle flexibility. In *Therapeutic exercise: Techniques for intervention*. eds. W.D. Bandy and B. Sanders, 37-62. Baltimore: Lippincott Williams & Wilkins.

Bandy, W.D., J.M. Irion, and M. Briggler. 1997. The effect of time and frequency of static stretch on flexibility of the hamstring muscles. *Physical Therapy* 77(5), S105.

Bandy, W.D., J.M. Irion, and M. Briggler. 1998. The effect of static stretch and dynamic range of motion training on the flexibility of the hamstring muscles. *Journal of Orthopaedic and Sport Physical Therapy* 27(4), 295-300.

Banker, I.A. 1980. The isolated mammalian muscle spindle. *Trends in Neuroscience* 3(11), 258-265.

Baratta, R., M. Solomonow, B.H. Zhou, E.D. Letson, R. Chuinard, and R. D'Ambrosia. 1988. *American Journal of Sports Medicine* 16(2), 113-122.

Barbizet, J. 1958. Yawning. *Journal Neurology, Neurosurgery and Psychiatry* 21(3), 203-209.

Barbosa, A.R., J.M. Santarém, W.J. Filho, M. Marucci. 2002. Effects of resistance training on the sit-and-reach test in elderly women. *Journal of Strength and Conditioning Research* 16(1), 14-18.

Barker, D. 1974. The morphology of muscle receptors. In *Handbook of sensory physiology. Muscle receptors* (Vol. 3, Part 2), ed. C.C. Hunt, 1-190. New York: Springer.

Barlow, J.C., B.W. Benjamin, P.J. Birt, and C.J. Hughes. 2002. Shoulder strength and range-of-motion characteristics in bodybuilders. *Journal of Strength and Conditioning Research* 16(3), 367-372.

Barnard, R.J., G.W. Gardner, N.V. Diaco, R.N. McAlpin, and A.A. Kattus. 1973a. Cardiovascular responses to sudden strenuous exercise—Heart rate, blood pressure and ECG. *Journal of Applied Physiology* 34(6), 833-837.

Barnard, R.J., R. McAlpin, A.A. Kattus., and G.D. Buckberg. 1973b. Ischemic response to sudden exercise in healthy men. *Circulation* 48(5), 936-942.

Barnes, J. 1999. Myofascial release. In *Functional soft tissue examination and treatment by manual methods*. 2nd ed, ed. W.I. Hammer, 533-548. Gaithersburg, MD: Aspen.

Barnett, C.H. 1971. The mobility of synovial joints. *Rheumatology and Physical Medicine* 11, 20-27.

Barnett, J.G., R.G. Holly, and C.R. Ashmore. 1980. Stretch-induced growth in chicken wing muscles: Biochemical and morphological characterization. *American Journal of Physiology* 239(1), C39-C46.

Barone, J.N. 1989. Topical analgesics: How effective are they? *The Physician and Sportsmedicine* 17(2), 162-166.

Barrack, R.L., H.B. Skinner, M.E. Brunet, and S.D. Cook. 1983. Joint laxity and proprioception in the knee. *The Physician and Sportsmedicine* 11(6), 130-135.

Barrett, C., and P. Smerdely. 2002. A comparison of community-based resistance exercise and flexibility exercise for seniors. *Australian Journal of Physiotherapy* 48(3), 215-219.

Barrett, J., L. Lack, and M. Morris. 1993. The sleep-evoked decrease of body temperature. *Sleep* 16(2), 93-99.

Barry, W., R. Cashman, S. Coote, B. Hastings, and M. Imperatrice. 1987. The relationship between lung function and thoracic mobility in normal subjects. *New Zealand Journal of Physiotherapy* 15(1), 9-11.

Bartelink, D.L. 1957. The role of abdominal pressure in relieving pressure on the lumbar intervertebral discs. *Journal of Bone and Joint Surgery* 39B(4), 718-725.

Basmajian, J.V. 1963. Control and training of individual motor units. *Science* 141(3579), 440-441.

Basmajian, J.V. 1967. Control of individual motor units. *American Journal of Physical Medicine* 46(1), 480-486.

Basmajian, J.V. 1972. Electromyography comes of age. *Science* 176(4035), 603-609.

Basmajian, J.V. 1975. Motor learning and control. *Archives of Physical Medicine and Rehabilitation* 58(1), 38-41.

Basmajian, J.V. 1998. Biofeedback in physical medicine and rehabilitation. In *Rehabilitation medicine: Principles and practices*. 3rd ed. eds. J.A. DeLisa and B.M. Gans, 505-520. Philadelphia: Lippincott-Raven.

Basmajian, J.V., M. Baeza, and C. Fabrigar. 1965. Conscious control and training of individual spinal motor neurons in normal human subjects. *Journal of New Drugs* 5(2), 78-85.

Bassey, E.J., K. Morgan, H.M. Dallosso, and S.B.J. Ebrahim. 1989. Flexibility of the shoulder joint measured as range of abduction in a large representative sample of men and women over 65 years of age. *European Journal of Applied Physiology* 58(4), 353-360.

Bates, R.A. 1971. *Flexibility training: The optimal time period to spend in a position of maximal stretch*. Master's thesis, University of Alberta.

Bates, R.A. 1976. Flexibility development: Mind over matter. In *The advanced study of gymnastics*, ed. J.H. Salmela, 233-241. Springfield, IL: Charles C Thomas.

Batson, G. 1993. Stretching technique: A somatic learning model: Part I: Training sensory responsivity. *Impulse* 1(2), 126-140.

Batson, G. 1994. Stretching technique: A somatic learning model: Part II: Training purposivity through Sweigard Ideokinesis. *Impulse* 2(1), 39-58.

Battié, M.C., S.J. Bigos, L.D. Fisher, D.M. Spengler, T.H. Hansson, A.L. Nachemson, and M.D. Wortley. 1990. The role of spinal flexibility in back pain complaints within industry: A prospective study. *Spine* 15(8), 768-773.

Battié, M.C., S.J. Bigos, A. Sheehy, and M.D. Wortley. 1987. Spinal flexibility and individual factors that influence it. *Physical Therapy* 67(5), 653-658.

Bauman, P.A., R. Singson, and W.G. Hamilton. 1994. Femoral neck anteversion in ballerinas. *Clinical Orthopaedics and Related Research* 302(May), 57-63.

Baxter, C., and T. Reilly, T. 1983. Influence of time of day on all-out swimming. *British Journal of Sports Medicine* 17(2), 122-127.

Baxter, D.E., and P.F. Davis. 1995. Rehabilitation of the elite athlete. In *The foot and ankle in sport*, ed. D.E. Baxter, 379-392. St. Louis: Mosby.

Baxter, M.P., and C. Dulberg. 1988. "Growing pains" in childhood: A proposed treatment. *Journal of Pediatric Orthopaedics* 8(4), 402-406.

Beach, M.L., S.L. Whitney, and S.A. Dickoff-Hoffman. 1992. Relationship of shoulder flexibility, strength, and endurance to shoulder pain in competitive swimmers. *Journal of Orthopaedic and Sports Physical Therapy* 16(6), 262-268.

Beaulieu, J.E. 1981. Developing a stretching program. *The Physician and Sportsmedicine* 9(11), 59-69.

Bechbache, R.R., and J. Duffin. 1977. The entrainment of breathing frequency by exercise rhythm. *Journal of Physiology* (London) 272(3), 553-561.

Becker, A.H. 1979. Traction for knee-flexion contractures. *Physical Therapy* 59(9), 1114.

Beekman, S., and B.H. Block. 1975. The relationship of calcaneal varus to hamstring tightening. *Current Podiatry* 24(11), 7-10.

Beel, J.A., D.E. Groswald, and M.W. Luttges. 1984. Alterations in the mechanical properties of peripheral nerve following crush injury. *Journal of Biomechanics* 17(3), 185-193.

Beel, J.A., L.S. Stodieck, and M.W. Luttges. 1986. Structural properties of spinal nerve roots: Biomechanics. *Experimental Neurology* 91(1), 30-40, 1986.

Behm, D.G., D.C. Button, and J.C. Butt. 2001. Factors affecting force loss with prolonged stretching. *Canadian Journal of Applied Physiology* 26(3), 262-272.

Beighton, P. 1971. How contortionists contort. *Medical Times* 99(4), 181-187.

Beighton, P., A. de Paepe, D. Danks, G. Finidori, T. Gedde-Dahl, R. Goodman, J.G. Hall, D.W. Hollister, W. Horton, V.A. McKusick, J.M. Opitz, F.M. Pope, R.E. Pyeritz, D.L. Rimoin, D. Sillence, J.W. Spranger, E. Thompson, D. Tsipouras, D. Viljoen, I. Winship, and I. Young. 1988. International nosology of heritable disorders of connective tissue, Berlin, 1986. *American Journal of Medical Genetics* 29(3), 581-594.

Beighton, P., A. de Paepe, B. Steinmann, P. Tsipouras, and R.J. Wenstrup. 1998. Ehlers-Danlos Syndromes: Revised nosology. Villefranche. *American Journal of Medical Genetics* 77(1), 31-37.

Beighton, P., R. Grahame, and H. Bird. 1983. *Hypermobility of joints.* London: Springer-Verlag.

Beighton, P., R. Grahame, and H. Bird. 1999. *Hypermobility of joints.* 3rd ed. London: Springer-Verlag.

Beighton, P., and F.T. Horan. 1969. Orthopaedic aspects of the Ehlers-Danlos syndrome. *Journal of Bone and Joint Surgery* 51B(3), 444-453.

Beighton, P., and F.T. Horan. 1970. Dominant inheritance in familial generalized articular hypermobility. *Journal of Bone and Joint Surgery* 52B(1), 145-147.

Beighton, P.H., L. Solomon, and C.L. Soskolne. 1973. Articular mobility in an African population. *Annals of the Rheumatic Diseases* 32(5), 413-418.

Bell, G.W., and W.E. Prentice. 1999. Infrared modalities (therapeutic heat and cold). In *Therapeutic modalities in sports medicine.* 4th ed, ed. W.E. Prentice, 173-199. Boston: WCB McGraw-Hill.

Bell, R.D., and T.B. Hoshizaki. 1981. Relationship of age and sex with range of motion of seventeen joint actions in humans. *Canadian Journal of Applied Sports Science* 6(4), 202-206.

Benjamin, B.E. 1978. *Are you tense?* New York: Pantheon Books.

Benjamin, M., and J.R. Ralphs. 2000. The cell and developmental biology of tendons and ligaments. *International Review of Cytology* 196, 85-130.

Bennell, K., E. Tully, and N. Harvey. 1999a. Does the toe-touch test predict hamstring injury in Australian rules footballers? *Australian Journal of Physiotherapy* 45(2), 103-109.

Bennell, K., S. White, and K. Crossley. 1999b. The oral contraceptive pill: A revolution for sportswomen? *British Journal of Sports Medicine* 33(4), 231-238.

Bennell, K.L., and K. Crossley. 1996. Musculoskeletal injuries in track and field: Incidence distribution and risk factors. *Australian Journal of Science and Medicine in Sport* 28(3), 69-75.

Benson, H. 1980. *The relaxation response.* New York: Avon Books.

Bentivoglio, M. 1998. 1898: The golgi apparatus emerges from nerve cells. *Trends in Neuroscience* 21(5), 195-200.

Berland, T., and R.G. Addison. 1972. *Living with your bad back.* New York: St. Martin's Press.

Bernstein, D.A., and T.D. Borkovec. 1973. *Progressive relaxation training.* Champaign, IL: Research Press.

Berque, P., and H. Gray. 2002. The influence of neck-shoulder pain on trapezius muscle activity among professional violin and viola players: An electromyographic study. *Medical Problems of Performing Artists* 17(2), 68-75.

Bertolasi, L., D. De Grandis, L.G. Bongiovanni, G.P. Zanette, and M. Gasperini. 1993. The influence of muscular lengthening on cramps. *Annals of Neurology* 33(2), 176-180.

Best, T.M., B. Loitz-Ramage, D.T. Corr, and R. Vanderby. 1998a. Hyperbaric oxygen in the treatment of acute muscle stretch injuries. *American Journal of Sports Medicine* 26(3), 367-372.

Best, T.M., R.P. McCabe, D. Corr, and R. Vanderby. 1998b. Evaluation of a new method to create a standardized muscle stretch injury. *Medicine and Science in Sports and Exercise* 30(2), 200-205.

Best, T.M., J.H. McElhaney, W.E. Garrett, and B.S. Myers. 1996. Axial strain measurements in skeletal muscle at various strain rates. *Journal of Biomechanical Engineering* 117(3), 262-265.

Bestcourses.com. 2002. Q & A.

Beynon, C., and T. Reilly. 2001. Spinal shrinkage during a seated break and standing break during simulated nursing tasks. *Applied Ergonomics* 32(6), 617-622.

Bick, E.M. 1961. Aging in the connective tissues of the human musculoskeletal system. *Geriatrics* 16(9), 448-453.

Biering-Sørensen, F. 1984. Physical measurements as risk indicators or low-back trouble over a one-year period. *Spine* 9(2), 106-119.

Biesterfeldt, H.J. 1974. Flexibility program. *International Gymnast* 16(3), 22-23.

Bigland-Ritchie, B., and J.J. Woods. 1976. Integrated electromyogram and oxygen uptake during positive and negative work. *Journal of Physiology* (London) 260(2), 267-277.

Bigliani, L.U., T.P. Codd, P.M. Connor, W.N. Levine, M.A. Littlefield, and S.J. Hershon. 1997. Shoulder motion and laxity in the professional baseball player. *American Journal of Sports Medicine* 25(5), 609-613.

Bilkey, W.J. 1992. Involvement of fascia in mechanical pain syndromes. *Journal of Manual Medicine* 6(5), 157-160.

Billig, H.E. 1943. Dysmenorrhea: The result of a postural defect. *Archives of Surgery* 46(5), 611-613.

Billig, H.E. 1951. Fascial stretching. *Journal of Physical and Mental Rehabilitation* 5(1), 4-8.

Billig, H.E., and E. Lowendahl. 1949. *Mobilization of the human body.* Stanford: Stanford University Press.

Bird, H. 1979. Joint laxity in sport. *MediSport: The Review of Sports Medicine* 1(5), 30-31.

Bird, H.A., D.A. Brodie, and V. Wright. 1979. Quantification of joint laxity. *Rheumatology and Rehabilitation* 18, 161-166.

Bird, H.A., M. Calguneri., and V. Wright. 1981. Changes in joint laxity occurring during pregnancy. *Annals of the Rheumatic Diseases* 40(2), 209-212.

Bird, H.A., A. Hudson, C.J. Eastmond, and V. Wright. 1980. Joint laxity and osteoarthritis: A radiological survey of female physical education specialists. *British Journal of Sports Medicine* 14(4), 179-188.

Biro, F., H.L. Gewanter, and J. Baum. 1983. The hypermobility syndrome. *Pediatrics* 72(5), 701-706.

Birrell, F.N., A.O. Adebajo, B.L. Hazleman, and A.J. Silman. 1994. High prevalence of joint laxity in West Africans. *British Journal of Rheumatology* 33(1), 56-59.

Bischoff, C., and D.H. Perrin. 1999. Injury prevention. In *Athletic training and sports medicine.* 3rd ed, ed. R.C. Schenck, 37-62. Rosemont, IL: American Academy of Orthopaedic Surgeons.

Bishop, D. 2003. Warm up I: Potential mechanisms and the effects of passive warm up on exercise performance. *Sports Medicine* 33(6), 439-454.

Bissell, M.J., H.G. Hall, and G. Parry. 1982. How does the extracellular matrix direct gene expression? *Journal of Theoretical Biology* 99(1), 31-68.

Bixler, B., and R.L. Jones. 1992. High-school football injuries: Effects of a post-halftime warm-up and stretching routine. *Family Practice Research Journal* 12(2), 131-139.

Björklund, K., S. Bergström, M-L. Nordström and U. Ulmsten. 2000. Symphyseal distention in relation to serum relaxin levels and pelvic pain in pregnancy. *Acta Obstetrica et Gynecologica Scandinavica* 79(4), 269-275.

Black, J.D.J., and E.D. Stevens. 2001. Passive stretching does not protect against acute contraction-induced injury in mouse EDL muscle. *Journal of Muscle Research and Cell Motility* 22(4), 301-310.

Blau, H. 1989. How fixed is the differentiated state? Lessons from heterokaryons. *Trends in Genetics* 5(8), 268-272.

Blecher, A.M., and J.C. Richmond. 1998. Transient laxity of an anterior cruciate ligament-reconstructed knee related to pregnancy. *Arthroscopy* 14(1), 77-79.

Bledsoe, J. 2003. The truth about stretching and why the Kenyan athletes always do it after their workouts are over. *Peak Performance.* [Online]. Available: www.pponline.co.uk/encyc/0250.htm [October 31, 2003].

Block, R.A., L.A. Hess, E.V. Timpano, and C. Serlo. 1985. Physiological changes in the foot in pregnancy. *Journal of the American Podiatric Medical Association* 75(6), 297-299.

Bloom, W., D.W. Fawcett, and E. Raviola. 1994. *A textbook of histology.* 12th ed. New York: Chapman Hall.

Bloomfield, J., T.R. Ackland, and B.C. Elliott. 1994. *Applied anatomy and biomechanics in sport.* Oxford: Blackwell Scientific.

Bloomfield, J., and B.A. Blanksby. 1971. Strength, flexibility and anthropometric measurements. *Australian Journal of Sports Medicine* 3(10), 8-15.

Bloomfield, J., B.A. Blanksby, T.R. Ackland, and B.C. Elliott. 1985. The anatomical and physiological characteristics of pre-adolescent swimmers, tennis players and non competitors. *The Australian Journal of Science and Medicine in Sport* 17(3), 19-23.

Blumenthal, J.A., C.F. Emery, D.J. Madden, L.K. George, R.E. Coleman, M.W. Riddle, D.C. McKee, J. Reasoner, and R.S. Williams. 1989. Cardiovascular and behavioral effects of aerobic exercise training in healthy older men and women. *Journal of Gerontology* 44(5), M147-M157.

Blumenthal, J.A., and E.C.D. Gullette. 2001. Exercise. In *The encyclopedia of aging. A comprehensive resource in gerontology and geriatrics*. 3rd ed, ed. G.L. Maddox, 371-373. New York: Springer.

Bobbert, M.F., A.P. Hollander, and P.A. Huijing. 1986. Factors in delayed onset muscular soreness of man. *Medicine and Science in Sports and Exercise* 18(1), 75-81.

Bogduk, N. 1984. Applied anatomy of the thoracolumbar fascia. *Spine* 9(9), 164-170.

Bohannon, R.W. 1982. Cinematographic analysis of the passive straight-leg-raising test for hamstring muscle length. *Physical Therapy* 62(9), 1269-1273.

Bohannon, R.W. 1984. Effect of repeated eight-minute muscle loading on the angle of straight-leg raising. *Physical Therapy* 64(4), 491-497.

Bohannon, R., R. Gajdovsik, and B. LeVeau. 1985. Contribution of pelvic and lower limb motion to increase in the angle of passive straight leg raising. *Physical Therapy* 65(4), 474-476.

Boland, R.A. and R.D. Adams. 2000. Effects of ankle dorsiflexion on range and reliability of straight leg raising. *Australian Journal of Physiotherapy* 46(3), 191-200.

Bompa, T. 1990. *Theory and methodology of training*. 2nd ed. Dubuque, IA: Kendall/Hunt.

Bonci, C.M., F.J. Hensal, and J.S. Torg. 1986. A preliminary study on the measurement of static and dynamic motion at the glenohumeral joint. *The American Journal of Sports Medicine* 14(1), 12-17.

Boocock, M.G., G. Garbutt, G. Linge, T. Reilly, and J.D.G. Troup. 1990. Changes in stature following drop jumping and post-exercise gravity inversion. *Medicine and Science in Sports and Exercise* 22(3), 385-390.

Boocock, M.G., G. Garbutt, T. Reilly, G. Linge, and J.D.G. Troup. 1988. The effects of gravity inversion on exercise-induced spinal loading. *Ergonomics* 31(11), 1631-1637.

Boone, D.C., and S.P. Azen. 1979. Normal range of motion of joints in male subjects. *Journal of Bone and Joint Surgery* 61A(5), 756-759.

Borg, G. 1998. *Borg's perceived exertion and pain scales*. Champaign, IL: Human Kinetics.

Borg, T.K., and J.B. Caulfield. 1980. Morphology of connective tissue in skeletal muscle. *Tissue & Cell* 12(1), 197-207.

Borkovec, T.D., and J.K. Sides. 1979. Critical procedural variables related to the physiological effects of progressive relaxation: A review. *Behaviour Research and Therapy* 17(2), 119-125.

Borms, J., P. Van Roy, J.P. Santens, and A. Haentjens. 1987. Optimal duration of static stretching exercises for improvement of coxofemoral flexibility. *Journal of Sports Sciences* 5(1), 39-47.

Boscardin, J.B., P. Johnson, and H. Schneider. 1989. The wind-up, the pitch, and pre-season conditioning. *SportCare & Fitness* 2(1), 30-35.

Boscoe, C., I. Tarkka, and P.V. Komi. 1982. Effects of elastic energy and myoelectrical potentiation of triceps surae during stretch-shortening cycle exercise. *International Journal of Sports Medicine* 3(3), 137-140.

Bosien, W.R., D.S. Staples, and S.W. Russell. 1955. Residual disability following acute ankle sprains. *Journal of Bone and Joint Surgery* 37A(6), 1237-1243.

Botsford, D.J., S.I. Esses, and D.J. Ogilvie-Harris. 1994. In vivo diurnal variation in intervertebral disc volume and morphology. *Spine* 19(8), 935-940.

Bouchard, C., R.M. Malina, and L. Pérusse. 1997. *Genetics of fitness and physical performance*. Champaign, IL: Human Kinetics.

Boulgarides, L.K., S.M. McGinty, J.A. Willett, and C.W. Barnes. 2003. Use of clinical and impairment-based tests to predict falls by community-dwelling older adults. *Physical Therapy* 83(4), 328-339.

Bovens, A.M.P.M., M.A van Baak, J.G.P.M. Vrencken, J.A.G.Wijnen, and F.T.J. Verstappen. 1990. Variability and reliability of joint

measurements. *American Journal of Sports Medicine* 18(1), 58-63.

Bowen, W.P. 1934. *Applied kinesiology*. 5th ed. Philadelphia: Lea & Febiger.

Bowker, J.H., and E.B. Thompson. 1964. Surgical treatment of recurrent dislocation of the patella. *Journal of Bone and Joint Surgery* 46A(7), 1451-1461.

Bowman, M.W. 2000. Athletic injuries to the midfoot and hindfoot. In *Principles and practices of orthopaedic sports medicine* eds. W.E. Garrett, K.P. Speer, and D.T. Kirkendall, 893-943. Philadelphia: Lippincott Williams & Wilkins.

Bozeman, M., J. Mackie, and D.A. Kaufmann. 1986. Quadriceps, hamstring strength and flexibility. *Track Technique* 96, 3060-3061.

Brainum, J. 2000. Stretching the truth. *Ironman* 59(6), 120-125.

Brand, R.A. 1986. Knee ligaments: A new view. *Journal of Biomechanical Engineering* 108(2), 106-110.

Brandfonbrener, A.G. 1990. Joint laxity in instrumental musicians. *Medical Problems of Performing Artists* 5(3), 117-119.

Brandfonbrener, A.G. 1997. Pathogenesis of medical problems of performing artists: General considerations. *Medical Problems of Performing Artists* 12(2), 45-50.

Brandfonbrener, A.G. 2000. Joint laxity and arm pain in musicians. *Medical Problems of Performing Artists* 15(2), 72-74.

Brandfonbrener, A.G. 2001. The medical problems of musicians. *American Music Teacher* 50(6), 21-25.

Brandon, R. 2003. Stretching flexibility exercises: What science has to say about the performance benefits of flexibility training. *Peak Performance*. [Online]. Available: www.pponline.co.uk/encyc/0203b.htm [October 31, 2003].

Brant, J. 1987. See Dick run: Videotape analysis of your running form can make you a more efficient runner. *Runner's World* 22(7), 28-35.

Breig, A. 1960. *Biomechanics of the central nervous system: Some basic normal and pathological phenomena*. Stockholm: Almquist and Wiksell.

Breig, A., and J.D.G. Troup. 1979. Biomechanical considerations in the straight-leg-raising test: Cadaveric and clinical studies of the effects of medial hip rotation. *Spine* 4(3), 242-250.

Brendstrup, P. 1962. Late edema after muscular exercise. *Archives of Physical Medicine and Rehabilitation* 43(8), 401-405.

Bressel, E., and P.J. McNair. 2002. Effect of prolonged static and cyclic stretching on ankle joint stiffness, torque relaxation, and gait in people with stroke. *Physical Therapy* 82(9), 880-887.

Brewer, B., R. Wubben, and G. Carrera. 1986. Excessive retroversion of the glenoid cavity. *Journal of Bone and Joint Surgery* 68A(5), 724-731.

Brewer, V., and M. Hinson. 1978. Relationship of pregnancy to lateral knee stability. *Medicine and Science in Sports* 10(1), 39.

Brill, P.A., and C.A. Macera. 1995. The influence of running patterns on running injuries. *Sports Medicine* 20(6), 365-368.

Brodelius, A. 1961. Osteoarthrosis of the talar joints in footballers and ballet dancers. *Acta Orthopaedica Scandinavica* 30(4), 309-314.

Brodie, D.A., H.A. Bird, and V. Wright. 1982. Joint laxity in selected athletic populations. *Medicine and Science in Sports and Exercise* 14(3), 190-193.

Brodowicz, G.R., R. Welsh, and J. Wallis. 1996. Comparison of stretching with ice, stretching with heat, or stretching alone on hamstring flexibility. *Journal of Athletic Training* 31(4), 324-327.

Brody, D.M. 1995. Running injuries. In *The lower extremity and spine in sports medicine*. 2nd ed., vol. 2. eds. J.A. Nicholas and E.B. Hershman, 1475-1507. St. Louis: Mosby.

Brody, L.T. 1999. Mobility impairment. In *Therapeutic exercise: Moving toward function*, eds. C.M. Hall and L.T. Brody, 87-111. Philadelphia: Lippincott, Williams & Wilkins.

Broer, M.R., and N.R. Gales. 1958. Importance of various body measurements in performance of toe touch test. *Research Quarterly* 29(3), 253-257.

Brooks, G.A., and T.D. Fahey. 1987. *Fundamentals of human performance*. New York: Macmillan.

Brooks, S.V., E. Zerba, and J.A. Faulkner. 1995. Injury to muscle fibres after single stretches of pasive and maximally stimulated muscles in mice. Journal of Physiology 488(Pt.2), 459-469.

Brown, L.E. 2002. Stretch or no stretch? *Strength and Conditioning Journal* 24(1), 20-21.

Brown, L.P., S.L. Niehues, A. Harrah, P. Yavorsky, and H.P. Hirschman. 1998. Upper extremity range of motion and isokinetic strength of the internal and external shoulder rotators in major league baseball players. *American Journal of Sports Medicine* 16(6), 577-585.

Brown, M., and J.O. Holloszy. 1991. Effects of a low-intensity exercise program on selected physical performance characteristics of 60-to-71-year-olds. *Aging* 3, 129-139.

Browne, A.O., P. Hoffmeyer, S. Tanaka, K.N. An, and B.F. Morrey. 1990. Glenohumeral elevation studied in three dimensions. *Journal of Bone and Joint Surgery* 72B(5), 843-845.

Browse, N.L., A.E. Young, and M.L. Thomas. 1979. The effect of bending on canine and human arterial walls and on blood flow. *Circulation Research* 45(1), 41-47.

Brukner, P., and K. Khan. 2002. *Clinical sports medicine*. 2nd ed. Sydney/New York: McGraw-Hill.

Bruser, M. 1997. *The art of practicing: A guide to making music from the heart*. New York: Bell Tower.

Bryant, S. 1984. Flexibility and stretching. *The Physician and Sportsmedicine* 12(2), 171.

Buckingham, R.B., T. Braun, D.A. Harinstein, D. Oral, D. Bauman, W. Bartynski, P.J. Killian, and L.P. Bidula. 1991. Temporomandibular joint dysfunction syndrome: A close association with systemic joint laxity (the hypermobile joint syndrome). *Oral Surgery, Oral Medicine, Oral Pathology* 72(5), 514-519.

Bulbena, A., J.C. Duro, M. Porta, R. Martin-Santos, A. Mateo, L. Molina, R. Vallescar, and J. Vallejo. 1993. Anxiety disorders in the joint hypermobility syndrome. *Psychiatry Research* 46(1), 59-68.

Bunch, M. 1997. *Dynamics of the singing voice*. New York: Springer-Verlag.

Bunn, J.W. 1972. *Scientific principles of coaching*. 2nd ed. Englewood Cliffs, NJ: Prentice-Hall.

Burgener, M. 1991. How to properly miss with a barbell. *National Strength and Conditioning Journal* 13(3), 24-25.

Burke, D., K.E. Hagbarth, and L. Lofstedt. 1978. Muscle spindle activity in man during shortening and lengthening contraction. *Journal of Physiology* (London) 277, 131-142.

Burke, D.G., L.E. Holt, R. Rasmussen, N.C. MacKinnon, J.F. Vossen, and T.W. Pelham. 2001. Effects of hot or cold water immersion and modified proprioceptive neuromuscular facilitation flexibility exercise on hamstring length. *Journal of Athletic Training* 36(1), 16-19.

Burke, R.E., and P. Rudomin. 1978. Spinal neurons and synapses. In *Handbook of physiology: The nervous system. Cellular biology of neurons*, ed. E.R. Kandel, 877-944. Baltimore, MD: Williams & Wilkins.

Burkett, L.N. 1970. Causative factors in hamstring strain. *Medicine and Science in Sports* 2(1), 39-42.

Burkett, L.N. 1971. Cause and prevention of hamstring pulls. *Athletic Journal* 51(6), 34.

Burkett, L.N. 1975. Investigation into hamstring strains: The case of the hybrid muscle. *The Journal of Sports Medicine and Physical Fitness* 3(5), 228-231.

Burkett, L.N., C.C. Seminoff, and B.A. Alvar. 1998. Comparison of the power stretch machine with traditional stretching techniques for increasing low back and hamstrings flexibility. *Isokinetics and Exercise Science* 7(2), 95-99.

Burley, L.R., H.C. Dobell, and B.J. Farrell. 1961. Relations of power, speed, flexibility and certain anthropometric measures of junior high school girls. *Research Quarterly* 32(4), 443-448.

Buroker, K.C., and J.A. Schwane. 1989. Does postexercise static stretching alleviate delayed muscle soreness? *The Physician and Sportsmedicine* 17(6), 65-83.

Burrows, N.P. 1999. The molecular genetics of the Ehlers-Danlos syndrome. *Clinical and Experimental Dermatology* 24(2), 99-105.

Burton, A.K., K.M. Tillotson, and J.D.G. Troup. 1989. Variation in lumbar sagittal mobility with low-back trouble. *Spine* 14(6), 584-590.

Butler, D.S., and L. Gifford. 1989. The concept of adverse mechanical tension in the nervous system. Part I. Testing for dural tension. *Physiotherapy* 75(11), 622-636.

Buxton, D. 1957. Extension of the Kraus-Weber test. *Research Quarterly* 28(3), 210-217.

Byers, P. 1995. Disorders of collagen biosynthesis and structure. In *The metabolic basis of inherited disease*. eds. C. Scriver, A. Beauder, W. Sly, and D. Valle, 4029-4075. New York: McGraw-Hill.

Byers, P.H., R.E. Pyeritz and J. Uitto 1992. Research perspectives in heritable disorders of connective tissue. *Matrix* 12(4), 333-342.

Byrd, R.J. 1973. The effect of controlled, mild exercise on the rate of physiological aging in rats. *Journal of Sports Medicine and Physical Fitness* 13(1), 1-3.

Byrd, S.K. 1992. Alterations in the sarcoplasmic reticulum: A possible link to exercise-induced muscle damage. *Medicine and Science in Sports and Exercise* 24(5), 531-536.

Byrnes, W.C., and P.M. Clarkson. 1986. Delayed onset muscle soreness and training. *Clinics in Sports Medicine* 5(3), 605-614.

Byrnes, W.C., P.M. Clarkson, J.S. White, S.S. Hsieh, P.N. Frykman, and R.J. Maughan. 1985. Delayed onset muscle soreness following repeated bouts of downhill running. *Journal of Applied Physiology* 59(3), 710-713.

Cailliet, R. 1966. *Shoulder pain*. Philadelphia: F.A. Davis.

Cailliet, R. 1977. *Soft tissue pain and disability*. Philadelphia: F.A. Davis.

Cailliet, R. 1981. *Low back pain syndrome*. 3rd ed. Philadelphia: F.A. Davis.

Cailliet, R. 1985. Gravity inversion therapy. *Postgraduate Medicine* 77(6), 270, 274.

Cailliet, R. 1988. *Low back pain syndrome*. 4th ed. Philadelphia: F.A. Davis.

Cailliet, R. 1991. *Shoulder pain*. 3rd ed. Philadelphia: F.A. Davis.

Cailliet, R. 1996. *Soft tissue pain and disability*. 3rd ed. Philadelphia: F.A. Davis.

Cailliet, R., and L. Gross. 1987. *The rejuvenation strategy*. Garden City, NY: Doubleday.

Calais-Germain, B. 1993. *Anatomy of movement*. Seattle: Eastland Press.

Caldwell, R., and Wall, J. 2001. *Excellence in singing*. Vol. 2. Redmond, WA: Caldwell Publishing Company.

Caldwell, W.E., and H.C. Moloy. 1933. Anatomical variations in the female pelvis and their effect in labor with a suggested classification. *American Journal of Obstetrics and Gynecology* 26(4), 479-505.

Calguneri, M., H.A. Bird, and V. Wright. 1982. Changes in joint laxity occurring during pregnancy. *Annals of the Rheumatic Diseases* 41(2), 126-128.

Campbell, E.J.M. 1970. Accessory muscles. In *The respiratory muscles mechanics and neural control*. eds. E.J.M. Campbell, E. Agostoni, and J.N. Davis, 181-193. Philadelphia: W.B. Saunders.

Campbell, K.S., and Lakie, M. 1998. A cross-bridge mechanism can explain the thixotropic short-range elastic component of relaxed frog skeletal muscle. *Journal of Physiology* 510(3), 941-962.

Campbell, R., M. Evans, M. Tucker, B. Quilty, P. Dieppe, and J.L. Donovan. 2001. Why don't patients do their exercises? Understanding non-compliance with physiotherapy in patients with osteoarthritis of the knee. *Journal of Epidemiology & Community Health* 55(2), 132-138.

Cantu, R.I., and A.J. Grodin. 2001. *Myofascial manipulation: Theory and clinical application*. 2nd ed. Gaithersburg, MD: Aspen.

Cao, X. 2002. Scientific bases of acupuncture analgesia. *Acupuncture & Electro-Therapeutics Research: The International Journal* 27(1), 1-14.

Capaday, C., and R.B. Stein. 1987a. Amplitude modulation of the soleus H-reflex in the human during walking and standing. *Journal of Neuroscience Methods* 21(2-4), 91-104.

Capaday, C., and R.B. Stein. 1987b. Difference in the amplitude of the human soleus H-reflex during walking and running. *Journal of Physiology* (London) 392, 513-522.

Carborn, D.N.M., T.D. Armsey, L. Grollman, J.A. Nyland, and J.A. Brosky. 2001. Running. In *Sports injuries: Mechanisms, prevention, treatment*. 2nd ed. eds. F.H. Fu and D.A. Stone, 665-689. Philadelphia: Lippincott Williams & Wilkins.

Carlson, F.D., and D.R. Wilkie. 1974. *Muscle physiology*. Englewood Cliffs, NJ: Prentice-Hall.

Carp, J.S., X.Y. Chen, H. Sheik, and J.R. Wolpaw. 2001. Motor unit properties after operant conditioning of rat H-reflex. *Experimental Brain Research* 140(3), 382-386.

Carr, G. 1997. *Mechanics of sport: A practitioner's guide.* Champaign, IL: Human Kinetics.

Carranza, J. 2002. Create power with proper posture. [Online]. Available: www.golfwashington.com/Instruction/20020410_Proper_Posture [October 31, 2003].

Carrico, M. 1986. Yoga with a chair. *Yoga Journal* 68, 45-51.

Carson, J.A., and F.W. Booth. 1998. Myogenin mRNA is elevated during rapid, slow, and maintenance phases of stretch-induced hypertrophy in chick slow-tonic muscle. *Pflügers Archiv: European Journal of Physiology* 453(6), 850-858.

Carter, C., and R. Sweetnam. 1958. Familial joint laxity and recurrent dislocation of the patella. *Journal of Bone and Joint Surgery* 40B(4), 664-667.

Carter, C., and R. Sweetnam. 1960. Recurrent dislocation of the patella and the shoulder. *Journal of Bone and Joint Surgery* 42B(4), 721-727.

Carter, C., and J. Wilkinson. 1964. Persistent joint laxity and congenital dislocation of the hip. *Journal of Bone and Joint Surgery* 46B(1), 40-45.

Carter, R.L. 2001. Competitive diving. In *Sports injuries: Mechanisms, prevention, treatment.* 2nd ed. eds. F.H. Fu and D.A. Stone, 352-371. Philadelphia: Lippincott Williams & Wilkins.

Cassidy, J.D., J.A. Quon, L.J. Lafrance, and K. Yong-Hing. 1992. The effect of manipulation on pain and range of motion in the cervical spine: A pilot study. *Journal of Manipulative and Physiological Therapeutics* 15(8), 495-500.

Cassidy, S.S., and F. Schwiep. 1989. Cardiovascular effects of positive end-expiratory pressure. In *Heart-lung interactions in health and disease.* eds. S.M. Scharf and S.S. Cassidy, 463-506. New York: Marcel Dekker.

Cavagna, G.A., B. Dusman, and R. Margaria. 1968. Positive work done by a previously stretched muscle. *Journal of Applied Physiology* 24(1), 21-32.

Cavagna, G.A., F.P. Saibene, and R. Margaria. 1965. Effect of negative work on the amount of positive work performed by an isolated muscle. *Journal of Applied Physiology* 20(1), 157-160.

Cerretelli, P., and P.E. di Prampero 1987. Gas exchange in exercise. In *Handbook of physiology a critical, comprehensive presentation of physiological knowledge and concepts. Section 3: The respiratory system.* ed. A.P. Fishman, 297-339. Bethesda, Maryland: American Physiological Society.

Chaitow, L. 1990. *Osteopathic self-treatment.* Rochester, VT: Thorsons.

Chaitow, L. 2002. *Positional release techniques.* Edinburgh: Churchill Livingstone.

Chan, S.P., Hong, Y, and P.D. Robinson. 2001. Flexibility and passive resistance of the hamstrings of young adults using two different static stretching protocols. *Scandinavian Journal of Medicine & Science in Sports* 11(2), 81-86.

Chandler, T.J., W.B. Kibler, T.L. Uhl, B. Wooten, A. Kiser, and E. Stone, E. 1990. Flexibility comparisons of junior elite tennis players to other athletes. *American Journal of Sports Medicine* 18(2), 134-136.

Chandler, T.J., G.D. Wilson, and M.H. Stone. 1989. The effect of the squat exercise on knee stability. *Medicine and Science in Sports and Exercise* 21(3), 299-303.

Chang, D.E., L.P. Buschbacher, and R.F. Edlich. 1988. Limited joint mobility in power lifters. *American Journal of Sports Medicine* 16(3), 280-284.

Chapman, E.A., H.A. de Vries, and R. Swezey. 1972. Joint stiffness: Effects of exercise on young and old men. *Journal of Gerontology* 27(2), 218-221.

Chapron, D.J., and R.W. Besdine. 1987. Drugs as obstacle to rehabilitation of the elderly: A primer for therapists. *Topics in Geriatric Rehabilitation* 2(3), 63-81.

Chatfield, S.J., W.C. Byrnes, D.A. Lally, and S.E. Rowe. 1990. Cross-sectional physiologic profiling of modern dancers. *Dance Research Journal* 22(1), 13-20.

Chatterjee, S., and N. Das. 1995. Physical and motor fitness in twins. *Japanese Journal of Physiology* 45(3), 519-534.

Chen, C-Y., P.S. Neufeld, C.A. Feely, and C.S. Skinner. 1999. Factors influencing compliance with home exercise programs among patients with upper-extremity impairment. *American Journal of Occupational Therapy* 53(2), 171-180.

Cheng, J.C.Y., P.S. Chan, and P.W. Hui. 1991. Joint laxity in children. *Journal of Pediatric Orthopaedics* 11(6), 752-756.

Cherry, D.B. 1980. Review of physical therapy alternatives for reducing muscle contracture. *Physical Therapy* 60(7), 877-881.

Chiarello, C.M., and R. Savidge. 1993. Interrater reliability of the Cybex EDI-320 and fluid goniometer in normals and patients with low back pain. *Archives of Physical Medicine and Rehabilitation* 74(1), 32-37.

Child, A.H. 1986. Joint hypermobility syndrome: Inherited disorder of collagen synthesis. *Journal of Rheumatology* 13(2), 239-243.

Chinn, C.J., J.D. Priest, and B.E. Kent. 1974. Upper extremity range of motion, grip strength, and girth in highly skilled tennis players. *Physical Therapy* 54(5), 474-483.

Chissell, J. 1967. *Schumann.* New York: Farrar, Straus and Giroux.

Cholewicki, J., and S.M. McGill. 1992. Lumbar posterior ligament involvement during extremely heavy lifts estimated from fluoroscopic measurements. *Journal of Biomechanics* 25(1), 17-28.

Cholewicki, J., and S.M. McGill. 1996. Mechanical stability of the in vivo lumbar spine: Implications for injury and chronic low back pain. *Clinical Biomechanics* 11(1), 1-15.

Cholewicki, J., S.M. McGill, and R.W. Norman. 1995. Comparison of muscle forces and joint load from an optimization and EMG assisted lumbar spine model: Towards development of a hybrid approach. *Journal of Biomechanics* 28(3), 321-331.

Christian, G.F., G.J. Stanton, D., Sissons, H.Y. How, J. Jamison, B. Alder, M. Fullerton, and J.W. Funder. 1988. Immunoreactive ACTH, β-endorphin, and cortisol levels in plasma following spinal manipulative therapy. *Spine* 13(12), 1411-1417.

Christiansen, C.H., and C.M. Baum. 1997. Glossary. In *Occupational therapy: Enabling function and well-being.* 2nd ed. eds. C.H. Christiansen and C.M. Baum. Thorofare, NJ: Slack.

Chujoy, A., and P.W. Manchester. eds. 1967. *The dance encyclopedia.* New York: Simon and Schuster.

Church, J.B., M.S. Wiggins, F.M. Moode, and R. Crist. 2001. Effect of warm-up and flexibility treatments on vertical jump perfromance. *Journal of Strength and Conditioning Research* 15(3), 332-336.

Cipriani, D., B. Abel, and D. Pirrwitz. 2003. A comparison of two stretching protocols on hip range of motion: Implications for total daily stretch duration. *Journal of Strength and Conditioning Research* 17(2), 274-278.

Ciullo, J.V., and B. Zarins. 1983. Biomechanics of the musculotendinous unit. *Clinics in Sports Medicine* 2(1), 71-85.

Clanton, T.O., and K.J. Coupe. 1998. Hamstring strains in athletes: Diagnosis and treatment. *Journal of the American Academy of Orthopaedic Surgeons* 6(4), 237-248.

Clark, J.M., F.C. Hagerman, and R. Gelfand. 1983. Breathing patterns during submaximal and maximal exercise in elite oarsmen. *Journal of Applied Physiology* 55(2), 440-446.

Clarke, H.H. 1975. Joint and body range of movement. *Physical Fitness Research Digest* 5: 16-18.

Clarkson, P.M., W.C. Byrnes, E. Gillison, and E. Harper. 1987. Adaptation to exercise-induced muscle damage. *Clinical Science* 73(4), 383-386.

Clarkson, P.M., K. Nosaka, and B. Braun. 1992. Muscle function after exercise-induced muscle damage and rapid adaptation. *Medicine and Science in Sports and Exercise* 24(5), 512-520.

Clarkson, P.M., and I. Tremblay. 1988. Rapid adaptation to exercise induced muscle damage. *Journal of Applied Physiology* 65(1), 1-6.

Cleak, M.J., and R.G. Eston. 1992. Delayed onset muscle soreness: Mechanisms and management. *Journal of Sports Sciences* 10(4), 325-341.

Clemente, C.D. 1985. *Anatomy of the human body.* 30th ed. Philadelphia: Lea & Febiger.

Cleveland, T.F. 1998a. A comparison of breath management strategies in classical and nonclassical singers Part 1. *Journal of Singing* 54(5), 47-49.

Cleveland, T.F. 1998b. A comparison of breath management strategies in classical and nonclassical singers Part 2. *Journal of Singing* 55(1), 45-46.

Cleveland, T.F. 1998c. A comparison of breath management strategies in classical and nonclassical singers. Part 3. *Journal of Singing* 55(2), 53-55.

Clippinger-Robertson, K. 1988. Understanding contraindicated exercises. *Dance Exercise Today* 6(1), 57-60.

Cohen, D.B., M.A. Mont, K.R. Campbell., B.N. Vogelstein, and J.W. Loewy. 1994. Upper extremity physical factors affecting tennis serve velocity. *American Journal of Sports Medicine* 22(6), 746-750.

Colachis, S.C., and B.R. Strohm. 1965. Relationship of time to varied tractive force with constant angle of pull. *Archives of Physical Medicine and Rehabilitation* 46(11), 815-819.

Comeau, M.J. 2002. Stretch or no stretch? Cons. *Strength and Conditioning Journal* 24(1), 20-21.

Comwell, D.B. 1941. *The championship technique in track and field.* New York: McGraw-Hill.

Concu, A., W. Ferrari, G.L. Gessa, F.P. Mercu, and A. Tagliamonte. 1974. EEG changes induced by the intraventricular injection of ACTH in cats. In *Sleep*, eds. P. Levin and W.P. Koella, 321. Basel: Karger.

Condon, S.A. 1983. *Resistance to muscle stretch induced by volitional muscle contraction.* Master's thesis, University of Washington.

Condon, S.A., and R.S. Hutton. 1987. Soleus muscle electromyographic activity and ankle dorsiflexion range of motion during four stretching procedures. *Physical Therapy* 67(1), 24-30.

Conroy, R.T.W.L., and J.N. Mills. 1970. *Human circadian rhythms.* London: Churchill.

A contortionist. 1882. *Lancet* 1, 576.

Cook, E.E., V.L. Gray, E. Savinar-Nogue, and J. Medeiros. 1987. Shoulder antagonistic strength ratios: A comparison between college level baseball pitchers and nonpitchers. *Journal of Orthopaedic and Sports Physical Therapy* 8(9), 451-461.

Cooper Fitness Center, The. 2002. Stretching FAQs. [online]. www.cooperfitness.com/contents/Story.asp?SID=1460.

Corbett, M. 1972. The use and abuse of massage and exercise. *The Practitioner* 208(1243), 136-139.

Corbin, C.B., L.J. Dowell, R. Lindsey, and H. Tolson. 1978. *Concepts in physical education.* 3rd ed. Dubuque, IA: Brown.

Corbin, C.B., and L. Noble. 1980. Flexibility: A major component of physical fitness. *Journal of Physical Education and Recreation* 51(6), 23-24, 57-60.

Cornbleet, S.L., and N.B. Woolsey. 1996. Assessment of hamstring muscle length in school-aged children using the sit-and-reach test and the inclinometer measure of hip joint angle. *Physical Therapy* 76(8), 850-855.

Cornelius, W.L. 1983. Stretch evoked EMG activity by isometric contraction and submaximal concentric contraction. *Athletic Training* 18(2), 106-109.

Cornelius, W.L. 1984. Exercise beneficial to the hip but questionable for the knee. *NSCA Journal* 6(5), 40-41.

Cornelius, W.L. 1989. Flexibility exercises: Effective practices. *NSCA Journal* 11(6), 61-62.

Cornelius, W.L., and K. Craft-Hamm. 1988. Proprioceptive neuromuscular facilitation techniques: Acute affects on arterial blood pressure. *Physician and Sportsmedicine* 16(4), 152-161.

Cornelius, W.L., R.W. Hagemann, and A.W. Jackson. 1988. A study on placement of stretching within a workout. *Journal of Sports Medicine and Physical Fitness* 28(3), 234-236.

Cornelius, W.L., and M.M. Hinson. 1980. The relationship between isometric contractions of hip extensors and subsequent flexibility in males. *Journal of Sports Medicine and Physical Fitness* 20(1), 75-80.

Cornelius, W.L., and A. Jackson. 1984. The effects of cryotherapy and PNF on hip extensor flexibility. *Athletic Training* 19, 183-199.

Cornelius, W.L., R.L. Jensen, and M.E. Odell. 1995. Effects of PNF stretching phases on acute arterial blood pressure. *Canadian Journal of Applied Physiology* 20(2), 222-229.

Couch, J. 1979. *Runner's World yoga book.* Mountain View, CA: World.

Cottrell, N.B. 1968. Performance in the presence of other human beings: Mere presence, audience, and affiliative effects. In *Social facilitation and imitative behavior*, eds. E.C. Simmell, R.A. Hoppe, and G.A. Milton, 91-110. Boston: Allyn and Bacon.

Cottrell, N.B., D.L. Wack, G.J. Sekerak, and R.H. Rittle. 1968. Social facilitation of dominanat response by the presence of an audience and the mere presence of others. *Journal of Personality and Social Psychology* 9(3), 245-250.

Coulter, D., 2001. *Anatomy of hatha yoga.* Honesdale, PA: Body and Breath.

Counsilman, J.E. 1968. *The science of swimming.* Englewood Cliffs, NJ: Prentice-Hall.

Counsilman, J.E. 1977. *The complete book of swimming.* New York: Antheneum.

Coville, C.A. 1979. Relaxation in physical education curricula. *The Physical Educator* 36(4), 176-181.

Coyle, E.F., D.L. Costill, and G.R. Lesmes. 1979. Leg extension power and muscle fiber composition. *Medicine and Science in Sports* 1(11), 12-15.

Craib, M.W., V.A. Mitchell, K.B. Fields, T.R. Cooper, R. Hopewell, and D.W. Morgan. 1996. The association between flexibility and running economy in sub-elite male distance runners. *Medicine and Science in Sports and Exercise* 28(6), 737-743.

Craig, E.J., and D. Kaelin. 2000. Physical modalities. In *Physical medicine and rehabilitation: The complete approach*, eds. M. Grabois, S.J. Garrison, K.A. Hart, and L.D. Lehmkuhl, 441-450. Oxford: Blackwell Science.

Cramer, L.M., and C.H. McQueen. 1990. Overuse injuries in figure skating. In *Winter sports medicine*, ed. M.J. Casey, C. Foster, and E.G. Hixson, 254-268. Philadelphia: Davis.

Crawford, H.J., and G.A. Jull. 1993. The influence of thoracic posture and movement on range of arm elevation. *Physiotherapy Theory and Practice* 9(3), 143-148.

Crisp, J. 1972. Properties of tendon and skin. In *Biomechanics: Its foundation and objectives.* eds. Y.C. Yung, N. Perrone, and M. Anliker, 141-180. Englewood Cliffs, NJ: Prentice-Hall.

Crosman, L.J., S.R. Chateauvert, and J. Weisberg. 1984. The effects of massage to the hamstring muscle group on the range of motion. *Journal of Orthopaedic and Sports Physical Therapy* 6(3), 168-172.

Cross, K.M., and T.W. Worrell. 1999. Effects of a static stretching program on the incidence of lower extremity musculotendinous strains. *Journal of Athletic Training* 34(1), 11-14.

Cummings, G.S. 1984. Comparison of muscle to other soft tissue in limiting elbow extension. *Journal of Orthopaedic and Sports Physical Therapy* 5(4), 170-174.

Cummings, G.S., and L.J. Tillman. 1992. Remodeling of dense connective tissue in normal adult tissues. In *Dynamics of human biologic tissues.* eds. D.P. Currier and R.M. Nelson, 45-73. Philadelphia: Davis.

Cummings, M.S., V.E. Wilson, and E.I. Bird. 1984. Flexibility development in sprinters using EMG biofeedback and relation training. *Biofeedback and Self-Regulation* 9(3), 395-405.

Cureton, T.K. 1930. Mechanics and kinesiology of swimming. *Research Quarterly* 1(4), 87-121.

Dahm, D.L., and C.M. Lajam. 2002. Shoulder instability in the female athlete. *Operative Techniques in Sports Medicine* 10(1), 5-9.

Daleiden, S. 1990. Prevention of falling: Rehabilitative or compensatory interventions? *Topics in Geriatric Rehabilitation* 5(2), 44-53.

Danforth, D.N. 1967. Pregnancy and labor: From the vantage point of the physical therapist. *American Journal of Physical Medicine* 46(1), 653-658.

Daniell, H.W. 1979. Simple cure for nocturnal leg cramps. *New England Journal of Medicine* 301(4), 216.

Danlos, P.M. 1908. Un cas de Cutis laxa avec tumeurs par contusion chronique des coudes et des genoux. *Bulletin de la Société De Dermatologie et de Syphiligraphie* 19(Janvier) 70-72.

Davies, A., K. Finlay, M. Hilly, and C. Purdam. 1992. A comparison of the effect of static and ballistic stretching on hamstring strength. Proceedings from the annual scientific conference in sports medicine, Australian Sports Medicine Federation, Perth.

Davies, C. 2002. Musculoskeletal pain from repetitive strain in musicians: Insights into an alternative approach. *Medical Problems of Performing Artists* 17(1), 42-49.

Davies, C.T.M., and C. Barnes. 1972. Negative (eccentric) work. 1. Effects of repeated exercise. *Ergonomics* 15(1), 3-14.

Davies, C.T.M., and K. Young. 1983. Effects of training at 30% and 100% maximal isometric force (MVC) on the contractile properties of the triceps surae in man (Abstract). *Journal of Physiology* (London) 336: 31P.

Davies, G.J., D.T. Kirkendall, D.H. Leigh, M.L. Lui, T.R. Reinbold, and P.K. Wilson. 1981. Isokinetic characteristics of professional football players: I. Normative relationships between quadriceps and hamstring muscle group and relative to body weight. *Medicine and Science in Sports and Exercise* 13(2), 76-77.

Davis, E.C., G.A. Logan, and W.C. McKinney. 1965. *Biophysical values of muscular activity with implications for research.* 2nd ed. Dubuque, IA: Brown.

Davis, L. 1988. Stretching a point. *Hippocrates* 2(4), 90-92.

Davison, S. 1984. Standing: A good remedy. *Journal of the American Medical Association* 252(24), 3367.

Davson, H. 1970. *A textbook of general physiology.* 4th ed. Baltimore: Williams & Wilkins.

Dawson, W.J. 1995. Experience with hand and upper-extremity problems in 1,000 instrumentalists. *Medical Problems of Performing Artists* 10(4), 128-133.

Dawson, W.J. 2001. Upper extremity difficulties in the dedicated amateur instrumentalist. *Medical Problems of Performing Artists* 16(4), 152-156.

Day, R.K., C.R. Ashmore, and Y.B. Lee. 1984. The effect of stretch removal on muscle weight and proteolytic enzyme activity in normal and dystrophic chicken muscles. *Muscle & Nerve* 7(6), 482-485.

Day, R.W., and B.P. Wildermuth. 1988. Proprioceptive training in the rehabilitation of lower extremity injuries. In *Advances in sports medicine and fitness*, ed. W.A. Grana, 241-258. Chicago: Year Book Medical.

Dean, E. 1988. Physiology and therapeutic implications of negative work: A review. *Physical Therapy* 68(2), 233-237.

Debevoise, N.T., G.W. Hyatt, and G.B. Townsend. 1971. Humeral torsion in recurrent shoulder dislocations: A technic of determination by x-ray. *Clinical Orthopaedics and Related Research*, 76(May): 87-93.

Debreceni, L. 1993. Chemical releases associated with acupuncture and electrical stimulation. *Critical Reviews in Physical and Rehabilitation Medicine* 5(3), 247-275.

Decoster, L.C., J.C. Vailas, R.H. Lindsay, and G.R. Williams. 1997. Prevalence and features of joint hypermobility among adolescent athletes. *Archives of Pediatrics & Adolescent Medicine* 151(10), 989-992.

de Jong, R.H. 1980. Defining pain terms. *Journal of the American Medical Association* 244(2), 143.

de Koninck, J., D. Lorrain, and P. Gagnon. 1992. Sleep positions and position shifts in five age groups: An ontogenetic picture. *Sleep* 15(2), 143-149.

de Lateur, B.J. 1994. Flexibility. *Physical Medicine and Rehabilitation Clinics of North America* 5(2), 295-307.

Delforge, G. 2002. *Musculoskeletal trauma: Implications for sports injury management.* Champaign, IL: Human Kinetics.

Delitto, R.S., S.J. Rose, and D.W. Apts. 1987. Electromyographic analysis of two techniques for squat lifting. *Physical Therapy* 67(9), 1329-1334.

DeLuca, C. 1985. Control properties of motor units. *Journal of Experimental Biology* 115, 125-136.

Denny-Brown, D., and M.M. Doherty. 1945. Effects of transient stretching of peripheral nerve. *Archives of Neurology and Psychiatry* 54(2), 116-122.

DePino, G.M., W.G. Webright, and B.L. Arnold. 2000. Duration of maintained hamstring flexibility after cessation of an acute stretching protocol. *Journal of Athletic Training* 35(1), 56-59.

DePriest, S.M., T.M. Adams, A. Byars, J.L. Stilwell, C. Albright, and P. Finnicum. 2002. An investigation of the effectiveness of The Rack on ankle plantar flexion. *Research Quarterly for Exercise and Sport* 70(1 Suppl.), A18-A19.

De Smet, A.A., and T.M. Best. 2000. MR imaging of the distribution and location of acute hamstring injuries in athletes. *American Journal of Roentgenology* 174(2), 393-399.

De Troyer, A., and S.H. Loring. 1986. Action of the respiratory muscles. In *Handbook of physiology: Sec. 3. The respiratory system: Vol. 3. Mechanics of breathing. Part 2*, ed. S.R. Geiger, 443-461. Bethesda, MD: American Physiological Society.

Devor, E.J., and M.H. Crawford. 1984. Family resemblance for neuromuscular performance in a Kansas Mennonite community. *American Journal of Physical Anthropology* 64(3), 289-296.

de Vries, H.A. 1961a. Electromyographic observation of the effect of static stretching upon muscular distress. *Research Quarterly* 32(4), 468-479.

de Vries, H.A. 1961b. Prevention of muscular distress after exercise. *Research Quarterly* 32(2), 177-185.

de Vries, H.A. 1962. Evaluation of static stretching procedures for improvement of flexibility. *Research Quarterly* 33(2), 222-229.

de Vries, H.A. 1963. The "looseness" factor in speed and O2 consumption of an anaerobic 100-yard dash. *Research Quarterly* 34(3), 305-313.

de Vries, H.A. 1966. Quantitative electromyographic investigation of the spasm theory of muscle pain. *American Journal of Physical Medicine* 45(3), 119-134.

de Vries, H.A. 1985. Inversion devices: Potential benefits and precautions. *Corporate Fitness & Recreation* 4(6), 24-27.

de Vries, H.A. 1986. *Physiology of exercise.* 4th ed. Dubuque, IA: Brown.

de Vries, H.A., and G.M. Adams. 1972. EMG comparison of single doses of exercise and meprobamate as to effects on muscular relaxation. *American Journal of Physical Medicine* 51(3), 130-141.

de Vries, H.A., and R. Cailliet. 1985. Vagotonic effect of inversion therapy upon resting neuromuscular tension. *American Journal of Physical Medicine* 64(3), 119-129.

de Vries, H.A., R.A. Wiswell, R. Bulbulion, and T. Moritani. 1981. Tranquilizer effect of exercise. *American Journal of Physical Medicine* 60(2), 57-66.

Deyo, R.A., N.E. Walsh, D.C. Martin, L.S. Schoenfeld, and S. Ramamurthy. 1990. A controlled trial of transcutaneous electrical nerve stimulation (TENS) and exercise for chronic low back pain. *New England Journal of Medicine*, 322(23), 1627-1634.

Dick, F.W. 1980. *Sports training principles.* London: Lepus Books.

Dick, R.W., and P.R. Cavanagh. 1987. An explanation of the upward drift in oxygen uptake during prolonged sub-maximal downhill running. *Medicine and Science in Sports and Exercise* 19(3), 310-317.

Dickenson, R.V. 1968. The specificity of flexibility. *Research Quarterly* 39(3), 792-794.

Dillman, C.J., G.S. Fleisig, and J.R. Andrews. 1993. Biomechanics of pitching with emphasis upon shoulder kinematics. *Journal of Orthopaedic and Sports Physical Therapy* 18(2), 402-408.

DiMatteo, M.R., and D.D. DiNicola. 1982. *Achieving patient compliance: The psychology of the medical practitioner's role.* New York: Pergamon.

DiMatteo, M.R., L.M. Prince, and A. Taranta. 1979. Patients' perceptions of physicians' behavior: Determinants of patient commitment to the therapeutic relationship. *Journal of Community Health* 4(4), 280-290.

Dintiman, G., and R. Ward. 1988. *Sport speed.* Champaign, IL: Human Kinetics.

DiRaimondo, C. 1991. Overuse conditions of the foot and ankle. In *Foot and ankle manual*, ed. G.J. Sammarco, 260-275. Philadelphia: Lea & Febiger.

Dishman, R.K, ed. 1988. *Exercise adherence: Its impact on public health.* Champaign, IL: Human Kinetics.

DiTullio, M., L. Wilczek, D. Paulus, A. Kiriakatis, M. Pollack, and J. Eisenhardt. 1989. Comparison of hip rotation in female classical ballet dancers versus female nondancers. *Medical Problems of Performing Artists* 4(4), 154-158.

Dix, D.J., and B.R. Eisenberg. 1990. Myosin mRNA accumulation and myofibrillogenesis at the myotendinous junction of stretched muscle fibers. *Journal of Cell Biology* 111(5, Pt. 1), 1885-1894.

Dix, D.J., and B.R. Eisenberg. 1991a. Distribution of myosin mRNA during development and regeneration of skeletal muscle. *Developmental Biology* 143(2), 422-426.

Dix, D.J., and B.R. Eisenberg. 1991b. Redistribution of myosin heavy chain mRNA in the midregion of stretched muscle fibers. *Cell and Tissue Research* 263(1), 61-69.

Dobeln. *See* Allander et al. 1974.

Dobrin, P.B. 1983. Vascular mechanics. In *The handbook of physiology: Sec. 2. The cardiovascular system III: Vol. 3. Peripheral circulation and organ blood flow, Pt. I.* eds. J.T. Shepherd and F.M. Abboud, 65-102. Bethesda, MD: American Physiological Society.

Docherty, D., and R.D. Bell. 1985. The relationship between flexibility and linearity measures in boys and girls 6-15 years of age. *Journal of Human Movement Studies* 11(5), 279-288.

Doherty, K. 1985. *Track and field omnibook.* 4th ed. Swarthmore, PA: Tafmop.

Dolan, P., and M.A. Adams. 1993. Influence of lumbar and hip mobility on the bending stresses acting on the lumbar spine. *Clinical Biomechanics* 8(4), 185-192.

Dominguez, R.H. 1980. Shoulder pain in swimmers. *The Physician and Sportsmedicine* 8(7), 36-42.

Dominguez, R.H., and R. Gajda. 1982. *Total body training.* New York: Warner.

Donatelli, R., and H. Owens-Burkhart. 1981. Effects of immobilization on the extensibility of periarticular connective tissue. *Journal of Orthopaedic and Sports Physical Therapy* 3(2), 67-72.

Donisch, E.W., and J.V. Basmajian. 1972. Electromyography of deep back muscles in man. *American Journal of Anatomy* 133(1), 25-36.

Donison, C. 1998. Small hands? Try this keyboard, you'll like it. *Piano & Keyboard* 193, 41-43.

DonTigny, R.L. 1985. Function and pathomechanics of the sacroiliac joint. *Physical Therapy* 65(1), 35-41.

Doran, D.M.L., and D.J. Newell. 1975. Manipulation in the treatment of low back pain: A multicentre study. *British Medical Journal* 2, 161-164.

Dorland's illustrated medical dictionary. 29th ed. 2000. Philadelphia: W.B. Saunders.

Doss, W.S., and P.V. Karpovich. 1965. A comparison of concentric, eccentric, and isometric strength of elbow flexors. *Journal of Applied Physiology* 20(2), 351-353.

Douglas, S. 1980. *Physical evaluation of the swimmer.* Presented at the First Annual Vail Sportsmedicine Symposium, Vail, CO.

Downer, A.H. 1996. *Physical therapy procedures: Selected techniques.* 5th ed. Springfield, IL: Charles C Thomas.

Dowsing, G.S. 1978. Partner exercise. *Coaching Women's Athletics* 4(2), 18-20.

Draper, D.O., C. Anderson, S.S. Schulthies, and M.D. Ricard. 1998. Immediate and residual changes in dorsiflexion range of motion using an ultrasound heat and stretch routine. *Journal of Athletic Training* 33(2), 141-144.

Draper, D.O., J.C. Castel, and D. Castel. 1995. Rate of temperature increase in human muscle during 1 MHz and 3MHz continuous ultrasound. *Journal of Orthopaedic and Sports Physical Therapy* 22(4), 142-150.

Draper, D.O., C. Hatheway, and D. Fowler. 1991. Methods of applying underwater ultrasound: Science versus folklore. *Athletic Training* 26(2), 152-154.

Draper, D.O., K.L. Knight, T. Fujiwara, and J.C. Castel. 1999. Temperature change in human muscle during and after pulsed shortwave diathermy. *Journal of Orthopaedic and Sports Physical Therapy* 29(1), 13-22.

Draper, D.O., and M.D. Ricard. 1995. Rate of temperature decay in human muscle following 3-MHz ultrasound: The stretching window revealed. *Journal of Athletic Training* 30(4), 304-307.

Draper, D.O., S. Sunderland, D.T. Kirkendall, and M. Ricard. 1993. A comparison of temperature rise in human calf muscles following applications of underwater and topical gel ultrasound. *Journal of Orthopaedic and Sports Physical Therapy* 17(5), 247-251.

Drezner, J.A. 2003. Practical management hamstring muscle injuries. *Clinical Journal of Sport Medicine* 13(1), 48-52.

Dubrovskii, V.I. 1990. The effect of massage on athletes' cardiorespiratory systems (clinico-physiological research). *Soviet Sports Review* 25(1), 36-38.

Dummer, G.M., P. Vaccaro, and D.H. Clarke. 1985. Muscular strength and flexibility of two female master swimmers in the eighth decade of life. *Journal of Orthopaedic and Sports Physical Therapy* 6(4), 235-237.

Dvorkin, L.S. 1986. The young weightlifter: Development of flexibility. *Soviet Sports Review* 21(3), 153-156.

Dye, A.A. 1939. *The evolution of chiropractic: Its discovery and development.* Philadelphia: Author.

Dyson, G.H.G. 1986. *The mechanics of athletics.* London: Hodder and Stoughton.

Ebbeling, C.B., and Clarkson, P.M. 1989. Exercise-induced muscle damage and adaptation. *Sports Medicine* 7(4), 207-234.

Ecker, T. 1971. *Track & field dynamics.* Los Altos, CA: Tafnews Press.

Edworthy, S.M. 1999. Morning stiffness: Sharpening an old saw? *Journal of Rheumatology* 26(5), 1015-1017.

Ehlers, E. 1901. Cutis laxa Neigung zu Haemorrhagien in der Haut, Lockerung mehrerer Artikulationen. (Case for Diagnosis). *Dermatologische Zeitschrift* 8(2), 173-174.

Ehrhart, B. 1976. Thirty Russian flexibility exercises for hurdlers. *Athletic Journal* 56(7), 38-39, 96.

Einkauf, D.K., M.L. Gohdes, G.M. Jensen, and M.J. Jewell. 1986. Changes in spinal mobility with increasing age in women. *Physical Therapy* 67(3), 370-375.

Eklund, J.A.E., and E.N. Corlett. 1984. Shrinkage as a measure of the effect of load on the spine. *Spine* 9(2), 189-194.

Ekman, B., K.-G. Ljungquist, and U. Stein. 1970. Roentgenologic-photometric method for bone mineral determinations. *Acta Radiologica* 10, 305-325.

Ekstrand, J., and J. Gillquist. 1982. The frequency of muscle tightness and injuries in soccer. *American Journal of Sports Medicine* 10(2), 75-78.

Ekstrand, J., and J. Gillquist. 1983. The avoidability of soccer injuries. *International Journal of Sports Medicine* 4(2), 124-128.

Eldred, E., R.S. Hutton, and J.L. Smith. 1976. Nature of the persisting changes in afferent discharge from muscle following its contraction. *Progressive Brain Research* 44, 157-170.

Eldren, H.R. 1968. Physical properties of collagen fibers. *International Review of Connective Tissue Research* 4, 248-283.

Ellenbecker, T.S., and E.P. Roetert. 2002. Effects of a 4-month season on glenohumeral joint rotational strength and range of motion in female collegiate tennis players. *Journal of Strength and Conditioning Research* 16(1), 92-96.

Ellenbecker, T.S., E.P. Roetert, P.A. Piorkowski, and D.A. Schultz. 1996. Glenohumeral joint internal and external rotation range of motion in elite junior tennis players. *Journal of Orthopaedic and Sports Physical Therapy* 24(6), 336-341.

Elliott, D.H. 1965. Structure and function of mammalian tendon. *Biological Review* 40(3), 392-421.

Elliott, J. 1993. Shoulder pain and flexibility in elite water polo players. *Physiotherapy* 79(10), 693-697.

Ellis, C.G., O. Mathieu-Costello, R.F. Potter, I. C. MacDonald, and A.C. Groom. 1990. Effect of sarcomere length on total capillary length in skeletal muscle: In vivo evidence for longitudinal stretching of capillaries. *Microvascular Research* 40(1), 63-72.

Ellis, J. 1986. Shinsplints too much, too soon. *Runners World* 21(3), 50-53, 86.

Elnaggar, I.M., M. Nordin, M.A. Sheikhzadeh, M. Parnianpour, and N. Kahanovitz. 1991. Effects of spinal flexion and extension exercises in low back pain and spinal mobility in chronic mechanical low back pain patients. *Spine* 16(8), 967-971.

el-Shahaly, H.A., and A.K. el-Sherif. 1991. Is the benign joint hypermobility syndrome benign? *Clinical Rheumatology* 10(3), 302-307.

Emery, C.A., W.H. Meeuwisse, and J.W. Powell. 1999. Groin and abdominal strain injuries in the National Hockey League. *Clinical Journal of Sport Medicine* 9(3), 151-156.

Emmons, M. 1978. *The inner source: A guide to meditative therapy.* San Luis Obispo, CA: Impact.

Ende, L.S., and J. Wickstrom. 1982. Ballet injuries. *The Physician and Sportsmedicine* 10(7), 101-118.

Engesvik, F. 1993. Leg movements in the breaststroke. *Swimming Technique* 29(4), 26-27.

Enoka, R.M. 2002. *Neuromechanics of human movement.* 3rd ed. Champaign, IL: Human Kinetics.

Ensink, F-B. M., P.M.M. Saur, K. Frese, D. Seeger, and J. Hildebrandt. 1996. Lumbar range of motion: Influence of time of day and individual factors on measurements. *Spine* 21(11), 1339-1343.

Eppel, W., E. Kucera, and C. Bieglmayer. 1999. Relationship of serum levels of endogenous relaxin to cervical size in the second trimester and to cervical ripening at term. *British Journal of Obstetrics and Gynecology* 106(9), 917-923.

Ernst, E. 1998. Does post-exercise massage treatment reduce delayed onset muscular soreness? A systematic review. *British Journal of Sports Medicine* 32(3), 212-214.

Esola, M.A., P.W. McClure, G.K. Fitzgerald, and S. Siegler. 1996. Analysis of lumbar spine and hip motion during forward bending in subjects with and without a history of significant low back pain. *Spine* 21(1), 71-78.

Etnyre, B., and L. Abraham. 1984. Effects of three stretching techniques on the motor pool excitability of the human soleus muscle (Abstract). In *Abstracts of research papers 1984*, ed. W. Roll, 90. Reston, VA: American Alliance of Health, Physical Education, and Recreation.

Etnyre, B.R., and D.L. Abraham. 1986a. Gains in range of ankle dorsiflexion using three popular stretching techniques. *American Journal of Physical Medicine* 65(4), 189-196.

Etnyre, B.R., and L.D. Abraham. 1986b. H-reflex changes during static stretching and two variations of proprioceptive neuromuscular facilitation techniques. *Electroencephalography and Clinical Neurophysiology* 63(2), 174-179.

Etnyre, B.R., and L.D. Abraham. 1988. Antagonist muscle activity during stretching: A paradox re-assessed. *Medicine and Science in Sports and Exercise* 20(3), 285-289.

Etnyre, B.R., and E.J. Lee. 1987. Comments on proprioceptive neuromuscular facilitation stretching techniques. *Research Quarterly for Exercise and Sport* 58(2), 184-188.

Evans, D.P., M.S. Burke, K.H. Lloyd, E.E. Roberts, and G.M. Roberts. 1978. Lumbar spinal manipulation on trial. 1. Clinical assessment. *Rheumatology and Rehabilitation* 17(1), 46-53.

Evans, G.A., P. Harcastle, and A.D. Frenyo. 1984. Acute rupture of the lateral ligament of the ankle. *Journal of Bone and Joint Surgery* 66B(2), 209-212.

Evans, S.A., T.J. Housh, G.O. Johnson, J. Beaird, D.J. Housh, and M. Pepper. 1993. Age-specific differences in the flexibility of high school wrestlers. *Journal of Strength and Conditioning Research* 7(1), 39-42.

Evans, W.J., C.N. Meredith, and J.C. Cannon, C.A. Dinarello, W.R. Frontera, V.A. Hughes, B.H. Jones, and H.G. Knuttgen. 1985. Metabolic changes following eccentric exercise in trained and untrained men. *Journal of Applied Physiology* 61(5), 1864-1868.

Evatt, M.L., S.L. Wolf, and R.L. Segal. 1989. Modification of human spinal stretch reflexes: Preliminary studies. *Neuroscience Letters* 105(3), 350-355.

Everly, G.S. 1989. *A clinical guide to the treatment of the human stress response.* New York: Plenum Press.

Everly, G.S., M. Spollen, A. Hackman, and E. Kobran. 1987. Undesirable side-effects and self-regulatory therapies. In *Proceedings of the eighteenth annual meeting of the Biofeedback Society of America,* 166-167. Boston.

Evjenth, O., and J. Hamberg. 1989. *Auto stretching.* Alfta, Sweden: Alfta Rehab Förlag.

Evjenth, O., and J. Hamberg. 1993. *Muscle stretching in manual therapy. A clinical manual.* 3rd ed. Alfta, Sweden: Alfta Rehab Förlag.

Fairbank, J.C.T., P.B. Pynsent, J.A. van Poortvliet, and H. Phillips. 1984. Influence of anthropometric factors and joint laxity in the incidence of adolescent back pain. *Spine* 9(5), 461-464.

Falkel, J.E. 1988. Swimming injuries. In *Shoulder injuries*, ed. J.E. Falkel and J.C. Murphy, 477-503. Baltimore: Williams & Wilkins.

Falls, H.B., and D. Humphrey. 1989. Dr. Falls and Dr. Humphrey reply. *The Physician and Sportsmedicine* 17(6), 20, 22.

Fardy, P.S. 1981. Isometric exercise and the cardiovascular system. *The Physician and Sportsmedicine* 9(9), 43-56.

Farfan, H.F. 1973. *Mechanical disorders of the low back.* Philadelphia: Lea & Febiger.

Farfan, H.F. 1978. The biomechanical advantage of lordosis and hip extension for upright activity. *Spine* 3(4), 336-342.

Farley, C.T., and O. Gonzalez. 1996. Leg stiffness and stride frequency in human running. *Journal of Biomechanics* 29(2), 181-186.

Farrell, J., and L. Twomey. 1982. Acute low back pain: Comparison of two consecutive treatment approaches. *Medical Journal of Australia* 1(4), 160-164.

Fatouros, I.G., K. Taxildaris, S.P. Tokmakidis, V. Kalapotharakos, N. Aggelousis, S. Athanasopoulos, I. Zeeris, and I. Katrabasas. 2002. The effects of strength training, cardiovascular training and their combination on flexibility of inactive older adults. *International Journal of Sports Medicine* 23(2), 112-119.

Faulkner, J.A., S.V. Brooks, and J.A. Opiteck. 1993. Injury to skeletal muscle fibers during contractions: Conditions of occurrence and prevention. *Physical Therapy* 73(12), 911-921.

Federation of Straight Chiropractic Organizations (FSCO) n.d. *Statement on chiropractic standard of care/patient safety.* Clifton, NJ: Author.

Federation of Straight Chiropractors and Organizations (FSCO) (12/13/2002). *FSCO fact sheet.* Hellertown, PA: Author. [Online]. www.straightchiropractic.com.

Feinberg, J. 1988. The effect of patient-practitioner interaction on compliance: A review of the literature and application in rheumatoid arthritis. *Patient Education and Counseling* 11(3), 171-187.

Feit, E.M., and R. Berenter. 1993. Lower extremity tennis injuries: Prevalence, etiology, and mechanisms. *Journal of the American Podiatric Medical Association* 83(9), 509-522.

Feland, J.B., J.W. Myrer, S.S. Schulthies, G.W. Fellingham, and G.W. Measom. 2001. The effect of duration of stretching of the hamstring muscle group for increasing range of motion in people aged 65 years or older. *Physical Therapy* 81(5), 1110-1117.

Feldman, D., I. Shrier, M. Rossignol, and L. Abenhaim. 1999. Adolescent growth is not associated with changes in flexibility. *Clinical Journal of Sport Medicine* 9(1), 24-29.

Fellabaum, J. 1993. The effect of eye positioning on bodily movement. *Digest of Chiropractic Economics* 36(1), 14-17.

Feltner, M., and J. Dapena. 1986. Dynamics of the shoulder and elbow joints of the throwing arm during a baseball pitch. *International Journal of Sport Biomechanics* 2, 235-259.

Ferlic, D. 1962. The range of motion of the "normal" cervical spine. *Bulletin of the Johns Hopkins Hospital* 110, 59-65.

Ferrari, W., G.L. Gessa, and L. Vargiu. 1963. Behavioral effects induced by intracisternally injected ACTH and MSH. *Annals of the New York Academy of Sciences* 104, 330-345.

Fick, R. 1911. *Handbuch der Anatomie und Mechanik der Gelenke* (Vol. 3). Jena: Gustav Fischer.

Fick, S., J.P. Albright, and B.P. Murray. 1992. Relieving painful 'shin splints'. *Physician and Sportsmedicine* 20(12), 105-113.

Finkelstein, H. 1916. Joint hypotonia. *New York Medical Journal* 104(20), 942-944.

Finkelstein, H., and R. Roos. 1990. Ontario study raises doubt about stretching. *The Physician and Sportsmedicine* 18(1), 48-49.

Finneson, B.E. 1980. *Low back pain*. Philadelphia: Lippincott.

Finsterbush, A., and H. Pogrund. 1982. The hypermobility syndrome: Musculoskeletal complaints in 100 consecutive cases of generalized joint hypermobility. *Clinical Orthopaedics and Related Research* 168, 124-127.

Fisher, A.C., M.A. Domm, and D.A. Wuest. 1988. Adherence to sports-injury rehabilitation programs. *The Physician and Sportsmedicine* 16(7), 47-51.

Fisk, J.W. 1975. The straight-leg raising test—Its relevance to possible disc pathology. *New Zealand Medical Journal* 81(542), 557-560.

Fisk, J.W. 1979. A controlled trial of manipulation in a selected group of patients with low back pain favoring one side. *New Zealand Journal of Medicine* 90(645), 288-291.

Fisk, J.W., and R.S. Rose. 1977. *A practical guide to management of the painful neck and back*. Springfield, IL: Charles C Thomas.

Fitness and Sports Review International 1992. The intricacies of stretching. *Fitness and Sports Review International* 27(1), 5-6.

Fitt, S.S. 1988. *Dance kinesiology*. New York: Schirmer Books.

Fixx, J. 1983. Is stretching (yawn) everything you hoped it would be? *Running Times* 80, 66.

Fleckenstein, J.L., P.T. Weatherall, E.W. Parkey, J.A. Payne, and R.M. Peshock. 1989. Sports-related muscle injuries: Evaluation with MR imaging. *Radiology* 172(3), 793-798.

Fleischman, E.A. 1964. *The structure and measurement of physical fitness*. Englewood Cliffs, NJ: Prentice-Hall.

Fleisig, G.S., J.R. Andrews, C.J. Dillman, and R.F. Escamilla. 1995. Kinetics of baseball pitching with implication about injury mechanisms. *American Journal of Sports Medicine* 23(2), 233-239.

Flint, M.M. 1963. Lumbar posture: A study of roentgenographic measurement and the influence of flexibility and strength. *Research Quarterly* 34(1), 15-22.

Flint, M.M. 1964. Selecting exercises. *Journal of Health, Physical Education, and Recreation* 35(2), 19-23, 74.

Flintney, F.W., and D.G. Hirst. 1978. Cross-bridge detachment and sarcomere "give" during stretch of active frog's muscle. *Journal of Physiology* (London) 276, 449-465.

Flood, J., and J. Nauert. 1973. Shin splints. *Scholastic Coach* 42(5), 28, 30, 102-103.

Floyd, W.F., and P.H.S. Silver. 1950. Electromyographic study of patterns of activity of the anterior abdominal wall muscles in man. *Journal of Anatomy* 84(2), 132-145.

Floyd, W.F., and P.H.S. Silver. 1951. Function of the erectores spinae in flexion of the trunk. *Lancet* 1, 133-134.

Floyd, W.F., and P.H.S. Silver. 1955. The function of the erectores spinae muscles in certain movements and postures in man. *Journal of Physiology* (London) 129, 184-203.

Follan, L.M. 1981. *Lilias and your life*. New York: Collier Books.

Found, E., R. Harney, and G.P. Whitelaw. 1986. Lower leg pain in athletes. *Journal of Musculoskeletal Medicine* 3(9), 60-65.

Fowler, A.W. 1973. Relief of cramp. *Lancet* 1(7794), 99.

Fowler, P.J., and S.S. Messieh. 1987. Isolated posterior cruciate ligament injuries in athletes. *American Journal of Sports Medicine* 15(6), 553-557.

Fowles, J.R., J.D. MacDougall, M.A. Tarnopolsky, D.G. Sale, B.D. Roy, and K.E. Yarasheski. 2000a. The effect of acute passive stretch on muscle protein synthesis in humans. *Canadian Journal of Applied Physiology* 25(3), 165-180.

Fowles, J.R., J.D. MacDougall, and D.G. Sale. 2000b. Reduced strength after passive stretch of the human plantary flexors. *Journal of Applied Physiology* 89(3), 1179-1188.

Fowles, J.R., and D.G. Sale. 1997. Time course strength deficit after maximal passive stretch in humans. *Medicine and Science in Sports and Exercise* 29, S26.

Fradkin, A.J., C.F. Finch, and C.A. Sherman. 2001. Warm up practices of golfers: Are they adequate? *British Journal of Sports Medicine* 35(2), 125-127.

Francis, K.T. 1983. Delayed muscle soreness: A review. *Journal of Orthopaedic and Sports Physical Therapy* 5(1), 10-13.

Frankeny, J.R., R.G. Holly, and C.R. Ashmore. 1983. Effects of graded duration of stretch on normal and dystrophic skeletal muscle. *Muscle & Nerve* 6(4), 269-277.

Franzblau, C., and B. Faru. 1981. Elastin. In *Cell biology of extracellular matrix*, ed. E.D. Hay, 75-78. New York: Plenum Press.

Franzini-Armstrong, C. 1970. Details of the I-band structure revealed by localization of ferritin. *Tissue Cell* 2(2), 327-338.

Frederick E.C. 1982. Stretching things a bit. *Running* 8(3), 65.

Frederickson, K.B. 2002. Fit to play: Musicians' health tips. *Music Educators Journal* 88(6), 38-44.

Fredette, D.M. 2001. Exercise recommendations for flexibility and range of motion. In American College of Sports Medicine. *ACSM's resource manual for guidelines for exercise testing and prescription*. 4th ed. ed. J.L. Roitman, 468-477. Baltimore: Lippincott Williams & Wilkins.

Freed, D.C. 1994. Breath management terminology: How far have we come? *The NATS Journal* 50(5), 15-28.

Freeman, M.A.R., M.R.E. Dean, and I.W.F. Hanham. 1965. The etiology and prevention of functional instability of the foot. *Journal of Bone and Joint Surgery* 47B(4), 678-685.

Freivalds, A. 1979. *Investigation of circadian rhythms on select psychomotor and neurological functions*. PhD diss. University of Michigan, Ann Arbor.

Frekany, G.A., and D.K. Leslie. 1975. Effects of an exercise program on selected flexibility measurements of senior citizens. *The Gerontologist* 15(2), 182-183.

Frey, C., and K.S. Feder. 1999. Foot and ankle injuries in sports. In *Orthopaedic knowledge update. Sports medicine* 2, ed. E.A. Arendt, 379-393. Rosmont, IL: American Academy of Orthopaedic Surgeons.

Friberg, T.R., and R.N. Weinreb. 1985. Ocular manifestations of gravity inversion. *Journal of the American Medical Association* 253(12), 1755-1757.

Fridén, J. 1984a. Changes in human skeletal muscle induced by long-term eccentric exercise. *Cell Tissue Research* 236(2), 365-372.

Fridén, J. 1984b. Muscle soreness after exercise: Implications of morphological changes. *International Journal of Sports Medicine* 5(2), 57-66.

Fridén, J., and R.L. Lieber. 1992. Structural and mechanical basis of exercise-induced muscle injury. *Medicine and Science in Sports and Exercise* 24(5), 521-530.

Fridén, J., and R.L. Lieber. 2001. Eccentric exercise-induced injuries to contractile and cytoskeletal muscle fibre components. *Acta Physiologica Scandinavica* 171(3), 321-326.

Fridén, J., and R.L. Lieber. 2003. Spastic muscle cells are shorter and stiffer than normal cells. *Muscle & Nerve* 27(2), 157-163.

Fridén, J., J. Seger, and B. Ekblom. 1988. Sublethal muscle fibre injuries after high-tension anaerobic exercise. *European Journal of Applied Physiology* 57(3), 360-368.

Fridén, J., M. Seger, M. Sjöström, and B. Ekblom. 1983. Adaptive response in human skeletal muscle subjected to prolonged eccentric training. *International Journal of Sports Medicine* 4(3), 177-184.

Fridén, J., P.N. Sfakianos, and A.R. Hargens. 1986. Muscle soreness and intramuscular fluid pressure: Comparison between eccentric and concentric load. *Journal of Applied Physiology* 61(6), 2175-2179.

Fridén, J., P.N. Sfakianos, A.R. Hargens, and W.H. Akeson. 1988. Residual muscular swelling after repetitive eccentric contractions. *Journal of Orthopaedic Research* 6(4), 493-498.

Fridén, J., M. Sjöström, and B. Ekblom. 1981. A morphological study of delayed muscle soreness. *Experimentia* 37(5), 506-507.

Fridén, J., M. Sjöström, and B. Ekblom. 1983. Myofibrillar damage following intense eccentric exercise in man. *International Journal of Sports Medicine* 4(3), 170-176.

Fried, R. 1987. *The hyperventilation syndrome*. Baltimore: Johns Hopkins University Press.

Friedman, L.M., C.D. Furberg, and D.L. Demets. 1998. *Fundamentals of clinical trials*. 3rd ed. New York: Springer-Verlag.

Friedmann, L.W., and L. Galton. 1973. *Freedom from backaches*. New York: Simon and Schuster.

Fry, A.C., R.S. Staron, C.B. James, R.S. Hikida, and F.C. Hagerman. 1997. Differential titin isoform expression in human skeletal muscle. *Acta Physiologica Scandinavica* 161(4), 473-479.

Fujiwara, M., and J.V. Basmajian. 1975. Electromyographic study of the two-joint muscles. *American Journal of Physical Medicine* 54(5), 234-242.

Fukashiro, S., T. Abe, A. Shibayama, and W.F. Brechue. 2002. Comparison of viscoelastic characteristics in triceps surae between black and white athletes. *Acta Physiologica Scandinavica* 175(3), 183-187.

Fulton, A.B., and W.B. Isaacs. 1991. Titin: A huge, elastic sarcomeric protein with a probable role in morphogenesis. *BioEssays* 13(4), 157-161.

Funatsu, T., H. Higuchi, and S. Ishiwata. 1990. Elastic filaments in skeletal muscle revealed by selective removal of titin filaments with plasma gelsolin. *Journal of Cell Biology* 110(1), 53-62.

Furst, D.O., M. Osborn, R. Nave, and K. Weber. 1988. The organization of titin filaments in the half-sarcomere revealed by monoclonal antibodies in immunoelectron microscopy: A map of ten nonrepetitive epitomes starting at the Z-line extends close to the M line. *Journal of Cell Biology* 106(5), 1563-1572.

Gabbard, C., and R. Tandy. 1988. Body composition and flexibility among prepubescent males and females. *Journal of Human Movement Studies* 14(4), 153-159.

Gajda, R. *See* D.R. Murphy (1991).

Gajdosik, R.L. 1991. Passive compliance and length of clinically short hamstring muscles of healthy men. *Clinical Biomechanics* 6(4), 239-244.

Gajdosik, R.L. 1995. Flexibility or muscle length? *Physical Therapy* 75(3), 238-239.

Gajdosik, R.L. 1997. Influence of age on calf muscle length and passive stiffness variables at different stretch velocities. *Isokinetics and Exercise Science* 6(3), 163-174.

Gajdosik, R.L. 2001. Passive extensibility of skeletal muscle: Review of the literature with clinical implications. *Clinical Biomechanics* 16(2), 87-101.

Gajdosik, R.L., C.R. Albert, and J.J. Mitman. 1994. Influence of hamstring length on standing position and flexion range of motion of the pelvic angle, lumbar angle, and thoracic angle. *Journal of Orthopaedic and Sport Physical Therapy* 20(4), 213-219.

Gajdosik, R.L., and R.W. Bohannon. 1987. Clinical measurement of range of motion: Review of goniometry emphasizing reliability and validity. *Physical Therapy* 67(12), 1867-1872.

Gajdosik, R.L., C.A. Giuliani, and R.W. Bohannon. 1990. Passive compliance and length of the hamstring muscles of healthy men and women. *Clinical Biomechanics* 5(1), 23-29.

Gajdosik, R., and G. Lusin. 1983. Hamstring muscle tightness: Reliability of an active-knee-extension test. *Physical Therapy* 63(7), 1085-1089.

Gajdosik, R.L., D.W. Vander Linden, and A.K. Williams. 1999. Influence of age on length and passive elastic stiffness characteristics of the calf muscle-tendon unit of women. *Physical Therapy* 79(9), 827-838.

Gál, J., W. Herzog, G. Kawchuk, P. Conway, and Y-T. Zhang. 1994. Biomechanical studies of spinal manipulative therapy (SMT): Quantifying the movements of vertebral bodies during SMT. *Journal of the Canadian Chiropractic Association* 38(1), 11-24.

Galin, M.A., J.W. McIvor, and G.B. Magruder. 1963. Influence of position on intraocular pressure. *American Journal of Ophthalmology* 55(4), 720-723.

Galley, P.M., and A.L. Forster. 1987. *Human movement: An introductory text for physiotherapy students.* Melbourne: Churchill Livingstone.

Galloway, M.T., and P. Jokl. 2000. Aging successfully: The importance of physical activity in maintaining health and function. *Journal of the American Academy of Orthopaedic Surgeons* 8(1), 37-44.

Gallup Organization. 2000. *International Musician* 98(9), 2.

Garamvölgyi, N. 1971. The functional morphology of muscle. In *Contractile proteins and muscle,* ed. K. Laki, 1-96. New York: Marcel Dekker.

Garde, R.E. 1988. Cervical traction: The neurophysiology of lordosis and the rheological characteristics of cervical curve rehabilitation. In *Chiropractic: The physics of spinal correction,* ed. D.D. Harrison, 535-659. Sunnyvale, CA: Author.

Garfin, S.R., C.M. Tipton, S.J. Mubarak, S.L.-Y. Woo, A.R. Hargens, and A.W.H. Akekeson. 1981. Role of fascia in maintenance of muscle tension and pressure. *Journal of Applied Physiology* 51(2), 317-320.

Garhammer, J. 1989a. Principles of training and development. In *Kinesiology and applied anatomy.* 7th ed, ed. P.J. Rasch, 258-265. Philadelphia: Lea & Febiger.

Garhammer, J. 1989b. Weight lifting and training. In *Biomechanics of sport,* ed C.L. Vaughan, 169-211. Boca Raton, FL: CRC Publishers.

Garrett, W.E. 1990. Muscle strain injuries: Clinical and basic aspects. *Medicine and Science in Sports and Exercise* 22(4), 436-443.

Garrett, W.E. 1993. Muscle flexibility and function under stretch. In *Sports and exercise in midlife,* ed. S.L. Gordon, X. Gonzalez-Mestre and W.E. Garrett, 105-116. Rosemont, IL: American Academy of Orthopaedic Surgeons.

Garrett, W.E. 1996. Muscle strain injuries. *American Journal of Sports Medicine* 24(6), S2-S8.

Garrett, W.E., W. Bradley, S. Byrd, V.R. Edgerton, and P. Gollnick. 1989. Basic science perspectives. In *New perspectives in low back pain,* ed. J.W. Frymoyer and S.L. Gordon, 335-372. Park Ridge, IL: American Academy of Orthopaedic Surgeons.

Garrett, W.E., J.C. Califf, and F.H. Bassett. 1984. Histochemical correlates of hamstring injuries. *American Journal of Sports Medicine* 12(2) 98-103.

Garrett, W.E., F.R. Rich, P.K. Nikolaou, J.B. Vogler. 1989. Computed tomography of hamstring muscle strains. *Medicine and Science in Sports and Exercise* 21(5), 506-514.

Garrett, W.E., M.R. Safran, A.V. Seaber, R.R. Glisson, and B.M. Ribbeck. 1987. Biomechanical comparison of stimulated and nonstimulated skeletal muscle pulled to failure. *American Journal of Sports Medicine* 15(5), 448-454.

Garrett, W.E., P.K. Nikolaou, B.M. Ribbeck, R.R. Glisson, A.V. Seaber. 1988. The effect of muscle architecture on the biomechanical failure properties of skeletal muscle under passive extension. *American Journal of Sports Medicine* 16(1), 7-11.

Garu, J. 1986. Exercise do's & don'ts: Side bends. *Dance Exercise Today* 4(4), 34-35.

Gaskell, W.H. 1877. On the changes of the bloodstream of the muscles through stimulation of their nerves. *Journal of Anatomy and Physiology* 11, 360-402.

Gatton, M.L., and M.J. Pearcy. 1999. Kinematics and movement sequencing during flexion of the lumbar spine. *Clinical Biomechanics* 14(6), 376-383.

Gaughran, J.A. 1972. *Advanced swimming.* Dubuque, IA: Brown.

Gaymans, F. 1980. Die Bedeutung der Atemtypen für Mobilisation der Wirbelsaule. *Manuelle Medizin* 18, 96.

Gedalia, A., and E.J. Brewer. 1993. Joint hypermobility in pediatric practice: A review. *Journal of Rheumatology* 20(2), 371-374.

Geisler, P.R. 2001. Golf. in *Sports injury prevention & rehabilitation,* ed. Shamus and J. Shamus, 185-225. New York: McGraw-Hill.

Gelabert, R. 1989. Classic lines: the ballet dancer's physique. *SportsCare & Fitness* 2(3) 46-50.

George, G.S. 1980. *Biomechanics of women's gymnastics.* Englewood Cliffs, NJ: Prentice-Hall.

Germain, N.W., and S.N. Blair. 1983. Variability of shoulder flexion with age, activity and sex. *American Corrective Therapy Journal* 37(6), 156-160.

Gibala, M.J., J.D. MacDougall, M.A. Tarnopolsky, W.T. Stauber, and A. Elorriaga. 1995. Changes in human skeletal muscle ultrastructure and force production after acute resistance exercise. *Journal of Applied Physiology* 78(2), 702-708.

Giel, D. 1988. Women's weightlifting: Elevating a sport to world-class status. *The Physician and Sportsmedicine* 16(4), 163-170.

Gifford, L.S. 1987. Circadian variation in human flexibility and grip strength. *Australian Journal of Physiotherapy* 33(1), 3-9.

Gilad, G.M., B.D. Mahon, Y. Finkelstein, B. Koffler, and V.H. Gilad. 1985. Stress-induced activation of the hippocampal cholingeric system and the pituitary-adrenocortical axis. *Brain Research* 347(2), 406-408.

Gilhoges, J.C., V.S. Gurfinkel, and J.P. Roll. 1992. Role of Ia muscle spindle afferents in post-contraction and post-vibration motor effect genesis. *Neuroscience Letters* 135(2), 247-251.

Gillberg, M., and T. Åkerstedt. 1982. Body temperature and sleep at different times of day. *Sleep* 5(4), 378-388.

Gillette, P.D., and R.D. Fell. 1996. Passive tension in rat hindlimb during suspension unloading and recovery: Muscle/joint contributions. *Journal of Applied Physiology* 81(2), 724-730.

Gilliam, T.B., J.F. Villanacci, P.S. Freedson, and S.P. Sady. 1979. Isokinetic torque in boys and girls age 7 to 13: Effect of age, height, and weight. *Research Quarterly* 50(4), 599-609.

Girouard, C.K., and B.F. Hurley. 1995. Does strength training inhibit gains in range of motion from flexibility training in older adults? *Medicine and Science in Sports and Exercise* 27(10), 1444-1449.

Glazer, R.M. 1980. Rehabilitation. In *Fracture treatment and healing*, ed. R.B. Happenstall, 1041-1068. Philadelphia: Saunders.

Gleim, G.W., and M.P. McHugh. 1999. Training and conditioning. In *Orthopaedic knowledge update. Sports medicine 2*, ed. E.A. Arendt, 57-63. Rosmont, IL: American Academy of Orthopaedic Surgeons.

Gleim, G.W., and M.P. McHugh. 1997. Flexibility and its effects on sports injury and performance. *Sports Medicine* 24(5), 289-299.

Gleim, G.W., N.S. Stachenfeld, and J.A. Nicholas. 1990. The influence of flexibility on the economy of walking and jogging. *Journal of Orthopaedic Research* 8(6), 350-357.

Goats, G.C. 1994. Massage—The scientific basis of an ancient art: Part 2: Physiological and therapeutic effects. *British Journal of Sports Medicine* 28 (3), 153-156.

Godges, J.J., H. Macrae, C. Longdon, C. Tinberg, and P. MacRae. 1989. The effects of two stretching procedures on hip range of motion and gait economy. *Journal of Orthopaedic and Sports Physical Therapy* 10(9), 350-357.

Goebel, H.H. 2002. Desmin-related disorders. In *Skeletal muscle pathology, diagnosis and management of disease*, ed. V.R. Preedy and T.J. Peters, 263-272. London: Greenwich Medical Media.

Göeken, L.N., and A.L. Hof. 1991. Instrumental straight-leg raising: Results in patients. *Archives of Physical Medicine and Rehabilitation* 72(12), 959-966.

Göeken, L.N., and A.L. Hof. 1994. Instrumental straight-leg raising: A new approach to Lasègue's test. *Archives of Physical Medicine and Rehabilitation* 75(4), 470-477.

Gold, R. 1987. *Album #1: The philosophy*. Gladwyne, PA: Chiro Products.

Goldberg, B., and M. Rabinovich. 1988. Connective tissue. In *Cell and tissue biology a textbook of histology*. 6th ed, ed. Weiss, 157-188. Baltimore: Urban & Schwarzenberg.

Goldspink, G. 1968. Sarcomere length during post-natal growth and mammalian muscle fibres. *Journal of Cell Science* 3(4), 539-548.

Goldspink, G. 1976. The adaptation of muscle to a new functional length. In *Mastication*, ed. D.J. Anderson and B. Matthews, 90-99. Bristol, England: Wright and Sons.

Goldspink, G. 1999. Changes in muscle mass and phenotype and the expression of autocrine and systemic growth factors by muscle in response to stretch and overload. *Journal of Anatomy* 194(3), 323-334.

Goldspink, G. 2002. Gene expression in skeletal muscle. *Biochemical Society Transaction* 39(2), 285-290.

Goldspink, G., A. Scutt., P.T. Loughna, D.J. Wells, T. Jaenicke, and G.F. Gerlach. 1992. Gene expression in skeletal muscle in response to stretch and force generation. *American Journal of Physiology* 262(31), R356-R363.

Goldspink, G., C. Tabary, J.C. Tabary, C. Tardieu, and G. Tardieu. 1974. Effect of denervation on the adaptation of sarcomere number and muscle extensibility to the functional length of the muscle. *Journal of Physiology* (London) 236(3), 733-742.

Goldspink, G., and P.E. Williams. 1979. The nature of the increased passive resistance in muscle following immobilization of the mouse soleus muscle. *Journal of Physiology* (London) 289, 55P (Proceedings of the Physiological Society December 15-16, 1978).

Goldstein, J.D., P.E. Berger, G.E. Windler, and D.W. Jackson. 1981. Spine injuries in gymnasts and swimmers. An epidemiologic investigation. *American Journal of Sports Medicine* 19(5), 463-468.

Goldthwait, J.E. 1941. *Body mechanics in health and disease*. Philadelphia: Lippincott.

Golub, L.J. 1987. Exercises that alleviate primary dysmenorrhea. *Contemporary Ob/Gyn* 29(5), 51-59.

Golub, L.J., and J. Christaldi. 1957. Reducing dysmenorrhea in young adolescents. *Journal of Health, Physical Education, and Recreation* 28(5), 24-25, 59.

Golub, L.J., W.R. Lang, and H. Menduke. 1958. Dysmenorrhea in high school and college girls: Relationship to sports participation. *Western Journal of Surgery, Obstetrics and Gynecology* 66(3), 163-165.

Golub, L.J., H. Menduke, and W.R. Lang. 1968. Exercise and dysmenorrhea in young teenagers: A 3-year study. *Obstetrics and Gynecology* 32(4), 508-511.

Goode, D.J., and J. Van Hoven. 1982. Loss of patellar and achilles tendon reflexes in classical ballet dancers. *Archives of Neurology* 39(5), 323.

Goode, J.D., and B.M. Theodore. 1983. Voluntary and diurnal variation in height and associated surface contour changes in spinal curves. *Engineering in Medicine* 12(2), 99-101.

Goodridge, J.P. 1981. Muscle energy technique: Definition, explanations, methods of procedure. *Journal of the American Osteopathic Association* 81(4), 67-72.

Gordon, A.M., A.F. Huxley, and F.J. Julian. 1966a. Tension development in highly stretched vertebrate muscle fibres. *Journal of Physiology (London)* 184 (1), 143-169.

Gordon, A.M., A.F. Huxley, and F.J. Julian. 1966b. The variation in isometric tension with sarcomere length in vertebrate muscle fibres. *Journal of Physiology (London)* 184(1), 170-192.

Gordon, G.M., and B.A. Klein. 1987. The benefits of weight training for hamstring strains. *Journal of the American Podiatric Medical Association* 77(10), 567-569.

Gordon, S.J., P. Trott, and K.A. Grimmer. 2002. Walking cervical pain and stiffness, headache, scapular or arm pain: Gender and age effects. *Australian Journal of Physiotherapy* 48(1), 9-15.

Gosline, J.M. 1976. The physical properties of elastic tissue. *International Review of Connective Tissue Research* 7, 211-257.

Gosselin, L.E., C. Adams, T.A. Cotter, R.J. McCormick, and D.P. Thomas. 1998. Effect of exercise training on passive stiffness in locomotor skeletal muscle: Role of extracellular matrix. *Journal of Applied Physiology* 85(3), 1011-1016.

Gosselin, L.E., D.A. Martinez, A.C. Vailas, and G.C. Sieck. 1994. Passive length-force properties of the senescent diaphragm: Relationship to collagen characteristics. *Journal of Applied Physiology* 76(6), 2680-2685.

Gould, D. 1987. Understanding attrition in children's sport. In *Advances in pediatric sport sciences*, ed. D. Gould and M.R. Weiss, 61-85. Champaign, IL: Human Kinetics.

Gould, G.M., and W.L. Pyle. 1896. *Anomalies and curiosities of medicine*. Philadelphia: Saunders.

Goulding, D., B. Bullard, and M. Gautel. 1997. A survey of in situ sarcomere extension in mouse skeletal muscle. *Journal of Muscle Research and Cell Motility*, 18(4), 465-472.

Gowitzke, B.A., M. Milner, and A.L. O'Connell. 1988. *Understanding the scientific bases of human movement*. 2nd ed. Baltimore: Williams & Wilkins.

Grace, T.G. 1985. Muscle imbalance and extremity injury: A perplexing relationship. *Sports Medicine* 2(2), 77-82.

Gracovetsky, S., H.F. Farfan, and C. Lamy. 1977. A mathematical model of the lumbar spine using an optimized system to control muscles and ligaments. *Orthopaedics Clinics of North America* 8(1), 135-153.

Gracovetsky, S., M. Kary, I. Pitchen, S. Levy, and R.B. Said. 1989. The importance of pelvic tilt in reducing compression stress in the spine during flexion-extension exercises. *Spine* 14(4), 412-417.

Grady, J.F., and A. Saxena. 1991. Effects of stretching the gastrocnemius muscle. *Journal of Foot & Surgery* 30 (5), 465-469.

Graham, C.E. 1987. Plantar fasciitis and the painful heel syndrome. *Medicine and Sport Science* 23, 99-104.

Graham, G. 1965. Cramp. *Lancet* 2, 537.

Grahame, R. 1971. Joint hypermobility—Clinical aspects. *Proceedings of the Royal Society of Medicine* 64(June), 692-694.

Grahame, R. 2000. Hypermobility-not a circus act. *International Journal of Clinical Practice* 54(5), 314-315.

Grahame, R. 1999. Joint hypermobility and genetic collagen disorders: Are they related? *Archives of Disease in Childhood* 80(2), 188-191.

Grahame, R., and H. Bird. 2001. British consultant rheumatologists' perceptions about the hypermobility syndrome: A national survey. *Rheumatology* 40(5), 559-562.

Grahame, R., and J.M. Jenkins. 1972. Joint hypermobility—Asset or liability? *Annals of the Rheumatic Diseases* 31(2), 109-111.

Grana, W.A., and J.A. Moretz. 1978. Ligamentous laxity in secondary school athletes. *Journal of the American Medical Association* 240(18), 1975-1976.

Granit, R. 1962. Muscle tone and postural regulation. In *Muscle as tissue*, ed. K. Rodahl and S.M. Horvath, 190-210. New York: McGraw-Hill.

Grant, M.E., P.D. Prockop, and J. Darwin. 1972. The biosynthesis of collagen. *New England Journal of Medicine* 286(4), 194-199.

Granzier, H., D. Labeit, Y. Wu, and S. Labeit. 2002. Titin as a modular spring: Emerging mechanisms for elasticity control by titin in cardiac physiology and pathophysiology. *Journal of Muscle Research and Cell Motility*. 23(5-6), 457-471.

Grassino, A., M.D. Goldman, J. Mead, and T.A. Sears. 1978. Mechanisms of the human diaphragm during voluntary contraction statics. *Journal of Applied Physiology* 44(6), 829-839.

Gray, M.L., A.M. Pizzanelli., A.J. Grodzinsky, and R.C. Lee. 1988. Mechanical and physiochemical determinants of the chondrocyte biosynthetic response. *Journal of Orthopaedic Research* 6(6), 777-792.

Gray, S.D., and N.C. Staub. 1967. Resistance to blood flow in leg muscles of dog during tetanic isometric contraction. *American Journal of Physiology* 213(3), 677-682.

Green, J.D. 1964. The hippocampus. *Physiological Reviews* 44(Oct), 561-608.

Green, J.D., and A.A. Arduini. 1954. Hippocapmal electrical activity of arousal. *Journal of Neurophysiology* 17(6), 533-557.

Greenberg, D. 2001. Psychology and the injured female athlete. In *Women's sports medicine and rehabilitation*. ed. N. Swedan. Gaithersburg, MD: Aspen.

Greene, W.B., and J.D. Heckman. 1994. *The clinical measurement of joint motion*. Rosemont, IL: American Academy of Orthopaedic Surgeons.

Greey, G.W. 1955. *A study of the flexibility in five selected joints of adult males ages 18 to 71*. Ph.D. diss. University of Michigan, Ann Arbor.

Gregory, J.E., A.K. Wise, S.A. Wood, A. Prochazka, and U. Proske. 1998. Muscle history, fusomotor activity and the human stretch reflex. *Journal of Physiology (London)* 513(3), 927-934.

Greipp, J.F. 1985. Swimmer's shoulder: The influence of flexibility and weight training. *The Physician and Sportsmedicine* 13(8), 92-105.

Greipp, J.F. 1986. The flex factor. *Swimming Technique* 22(3), 17-24.

Grewal, R., J. Xu, D.G. Sotereanos, and S.L-Y. Woo. 1996. Biomechanical properties of peripheral nerves. *Hand Clinics* 12(2), 195-204.

Gribble, P.A., K.M. Guskiewicz, W.E. Prentice, and E.W. Shields. 1999. Effects of static and hold-relax stretching on hamstring range of motion using the FlexAbility LE1000. *Journal of Sport Rehabilitation* 8(3), 195-208.

Grieve, D.W. 1970. Stretching active muscles. *Track Technique* 42(December), 1333-1335.

Grieve, G.P. 1988. *Common vertebral joint problems*. 2nd ed. London: Churchill Livingstone.

Grodzinsky, A.J. 1983. Electromechanical and physiochemical properties of connective tissue. *CRC Critical Reviews in Biomedical Engineering* 9(2), 133-199.

Grodzinsky, A.J. 1987. Electromechanical transduction and transport in the extracellular matrix. *Advances in Microcirculation* 13, 35-46.

Grodzinsky, A.J., H. Lipshitz, and M.J. Glimcher. 1978. Electromechanical properties of articular cartilage during compression and stress relaxation. *Nature* 275(5679), 448-450.

Groth, G.N., and M.B. Wulf. 1995. Compliance with hand rehabilitation: Health beliefs and strategies. *Journal of Hand Therapy* 8(1), 18-22.

Guissard, N., J. Duchateau, and K. Hainaut. 1988. Muscle stretching and motor neuron excitability. *European Journal of Applied Physiology and Occupational Physiology* 58(1/2), 47-52.

Gulick, D.T., I.F. Kimura, M. Sitler, A. Paolone, and J.D. Kelly. 1996. Various treatment techniques on signs and symptoms of delayed onset muscle soreness. *Journal of Athletic Training* 31(2), 145-152.

Gurewitsch, A.D., and M. O'Neill. 1944. Flexibility of healthy children. *Archives of Physical Therapy* 25(4), 216-221.

Gurry, M., A. Pappas, J. Michaels, P. Maher, A. Shakman, R. Goldberg, and J. Rippe. 1985. A comprehensive preseason fitness evaluation for professional baseball players. *The Physician and Sportsmedicine* 13(6), 63-74.

Gustavsen, R. 1985. *Training therapy prophylaxis and rehabilitation*. New York: Thieme.

Gutman, G.M., C.P. Herbert, and S.R. Brown. 1977. Feldenkrais versus conventional exercises for elderly. *Journal of Gerontology* 32(5), 562-572.

Gutmann, E. 1977. Muscle. In *Handbook of the biology of aging*, ed. C.E. Finch and L. Hoyflick, 445-469. New York: Van Nostrand Reinhold.

Gutmann, E., S. Schiaffino, and V. Hanzlikavá. 1971. Mechanism of compensatory hypertrophy in skeletal muscle of the rat. *Experimental Neurology* 31(3), 451-464.

Gutmann, G. 1983. Injuries to the vertebral artery caused by manual therapy. *Manuelle Medizin* 21, 2-14.

Guyton, A.C., and J.E. Hall. 1997. *Textbook of Medical Physiology*. Philadelphia: W.B. Saunders.

Haftek, J. 1970. Stretch injury of peripheral nerve: Acute effects of stretching on rabbit nerve. *Journal of Bone and Joint Surgery* 52B(2), 354-365.

Hagbarth, K.-E., J.V, Hägglund, M. Nordin, and E.U. Wallin. 1985. Thixotropic behaviour of human finger flexor muscles with accompanying changes in spindle and reflex responses to stretch. *Journal of Physiology (London)* 368(November), 323-342.

Hagbarth, K-E., and M. Nordin. 1998. Postural after-contractions in man attributed to muscle spindle thixotropy. *Journal of Physiology* 506(3), 875-883.

Hagbarth, K-E., M. Nordin, and G. Bongiovanni. 1995. After-effects on stiffness and stretch reflexes of human finger flexor muscles attributed to muscle thixotropy. *Journal of Physiology (London)* 482(1), 215-223.

Hagerman, P. 2001. Warm-up or no warm up: Cons. *National Strength and Conditioning Association* 23(6), 36.

Halbertsma, J.P.K., A.I. van Bolhuis, and L.N.H. Göeken. 1996. Sport stretching: Effect on passive muscle stiffness of short hamstrings. *Archives of Physical Medicine and Rehabilitation* 77(7), 688-692.

Halbertsma, J.P.K., and L.N.H. Göeken. 1994. Stretching exercises: Effect on passive extensibility and stiffness in short hamstrings of healthy subjects. *Archives of Physical Medicine and Rehabilitation* 75(9), 976-981.

Hald, R.D. 1992. Dance injuries. *Primary Care* 19(2), 393-411.

Haldeman, S., F.J. Kohlbeck, and M. McGregor. 1999. Risk factors and precipitating neck movements causing vertebrobasilar artery dissection after cervical trauma and spinal manipulation. *Spine* 24(8), 785-794.

Haley, S.M., W.L. Tada, and E.M. Carmichael. 1986. Spinal mobility in young children: A normative study. *Physical Therapy* 66(11), 1697-1703.

Haley, T.L. 2000. Percussionist's common back injuries. *Percussive Notes* 38(2), 60-65.

Hall, A.C., J.P.G. Urban, and K.A. Gehl. 1991. Effects of compression on the loss of newly synthesized proteoglycans and proteins from cartilage explants. *Archives of Biochemistry and Biophysics* 286, 20-29.

Hall, D.A. 1981. Gerontology: Collagen disease. *Clinical Endocrinology and Metabolism* 10(1), 23-55.

Hall, T., M. Zusman, and R. Elvey. 1998. Adverse mechanical tension in the nervous system? Analysis of straight leg raise. *Manual Therapy* 3(3), 140-146.

Halvorson, G.A. 1990. Therapeutic heat and cold for athlete injuries. *The Physician and Sportsmedicine* 18(5), 87-92.

Halvorson, G.A. 1989. Principles of rehabilitating sports injuries. In *Scientific foundations of sports medicine*, ed. C.C. Teitz, 345-371. Philadelphia: Decker.

Hamberg, J., M. Björklund, B. Nordgren, and B. Sahlstedt. 1993. Stretchability of the rectus femoris muscle: Investigation of validity and intratester reliability of two methods including X-ray analysis of pelvic tilt. *Archives of Physical Medicine and Rehabilitation* 74(3), 263-270.

Hamill, J., and K.M. Knutzen. 1995. *Biomechanical basis of human movement*. Baltimore: Williams & Wilkins.

Hamilton, L.H. 2002. Stress management: A significant factor in injury prevention. *International Association for Dance Medicine & Science* 9(3), 2.

Hamilton, W.G. 1978a. Ballet and your body: An orthopedist's view. *Dance Magazine* 52(2), 79.

Hamilton, W.G. 1978b. Ballet and your body: An orthopedist's view. *Dance Magazine* 52(4), 126-127.

Hamilton, W.G. 1978c. Ballet and your body: An orthopedist's view. *Dance Magazine* 52(7), 86-87.

Hamilton, W.G. 1978d. Ballet and your body: An orthopedist's view. *Dance Magazine* 52(8), 84-85.

Hamilton, W.G., L.H. Hamilton, P. Marshall, and M. Molnar. 1992. A profile of the musculoskeletal characteristics of elite professional ballet dancers. *American Journal of Sports Medicine* 20(3), 267-273.

Hammer, W.I. 1999. *Functional soft tissue examination and treatment by manual methods: New perspectives*. 2nd ed. Gaithersburg, MD: Aspen.

Han, J-S. 2003. Acupuncture: Neuropeptide release produced by electrical stimulation of different frequencies. *Trends in Neurosciences* 26(1), 17-22.

Handel, M., T. Horstmann, H.-H. Dickhuth, and R.W. Gülch. 1997. Effects of contract-relax stretching training on muscle performance in athletes. *European Journal of Applied Physiology and Occupational Physiology* 76(5), 400-408.

Hansson, L. 2002. 'Why don't you do as I tell you?' compliance and antihypertensive regimens. *International Journal of Clinical Practice* 56(3), 191-196.

Hanus, S.H., T.D. Homer, and D.H. Harter. 1977. Vertebral artery occlusion complicating yoga exercises. *Archives of Neurology* 34(September), 574-575.

Haravuori, H., A. Vihola, V. Straub, M. Auranen, I. Richard, S. Marchand, T. Voit, S. Albeit, H. Somer, L. Peltonen, J.S. Beckmann, and B. Udd. 2001. Secondary calpain 3 deficiency in 2q-linked muscular dystrophy-titin is the candidate gene. *Neurology* 56(7), 869-877.

Hardaker, W.T., L. Erickson, and M. Myers. 1984. The pathogenesis of dance injury. In *The dancer as athlete*, ed. C.G. Shell, 12-13. Champaign, IL: Human Kinetics.

Hardy, L. 1985. Improving active range of hip flexion. *Research Quarterly for Exercise and Sport* 56(2), 111-114.

Hardy, L., R. Lye, and A. Heathcote. 1983. Active versus passive warm up regimes and flexibility. *Research Papers in Physical Education* 1(5), 23-30.

Hardy, M., and W. Woodall. 1998. Therapeutic effects of heat, cold, and stretch on connective tissue. *Journal of Hand* 11(2), 148-156.

Harmer, P. 1991. The effect of pre-performance massage on stride frequency in sprinters. *Athletic Training* 26(1), 55-59.

Harris, F.A. 1978. Facilitation techniques in therapeutic exercise. In *Therapeutic exercise*. 3rd ed, ed. J.V. Basmajian, 93-137. Baltimore: Williams & Wilkins.

Harris, H., and J. Joseph. 1949. Variation in extension of the metacarpophalangeal and interphalangeal joints of the thumb. *Journal of Bone and Joint Surgery* 31B(4), 547-559.

Harris, M.L. 1969a. A factor analytic study of flexibility. *Research Quarterly* 40(1), 62-70.

Harris, M.L. 1969b. Flexibility. *Physical Therapy* 49(6), 591-601.

Harris, P.M. 1991. *The effects of muscle energy techniques on range of motion of the cervical spine*. Master's thesis. D'Youville College, Buffalo, New York.

Harryman, D.T., J.A. Sidles, J.M. Clark, K.J. McQuade, T.D. Gibb, and F.A. Matsen. 1990. Translation of the humeral head on the glenoid with passive glenohumeral motion. *Journal of Bone and Joint Surgery* 72A(9), 1334-1343.

Hartig, D.E., and J.M. Henderson. 1999. Increasing hamstring flexibility decreases lower extremity overuse injuries in military basic trainees. *American Journal of Sports Medicine* 27(2), 173-176.

Hartley-O'Brien, S.J. 1980. Six mobilization exercises for active range of hip flexion. *Research Quarterly for Exercise and Sport* 51(4), 625-635.

Harvey, C., L. Benedetti, L. Hosaka, and R.L. Valmassy. 1983. The use of cold spray and its effect on muscle length. *Journal of the American Podiatry Association* 73(12), 629-632.

Harvey, L.A., and R.D. Herbert. 2002. Muscle stretching for treatment and prevention of contracture in people with spinal cord injury. *Spinal Cord* 40(1), 1-9.

Harvey, L., R. Herbert, and J. Crosbie. 2002. Does stretching induce lasting increases in joint ROM? A systematic review. *Physiotherapy Research International* 7(1), 1-13.

Harvey, V.P., and F.P. Scott. 1967. Reliability of a measure of forward flexibility and its relation to physical dimensions of college women. *Research Quarterly* 38(1), 28-33.

Hasan, Z. 1986. Optimized movement trajectories and joint stiffness in unperturbed, inertially loaded movements. *Biological Cybernetics* 53(6), 373-382.

Hasselman, C.T., T.M. Best, A.V. Seaber, and W.E. Garrett. 1995. Threshold and continuum of injury during active stretch of rabbit skeletal muscle. *American Journal of Sports Medicine* 23(1), 65-73.

Hatfield, F.C. 1982. Learning to stretch for strength and safety. *Muscle Fitness* 43(12), 24-25, 193-194.

Hay, J.G. 1993. *The biomechanics of sports techniques*. 3rd ed. Englewood Cliffs, NJ: Prentice-Hall.

Haynes, R.B., D.W. Taylor, and D.L. Sackett. eds. 1979. *Compliance in health care*. Baltimore: John Hopkins Press.

Haynes, S.C., and D.H. Perrin. 1992. Effect of a counterirritant on pain and restricted range of motion associated with delayed onset muscle soreness. *Journal of Sport Rehabilitation* 1(1), 13-18.

Haywood, K.M. 1980. Strength and flexibility in gymnasts before and after menarche. *British Journal of Sports Medicine* 14(4), 189-192.

Hebbelinck, M. 1988. Flexibility. In *The Olympic book of sports medicine*, eds. A. Dirix, H.G. Knuttgen, and K. Tittel, 213-217. Oxford: Blackwell Scientific.

Hedricks, A. 1993. Flexibility and the conditioning program. *National Strength and Conditioning Association Journal* 15(4), 62-66.

Heil, J. 1993. Specialized treatment approaches: Problems in rehabilitation. In *Psychology of sport injury*, ed. J. Heil, 195-218. Champaign, IL: Human Kinetics.

Heil, J.O., and O'Connor, A. 2001. Psychological impact of injury and rehabilitation. In *Principles and practice of primary care sports medicine*, ed. W.E. Garrett, D.T. Kirkendahl and D.L. Squire, 191-204. Philadelphia: Lippincott Williams & Wilkins.

Heino, J.G., J.J. Godges, and C.L. Carter. 1990. Relationship between hip extension range of motion and posture alignment. *Journal of Orthopaedic and Sports Physical Therapy* 12(6), 243-247.

Heiser, T.M., J. Weber, G. Sullivan, P. Clare, and R.R. Jacobs. 1984. Prophylaxis and management of hamstring muscle injuries in intercollegiate football players. *American Journal of Sports Medicine* 12(5), 368-370.

Helin, P. 1985. Physiotherapy and electromyography in muscle cramp. *British Journal of Sports Medicine* 19(4), 230-231.

Hellig, D. 1969. Illustrative points in technique. In *Osteopathic medicine*, ed. J.M. Hoag, W.V. Cole, and S.G. Bradford, 197-218. New York: McGraw-Hill.

Helliwell, P.S. 1993. Joint stiffness. In *Mechanics of human joints*, ed. V. Wright and E.L. Radin, 203-218. New York: Marcel Dekker.

Hemmings, B., M. Smith, J. Graydon, and R. Dyson. 2000. Effects of massage on physiological restoration, perceived recovery, and repeated sports performance. *British Journal of Sports Medicine* 34(2), 109-115.

Heng, M.K., J.X. Bai, N.J. Talian, W.J. Vincent, S.S. Reese, S. Shaw, and G.J. Holland. 1992. Changes in cardiovascular function during inversion. *International Journal of Sports Medicine* 13(1), 69-73.

Hennessy, L., and A.W.S. Watson. 1993. Flexibility and posture assessment in relation to hamstring injury. *British Journal of Sports Medicine* 27(4), 243-246.

Henricson, A.S., K. Fredriksson, I. Persson, R. Pereira, Y. Rostedt, E. Nils, and M.D. Westlin. 1984. The effect of heat and stretching on the range of hip motion. *Journal of Orthopaedic and Sports Physical Therapy* 6(2), 110-115.

Henry, J.H. 1986. Commentary. *American Journal of Sports Medicine* 14(1), 17.

Henry, J.P. 1951. *Studies of the physiology of negative acceleration* (AF Tech. Report #5953). Dayton, OH: U.S. Air Force Air Material Command, Wright-Patterson AFB.

Henry, K.D., C. Rosemond, and L.B. Eckert. 1998. Effect of number of home exercise exercises on compliance and performance in adults over 65 years of age. *Physical Therapy* 78(3), 270-277.

Herbert, R.D., and M. Gabriel. 2002. Effects of stretching before and after exercising on muscle soreness and risk of injury: Systematic review. *British Medical Journal* 325(7362), 468-470.

Herbison, G.J., and V. Graziani. 1995. Neuromuscular disease: Rehabilitation and electrodiagnosis. 1. Anatomy and physiology of nerve and muscle. *Archives of Physical Medicine and Rehabilitation* 76(5), S3-S9.

Herrington, L. 1998. Glenohumeral joint: Internal and external rotation range of motion in Javelin throwers. British *Journal of Sports Medicine* 32(3), 226-228.

Hertling, D.M., and D. Jones. 1996. Relaxation. In *Management of common musculoskeletal disorders*. 2nd ed, ed. D. Hertling and R.M. Kessler, 140-162. Philadelphia: Lippincott.

Herzog, W. 1991. Biomechanical studies of spinal manipulative therapy. *Journal of the CCA* 35(3), 156-164.

Herzog. W. 1994. The biomechanics of spinal manipulative treatments. *Journal of the CCA* 38(4), 216-222.

Hesselink, M.K.C., H. Kuipers, P. Geurten, and H. van Straaten. 1996. Structural muscle damage and muscle strength after incremental number of isometric and forced lengthening contractions. *Journal of Muscle Research and Cell Motility* 17(3), 335-341.

Heusner, A.P. 1946. Yawning and associated phenomena. *Physiological Reviews* 26(1), 157-168.

Hewett, T.E. 2000. Neuromuscular and hormonal factors associated with knee injuries in female athletes. *Sports Medicine* 29(5), 313-327.

High, D.M, E.T. Howley, and B.D. Franks. 1989. The effects of static stretching and warm-up on prevention of delayed-onset muscle soreness. *Research Quarterly for Exercise and Sport* 69(4), 357-361.

Highet, W.B., and F.K. Sanders. 1943. The effects of stretching nerves after suture. *British Journal of Surgery* 30(120), 355-371.

Hill, A.R., J.M. Adams, B.E. Parker, and D.F. Rochester. 1988. Short-term entrainment of ventilation to the walking cycle in humans. *Journal of Applied Physiology* 65(2), 570-578.

Hill, A.V. 1948. The pressure developed in muscle during contraction. *Journal of Physiology* (London) 107, 518-526.

Hill, A.V. 1961. The heat produced by a muscle after the last shock of tetanus. *Journal of Physiology* (*London*) 159(3), 518-545.

Hill, C., and K. Weber. 1986. Monoclonal antibodies distinguish titins from heart and skeletal muscle. *Journal of Cell Biology* 102(3), 1099-1108.

Hill, D.K. 1968. Tension due to interaction between the sliding filaments in resting striated muscle. The effect of stimulation. *Journal of Physiology (London)* 199(3), 637-684.

Hilyer, J.C., K.C. Brown, A.T. Sirles, and L. Peoples. 1990. A flexibility intervention to reduce the incidence and severity of joint injuries among municipal firefighters. *Journal of Occupational Medicine* 32(7), 631-637.

Hinrichs, R.N. 1990. Whole body movement: Coordination of arms and legs in walking and running. In *Multiple muscle systems: Biomechanics and movement organization*, ed. J.M. Winters and S.L.-Y. Woo, 694-705. New York: Springer-Verlag.

Hinrichs, R.N. 1992. Case studies of asymmetrical arm action in running. *International Journal of Sport Biomechanics* 8(2), 111-128.

Hinterbuchner, C. 1985. Traction. In *Manipulation, traction and massage*. 3rd ed, ed. J.V. Basmajian, 172-200. Baltimore: Williams & Wilkins.

Hirche, H., W.K. Raff, and D. Grün. 1970. The resistance to blood flow in the gastrocnemius of the dog during sustained and rhythmical isometric and isotonic contractions. *European Journal of Physiology* 314, 97-112.

Hoeger, W.W.K. 1991. *Principles and labs for physical fitness and wellness*. Englewood, CO: Morton.

Hoeger, W.W.K., and D.R. Hopkins. 1992. A comparison of the sit and reach and the modified sit and reach in the measurement of flexibility in women. *Research Quarterly for Exercise and Sport* 63(2), 191-195.

Hoeger, W.W.K., D.R. Hopkins, S. Button, and T.A. Palmer. 1990. Comparing the sit and reach with the modified sit and reach in measuring flexibility in adolescents. *Pediatric Exercise Science* 2(2), 156-162.

Hoeger, W.W.K., D.R. Hopkins, and L.C. Johnson. 1991. *Muscular flexibility: Test protocols and national flexibility norms for the modified sit-and-reach test, total body rotation test, and shoulder rotation test.* Addison, IL: Novel Products Figure Finder Collection.

Hoehler, F.K., and J.S. Tobis. 1982. Low back pain and its treatment by spinal manipulation: Measures of flexibility and asymmetry. *Rheumatology and Rehabilitation* 21(1), 21-26.

Hoehler, F.K., J.S. Tobis, and A.A. Buerger. 1981. Spinal manipulation for low back pain. *Journal of the American Medical Association* 245(18), 1836-1838.

Hoen, T.I., and C.E. Brackett. 1970. Peripheral nerve lengthening. I. Experimental. *Journal of Neurosurgery* 13(1), 43-62.

Hoeve, C.A.J., and P.J. Flory. 1974. The elastic properties of elastin. *Biopolymers* 13(4), 677-686.

Hogg, J.M. 1978. Flexibility training. *Coaching Review* 1(3), 38-45.

Holcomb, W.R. 2000. Stretching and warm-up. In *Essentials of strength training and conditioning*. 2nd ed, ed. T.R. Baechle and R.W. Earle, 321-342. Champaign, IL: Human Kinetics.

Holland, G.J. 1968. The physiology of flexibility. A review of the literature. *Kinesiology Review* 1, 49-62.

Holly, R.G., J.G. Barnett, C.R. Ashmore, R.G. Taylor, and P.A. Mole. 1980. Stretch-induced growth in chicken wing muscles: A new model of stretch hypertrophy. *American Journal of Physiology* 238(Cell Physiology 7), C62-C71.

Holmer, I., and L. Gullstrand. 1980. Physiological responses to swimming with a controlled frequency of breathing. *Scandinavian Journal of Sports Sciences* 2(1), 1-6.

Hölmich, P., P. Uhrskou, L. Ulnits, I-L. Kanstrup, M.B. Nielsen, A.M. Bjerg, and K. Krogsgaard. 1999. Effectiveness of active physical training as treatment for long-standing adductor-related groin pain in athletes: Randomised trial. *Lancet* 353(9151), 439-443.

Holt, L.E. n.d. *Scientific stretching for sport (3-s)*. Halifax, Nova Scotia: Sport Research.

Holt, L.E., T.W. Pelham, and P.D. Campagna. 1995. Hemodynamics during a machine-aided flexibility protocol. *Canadian Journal of Applied Physiology* 20(4), 407-416.

Holt, L.E., and R.K. Smith. 1983. The effects of selected stretching programs on active and passive flexibility. In *Biomechanics in sport*, ed. J. Terauds, 54-67. Del Mar, CA: Research Center for Sports.

Holt, L.E., T.M. Travis, and T. Okita. 1970. Comparative study of three stretching techniques. *Perceptual and Motor Skills* 31(2), 611-616.

Hong, Y., J.X. Li, and P.D. Robinson. 2000. Balance control, flexibility, and cardiorespiratory fitness among older tai chi practitioners. *British Journal of Sports Medicine* 34(1), 29-34.

Hooker, D.N. 1999. Spinal traction. In *Therapeutic modalities in sports medicine*. 4th ed. ed. W.E. Prentice, 284-305. Boston: WCB McGraw-Hill.

Hooper, A.C.B. 1981. Length, diameter and number of ageing skeletal muscle fibres. *Gerontology* 27(3), 121-126.

Hoover, H.V. 1958. Functional technic. *Academy of Applied Osteopathy Yearbook 1958*, 47-51.

Hopkins, D.R. 1981. *The relationship between selected anthropometric measures and sit-and-reach performance*. Paper presented at the American Alliance for Health, Physical Education, Recreation and Dance National Measurement Symposium, Houston, TX.

Hopkins, D.R., and W.W.K. Hoeger. 1986. The modified sit and reach test. In *Lifetime physical fitness and wellness: A personalized program*, ed. W.W.K. Hoeger, 47-48. Englewood, CO: Morton.

Hopkins, D.R., B. Murrah, W.W. Hoeger, and R.C. Rhodes. 1990. Effects of low-impact aerobic dance on the functional fitness of elderly women. *The Gerontologist* 30(2), 189-192.

Horowits, R. 1992. Passive force generation and titin isoforms in mammalian skeletal muscle. *Biophysical Journal* 61(2), 392-398.

Horowits, R., E.S. Kempner, M.E. Bisher, and R.J. Podolsky. 1986. A physiological role for titin and nebulin in skeletal muscle. *Nature* 323(6084), 160-163.

Horowits, R., and R.J. Podolsky. 1987a. The positional stability of thick filaments in activated skeletal muscle depends on sarcomere length: Evidence for the role of titin filaments. *Journal of Cell Biology*, 105(5), 2217-2223.

Horowits, R., and R.J. Podolsky. 1987b. Thick filament movement and the effect of titin filaments in activated skeletal muscle. (Abstract). *Biophysical Journal* 51(2, Pt. 2), 219a.

Hosea, T.M., and C.J. Gatt. 1996. Back pain in golf. *Clinics in Sports Medicine* 15(1), 37-53.

Hosea, T. M., C.J. Gatt, N.A. Langrana, and J.P. Zawadsky. 1990. Biomechanical analysis of the golfer's back. In *Science and Golf*, ed. A.J. Cochran, 43-48. Glasgow: E & FN Spon.

Hossler, P. 1989. To bend or not to bend. *The Physician and Sportsmedicine* 17(6), 20.

Hough, T. 1902. Ergographic studies in muscular soreness. *American Journal of Physiology* 7(1), 76-92.

Houglum, P.A. 1992. Soft tissue healing and its impact on rehabilitation. *Journal of Sport Rehabilitation* 1(1), 19-39.

Houglum, P.A. 2001. *Therapeutic exercise for athletic injuries*. Champaign, IL: Human Kinetics.

Houk, J.C., and E. Henneman. 1967. Responses of Golgi tendon organs to forces applied to muscle tendon. *Journal of Neurophysiology* 30(6), 1466-1481.

Houk, J.C., J.J. Singer, and M.R. Goldman. 1971. Adequate stimulus for tendon organs with observations on mechanics of ankle joint. *Journal of Neurophysiology* 34(6), 1051-1065.

Howard, B.K., J.H. Goodsen, and W.J. Mengert. 1953. Supine hypotensive syndrome in late pregnancy. *Obstetrics and Gynecology* 1, 371.

Howell, J.N., A.G. Chila, G. Ford, D. David, and T. Gates. 1985. An electromyographic study of elbow motion during postexercise muscle soreness. *Journal of Applied Physiology* 58(5), 1713-1718.

Howes, R.G., and I.C. Isdale. 1971. The non-myotendinous force transmission. *Rheumatology and Physical Medicine* 11(2), 72-77.

Howse, A.J. 1972. Orthopedists aid ballet. *Clinical Orthopaedics and Related Research* 89, 52-63.

Howse, A.J.G. 1987. The young ballet dancer. In *Dance medicine: A comprehensive guide*. eds. A.J. Ryan and R.E. Stephens, 107-114. Chicago: Pluribus.

Hsieh, C., J.M. Walker, and K. Gillis. 1983. Straight-leg raising test: Comparison of three instruments. *Physical Therapy* 63(9), 1429-1433.

Hu, D.H., S. Kimura, and K. Maruyama. 1986. Sodium dodecyl sulfate gel electrophoresis studies of connectin-like high molecular weight proteins of various types of vertebrate and invertebrate muscles. *Journal of Biochemistry* (Tokyo) 99(5), 1485-1492.

Huang, Q-M., E. Andersson, and A. Thorstensson. 2001. Intramuscular myoelectric activity and selective coactivation of trunk muscles during lateral flexion with and without load. *Spine* 26(13), 1465-1472.

Hubley, C.L., J.W. Kozey, and W.D. Stanish. 1984. The effects of static stretching exercises and stationary cycling on range of motion at the hip joint. *Journal of Orthopaedic and Sports Physical Therapy* 6(2), 104-109.

Hubley-Kozey, C.L. 1991. Testing flexibility. In *Physiological testing of the high-performance athlete*. 2nd ed. eds. E.D. MacDougall, H.A. Wenger, and H.J. Green, 309-359. Champaign, IL: Human Kinetics.

Hubley-Kozey, C.L., and W.D. Stanish. 1990. Can stretching prevent athletic injuries? *Journal of Musculoskeletal Medicine* 7(3), 21-31.

Huijing, P.A. 1999. Muscular force transmission: A unified, dual or multiple system? A review and some explorative experimental results. *Archives of Physiology and Biochemistry* 107(4), 292-311.

Huijing, P.A., and G.C. Baan 2001. Extramuscular myofascial force transmission within the rat anterior tibial compartment: Proximodistal differences in muscular force. *Acta Physiologica Scandinavica* 173(3), 297-311.

Huijing, P.A., G.C. Baan, and G. Rebel. 1998. Non-myotendinous force transmission in rat extensor digitorum longus muscle. *Journal of Experimental Biology* 201(5), 683-691.

Hull, M. 1990-1991. Flexible ankles: Faster swimming. *Swimming Technique* 27(3), 23-24.

Hull, M. 2002. *The kick*. [Online]. Available: www.zoomers.net/new-thekick.htm [October 31, 2003].

Hulliger, J. 2003. Connective tissue polarity unraveled by a Markov-chain mechanism of collagen fibril segment self-assembly. *Biophysical Journal* 84(6), 3501-3507.

Hunt, D.G., O.A. Zuberbier, A.J. Kozlowski, J. Robinson, J. Berkowitz, I.Z. Schultz, R.A. Milner, J.M. Crook, and D.C. Turk. 2001. Reliability of the lumbar flexion, lumbar extension, and passive straight leg raise test in normal populations embedded within a complete physical examination. *Spine* 26(24), 2714-2718.

Hunter, D.G., and J. Spriggs. 2000. Investigation into the relationship between the passive flexibility and active stiffness of the ankle plantar-flexor muscles. *Clinical Biomechanics* 15(8), 600-606.

Hunter, G. 1998. Specific soft tissue mobilization in the management of soft tissue dysfunction. *Manual Therapy* 3(1), 2-11.

Hunter, J.P., and R.N. Marshall. 2002. Effects of power and flexibility training on vertical jump technique. *Medicine and Science in Sports and Exercise* 34(3), 476-486.

Hunter, S.C. 1994. Participation physical examination. In *Orthopaedic Knowledge Update Sports Medicine*, ed. by L. Y. Griffin, 127-132. Rosemont, IL: American Academy of Orthopaedic Surgeons.

Hupprich, F.L., and P.O. Sigerseth. 1950. The specificity of flexibility in girls. *Research Quarterly* 21(1), 25-33.

Hussain, S.N.A., B. Rabinovitch, P.T. Macklem, and R.L. Pardy. 1985. Effects of separate rib cage and abdominal restriction on exercise performance in normal humans. *Journal of Applied Physiology* 58(6), 2020-2026.

Hutson, M.A. 2001. Prevention of injury. In *Sports injuries recognition and management*. 3rd ed, ed. M.A. Hutson, 194-212. Oxford: Oxford University Press.

Hutton, R.S., K. Kaiya, S. Suzuki, and S. Watanabe. 1987. Post-contraction errors in human force production are reduced by muscle stretch. *Journal of Physiology* (London) 393(1), 247-259.

Huwyler, J. 1989. Physical examination to determine suitability for a career as a professional dancer. *Dance Medicine-Health Newsletter* 7(4), 5-11.

Huxley, H.E. 1957. The double array of filaments in cross-striated muscle. *Journal of Biophysics and Biochemical Cytology* 3(5), 631-648.

Huxley, H.E. 1965. The mechanism of muscular contraction. *Scientific American* 213(6), 18-27.

Huxley, H.E. 1967. Muscle cells. In *The cell*, ed. J. Brachet and A. Mirsky, 367-481. New York: Academic Press.

Huxley, H.E., and J. Hanson. 1954. Changes in the cross-striations of muscle during contraction and stretch and their structural interpretation. *Nature* 173(4412), 973-976.

Hyman, J., and S.A. Rodeo. 2000. Injury and repair of tendons and ligaments. *Physical Medicine and Rehabilitation Clinics of North America* 11(2), 267-288.

Iashvili, A.V. 1983. Active and passive flexibility in athletes specializing in different sports. *Soviet Sports Review* 18(1), 30-32.

Ice, R. 1985. Long-term compliance. *Physical Therapy* 65(12), 1832-1839.

Ichiyama, R.M., B.G. Ragan, G.W. Bell, and G.A. Iwamoto. 2002. Effects of topical analgesics on the precessor response evoked by muscle afferents. *Medicine and Science in Sports and Exercise* 34(9), 1440-1445.

Ikai, M., and T. Fukunaga. 1970. A study on training effect on strength per unit cross-sectional area of muscle by means of ultrasonic measurement. *European Journal of Applied Physiology* 28(3), 173-180.

Ingber, D.E. 1997. Tensegrity: The architectural basis of cellular mechanotransduction. *Annual Review of Physiology* 59:575-599.

Ingber, D.E., D. Prusty, J.V. Frangioni, E.J. Cragoe, C. Lechene, and M.A. Schwartz. 1990. Control of intracellular pH and growth by fibronectin in capillary endothelial cells. *Journal of Cell Biology* 110(5), 1803-1811.

Inman, V.T., J.B. Saunders, and L.C. Abbot. 1944. Observations on the functions of the shoulder joint. *The Journal of Bone and Joint Surgery* 26(1), 1-30.

Inoué, S., and C.P. Leblond. 1986. The microfibrils of connective tissue: I. Ultrastructure. *American Journal of Anatomy* 176(2), 121-138.

International Chiropractors Association. 1993. *Policy handbook & code of ethics.* Arlington, VA: Author.

International Dance-Exercise Association. n.d. *Guidelines for convention presenters.* San Diego: Author.

Irvin, R., D. Iversen, and S. Roy. 1998. *Sports medicine: Prevention, assessment, management.* 2nd ed. Boston: Allyn & Bacon.

Itay, S., A. Ganel, H. Horoszowski, and I. Farine. 1982. Clinical and functional status following lateral ankle sprains. *Orthopaedic Review* 11(5), 73-76.

Itoh, Y., T. Susuki, S. Kimura, K. Ohashi, H. Higuchi, H. Sawada, T. Shimizu, M. Shibata, and K. Maruyama. 1988. Extensible and less-extensible domains of connectin filaments in stretched vertebrate skeletal muscle as detected by immunofluorescence and immunoelectron microscopy using monoclonal antibodies. *Journal of Biochemistry* (Tokyo) 104(4), 504-508.

Iyengar, B.K.S. 1979. *Light on yoga.* New York: Schocken Books.

Jackman, R.V. 1963. Device to stretch the Achilles tendon. *Journal of the American Physical Therapy Association* 43(10), 729.

Jackson, A.W., and A.A. Baker. 1986. The relationship of the sit and reach test to criterion measures of hamstring and back flexibility in young females. *Research Quarterly for Exercise and Sport* 57(3), 183-186.

Jackson, A.W., and N.J. Langford. 1989. The criterion-related validity of the sit and reach test: Replication and extension of previous findings. *Research Quarterly for Exercise and Sport* 60(4), 384-385.

Jackson, A.W., J.R. Morrow, P.A. Brill, H.W. Kohl, N.F. Gordon, and S.N. Blair. 1998. Relations of sit-up and sit-and-reach tests to low back pain in adults. *Journal of Orthopaedic and Sports Physical Therapy* 27(1), 22-26.

Jackson, C.P., and M.D. Brown. 1983. Is there a role for exercise in the treatment of patients with low back pain? *Clinical Orthopedics and Related Research* 179(October), 39-45.

Jackson, D.W., L.L. Wiltse, and R.J. Cirincione. 1976. Spondylolysis in the female gymnast. *Clinical Orthopaedics and Related Research* 117(June), 68-73.

Jackson, M., M. Solomonow, B. Zhou, R. Baratta, and M. Harris. 2001. Multifidus EMG and tension-relaxation recovery after prolonged static lumbar flexion. *Spine* 26(7), 715-723.

Jacobs, M. 1976. Neurophysiological implications of slow, active stretching. *American Corrective Therapy Association* 30(8), 151-154.

Jacobs, S.J., and B.L. Berson. 1986. Injuries to runners: A study of entrants to a 10,000 meter race. *American Journal of Sports Medicine* 14(2), 151-155.

Jacobson, E. 1929. *Progressive relaxation.* Chicago: University of Chicago Press.

Jacobson, E. 1938. *Progressive relaxation.* 2nd ed. Chicago: University of Chicago Press.

Jaeger, B., and J.L. Reeves. 1986. Quantification of changes in myofascial trigger point sensitivity with the pressure algometer following passive stretch. *Pain* 27(2), 203-210.

Jahnke, M.T., U. Proske, and A. Struppler. 1989. Measurements of muscle stiffness, the electromyogram and activity in single muscle spindles on human flexor muscles following conditioning by passive stretch or contraction. *Brain Research* 493(1), 103-112.

Jahss, S.A. 1919. Joint hypotonia. *New York Medical Journal* 109(2106), 638-639.

Jami, L. 1992. Golgi tendon organs in mammalian skeletal muscle: Functional properties and central actions. *Physiological Reviews* 72(3), 623-666.

Jamieson, A.H., C.A. Alford, H.A. Bird, I. Hindmarch, and W. Wright. 1995. The effect of sleep and nocturnal movement on stiffness, pain, and psychomotor performance in ankylosing spondylitis. *Clinical and Experimental Rheumatology* 13(1), 73-78.

Japan Information Network. 2002. www.jinjapan.org.

Järvinen, T.A.H., L. Józsa, P. Kannus, T.L.N. Järvinen, and M. Järvinen. 2002. Organization and distribution of intramuscular connective tissue in normal and immobilized skeletal muscles. *Journal of Muscle Research and Cell Motility* 23(3), 245-254.

Järvinen, T.A.H., M. Kääriäinen, M. Järvinen, and H. Kalimo. 2000. Muscle strain injuries. *Current Opinions in Rheumatology* 12(2), 155-161.

Javurek, I. 1982. Experience with hypermobility in athletes. *Theorie A Praxe Telesne Vychovy* 30(3), 185.

Jay, I., and S. Rappaport. 1983. *Hanging out, the upside down exercise book.* Mill Valley, CA: Jay Ra Productions.

Jayson, M., H. Sims-Williams, S. Young, H. Baddeley, and E. Collins. 1981. Mobilization and manipulation for the low back pain. *Spine* 6(4), 409-416.

Jenkins, R., and R.W. Little. 1974. A constitutive equation for parallel-fibered elastic tissue. *Journal of Biomechanics* 7(5), 397-402.

Jerome, J. 1988. The pleasures of stretching. *Strings* 3(1), 14-21.

Jervey, A.A. 1961. *A study of the flexibility of selected joints in specified groups of adult females.* Ph.D. diss., University of Michigan, Ann Arbor.

Jesse, E.F., D.S. Owen, and K.B. Sagar. 1980. The benign hypermobile joint syndrome. *Arthritis and Rheumatism* 23(9), 1053-1056.

Jette, A.M., D. Rooks, M. Lachman, T.H. Lin, C. Levenson, D. Heislein, M.M. Giorgetti, and B.A. Harris. 1998. Home-based resistance training: Predictors of participation and adherence. *The Gerontologist* 38(4), 412-421.

Jobbins, B., H.A. Bird, and V. Wright. 1979. A joint hyperextensometer for the quantification of joint laxity. *Engineering in Medicine* 8(2), 103-104.

Johansson, P.H., L. Lindström, G. Sundelin, and B. Lindström. 1999. The effects of preexercise stretching on muscular soreness, tenderness and force loss following heavy eccentric exercise. *Scandinavian Journal of Medicine & Science in Sports* 9(4), 219-225.

Johns, R.J., and V. Wright. 1962. Relative importance of various tissues in joint stiffness. *Journal of Applied Physiology* 17(5), 824-828.

Johnson, J.E., F.H. Sim, and S.G. Scott. 1987. Musculoskeletal injuries in competitive swimmers. *Mayo Clinic Proceedings* 62(4), 289-304.

Johnson, J.N., J. Gauvin, and M. Fredericson. 2003. Swimming biomechanics and injury prevention: New stroke techniques and medical considerations. *The Physician and Sportsmedicine* 31(1), 41-46.

Johnson, R.J. 1991. Help your athletes heal themselves. *The Physician and Sportsmedicine* 19(5), 107-110.

Jones, A. 1975. Flexibility and metabolic condition. *Athletic Journal* 56(2), 56-61, 80-81.

Jones, A.M. 2002. Running economy is negatively related to sit-and-reach test performance in international-standard distance runners. *International Journal of Sports Medicine* 23(1), 40-43.

Jones, B.H., D.N. Cowan, J.P. Tomlinson, J.R. Robinson, D.W. Polly, and P.N. Frykman. 1993. Epidemiology of injuries associated with physical training among young men in the army. *Medicine and Science in Sports and Exercise* 25(2), 197-203.

Jones, C.J., R.R. Rikli, J. Max, and G. Noffal. 1998. The reliability and validity of a chair sit-and reach test as a measure of hamstring flexibility in older adults. *Research Quarterly for Exercise and Sport* 69(4), 338-343.

Jones, D. 1999. The effects of proprioceptive neuromuscular facilitation flexibility training on the clubhead speed of recreational golfers. In *Science and Golf III: Proceedings of the World Scientific Congress of Golf*, ed. M.R. Farrally and A.J. Cochran, 46-50. Champaign, IL: Human Kinetics.

Jones, D.A., and D.J. Newham. 1985. The effect of training on human muscle pain and damage. *Journal of Physiology (London)* 365(August), 76P.

Jones, D.A., D.J. Newham, and P.M. Clarkson. 1987. Skeletal muscle stiffness and pain following eccentric exercise of the elbow flexors. *Pain* 30(2), 233-242.

Jones, D.A., D.J. Newham, G. Obletter, and M.A. Giamberardino. 1987. Nature of exercise-induced muscle pain. *Advances in Pain and Therapy* 10, 207-218.

Jones, D.A., D.J. Newham, and C. Torgan. 1989. Mechanical influences on long-lasting human muscle fatigue and delayed-onset pain. *Journal of Physiology* 412(May), 415-427.

Jones, D.A., and O.M. Rutherford. 1987. Human muscle strength training: The effects of three different training regimes and the nature of the resultant changes. *Journal of Physiology (London)* 391(October), 1-11.

Jones, H.H. 1965. The Valsalva procedure. *Journal of the American Physical Therapy Association* 45(6), 570-572.

Jones, L.H. 1995. *Strain and counterstrain*. Boise, ID: Jones Strain-CounterStrain.

Jones, M.A., J.M. Buis, and I.D. Harris. 1986. Relationship of race and sex to physical and motor measures. *Perceptual and Motor Skills* 63(1), 169-170.

Jones, R.E. 1970. A kinematic interpretation of running and its relationship to hamstrings injury. *Journal of Health, Physical Education and Recreation* 41(8), 83.

Józsa, L.G., and P. Kannius. 1997. *Human tendons: Anatomy, physiology, and pathology*. Champaign, IL: Human Kinertics.

Jungueira, L.C., J. Carneiro, and J.A. Long. 1989. *Basic histology*. 6th ed. Los Altos, CA: Lange Medical.

Kabat, H., M. McLeod, and C. Holt. 1959. The practical application of proprioceptive neuromuscular facilitation. *Physiotherapy* 45(4), 87-92.

Kadi, F. 2000. Adaptation of human skeletal muscle to training and anabolic steroids. *Acta Physiologica Scandinavica* 168 (Suppl 646), 1-52.

Kadler, K., and G. Wallis. 1999. The molecular basis of joint hypermobility. In *Hypermobility of joints*. 3rd ed, ed. P. Beighton, R. Grahame and H. Bird, 23-37. London: Springer Verlag.

Kaigle, A.M., P. Wessberg, and T.H. Hansson. 1998. The muscular and kinematic behavior of the lumbar spine during flexion-extension. *Journal of Spinal Disorders* 11(2), 163-174.

Kalenak, A., and C. Morehouse. 1975. Knee stability and knee ligament injuries. *Journal of the American Medical Association* 234(11), 1143-1145.

Kammer, C.S., C.C. Young, and M.W. Niedfeldt. 1999. Swimming injuries and illnesses. *The Phyiscian and Sportsmedicine* 27(4), 51-60.

Kanamaru, A., M. Sibuya, T. Nagai, K. Inoue, and I. Homma. 1990. Stretch gymnastics training in asthmatic children. In *International series on sport sciences: Vol. 20. Fitness for the aged, disabled, and industrial worker*, ed. M. Kaneko, 178-181. Champaign, IL: Human Kinetics.

Kane, M.D., R.D. Karl, and J.H. Swain. 1985. Effects of gravity-facilitated traction on intervertebral dimensions of the lumbar spine. *Journal of Orthopaedic and Sports Physical Therapy* 6(5), 281-288.

Kannus, P. 2000. Structure of the tendon connective tissue. *Scandinavian Journal of Medicine and Science in Sports* 10(6), 312-320.

Kapandji, I.A. 1974. *The physiology of the joints: Vol. 3. The trunk and the vertebral column*. 2nd ed. Edinburgh: Churchill Livingstone.

Kapandji, I.A. 1982. *The physiology of the joints: Vol. 1. Upper limb*. 2nd ed. Edinburgh: Churchill Livingstone.

Kapandji, I.A. 1987. *The physiology of the joints: Vol. 2. Lower limb*. 5th ed. Edinburgh: Churchill Livingstone.

Karmenov, B. 1990. Knee-joint mobility. *Soviet Sports Review* 25(4), 200-2001.

Karpovich, P.V., P.V.M. Singh, and C.M. Tipton. 1970. The effect of deep knee squats upon knee stability. *Teor. Praxe tel Vych* 8, 112-122.

Karvonen, J. 1992. Importance of warm-up and cool-down on exercise performance. *Medicine in Sport Science* 35, 189-214.

Kasteler, J., R.L. Kane, D.M. Olse, and C. Thetford. 1976. Issues underlying prevalence of "doctor-shopping" behavior. *Journal of Health and Social Behavior* 17(4), 328-339.

Kastelic, J., A. Galeski, and E. Baer, E. 1978. The multicomposite structure of tendon. *Connective Tissue Research* 6(1), 11-23.

Kattenberg, B. 1952. Famous rubber men and limber jims are filed for future by a contortionist fan. *Life* 32(23), 18-19.

Kattenberg, B. 1963. Forgotten acrobats of the arena. *Muscle Power Magazine* Summer, 18-19, 42-43.

Kauffman, T. 1987. Posture and age. *Topics in Geriatric Rehabilitation* 2(4), 13-28.

Kauffman, T. 1990. Impact of aging-related musculoskeletal and postural changes on fall. *Topics in Geriatric Rehabilitation* 5(2), 34-43.

Kawashima, K., S. Takeshita, H. Zaitsu, and T. Meshizuka. 1994. A biomechanical analysis of the respiratory pattern during the golf swing. In *Science and golf II: Proceedings of the world scientific congress of golf* (46-49). edited by A.J. Cochran and M.R. Farrally. London: E. & FN Spon.

Keating, J.C. 1995. Purpose—straight chiropractic: Not science, not health care. *Journal of Manipulative and Physiological Therapeutics* 18(6), 416-418.

Kegerreis, S. 2001. Myofascial therapy. In C. Manheim. *The myofascial release manual*. 3rd ed., 2-6. Thorofare, New Jersey: Slack.

Keirns, M. 2000. *Myofascial release in sports medicine*. Champaign, IL: Human Kinetics.

Kellermayer, M.S.Z., and H.L. Granzier. 1996. Elastic properties of single titin molecules made visible through fluorescent F-actin binding. *Biochemical and Biophysical Research Communications* 221(3), 491-497.

Kellett, J. 1986 Acute soft tissue injuries—A review of the literature. *Medicine and Science in Sports and Exercise* 18(5), 489-500.

Kendall, F.P., and E.K. McCreary. 1983. *Muscles: Testing and function*. 3rd ed. Baltimore: Williams & Wilkins.

Kendall, H.O., and F.P. Kendall. 1948. Normal flexibility according to age groups. *Journal of Bone and Joint Surgery* 30A(3), 690-694.

Kendall, H.O., F.P. Kendall, and D.A. Boynton. 1970. *Posture and pain*. New York: Krieger.

Kendall, H.O., F.P. Kendall, and G.E. Wadsworth. 1971. *Muscles testing and function*. Baltimore: Williams & Wilkins.

Kent, M. 1998. *The Oxford dictionary of sports science and medicine*. 2nd ed. Oxford: Oxford University Press.

Kerner, J.A., and J.C. D'Amico. 1983. A statistical analysis of a group of runners. *Journal of the American Podiatry Association* 73(3), 160-164.

Kerr, K. 2000. Relaxation techniques: A critical review. *Critical Reviews in Physical and Rehabilitation Medicine* 12(1), 51-89.

Keskinen, K.L., and P.V. Komi. 1991. Breathing patterns of elite swimmers in aerobic/anaerobic loading. *Journal of Biomechanics* 215(7), 709.

Kettunen, J.A., U.M. Kujala, H. Räty, T. Videman, S. Sarna, O. Impivaara, and S. Koskinen. 2000. Factors associated with hip joint rotation in former elite athletes. *British Journal of Sports Medicine* 34(1), 44-48.

Key, J.A. 1927. Hypermobility of joints as a sex linked hereditary characteristic. *Journal of the American Medical Association* 88(22), 1710-1712.

Khalil, T.M., S.S. Asfour, L.M. Martinez, S.M. Waly, R.S. Rosomoff, and H.L. Rosomoff. 1992. Stretching in rehabilitation of low-back pain patients. *Spine* 17(3), 311-317.

Khan, K.M., K. Bennell, S. Ng, B. Matthews, P. Roberts, C. Nattrass, S. Way, and J. Brown. 2000. Can 16–18-year-old elite ballet dancers improve their hip and ankle range of motion over a 12-month period? *Clinical Journal of Sport Medicine* 10(2), 98-103.

Kibler, W.B., J. Chandler, B.P. Livingston, and E.P. Roetert. 1996. Shoulder range of motion in elite tennis players: Effect of age and years of tournament play. *American Journal of Sports Medicine* 24(3), 279-285.

Kihira, M., J. Ryu, J.S. Han, and B. Rowen. 1995. Wrist motion analysis in violinists. *Medical Problems of Performing Artists* 10(3), 79-85.

Kim, P.S., D.D. Santos, G. O'Neill, S. Julien, D. Kelm, and M. Dube. 1992. The effect of single chiropractic manipulation on sagittal mobility of the lumbar spine in symptomatic low back pain patients. In *Proceedings of the 1992 International Conference on Spinal Manipulation.* Chicago.

Kim, Y.-J., R.L.Y. Sah, A.J. Grodzinsky, A.H.K. Plaas, and J.D. Sandy. 1994. Mechanical regulation of cartilage biosynthetic behavior: Physical stimuli. *Archives of Biochemistry and Biophysics* 311(1), 1-12.

Kimberly, P.E. 1980. Formulating a prescription for osteopathic manipulative treatment. *Journal of the American Osteopathic Association* 79(8), 146-152.

Kindig, C.A., and D.C. Poole. 1999. Effects of skeletal muscle sarcomere length on in vivo capillary distensibility. *Microvascular Research* 57(2), 144-152.

King, J.W., H.J. Brelsford, and H.S Tullos. 1969. Analysis of the pitching arm of the professional baseball pitcher. *Clinical Orthopaedics and Related Research* 67(November-December), 116-123.

King, N.J. 1980. The therapeutic utility of abbreviated progressive relaxation: A critical review with implications for clinical practice. In *Progress in behavior modification* (Vol. 10), ed. M. Hersen, R. Eisler and P. Miller. New York: Academic Press.

Kippers, V., and A.W. Parker. 1984. Posture related to myoelectric silence of erectores spinae during trunk flexion. *Spine* 9(7), 740-745.

Kirk, J.A., B.M. Ansell, and E.G.L. Bywaters. 1967. The hypermobility syndrome. *Annals of the Rheumatic Diseases* 26(5), 419-425.

Kirkebø, A., and A. Wisnes. 1982. Regional tissue fluid pressure in rat calf muscle during sustained contraction or stretch. *Acta Physiologica Scandinavica* 114(4), 551-556.

Kirkendall, D.T., W.E. Prentice, and W.E. Garrett. 2001. Rehabilitation of muscle injuries. In *Rehabilitation of sports injuries*, ed. G. Pudda, A. Giombini, and A. Selvanetti, 185-193. Berlin: Spinger Verlag.

Kirstein, L. 1939. *Ballet alphabet; A primer for laymen.* New York: Kamin.

Kirwan, T., L. Tooth, and C. Harkin. 2002. Compliance with hand therapy programs: Therapists' and patients' perceptions. *Journal of Hand Therapy* 15(1), 31-40.

Kisner, C., and L.A. Colby. 1996. *Therapeutic exercise foundations and techniques.* 3rd ed. Philadelphia: F.A. Davis.

Kisner, C., and L.A. Colby. 2002. *Therapeutic exercise foundations and techniques.* 4th ed. Philadelphia: F.A. Davis.

Klatz, R.M., B.G. Goldman, B.G., Pinchuk, K.E., Nelson, and R.S. Tarr. 1983. The effects of gravity inversion procedures on systemic blood pressure, and central retinal arterial pressure. *Journal of American Osteopathic Association* 82(11), 111-115.

Klee, A., T. Jöllenbeck, and K. Wiemann. 2002. The significance of titin filaments to resting tension and posture. In *International research in sports biomechanics*, ed. Y. Hong, 90-97. London: Routledge.

Klein, K.K. 1961. The deep squat exercise as utilized in weight training for athletics and its effect on the ligaments of the knee. *Journal of the Association for Physical and Mental Rehabilitation* 15(1), 6-11.

Klein, K.K., and C.A. Roberts. 1976. Mechanical problems of marathoners and joggers: Cause and solution. *American Corrective Therapy Journal* 30(6), 187-191.

Klemp, P., and I.D. Learmonth. 1984. Hypermobility and injuries in a professional ballet company. *British Journal of Sports Medicine* 18(3), 143-148.

Klemp, P., J.E. Stevens, and S. Isaacs. 1984. A hypermobility study in ballet dancers. *Journal of Rheumatology* 11(5), 692-696.

Klemp, P., S.M. Williams, and S.A. Stansfield. 2002. Articular mobility in Maori and European New Zealanders. *Rheumatology* 41(5), 554-557.

Kleynhans, A.M. 1980. Complications and contraindications to spinal manipulative therapy. In *Modern developments in the principles and practice of chiropractic*, ed. S. Haldeman, 359-384. New York: Appleton-Century-Crofts.

Klinge, K., S.P. Magnusson, E.B. Simonsen, P. Aagaard, K. Klausen, and M. Kjær, M. 1997. The effect of strength and flexibility training on

skeletal muscle, EMG, stiffness and viscoelastic response. *American Journal of Sports Medicine* 25(5), 710-716.

Kloeppel, R. 2000. Do the "speadability" and finger length of cellists and guitarists change due to practice? *Medical Problems of Performing Artists* 15(1), 23-30.

Knapik, J.J., B.H. Jones, C.L. Bauman, and J.M. Harris. 1992. Strength, flexibility and athletic injuries. *Sports Medicine* 14(5), 277-288.

Knapp, M.E. 1990. Massage. In *Krusen's handbook of physical medicine and rehabilitation.* 4th ed, ed. J.F. Lehmann and B.J. de Lateur, 433-435. Philadelphia: Saunders.

Knight, E.L., and J.B. Davis. 1984. *Flexibility: The concept of stretching and exercise.* Dubuque, IA: Kendall/Hunt.

Knight, K.L. 1995. *Cryotherapy in sport injury management.* Champaign, IL: Human Kinetics.

Knott, M., and D.E. Voss. 1968. *Proprioceptive neuromuscular facilitation.* New York: Harper & Row.

Knudson, D. 1998. Stretching: From science to practice. *Journal of Physical Education, Recreation and Dance* 69(3), 38-42.

Knudson, D. 1999. Stretching during warm-up: Do we have enough evidence? *Journal of Physical Education, Recreation and Dance* 70(7), 24-27, 51.

Knudson, D.V., P. Magnusson, and M. McHugh. 2000. Current issues in flexibility fitness. *President's Council on Physical Fitness and Sports Research Digest* 3(10), 1-19.

Knuttgen, H.G. 1986. Human performance in high-intensity exercise with concentric and eccentric muscle contractions. *International Journal of Sports Medicine* 7(Suppl. 1), 6-9.

Knuttgen, H.G., J.F. Patton, and J.A. Vogel. 1982. An ergometer for concentric and eccentric muscular exercise. *Journal of Applied Physiology* 53(3), 784-788.

Kobet, K.A. 1985. Retinal tear associated with gravity boot use. *Annals of Ophthalmology* 17(4), 308-310.

Koceja, D.M., J.R. Burke, and G. Kamen. 1991. Organization of segmental reflexes in trained dancers. *International Journal of Sports Medicine* 12(3), 285-289.

Kokjohn, K., D.M. Schmid, J.J., Triano, and P.C. Brennan. 1992. The effect of spinal manipulation on pain and prostaglandin levels in women with primary dysmenorrhea. *Journal of Manipulative and Physiological Therapeutics* 15(5), 279-285.

Kokkonen, J., A.G. Nelson, and A. Cornwell. 1998. Acute muscle stretching inhibits maximal strength performance. *Research Quarterly for Exercise and Sport* 69(4), 411-415.

Komi, P.V. 1984. Physiological and biomechanical correlates of muscle function effects of muscle structure and stretch-shortening cycle on force and speed. *Exercise and Sport Science Reviews* 12, 81-121.

Komi, P.V. 1986. Training of muscle strength and power: Interaction of neuromotoric, hypertrophic, and mechanical factors. *Journal of Sports Medicine* 7(1), 10-15.

Komi, P.V., and C. Boscoe. 1978. Utilization of stored elastic energy in men and women. *Medicine and Science in Sport* 10(4), 261-265.

Komi, P.V., and E.R. Buskirk. 1972. Effect of eccentric and concentric conditioning on tension and electrical activity in human muscle. *Ergonomics* 15(4), 417-434.

Kopell, H.P. 1962. The warm-up and autogenous injury. *New York State Journal of Medicine* 62(20), 3255-3258.

Kornberg, L., and R.L. Juliano. 1992. Signal transduction from the extracellular matrix: The integrin-tyrosine kinase connection. *Trends in Pharmacological Sciences* 13(3), 93-95.

Kornecki, S. 1992. Mechanism in muscular stabilization process in joints. *Journal of Biomechanics* 25(3), 235-245.

Korr, I.M. 1975. Proprioceptors and somatic dysfunction. *Journal of the American Osteopathic Association* 74(7), 638-650.

Koslow, R.E. 1987. Bilateral flexibility in the upper and lower extremities as related to age and gender. *Journal of Human Movement Studies* 13(9), 467-472.

Kottke, F.J., D.L. Pauley, and K.A. Ptak. 1966. Prolonged stretching for correction of shortening of connective tissue. *Archives of Physical Medicine and Rehabilitation* 47(6), 345-352.

Koutedakis, Y., L. Myszkewycz, D. Soulas, V. Papapostolou, I. Sullivan, and N.C.C. Sharp. 1999. The effects of rest and subsequent training on selected physiological parameters in professional female classical dancers. *International Journal of Sports Medicine* 20(6), 379-383.

Kotoulas, M. 2002. The use and misuse of the terms "manipulation" and "mobilization" in the literature establishing their efficacy in the treatment of lumber spine disorders. *Physiotherapy Canada* 54(1), 53-61.

Kovanen, V., H. Suominem, and E. Heikkinem. 1984a. Collagen of slow twitch and fast twitch muscle fibres in different types of rat skeletal muscle. *European Journal of Applied Physiology* 52(2), 235-242.

Kovanen, V., H. Suominem, and E. Heikkinem. 1984b. Mechanical properties of fast twitch and slow twitch skeletal muscle with special reference to collagen and endurance training. *Journal of Biomechanics* 17(10), 725-735.

Kovar, R. 1974. Prispevek ke studiu geneticke podminenosti lidske motiriky. PhD diss. Charles University (Prague).

Kovar, R. 1981. *Human variation in motor abilities and genetic analysis.* Prague: Charles University.

Krabak, B.J., E.R. Laskowski, J. Smith, M.J. Stuart, and G.Y. Wong. 2001. Neurophysiologic influences on hamstring flexibility: A pilot study. *Clinical Journal of Sport Medicine* 11(4), 241-246.

Kraeger, D.R. 1993. Foot injuries. In *Handbook of sportsmedicine: A symptom-oriented approach*, ed. W.A. Lillegard and K.S. Rucker, 159-171. Boston: Andover Medical.

Kraemer, W.J., N.T. Triplett, A.C. Fry, L.P. Koziris, J.E. Bauer, J.M. Lynch, T. McConnell, R.U. Newton, S.E. Gordon, R.C. Nelson, and H.G. Knuttgen. 1995. An in-depth sports medicine profile of women college tennis players. *Journal of Sports Rehabilitation* 4(2), 79-98.

Krahenbuhl, G.S., and S.L. Martin. 1977. Adolescence body size and flexibility. *Research Quarterly* 48(4), 797-799.

Kramer, A.M., and R.W. Schrier. 1990. Demographic, social, and economic issues. In *Geriatric medicine*, ed. R.W. Schrier, 1-11. Philadelphia: Saunders.

Kranz, K.C. 1988. Chiropractic treatment of low-back pain. *Topics in Acute Care and Trauma Rehabilitation* 2(4), 47-62.

Kraus, H. 1965. *Backache stress and tension: Their cause, prevention and treatment.* New York: Simon and Schuster.

Kraus, H. 1970. *Clinical treatment of back and neck pain.* New York: McGraw-Hill.

Kraus, H. and R.P. Hirschland. 1954. Minimum muscular fitness in school children. *Research Quarterly* 25(2), 178-187.

Kreighbaum, E., and K.M. Barthels. 1985. *Biomechanics: A qualitative approach for studying human movement.* 2nd ed. Minneapolis: Burgess.

Krejci, V., and P. Koch. 1979. *Muscle and tendon injuries in athletes.* Stuttgart: Georg Thieme.

Krieglstein, G.K., and M.E. Langham. 1975. Influence of body position on the intraocular pressure of normal and glaucomatous eyes. *Ophthalmologica* 171(2), 132-145.

Krivickas, L.S. 1999. Training flexibility. In *Exercise in rehabilitation medicine*, eds. W.R. Frontera, D.M. Dawson, and D.M. Slovik, 83-102. Champaign, IL: Human Kinetics.

Kroll, P.G., R.W. Muhlhauser, N.C. Parsons, and C.D. Taylor. 1997. The effect of increased straight leg raise on work production in subjects with tight hamstrings. *Isokinetics and Exercise Science* 6(3), 181-185.

Kroll, P.G., and M.A. Raya. 1997. Hamstring muscles: An overview of anatomy, biomechanics and function, injury etiology, treatment, and prevention. *Critical Reviews in Physical and Rehabilitation Medicine* 9(3 & 4), 191-203.

Kronberg, M., L-A. Brostrom, and V. Soderlund. 1990. Retroversion of the humeral head in the normal shoulder and its relationship to the normal range of motion. *Clinical Orthopaedics and Related Research* 253(April), 113-117.

Krugman, M. 1995. Posture. [Online]. Available: www.tifaq.com/archive/piano-posture.txt [August 8, 2002].

Kubo, K., H. Kanehisa, and T. Fukunaga. 2002a. Effects of resistance and stretching training programmes on the viscoelastic properties of human tendon structures in vivo. *Journal of Physiology* 538(1), 219-226.

Kubo, K., H. Kanehisa, and T. Fukunaga. 2002b. Effects of transient muscle contractions and stretching on the tendon structures on the tendon structures in vivo. *Acta Physiologica Scandinavica* 175(2), 157-164.

Kubo, K., H. Kanehisa, M. Ito, and T. Fukunaga. 2001a. Effects of isometric training on the elasticity of human tendon structures in vivo. *Journal of Applied Physiology* 91(1), 26-32.

Kubo, K., H. Kanehisa, M. Ito, and T. Fukunaga. 2001b. Is passive stiffness in human muscles related to the elasticity of tendon structure? *European Journal of Applied Physiology* 85(3-4), 226-232).

Kubo, K., H. Kanehisa, Y. Kawakami, and T. Fukunaga. 2000. Elasticity of tendon structures of the lower limbs in sprinters. *Acta Physiologica Scandinavica* 168(2), 327-335.

Kubo, K., H. Kanehisa, Y. Kawakami, and T. Fukunaga. 2001a. Growth changes in the elastic properties of human tendon structures. *International Journal of Sports Medicine* 22(2), 138-143.

Kubo, K., H. Kanehisa, Y. Kawakami, and T. Fukunaga. 2001b. Influence of static stretching on viscoelastic properties of human tendon structures in vivo. *Journal of Applied Physiology* 90(2), 520-527.

Kubo, K., H. Kanehisa, Y. Kawakami, and T. Fukunaga. 2002. Effects of stretching training on the viscoelastic properties of human tendon structures in vivo. *Journal of Applied Physiology* 92(2), 595-601.

Kubo, K., Y. Kawakami, and T. Fukunaga. 1999. The influence of elastic properties of tendon structures on jump performance in humans. *Journal of Applied Physiology* 87(6), 2090-2096.

Kuchera, W.A., and M.L. Kuchera. 1992. *Osteopathic principles in practice.* Kirksville, MO: Kirksville College of Osteopathic Medicine.

Kudina, L. 1980. Reflex effects of muscle afferents on antagonists studies on single firing motor units in man. *Electroencephalography and Clinical Neurophysiology* 50(3-4), 214-221.

Kuipers, H.J., P.M. Drukker, P.M. Frederik, P. Guerten, and G.V. Kranenburg. 1983. Muscle degeneration after exercise in rats. *International Journal of Sports Medicine* 4(1), 45-51.

Kulakov, V. 1989. The harmony of training: The training of long-distance runners. *Soviet Sport Review* 24(4), 164-168.

Kulkarni, J., C. Hale, C. and L. Reilly. 1999. Review of falls-related injuries. *Critical Reviews in Physical and Rehabilitation Medicine* 11(1), 63-74.

Kulund, D.N. 1980. The foot in athletics. In *Disorders of the foot*, ed. A.J. Helfet and D.M.G. Lee, 58-79. Philadelphia: Lippincott.

Kulund, D.N., J.B. Dewey, C.E. Brubaker, and J.R. Roberts. 1978. Olympic weight-lifting injuries. *The Physician and Sportsmedicine* 6(11), 111-119.

Kulund, D.N., and M. Töttössy. 1983. Warm-up, strength, and power. *Orthopaedic Clinics of North America* 14(2), 427-448.

Kunz, H., and D.A. Kaufmann. 1980. How the best sprinters differ. *Track & Field Quarterly Review* 80(2).

Kuo, P.-L., P-C. Li, and M.L. Li. 2001. Elastic properties of tendon measured by two different approaches. *Ultrasound in Medicine & Biology* 27(9), 1275-1284.

Kurzban, G.P., and K. Wang. 1988. Giant polypeptides of skeletal muscle titin: Sedimentation equilibrium in guanidine hydrochloride. *Biochemical and Biophysical Research Communications* 150(3), 1155-1161.

Kushner, S., L. Saboe, D. Reid, T. Penrose, and M. Grace. 1990. Relationship of turnout to hip abduction in professional ballet dancers. *American Journal of Sports Medicine* 18(3), 286-291.

Kuukkanen, T., and E. Mälkiä. 2000. Effects of a three-month therapeutic exercise programme on flexibility in subjects with low back pain. *Physiotherapy Research International* 5(1), 46-61.

Laban, M.M. 1962. Collagen tissue: Implications of its response to stress in vitro. *Archives of Physical Medicine and Rehabilitation* 43(9), 461-465.

Labeit, S., and B. Kolmerer. 1995. Titins: Giant proteins in charge of muscle ultrastructure and elasticity. *Science* 270 (5234), 293-296.

LaFreniere, J.G. 1979. *The low back patient: Procedures for treatment by physical therapy.* New York: Mason.

Lakie, M., and L.G. Robson. 1988. Thixotropic changes in human muscle stiffness and the effects of fatigue. *Quarterly Journal of Experimental Physiology* 73(4), 487-500.

Lakie, M., E.G. Walsh, and G.W. Wright. 1984. Resonance at the wrist demonstrated by the use of a torque motor: An instrumental analysis of muscle tone in man. *Journal of Physiology* 353(Aug), 265-285.

Lal, K. 1966. *The cult of desire*. Delhi: Asia Press.

Lan, C., J-S. Lai, M-K. Wong, and M-L. Yu. 1996. Cardiorespiratory function, flexibility and body composition among geriatric tai chi chuan practitioners. *Archives of Physical Medicine and Rehabilitation* 77(6), 612-616.

Langeland, R.H., and R.J. Carangelo. 2000. Injuries to the thigh and groin. In *Principles and practice of orthopaedic sports medicine*, ed. W.E. Garrett, K.P. Speer and D.T. Kirkendall, 583-611. Philadelphia: Lippincott Williams & Wilkins.

Lankhorst, G.J., R.J. Van de Stadt, and J.K. Van der Korst. 1985. The natural history of idiopathic low back pain: A 3 year follow-up study of spinal motion, pain and functional capacity. *Scandinavian Journal of Rehabilitation Medicine* 17(1), 1-4.

Larsson, L.-G., J. Baum and G.S. Mudholkar. 1987. Hypermobility: Features and differential incidence between sexes. *Arthritis and Rheumatism* 30(12), 1426-1430.

Larsson, L.-G., J. Baum, G.S. Mudholkar, and G. Kollia. 1993. Benefits and disadvantages of joint hypermobility among musicians. *New England Journal of Medicine* 329(15), 1079-1082.

Larsson, R., P.A. Öberg, and S.E. Larsson. 1999. Changes of trapezius muscle blood flow and electromyography in chronic neck pain due to trapezius myalgia. *Pain* 79(1), 45-50.

Larsson, S.-E., R. Larsson, Q. Zhang, H. Cai, and P.A. Öberg. 1995. Effects of psychophysiological stress on trapezius muscles blood flow and electromyography during static load. *European Journal of Applied Physiology* 71(6), 493-498.

Lasater, J. 1983. Asana triang mukhaikapada paschimottanasana. *Yoga Journal* 52(September-October), 9-11.

Lasater, J. 1986. Supta virasana: Reclining hero pose. *Yoga Journal* 67(March-April), 23-24.

Lasater, J. 1988a. Janu Sirsasana: Head of the knee pose. *Yoga Journal* 83(November-December), 35-40.

Lasater, J. 1988b. Uttanasana intense stretch pose. *Yoga Journal* 79(March-April), 30-35.

Laskowski, E.R. 1994. Rehabilitation of the physically challenged athlete. *Sports Medicine* 5(1), 215-233.

Laubach, L.C., and J.T. McConville. 1966a. Muscle strength, flexibility, and bone size of adult males. *Research Quarterly* 37(3), 384-392.

Laubach, L.C., and J.T. McConville. 1966b. Relationship between flexibility, anthropometry, and somatotype of college men. *Research Quarterly* 37(2), 241-251.

Laughlin, K. 2002a. *Thinking about posture*. [Online]. Available: www.posture-and-flexibility.com.au/pages/thinkingaboutstr.html [October 31, 2003].

Laughlin, K. 2002b. *Stretching is a waste of time*. [Online]. Available: www.posture-and-flexibility.com.au/pages/stretchingisawas.html [October 31, 2003].

Lavender, S.A., G.A. Mirka, R.W. Schoenmarklin, C.M. Sommerich, L.R. Sudhakar, and W.S. Marras. 1989. The effects of preview and task symmetry on trunk muscle response to sudden loading. *Human Factors* 31(1), 101-115.

Lawton, R.W. 1957. Some aspects of research in biological elasticity. In *Tissue elasticity*, ed. J.W. Remington, 1-11. Washington DC: American Physiological Society.

Laxton, A.H. 1990. Practical approaches to the normalization of muscle tension. *Journal of Manual Medicine* 5(3), 115-120.

Leard, J.S. 1984. Flexibility and conditioning in the young athlete. In *Pediatric and adolescent sports medicine*, ed. L.J. Micheli, 194-210. Boston: Little, Brown.

Leardini, A., J.J. O'Connor, F. Catani, and S. Giannini. 2000. The role of the passive structures in the mobility and stability of the human ankle joint: A literature review. *Foot & Ankle International* 21(7), 602-615.

Leboeuf, C., R.A. Ames, C.W. Budich, and A.F. Vincent. 1987. Changes in blood pressure and pulse rate following exercise in the inverted position. *Journal of the Australian Chiropractic Association* 17(2), 60-62.

Lebrun, C.M. 1993. Effects of the different phases of the menstrual cycle and oral contraceptives on athletic performance. *Sports Medicine* 16(6), 400-430.

Lederman, E. 1997. *Fundamentals of manual therapy*. New York: Churchill Livingstone.

Lee, D. 1989. *The pelvic girdle*. Edinburgh: Churchill Livingstone.

Lee, E.J., B.R. Etnyre, B.W. Poindexter, D.B. Sokol, and T.J. Toon. 1989. Flexibility characteristics of elite female and male volleyball players. *Journal of Sports Medicine and Physical Fitness* 29(1), 49-51.

Lee, G.C. 1980. Finite element analysis in soft tissue mechanics. In *Vol. 1. International conference on finite elements in biomechanics*, ed. B.R. Simon, 27-37. Tucson, AZ: National Science Foundation and the University of Arizona College of Engineering.

Lee, J. and G.W. Schmid-Schönbein. 1995. Biomechanics of skeletal muscle capillaries: Hemodynamic resistance, endothelial distensibility, and pseudoformation. *Annals of Biomedical Engineering* 23, 226-246.

Lee, M., J. Gal, and W. Herzog. 2000. Biomechanics of manual therapy. In *Clinical biomechanics*, ed. by Z. Dvir, 209-238. New York: Churchill Livingstone.

Lee, M.A., and N. Kleitman. 1923. Studies on the physiology of sleep. II. Attempts to demonstrate functional changes in the nervous system during experimental insomnia. *American Journal of Physiology* 67(1), 141-152.

Lee, R.Y.W., and J. Munn. 2000. Passive moment about the hip in straight leg raising. *Clinical Biomechanics* 15(5), 330-334.

Lehmann, J.F., A.J. Masock, C.G., Warren, and J.N. Koblanski. 1970. Effect of therapeutic temperature on tendon extensibility. *Archives of Physical Medicine and Rehabilitation* 51(8), 481-487.

Lehmann, J.F., D.R. Silverman, B.A. Baum, N.L. Kirk, and V.C. Johnson. 1966. Temperature distributions in the human thigh, produced by infrared, hot pack and microwave applications. *Archives of Physical Medicine and Rehabilitation* 47(5), 291-299.

Lehmann, J.P., and B.J. de Lateur. 1990. Diathermy and superficial heat, laser, and cold therapy. In *Krusen's handbook of physical medicine and rehabilitation*. 4th ed, ed. J.F. Lehmann and B.J. de Lateur, 285-367. Philadelphia: Saunders.

Lehrer, P.M., and R.L. Woolfolk. 1984. Are stress reduction techniques interchangeable, or do they have specific effects? A review of the comparative empirical literature. In *Principles and practices of stress management*, ed. R.L. Woolfolk and P.M. Lehrer. New York: Guilford Press.

Leighton, J.R. 1956. Flexibility characteristics of males ten to eighteen years of age. *Archives of Physical and Mental Rehabilitation* 37(8), 494-499.

Le Marr, J.D., I.A. Golding, and J.G. Adler. 1984. Intraocular pressure responses to inversion. *American Journal of Optometry and Physiological Optics* 61(11), 679-682.

Lentell, G., T. Hetherington, J. Eagan, and M. Morgan. 1992. The use of thermal agents to influence the effectiveness of a low-load prolonged stretch. *Journal of Orthopaedic and Sports Physical Therapy* 16(5), 200-207.

Leonard, T.J.K., M.G. Muir, G.R. Kirkby, and R.A. Hitchings. 1983. Ocular hypertension and posture. *British Journal of Ophthalmology* 67(6), 362-366.

Lepique, G., and G. Sell. 1962. Der Gelenk binnendruck im normalen und geshadigten Gelenk [Internal pressure in the normal and pathological joint]. *Zeitschrift Orthopaedie und Ihre Grenzgebiete* 96(July), 235-238.

Lerda, R., and C. Cardelli. 2003. Breathing and propelling in crawl as a function of skill and swim velocity. *International Journal of Sports Medicine* 24(1), 75-81.

Levin, R.M., and S.L. Wolf. 1987. Preliminary analysis on conditioning of exaggerated triceps surae stretch reflexes among stroke patients. *Biofeedback and Self-Regulation* 12(2), 153.

Levine, M., J. Lombardo, J. McNeeley, and T. Anderson, T. 1987. An analysis of individual stretching programs of intercollegiate athletes. *The Physician and Sportsmedicine* 15(3), 130-136.

Levine, M.G., and H. Kabat. 1952. Cocontraction and reciprocal innervation in voluntary movement in man. *Science* 116(3005), 115-118.

Levtov, V.A., N.Y. Shushtova, S.A. Regirer, N.K. Shadrina, N.A. Maltsev, and Y.I. Levkovich. 1985. Topographic and hydrodynamic heterogeneity of the terminal bed of the cat gastrocnemius muscle vessel. *Fiziologicheski Zhurnal SSR Imeni I.M. Sechenova* 71(9), 1105-1111. (In *Biological Abstracts* 81(9), AB-164, #79767.)

Lew, P.C., C.J. Morrow, and A.M. Lew. 1994. The effect of neck and leg flexion and their sequence on the lumbar spinal cord. *Spine* 19(21), 2421-2425.

Lewin, G. 1979. *Swimming*. Berlin: Sportverlag.

Lewit, K. 1999. *Manipulative therapy in rehabilitation of the locomotor system*. 3rd ed. Oxford: Buttersworth-Heinemann.

Ley, P. 1977. Psychological studies of doctor-patient communication. In *Contributions to medical psychology*. ed. S. Rachman. Oxford: Pergamon.

Ley, P. 1988. *Communicating with patient: Improving communication, satisfaction and compliance*. London: Croom Helm.

Li, B., and V. Daggett. 2002. Molecular basis for the extensibility of elastin. *Journal of Muscle Research and Cell Motility*. 23(5-6), 561-573.

Li, Y., P.W. McClure, and N. Pratt. 1996. The effect of hamstring muscle stretching on standing posture and on lumbar and hip motions during forward bending. *Physical Therapy* 76(8), 837-849.

Liberson, W.T., and M.M. Asa. 1959. Further studies of brief isometric exercises. *Archives of Physical Medicine* 40(8), 330-336.

Lichtor, J. 1972. The loose-jointed young athlete. *American Journal of Sports Medicine* 1(1), 22-23.

Lieber, R.L. 2002. *Skeletal muscle: Structure, function, & plasticity*. 2nd ed. Philadelphia: Lippincott Williams & Wilkins.

Lieber, R.L., and J. Fridén. 1993. Muscle damage is not a function of muscle force but active muscle strain. *Journal of Applied Physiology* 74(2), 520-526.

Liemohn, W. 1978. Factors related to hamstring strains. *Journal of Sports Medicine and Physical Fitness* 18(1), 71-75.

Liemohn, W. 1988. Flexibility and muscular strength. *Journal of Physical Education, Recreation and Dance* 59(7), 37-40.

Liemohn, W., G.L. Sharpe, and J.F. Wasserman. 1994. Criterion related validity of the sit-and-reach test. *Journal of Strength and Conditioning Research* 8(2), 91-94.

Light, K.E., S. Nuzik, W. Personius, and A. Barstrom. 1984. A low-loading prolonged stretch vs. high-low brief stretch in treating knee contractures. *Physical Therapy* 64(3), 330-333.

Lin, D.C., and W.Z. Rymer. 1993. Mechanical properties of cat soleus muscle elicited by sequential ramp stretches: Implications for control of muscle. *Journal of Neurophysiology* 70(3), 997-1008.

Lindesmith, A.R. 1968. Punishment. In *International encyclopedia of the social sciences* Vol. 13, ed. D.L. Sills, 217-222. New York: Macmillan Company and the Free Press.

Lindner, E. 1971. The phenomenon of the freedom of lateral deviation in throwing (Wurfseitenfreiheit). In *Medicine and sport: Vol. 6. Biomechanics II*, ed. J. Vredenbregt and J. Wartenwiller, 240-245. Basel: Karger.

Lindsay, D., and J. Horton. 2002. Comparison of spine motion in elite golfers with and without low back pain. *Journal of Sports Sciences* 20(8), 599-605.

Lineker, S., E. Badley, C. Charles, L. Hart, and D. Streiner. 1999. Defining morning stiffness in rheumatoid arthritis. *Journal of Rheumatology* 26(5), 1052-1057.

Linke, W.A., M. Kulke, H. Li, S. Fujita-Becker, C. Neagoe, D.J. Manstein, M. Gautel, and J.M. Fernandez. 2002. PEVK domain of titin: An entropic spring with actin-binding properties. *Journal of Structual Biology* 137(1-2), 194-205.

Linz, J.C., S.F. Conti, and D.A. Stone. 2001. Foot and ankle injuries. In *Sports injuries, mechanisms, prevention, treatment*. 2nd ed, ed. F.H. Fu and D.A. Stone, 1135-1163. Philadelphia: Lippincott Williams & Wilkins.

Litchfield, R., C. Hawkins, C. Dillman, G. Hagerman, and J.W. Atkins. 1995. Rehabilitation for the overhead athlete. *Sports Medicine and Arthroscopy Review* 3(1), 49-59.

Liu, J.X., P.O. Eriksson, L.E. Thornell, and F. Pedrosa-Domellof. 2002. Myosin heavy chain composition of muscle spindles in human biceps brachii. *Journal of Histochemistry and Cytochemistry* 50(2), 171-183.

Liu, S.H., R.A. Al-Shaikh, V. Panossian, G.A.M. Finerman, and J.M. Lane. 1997. Estrogen affects the cellular metabolism of the anterior cruciate ligament: A potential explanation for female athletic injury. *American Journal of Sports Medicine* 25(5), 704-709.

Liu, S.H., R.A. Al-Shaikh, V. Panossian, R.S. Yang, S.D. Nelson, N. Soleiman, G.A.M. Finerman, and J.M. Lane. 1996. Preliminary immunolocalization of estrogen and progesterone target cells in the human anterior cruciate ligament. *Journal of Orthopaedic Research* 14(4), 526-533.

Liu, W., S. Siegler, and L. Techner, L. 2001. Quantitative measurement of ankle passive flexibility using an arthrometer on sprained ankles. *Clinical Biomechanics* 16(3), 237-244.

Liversage, A.D., D. Holmes, P.J. Knight, L. Tskhovrebova, and J. Trinick. 2001. Titin and sarcomere symmetry paradox. *Journal of Molecular Biology* 305(3), 401-409.

Locke, J.C. 1983. Stretching away from back pain injury. *Occupational Health and Science* 52(7), 8-13.

Logan, G.A., and G.H. Egstrom. 1961. Effects of slow and fast stretching on the sacro-femoral angle. *Journal Association for Physical and Mental Rehabilitation* 15(3), 85-89.

Long, P.A. 1971. *The effects of static, dynamic, and combined stretching exercise programs on hip joint flexibility*. Master's thesis, University of Maryland.

Longworth, J.C. 1982. Psychophysiological effects of slow stroke back massage on normotensive females. *Advances in Nursing Science* 4(4), 44-61.

Loughna, P.T., and M.J. Morgan. 1999. Passive stretch modulates denervation induced alterations in skeletal muscle myosin heavy chain mRNA levels. *Pflügers Archiv: European Journal of Physiology* 439(1-2), 52-55.

Louttit, C.M., and J.F. Halford. 1930. The relationship between chest girth and vital capacity. *Research Quarterly* 1(4), 34-35.

Louis, M. n.d. *Contortionists*. West Germany: Europa Verlag.

Low, F.N. 1961a. The extracellular portion of the human blood-air barrier and its relation to tissue space. *Anatomical Record* 139(2), 105-122.

Low, F.N. 1961b. Microfibrils, a small extracellular component of connective tissue. *Anatomical Record* 139(2), 250.

Low, F.N. 1962. Microfibrils, fine filamentous components of the tissue space. *Anatomical Record* 142(2), 131-137.

Lowe, D.A., and S.E. Always. 2002. Animal models for inducing muscle hypertrophy: Are they relevant for clinical applications in humans? *Journal of Orthopaedic and Sports Physical Therapy* 32(2), 36-43.

Lubell, A. 1989. Potentially dangerous exercises: Are they harmful to all? *The Physician and Sportsmedicine* 17(1), 187-192.

Luby, S., and R.A. St. Onge. 1986. *Bodysense*. Winchester, MA: Faber and Faber.

Lucas, G.L., F.W. Cooke, and E.A. Friis. 1999. *A primer on biomechanics*. New York: Springer Verlag.

Lucas, R.C., and R. Koslow. 1984. Comparative study of static, dynamic, and proprioceptive neuromuscular facilitation stretching techniques on flexibility. *Perceptual and Motor Skills* 58(2), 615-618.

Lund, H., P. Vestergaard-Poulsen, I.-L.Kanstrup, and P. Sejrsen. 1998. The effect of passive stretching on delayed onset muscle soreness, and other detrimental effects following eccentric exercise. *Scandinavian Journal of Medicine & Science in Sports* 8(4), 216-221.

Lund, J.P., R. Donga, C.G. Widmer, and C.S. Stohler, C.S. 1991. The pain-adaptation model: A discussion of the relationship between chronic musculoskeletal pain and motor activity. *Canadian Journal of Physiological Pharmacology* 69(5), 683-694.

Lundberg, G., and B. Gerdle. 2000. Correlations between joint and spinal mobility, spinal sagittal configuration, segmental mobility, segmental pain, symptoms and disabilities in female homecare personnel. *Scandinavian Journal of Rehabilitation Medicine* 32(3), 124-133.

Lundberg, U., R. Kadefors, B. Melin, G. Palmerud, N.P. Hassmè, M. Engström, and I. Elfsberg. 1994. Psychophysiological stress and EMG activity of the trapezius muscle. *International Journal of Behavioral Medicine* 1, 354-370.

Lundborg, G. 1975. Structure and function of the intraneural microvessels as related to trauma, edema formation and nerve function. *Journal of Bone and Joint Surgery* 57A(7), 938-948.

Lundborg, G., and B. Rydevik. 1973. Effects of stretching the tibial nerve of the rabbit. *Journal of Bone and Joint Surgery* 55B(2), 390-401.

Lunde, B.K., W.D. Brewer, and P.A.Garcia. 1972. Grip strength of college women. *Archives of Physical Medicine and Rehabilitation* 53(10), 491-493.

Lung, W.W., H.D. Hartsell, and A.A. Vandervoort. 1996. Effects of aging on joint stiffnes: Implications for exercise. *Physiotherapy Canada* 48(2), 96-106.

Lustig, S.A., T.E. Ball, and M. Looney. 1992. A comparison of two proprioceptive neuromuscular facilitation techniques for improving range of motion and muscular strength. *Isokinetics and Exercise Science* 2(4), 154-159.

Luthe, W. 1969. *Psychosomatic medicine.* New York: Harper & Row.

Lysens, R.J., W. deWeerdt, and A. Nieuwboer. 1991. Factors associated with injury proneness. *Sports Medicine* 12(5), 281-289.

Lysens, R.J., J. Lefevre, M.S. Ostyn, and L. Renson. 1984. Study of the evaluation of joint flexibility as a risk factor in sports injuries. The CIBA-GEIGY Award of the Belgium Society of Sports Medicine and Sports Science, Leuven: University Press.

Lysens, R.J., M.S. Ostyn, Y.V. Auweele, J. Lefevre, M. Vuylsteke, and L. Renson. 1989. The accident-prone and overuse-prone profiles of the young athlete. *American Journal of Sports Medicine* 17(5), 612-619.

MacAuley, D. 2001. Do textbooks agree on their advice on ice? *Clinical Journal of Sports Medicine* 11(2), 67-72.

MacDonald, J. 1985. Falls in the elderly: The role of drugs in the elderly. *Clinical Geriatric Medicine* 1(3), 621-636.

MacDonald, J.B., and E.T. MacDonald. 1977. Nocturnal femoral fracture and continuing widespread use of barbiturate hypnotics. *British Medical Journal* 2(6085), 483-485.

MacFadden, G. 1912. *MacFaddens' encyclopedia of physical culture.* New York: Physical Culture Publishing.

Macera, C.A., R.P. Pate, K.E. Powell, K.L. Jackson, J.S. Kendrick, and T.E. Craven. 1989. Predicting lower-extremity injuries among habitual runners. *Archives of Internal Medicine* 149(11), 2565-2568.

Macintosh, J.E., N. Bogduk, and M.J. Pearcy. 1993. The effects of flexion on the geometry and actions of the lumbar erector spinae. *Spine* 18(7), 884-893.

Maclennan, S.E., G.A. Silvestri, J. Ward, and D.A. Mahler. 1994. Does entrainment breathing improve the economy of rowing? *Medicine and Science in Sport and Exercise* 26(5), 610-614.

Maddalozzo, G.F.J. 1987. An anatomical and biomechanical analysis of the full golf swing. *NSCA Journal* 9(4), 6-8, 77-79.

Madding, S.W., J.G. Wong, A. Hallum, and J.M. Medeiros. 1987. Effects of duration of passive stretch on hip abduction range of motion. *Journal of Orthopaedic Sports Physical Therapy* 8(8), 409-416.

Magder, R., M.L. Baxter, and Y.B Kassam. 1986. Does a diuretic improve morning stiffness in rheumatoid arthritis? *British Journal of Rheumatology* 25(3), 318-319.

Magee, D.J. 2002. *Orthopaedic physical assessment.* 4th ed. Philadelphia: Saunders.

Magid, A., H.P. Ting-Beall, M. Carvell, T. Kontis, and C. Lucaveche. 1984. Connecting filaments, core filaments, and side struts: A proposal to add three new load bearing structures to the sliding filament model. In *Contractile mechanisms in muscle,* ed. G.H. Pollack and H. Sugi, 307-323. New York: Plenum.

Magnusson, M., and M.H. Pope. 1996. Body height changes with hyperextension. *Clinical Biomechanics* 11(4), 236-238.

Magnusson, M., M.H. Pope, and T. Hansson. 1995. Does hyperextension have an unloading effect on the intervertebral disc? *Scandinavian Journal of Rehabilitation and Medicine* 27(1), 5-9.

Magnusson, S.P. 1998. Passive properties of human skeletal muscle during stretch maneuvers: A review. *Scandinavian Journal of Medicine & Science in Sports* 8(2), 65-77.

Magnusson, S.P., P. Aagaard, and J.J. Nielson. 2000. Passive energy return after repeated stretches of the hamstring muscle-tendon unit. *Medicine and Science in Sports and Exercise* 32(6), 1160-1164.

Magnusson, S.P., P. Aagaard, E.B. Simonsen, and F. Bojsen-Møller. 2000. Passive tensile stress and energy of the human hamstring muscles in vivo. *Scandinavian Journal of Medicine & Science in Sports* 10(6), 323-328.

Magnusson, S.P., G.W. Gleim, and J.A. Nicholas. 1994. Shoulder weakness in professional baseball pitchers. *Medicine and Science in Sports and Exercise* 26(1), 5-9.

Magnusson, S.P., C. Julsgaard, P. Aagaard, C. Zacharie, S. Ullman, T. Kobayasi, and M. Kjær. 2001. Viscoelastic properties and flexibility of the human muscle-tendon unit in benign joint hypermobility syndrome. *Journal of Rheumatology* 28(12), 2720-2725.

Magnusson, S.P., E.B. Simonsen, P. Aagaard, J. Boesen, F. Johannsen, and M. Kjær. 1997. Determinants of musculoskeletal flexibility: Viscoelastic properties, cross-sectional area, EMG and stretch tolerance. *Scandinavian Journal of Medicine and Science in Sports* 7(4), 195-202.

Magnusson, S.P., E.B. Simonsen, P. Aagaard, J. Boesen, C. Julsgaard, and M. Kjær. 2001. Determinants of musculoskeletal flexibility: Viscoelastic properties, cross-sectional area, EMG and stretch tolerance. *Scandinavian Journal Medical Science Sport* 7(4), 195-202.

Magnusson, S.P., E.B. Simonsen, P. Aagaard, P. Dyhre-Poulsen, M.P. McHugh, and M. Kjær. 1996a. Mechanical and physiological responses to stretching with and without preisometric contraction in human skeletal muscle. *Archives of Physical Medicine and Rehabilitation* 77(4), 373-378.

Magnusson, S.P., E.B. Simonsen, P. Aagaard, G.W. Gleim, M.P. McHugh, and M. Kjær. 1995. Viscoelastic response to repeated static stretching in the human hamstring muscle. *Scandinavian Journal of Medicine and Science in Sports* 5(6), 342-347.

Magnusson, S.P., E.B. Simonsen, P. Aagaard, and M. Kjær. 1996b. Biomechanical responses to repeated stretches in human hamstring muscle in vivo. *American Journal of Sports Medicine* 24(5), 622-628.

Magnusson, S.P., E.B. Simonsen, P. Aagaard, H. Sørensen, and M. Kjær. 1996c. A mechanism for altered flexibility in human skeletal muscle. *Journal of Physiology* 497(1), 291-298.

Maher, C. 1995. Perception of stiffness in manipulative physiotherapy. *Physiotherapy Theory and Practice* 11(1), 35-44.

Magnusson, S.P., E.B. Simonsen, P. Dyhre-Poulsen, P. Aagaard, T. Mohr, and M. Kjær. 1996d. Viscoelastic stress relation during static stretch in human skeletal muscle in the absence of EMG activity. *Scandinavian Journal of Medicine and Science in Sports* 6(6), 323-328.

Mahler, D.A., B. Hunter, T. Lentine, and J. Ward. 1991. Locomotor-respiratory coupling develops in novice female rowers with training. *Medicine and Science in Sports and Exercise* 23(12), 1362-1366.

Mair, S.D., A.V. Seaber, R.R. Glisson, and W.E. Garrett. 1996. The role of fatigue in susceptibility to acute muscle strain injury. *American Journal of Sports Medicine* 24(2), 137-143.

Maitland, G.D. 2001. *Maitland's vertebral manipulation* 6th ed. Oxford: Butterworth Heinemann.

Malina, R.M. 1988. Physical anthropology. In *Anthropometric standardization reference manual,* ed. T.G. Lohman, A.F. Roche, and R. Martorell, 99-102. Champaign, IL: Human Kinetics.

Mallac, C. 2003. Two sports physiotherapists show why flexibility is so important, and explain the science behind it. *Peak Performance.* Available: www.pponline.co.uk/ency/0833.htm [October 31, 2003].

Mallik, A.K., W.R. Ferrell, A.G. McDonald, and R.D.Sturrock. 1994. Impaired proprioceptive acuity at the proximal interphalangeal joint in patients with the hypermobility syndrome. *British Journal of Rheumatology* 33(7), 631-637.

Malm, C. 2001. Exercise-induced muscle damage and inflammation: Fact or fiction? *Acta Physiologica Scandinavica* 171(3), 233-239.

Maltz, M. 1970. *Psycho-Cybernetics.* New York: Simon and Schuster.

Manheim, C.J. 2001. *The myofascial release manual.* 3rd ed. Thorofare, NJ: Slack.

Manheim, C.J., and D.K. Lavett. 1989. *The myofascial release manual.* Thorofare, NJ: Slack.

Mann, R.A., D.E. Baxter, and L.D. Lutter. 1981. Running symposium. *Foot and Ankle* 1(4), 190-224.

Mantel, G. 1995. *Cello technique: Principles and forms of movement.* Translated by B.H. Thiem. Bloomington, IN: Indiana University Press.

Mao, J-R., and J. Bristow. 2001. The Ehlers-Danlos syndrome: On beyond collagens. *Journal of Clinical Investigation* 107(9), 1063-1069.

Marino, M. 1984. Profiling swimmers. *Clinics in Sports Medicine* 3(1), 211-229.

Markee, J.E., J.T. Logue, M. Williams, W.B. Stanton, R.N. Wrenn, and L.B. Walker. 1955. Two-joint muscles of the thigh. *Journal of Bone and Joint Surgery* 37A(1), 125-145.

Marras, W.S., S.L. Rangarajulu, and S.A. Lavender. 1987. Trunk loading and expectation. *Ergonomics* 30(3), 551-562.

Marras, W.S., and P.E. Wongsam. 1986. Flexibility and velocity of the normal and impaired lumbar spine. *Archives of Physical Medicine and Rehabilitation* 67(4), 213-217.

Marshall, J.L., N. Johanson, T.L. Wickiewicz, H.M. Tischler, B.L. Koslin, S. Zeno, and A. Meyers. 1980. Joint looseness: A function of the person and the joint. *Medicine and Science in Sports and Exercise* 12(3), 189-194.

Martin, D.E., and P.N. Coe. 1997. *Better training for distance runners*. 2nd ed. Champaign, IL: Human Kinetics.

Martin, P.E., and D.W. Morgan. 1992. Biomechanical considerations for economical walking and running. *Medicine and Science in Sports and Exercise* 24(4), 467-474.

Martin, R.B., D.B. Burr, and N.A. Sharkey. 1998. *Skeletal tissue mechanics*. New York: Springer.

Martin, R.M. 1982. *The gravity guiding system*. Pasadena, CA: Gravity Guidance.

Martín-Santos, R., A. Bulbena, M. Porta, J. Gago, L. Molina, and J.C. Duró. 1998. Association between joint hypermobility syndrome and panic disorder. *American Journal of Psychiatry* 155(11), 1578-1583.

Maruyana, K., S. Kimura, H. Yoshidomi, H. Sawada, and M. Kikuchi. 1984. Molecular size and shape of B-connectin, an elastic protein of muscle. *Journal of Biochemistry* (Tokyo) 95(5), 1423-1433.

Marvey, D. 1887. Recherces experimentales sur la morphologie de muscles [Experimental research on the morphology of muscles]. *Comptes Rendus Hebdomadaires du Seances de l'Academie des Sciences* (Paris) 105, 446-451.

Marx, R.G., J.W. Sperling, and F.A. Cordasco. 2001. Overuse injuries of the upper extremity in tennis players. *Clinics in Sports Medicine* 20(3), 439-451.

Mason, T., and B.J. Rigby. 1963. Thermal transition in collagen. *Biochemica et Biophysica Acta* 79(PN1254), 448-450.

Massey, B.A., and N.L. Chaudet. 1956. Effects of systematic, heavy resistance exercise on range of joint movement in young adults. *Research Quarterly* 27(1), 41-51.

Massie, W.K., and M.B. Howarth. 1951. Congenital dislocation of the hip. *Journal of Bone and Joint Surgery* 33A, 171-198.

Matchanov, A.T., V.A. Levtov, and V.V. Orlov. 1983. Changes of the blood flow in longitudinal stretch of the cat gastrocnemius muscle. *Fiziologicheskii Zhurnal SSSR Imeni I.M. Sechenova* 69(1), 74-83. (In *Biological Abstracts* 77(9), p. 7196 #65430, May 1984.)

Matchanov, A.T.N., N.Y. Shustova, V.N. Shuvaeva, L.I. Vasil'eva, and V.A. Levtov. 1983. Effects of stretch of the cat gastrocnemius muscle on its tetani, postcontraction hyperemia and parameters of energy metabolism. *Fiziologicheskii Zhurnal SSSR Imeni I.M. Sechenova* 69(2), 210-219. (In *Biological Abstracts* 77(6), p. 4883, #44673, March 1984.)

Mathews, D.K., V. Shaw, and M. Bohnen. 1957. Hip flexibility of college women as related to body segments. *Research Quarterly* 28(4), 352-356.

Mathews, D.K., V. Shaw, and J.W. Woods. 1959. Hip flexibility of elementary school boys as related to body segments. *Research Quarterly* 31(3), 297-302.

Mathews, D.K., R.W. Stacy, and G.N. Hoover. 1964. *Physiology of muscular activity and exercise*. New York: Ronald Press.

Mathieu-Costello, O. 1987. Capillary tortuosity and degree of contraction or extension of skeletal muscles. *Microvascular Research* 33(1), 98-117.

Mathieu-Costello, O., C.G. Ellis, R.F. Potter, I.C. Macdonald, and A.C. Groom. 1991. Muscle capillary-to-fiber perimeter ratio: Morphometry. *American Journal of Physiology* 261 (Heart Circulation Physiology 30), H1617-H1625.

Mathieu-Costello, O., H. Hoppeler, and E. Weibel. 1989. Capillary tortuosity in skeletal muscles of mammals depends on muscle contraction. *Journal of Applied Physiology* 66(5), 1436-1442.

Matsumura, K., T. Shimizu, I. Nonaka, and T. Mannen. 1989. Immunochemical study of connectin (titin) in neuromuscular diseases using a monoclonal antibody: Connectin is degraded extensively in Duchenne muscular dystrophy. *Journal of the Neurological Sciences* 93(2-3), 147-156.

Mattes, A.L. 1990. *Flexibility active and assisted stretching*. Sarasota, FL: Author.

Matveyev, L. 1981. *Fundamentals of sports training*. Moscow: Progress.

Matvienko, L.A., and M.V. Kartasheva. 1990. Treating calf-muscle cramps with a simple physical exercise. *Soviet Sport Review* 25(4), 162-163.

Maud, P.J., and M.Y. Cortez-Cooper. 1995. Static techniques for the evaluation of joint range of motion. In *Physiological assessment of human fitness*, ed. P.J. Maud and C. Foster, 221-243. Champaign, IL: Human Kinetics.

May, B.J. 1990. Principles of exercise for the elderly. In *Therapeutic exercise*. 5th ed, ed. J.V. Basmajian and S.L. Wolf, 279-298. Baltimore: Williams & Wilkins.

Mayer, T.G., R.J. Gatchel, N. Kishino, N. Keeley, P. Capra, H. Mayer, J. Barnett, and V. Mooney. 1985. Objective assessment of spine function following industrial injury. A prospective study with comparison group and one-year follow-up. *Spine* 10(6), 482-493.

Mayer, T.G., R.J. Gatchel, H. Mayer, N.D. Kishino, and J. Keeley. 1987. A prospective two-year study of functional restoration in industrial low back injury. An objective assessment procedure. *Journal of the American Medical Association* 258(13), 1763-1767.

Mayer, T.G., J. Tabor, E. Bovasso, and R.J. Gatchel. 1994. Physical progress and impairment quantification after functional restoration. Part I: Lumbar mobility. *Spine* 19(4), 389-394.

Mayer, T.G., A.F. Tencer, S. Kristoferson, and V. Mooney. 1984. Use of noninvasive techniques for quantification of spinal range-of-motion in normal subjects and chronic low-back dysfunction patients. *Spine* 9(6), 588-595.

Mayhew, T.P., B.J. Norton, and S.A. Sahrmann. 1983. Electromyographic study of the relationship between hamstring and abdominal muscles during unilateral straight leg raise. *Physical Therapy* 63(11), 1769-1773.

McAtee, R.E., and J. Charland. 1999. *Facilitated stretching*. 2nd ed. Champaign, IL: Human Kinetics.

McBride, J.M., T. Triplett-McBride, A.J. Davie, P.J. Abernethy, and R.U. Newton. 2003. Characteristics of titin in strength and power athletes. *European Journal of Applied Physiology* 88(6), 553-557.

McCarroll, J.R. 1986. Golf: Common injuries from a supposedly benign activity. *Journal of Musculoskeletal Medicine* 13(5), 9-16.

McCarroll, J.R., A.C. Rettig, and K.D. Shelbourne. 1982. Injuries in the amateur golfer. *The Physician and Sportsmedicine* 18(3), 122-126, 1990.

McComas, A.J. 1996. *Skeletal muscle*. Champaign, IL: Human Kinetics.

McCue, B.F. 1963. Flexibility measurements of college women. *Research Quarterly* 24(3), 316-324.

McCully, K.K., and J.A. Faulkner. 1985. Injury to skeletal muscle fibers of mice following lengthening contractions. *Journal of Applied Physiology* 59(1), 119-126.

McCully, K.K., and J.A. Faulkner. 1986. Characteristics of lengthening contractions associated with injury to skeletal muscle fibers. *Journal of Applied Physiology* 61(1), 293-299.

McCune, D.A., and R.B. Sprague. 1990. Exercise for low back pain. In *Therapeutic exercise*. 5th ed, ed. J.V. Basmajian and S.L. Wolf, 299-320. Baltimore: Williams & Wilkins.

McCutcheon, L.J., S.K. Byrd, and D.R. Hodgson. 1992. Ultrastructural changes in skeletal muscle after fatiguing exercise. *Journal of Applied Physiology* 72(3), 1111-1117.

McDonagh, M.J.N., and C.T.M. Davies. 1984. Adaptive response of mammalian skeletal muscle to exercise with high loads. *European Journal of Applied Physiology* 52(2), 139-155.

McDonagh, M.J.N., C.M. Hayward, and C.T.M. Davies. 1983. Isometric training in human elbow flexor muscles: The effects on voluntary and electrically evoked forces. *Journal of Bone and Joint Surgery* 65B(3), 355-358.

McDonough, A.L. 1981. Effects of immobilization and exercise on articular cartilage—A review of the literature. *The Journal of Orthopaedic and Sports Physical Therapy* 3(1), 2-5.

McEwen, B.S. 1980. The brain as a target organ of endocrine hormones. In *Neuroendocrinology*, eds. D.T. Krieger and J.C. Hughes, 33-42. Sunderlund, MA: Sinauer Associates.

McFarlane, A.C., R.S. Kalucy, and P.M. Brooks. 1987. Psychological predictor of disease course in rheumatoid arthritis. *Journal of Psychosomatic Research* 31(6), 757-764.

McFarlane, B. 1987. A look inside the biomechanics and dynamics of speed. *NSCA Journal* 9(5), 35-41.

McGee, S.R. 1990. Muscle cramps. *Archives of Internal Medicine* 150(3), 511-518.

McGill, S.M. 1997. The biomechanics of low back injury: Implications on current practice in industry and the clinic. *Journal of Biomechanics* 30(5), 465-475.

McGill, S.M. 1998. Low back exercises: Evidence for improving exercise regimens. *Physical Therapy* 78(7), 755-765.

McGill, S.M. 1999. Stability: From biomechanical concept to chiropractic practice. *Journal of the Canadian Chiropractic Association* 43(2), 75-88.

McGill, S.M., and S. Brown. 1992. Creep response of the lumbar spine to prolonged full flexion. *Clinical Biomechanics* 7(1), 43-46.

McGill, S.M., and V. Kippers. 1994. Transfer of loads between lumbar tissues during the flexion-relaxation phenomenon. *Spine* 19(9), 2190-2196.

McGlynn, G.H., and N. Laughlin. 1980. The effect of biofeedback and static stretching on muscle pain. *Athletic Training* 15(1), 42-45.

McGlynn, G.H., N.T. Laughlin, and S.P. Filios. 1979a. The effect of electromyographic feedback on EMG activity and pain in the quadriceps muscle group. *The Journal of Sports Medicine and Physical Fitness* 19(3), 237-244.

McGlynn, G.H., N.T. Laughlin, and V. Rowe. 1979b. Effect of electromyographic feedback and static stretching on artificially induced muscle soreness. *American Journal of Physical Medicine* 58(3), 139-148.

McGonigle, T., and K.W. Matley. 1994. Soft tissue treatment and muscle stretching. *Journal of Manual & Manipulative Therapy* 2(2), 55-62.

McGorry, R.W., S.M. Hsiang, F.A. Fathallah, and E.A. Clancy. 2001. Timing of activation of the erector spinae and hamstrings during a trunk flexion and extension task. *Spine* 26(4), 418-425.

McHugh, M.P., D.A. Connolly, R.G. Eston, I.J. Kremenic, S.J. Nicholas, and G.W. Gleim. 1999. The role of passive muscle stiffness in symptoms of exercise-induced muscle damage. *American Journal of Sports Medicine* 27(5), 594-599.

McHugh, M.P., I.J. Kremenic, M.B. Fox, and G.W. Gleim. 1996. The relationship of linear stiffness of human muscle to maximum joint range of motion. *Medicine and Science in Sports and Exercise* 28(5 Suppl.), S77.

McHugh, M.P., I.J. Kremenic, M.B. Fox, and G.W. Gleim. 1998. The role of mechanical and neural restraints to joint range of motion during passive stretch. *Medicine and Science in Sports and Exercise* 30(6), 928-932.

McHugh, M.P., S.P. Magnusson, G.W. Gleim, and J.A. Nicholas. 1992. Viscoelastic stress relaxation in human skeletal muscle. *Medicine and Science in Sports and Exercise* 24(12), 1375-1382.

McKenzie, R. 1981. *Mechanical diagnosis and treatment of the lumbar spine*. New Zealand: Spinal.

McKenzie, R. 1983. *Treat your own neck*. New Zealand: Spinal.

McKusick, V.A. 1956. *Heritable disorders of connective tissue*. St. Louis: Mosby.

McLaughlin, P.A., and R.J. Best. 1994. Three-dimensional kinematic analysis of the golf swing. In *Science and Golf II: Proceedings of the World Scientific Congress of Golf*, ed. A.J. Cochran and M.R. Farrally, 91-96. London: E & FN Spon.

McMaster, W. 1986. Painful shoulder in swimmers: A diagnostic challenge. *The Physician and Sportsmedicine* 14(12), 108-122.

McMaster, W.C., J.P. Troup, and S. Arredondo. 1989. The incidence of shoulder problems in developing elite swimmers. *Journal of Swimming Research* 5(1), 11-16.

McNair, P.J., and S.N. Stanley. 1996. Effect of passive stretching and jogging on the series elastic muscle stiffness and range of motion of the ankle joint. *British Journal of Sports Medicine* 30(4), 313-318.

McNeal, J.R., and W.A. Sands. 2001. Static stretching reduces power production in gymnasts. *USA Gymnastics Online*. 21(10). [Online]. Available: www.usa-gymnastics.org/publications/technique/2001/10/stretching.html [May 1, 2003].

McNitt-Gray, J.L. 1991. Biomechanics related to exercise and pregnancy. In *Exercise in pregnancy*. 2nd ed, ed. R. Artal, R.A. Wiswell, and B.L. Drinkwater, 133-140. Philadelphia: Williams & Wilkins.

McPoil, T.G., and T.C. McGarvey. 1995. The foot in athletics. In *Physical therapy of the foot and ankle*. 2nd ed, ed. G.C. Hunt and T.G. McPoil, 207-236. New York: Churchill Livingstone.

McTeigue, M., S.R. Lamb, R. Mottram, and F. Pirozzolo. 1994. Spine and hip motion analysis during the golf swing. In *Science and Golf II: Proceedings of the World Scientific Congress of Golf*, ed. A.J. Cochran and M.R. Farrally, 50-58. London: E & FN Spon.

Mead, N. 1994. Eating for flexibility. *Yoga Journal* 117 (July-August), 91-98.

Meal, G.M., and R.A. Scott. 1986. Analysis of the joint crack by simultaneous recording of sound and tension. *Journal of Manipulative and Physiological Therapeutics* 9(3), 189-195.

Medeiros, J.M., G.L. Smidt, L.F. Burmeister, and G.L. Soderberg. 1977. The influence of isometric exercise and passive stretch on hip joint motion. *Physical Therapy* 57(5), 518-523.

Medoff, L.E. 1999. The importance of movement education in the training of young violinists. *Medical Problems of Performing Artists* 14(4), 210-219.

Meichenbaum, D., and D.C. Turk. 1987. *Facilitating treatment adherence: A practitioner's guidebook*. New York: Plenum Press.

Mellin, G. 1985. Physical therapy for chronic low back pain: Correlations between spinal mobility and treatment outcome. *Scandinavian Journal of Rehabilitation Medicine* 17(4), 163-166.

Mellin, G. 1987. Correlations of spinal mobility with a degree of low back pain after correction for age and anthropometric factors. *Spine* 12(5), 464-468.

Mellin, G., and M. Poussa. 1992. Spinal mobility and posture in 8- to 16-year-old children. *Journal of Orthopaedic Research* 19(2), 211-216.

Mens, J.M.A., A. Vleeming, C.J. Snijders, B.W. Koes, and H.J. Stam. 2002. Validity of the active straight leg raise test for measuring disease severity in patients with posterior pelvic pain and pregnancy. *Spine* 27(2), 196-200.

Mens, J.M.A., A. Vleeming, C.J. Snijders, H.J. Stam, and A.Z. Ginai. 1999. The active straight leg raising test and mobility of the pelvic joints. *European Spine* 8(6), 468-473.

Merletti, R., F. Repossi, E. Richetta, C. Mathis, and C.R. Saracco. 1986. Size and x-ray density of normal and denervated muscles of the human legs and forearms. *International Rehabilitation Medicine* 8(2), 82-89.

Merni, F., M. Balboni, S. Bargellini, and G. Menegatti. 1981. Differences in males and females in joint movement range during growth. *Medicine and Sport* 15, 168-175.

Mersky, H., and N. Bogduk. eds. 1994. *Classification of chronic pain. Descriptions of chronic pain syndromes and definitions of pain terms*. 2nd ed. Seattle: IASP.

Metheny, E. 1952. *Body dynamics*. New York: McGraw-Hill.

Mewis, J. 1979. Thixotropy—A general review. *Journal of Non-Newtonian Fluid Mechanics* 6, 1-20.

Meyer, J.J., R.J. Berk, and A.V. Anderson. 1993. Recruitment patterns in the cervical paraspinal muscles during cervical forward flexion: Evidence of cervical flexion-relaxation. *Electromyography and Clinical Neurophysiology* 33(304), 217-223.

Meyers, E.J. 1971. Effect of selected exercise variables on ligament stability and flexibility of the knee. *Research Quarterly* 42(4), 411-422.

Michael, R.H., and L.E. Holder. 1985. The soleus syndrome. A cause of medial tibial stress (shin splints). *American Journal of Sports Medicine* 13(2), 87-94.

Michaud, T. 1990. Biomechanics of unilateral overhand throwing motion: An overview. *Chiropractic Sports Medicine* 4(1), 13-26.

Micheli, L.J. 1983a. Back injuries in dancers. *Clinics in Sports Medicine* 2(3), 473-484.

Micheli, L.J. 1983b. Overuse injuries in children's sport: The growth factor. *Orthopaedic Clinics of North America* 14(2), 337-360.

Micheli, L.J. 2000. Is adolescent growth associated with changes in flexibility? *Clinical Journal of Sports Medicine* 10(1), 76.

Michelson, L. 1987. Cognitive-behavioral assessment and treatment of agoraphobia. In *Anxiety and stress disorders*, ed. L. Michelson and L.M. Ascher, 213-279. New York: Guilford Press.

Mikawa, Y., R. Watanabe, Y., Yamano, and S. Miyake. 1988. Stress fracture of the body of pubis in a pregnant woman. *Archives of Orthopaedic and Traumatic Surgery* 107(3), 193-194.

Mikula, P.J. 1998. Health precautions for percussionists. *Percussive Notes* 36(6), 51-53.

Milberg, S., and M.S. Clark. 1988. Moods and compliance. *British Journal of Social Psychology* 27(Pt. I, March), 79-90.

Miller, E.H., H.J. Schneider, J.L. Bronson, and D. McClain. 1975. The classical ballet dancer: A new consideration in athletic injuries. *Clinical Orthopaedics and Related Research* 111(September), 181-191.

Miller, G., F. Boster, M. Roloff, and D. Seibold. 1977. Compliance-gaining message strategies: A typology and some findings concerning effects of situational differences. *Communication Monographs* 44(1), 37-51.

Miller, G., A. Wilcox, and J. Schwenkel. 1988. The protective effect of a prior bout of downhill running on delayed onset muscular soreness (DOMS). *Medicine and Science in Sports and Exercise* 20(2 Suppl.), S75.

Miller, J. 2002. Stretch or no stretch? Pros. *Strength and Conditioning Journal* 24(1), 20.

Miller, M.D., and M.D. Major. 1994. Posterior cruciate ligament injuries: History, examination, and diagnostic testing. *Sports Medicine and Arthroscopy Review* 2(2), 100-105.

Miller, W.A. 1977. Rupture of the musculotendinous juncture of the medial head of the gastrocnemius muscle. *American Journal of Sports Medicine* 5(5), 191-193.

Milne, C., V. Seefeldt, and P. Reuschlein. 1976. Relationship between grade, sex, race, and motor performance in young children. *Research Quarterly* 47(4), 726-730.

Milne, R.A., and D.R. Mierau. 1979. Hamstring distensibility in the general population: Relationship to pelvic and low back stresses. *Journal of Manipulative and Physiological Therapeutics* 2(1), 146-150.

Milne, R.A., D.R. Mierau, and J.D. Cassidy. 1981. Evaluation of sacroiliac joint movement and its relationship to hamstring distensibility (Abstract). *International Review of Chiropractic* 35(2), 40.

Milner-Brown, H.S., R.B. Stein, and R.G. Lee. 1975. Synchronization of human motor units: Possible roles of exercise and supraspinal reflexes. *Electroencephalography and Clinical Neurophysiology* 38(3), 245-254.

Minton, J. 1993. A comparison of thermotherapy and cryotherapy in enhancing supine extended-leg, hip flexion. *Journal of Athletic Training* 28(2), 172-176.

Mironov, V.M. 1969a. Correlation of breathing and movement in male gymnasts during execution of routines on the apparatus. *Theory and Practice of Physical Culture* 7, 23-26. (In *Yessis Review* 5(1), 14-19, 1970.)

Mironov, V.M. 1969b. The relationship between breathing and movement in masters of sport in gymnastics. *Theory and Practice of Physical Culture* 7, 14-16. (In *Yessis Review* 4(2), 35-40, 1969.)

Mishra, M.B., P. Ryan, P. Atkinson, H. Taylor, J. Bell, D. Calver, I. Fogelman, A. Child, G. Jackson, J.B. Chambers, and R. Grahame. 1996. Extra-articular features of benign joint hypermobility syndrome. *British Journal of Rheumatology* 35(9), 861-866.

Misner, J.E., B.H. Massey, M.G. Bemben, S.B. Going, and J. Patrick. 1992. Long-term effects of exercise on the range of motion of aging women. *Journal of Orthopaedic and Sports Physical Therapy* 16(1), 37-42.

Mitchell, F.L., and N. A. Pruzzo. 1971. Investigation of voluntary and primary respiratory mechanisms. *Journal of the American Osteopathic Association* 70(June), 149-153.

Mittelmark, R.A., R.A. Wiswell, B.L. Drinkwater, and W.E. St. Jones-Repovich. 1991. Exercise guidelines for pregnancy. In *Exercise in pregnancy*. 2nd ed, ed. R.A. Mittelmark, R.A. Wiswell, and B.L. Drinkwater, 299-312. Philadelphia: Williams & Wilkins.

Modis, L. 1991. *Organization of the extracellular matrix: A polarization microscopic approach*. Boca Raton, FL: CRC Press.

Mohan, S., and E. Radha. 1981. Age related changes in muscle connective tissue: Acid mucopolysaccharides and structural glycoprotein. *Experimental Gerontology* 16(5), 385-392.

Mohr, K.J., M.M. Pink, C. Elsner, and R.S. Kvitne. 1998. Electromyographic investigation of stretching: The effect of warm-up. *Clinical Journal of Sport Medicine* 8(3), 215-220.

Moll, J.M.H., S.L. Liyanage, and V. Wright. 1972. An objective clinical method to measure lateral spinal flexion. *Rheumatology and Physical Medicine* 11(5), 225-239.

Möller, M., J. Ekstrand, B. Öberg, and J. Gillquist. 1985. Duration of stretching effect on range of motion in lower extremities. *Archives of Physical Medicine and Rehabilitation* 66(3), 171-173.

Möller, M.H.L., B.E. Öberg, and J. Gillquist. 1985. Stretching exercise and soccer: Effect of stretching on range of motion in the lower extremity in connection with soccer training. *International Journal of Sports Medicine* 6(1), 50-52.

Möller-Nielsen, J., and M. Hammar. 1989. Women's soccer injuries in relation to the menstrual cycle and oral contraceptive use. *Medicine and Science in Sports and Exercise* 21(2), 126-129.

Möller-Nielsen, J., and M. Hammar. 1991. Sports injuries in relation to the menstrual cycle and oral contraceptive use. *Sports Medicine* 12(3), 152-160.

Montgomery, L.C., F.R. Nelson, J.P. Norton, and P.A. Deuster. 1989. Orthopedic history and examination in the etiology of overuse injuries. *Medicine and Science in Sports and Exercise* 21(3), 237-243.

Moore, J.C. 1984. The Golgi tendon organ: A review and update. *American Journal of Occupational Therapy* 38(4), 227-236.

Moore, J.S. 1992. Function, structure, and responses of components of the muscle tendon unit. *Occupational Medicine* 7(4), 713-740.

Moore, J.S. 1993. *Chiropractic in America: The history of a medical alternative*. Baltimore: Johns Hopkins University Press.

Moore, M.A. 1979. *An electromyographic investigation of muscle stretching techniques*. Master's thesis, University of Washington, Seattle, Washington.

Moore, M.A. 2003. Personal correspondence.

Moore, M.A., and R.S. Hutton. 1980. Electromyographic investigation of muscle stretching techniques. *Medicine and Science in Sports and Exercise* 12(5), 322-329.

Mora, J. 1990. Dynamic stretching. *Triathlete* 84, 28-31.

Moran, H.M., M.A. Hall, A. Barr, and B.M. Ansell. 1979. Spinal mobility in the adolescent. *Rheumatology and Rehabilitation* 18(3), 181-185.

Morelli, M., D.E. Seaborne, and S.J. Sullivan. 1989. Motoneurone excitability changes during massage of the triceps sura (Abstract). *Canadian Journal of Sport Sciences* 14(4), 129P.

Moreno, A., and M. Grodin. 2002. Tortue and its neurological sequelae. *SpinalCord* 40(5), 213-223.

Moreno, A. L. Piwowarczyk, and M. Grodin. 2001. Human rights violations and refugee health. *Journal of the Amercian Medical Association* 285(9), 1215.

Moretz, A.J., R. Walters, and L. Smith. 1982. Flexibility as a predictor of knee injuries in college football players. *The Physician and Sportsmedicine* 10(7), 93-97.

Morey, M.C., P.A. Cowper, J.R. Feussner, R.C. Dipasquale, G.M. Crowley, D.W. Kitzman, and R.J. Sullivan. 1989. Evaluation of a supervised exercise program in a geriatric population. *Journal of the American Geriatrics Society* 37(4), 348-354.

Morey, M.C., P.A. Cowper, J.R. Feussner, R.C. DiPasquale, G.M. Crowley, G.P. Samsa, and R.J. Sullivan. 1991. Two-year trends in physical performance following supervised exercise among community-dwelling older veterans. *Journal of the American Geriatrics Society* 39(10), 986-992.

Morgan, Dennis. 1994. Principles of soft tissue treatment. *Journal of Manual & Manipulative Therapy* 2(2), 63-65.

Morgan, D.L. 1990. New insights into the behavior of muscle during active lengthening. *Biophysical Journal* 57(2), 209-221.

Morgan, D.L. 1994. An explanation for residual increased tension in striated muscle after stretch during contraction. *Experimental Physiology* 79(5), 831-838.

Morgan, D.L., and D.G. Allen. 1999. Early events in stretch-induced muscle damage. *Journal of Applied Physiology* 87(6), 2007-2015.

Morgan, D., H. Sugaya, S. Banks, and F. Cook. 1997. A new 'twist' on golf kinematics and low back injuries: The Crunch Factor. American Society of Biomechanics. Presented at the Twenty-First Annual Meeting of the American Society of Biomechanics, Clemson University, South Carolina, September 24-27, 1997.

Morgan-Jones, R.L., T. Cross, and M.J. Cross. 2000. Hamstring injuries. *Critical Reviews in Physical and Rehabilitation Medicine* 12(4), 277-282.

Moritani, T., and H.A. de Vries. 1979. Neural factors versus hypertrophy in time course of muscle strength gain. *American Journal of Physical Medicine* 58(3), 115-130.

Morris, J.M., G. Brenner, and D.B. Lucas. 1962. An electromyographic study of the intrinsic muscles of the back in man. *Journal of Anatomy* 96(4), 509-520.

Morrissey, M. 1999. Active exercise is much more effective than passive therapies for athletes with chronic adductor-related groin pain: Commentary. *Australian Journal of Physiotherapy* 45(3), 241.

Mortimer, J.A., and D.D. Webster, D.D. 1983. Dissociated changes of short- and long-latency myotatic responses prior to a brisk voluntary movement in normals, in karate experts, and in Parkinsonian patients. In *Advances in Neurology, Vol. 39: Motor Control Mechanisms in Health and Disease*, ed. J.E. Desmedt, 541-554. New York: Raven.

Moseley, A.M., J. Crosbie, and J. Adams. 2001. Normative data for passive ankle plantarflexion-dorsiflexion flexibility. *Clinical Biomechanics* 16(6), 514-521.

Moss, F.P., and C.P. Leblond. 1971. Satellite cells as the source of nuclei in muscles of growing rats. *Anatomical Record* 170(4), 421-436.

Moulton, B., and S.H. Spence. 1992. Site-specific muscle hyper-reactivity in musicians with occupational upper limb pain. *Behavioral Research Therapy* 39(4), 375-386.

Mow, V.C., E.L. Flatow, and G.A. Ateshian. 2000. Biomechanics. In *Orthopaedic basic science: Biology and biomechanics of the musculoskeletal system*. 2nd ed, ed. J.A. Buckwalter, T.A. Einhorn and S.R. Simon, 133-180. Rosemont, IL: American Academy of Orthopaedic Surgeons.

Muckle, D.S. 1982. Associated factors in recurrent groin and hamstring injuries. *British Journal of Sports Medicine* 16(1), 37-39.

Mühlemann, D., and J.A. Cimino. 1990. Therapeutic muscle stretching. In *Functional soft tissue examination and treatment by manual methods. The extremities*, ed. W.I. Hammer, 251-275. Gaithersburg, MD: Aspen.

Muir, H. 1983. Proteoglycans as organizers of the intercellular matrix. *Biochemical Society Transactions* 11(6), 613-622.

Muir, L.W., B.M. Chesworth, and A.A. Vandervoort. 1999. Effect of a static stretching calf-stretching exercise on the resistive torque during passive ankle dorsiflexion in healthy subjects. *Journal of Orthopaedic and Sports Physical Therapy* 29(2), 106-115.

Müller, G.E., and Schumann, F. 1899. Uber die psychologischen Grundlagen der Vergleichung gehobener Gewichte. *Pflügers Archiv für die gesamte Physiologie* 45: 37-112.

Munns, K. 1981. Effects of exercise on the range of joint motion in elderly subjects. In *Exercise and aging: The scientific basis*, ed. E.L. Smith and R.C. Serfass, 167-178. Hillsdale, NJ: Enslow.

Munroe, R.A., and T.J. Romance. 1975. Use of the leighton flexometer in the development of a short flexibility test battery. *American Corrective Therapy Journal* 29(1), 22-25.

Murphy, D.R. 1991. A critical look at static stretching: Are we doing our patients harm? *Chiropractic Sports Medicine* 5(3), 67-70.

Murphy, P. 1986. Warming up before stretching advised. *The Physician and Sportsmedicine* 14(3), 45.

Murray, M.P., and S.B. Sepic. 1968. Maximum isometric torque of hip abductor and adductor muscles. *Physical Therapy* 48(12), 1327-1335.

Murray, P.M., and W.P. Cooney. 1996. Golf-induced injuries of the wrist. *Clinics in Sports Medicine* 15(1), 85-109.

Mutungi, G., and K.W. Ranatunga. 1996. The viscous and elastic characteristics of resting fast and slow mammalian (rat) muscle fibres. *Journal of Physiology (London)* 496(3), 827-836.

Myers, E.J. 1971. Effect of selected exercise variables on ligament stability and flexibility of the knee. *Research Quarterly* 42(2), 411-422.

Myers, E.R., C.G. Armstrong, and V.C. Mow. 1984. Swelling, pressure, and collagen tension. In *Connective tissue matrix*, ed. D.W.L. Hukin, 161-186. Deerfield Beach, FL: Verlag Chemie.

Myers, M. 1983. Stretching. *Dance Magazine* 57(6), 66-68.

Myklebust, B.M., G.L. Gottlieb, and G.C. Agarwal. 1986. Stretch reflexes of the normal human infant. *Developmental Medicine and Child Neurology* 28(4), 440-449.

Myllyharju, J., and K.I. Kivirikko. 2001. Collagen and collagen-related diseases. *Annals of Medicine* 33(1), 7-21.

Mysorekar, V.R., and A.N. Nandedkar. 1986. Surface area of the atlanto-occipital articulations. *Acta Anatomica* 126(4), 223-225.

Nadler, S.F., Malanga, Feinberg, J.H., Prybicien, M., Stitik, T.P., and DePrince, M. 2001. Relationship between hip muscle imbalance and occurrence of low back pain in collegiate athletes. *American Journal of Physical Medicine and Rehabilitation* 80(8), 572-577.

Nadler, S.F., K.D. Wu, T. Galski, and J.H. Feinberg. 1998. Low back pain in college athletes: A prospective study correlating lower extremity overuse or acquired ligamentous laxity with low back pain. *Spine* 23(7), 828-833.

Nagler, W. 1973a. Mechanical obstruction of vertebral arteries during hyperextension of neck. *British Journal of Sports Medicine* 7(1-2), 92-97.

Nagler, W. 1973b. Vertebral artery obstruction by hyperextension of the neck: Report of three cases. *Archives of Physical Medicine and Rehabilitation* 54(5), 237-240.

Naish, J.M., and J. Apley. 1951. "Growing pains": A clinical study of non-arthritic limb pains in children. *Archives of Disease in Childhood* 126(April), 134-140.

Nakazawa, K., Yamamoto, S-I., Ohtsuki, T., Yano, H., and Fukunaga, T. 2001. Neural control: Novel evaluation of stretch reflex sensitivity. *Acta Physiologica Scandinavica* 172(4), 257-268.

Nako, M., and S.S. Segal. 1995. Muscle length alters geometry of arterioles and venules in hamster retractor. *American Journal of Physiology* 268 (Heart Circulation Physiology) 37(1), H336-H344.

Nansel, D., and M. Szlazak. 1994. Findings on the relationship between spinal manipulation and cervical passive end-range capability. In *Advances in Chiropractic* Volume I, ed. D.J. Lawrence, 373-414. St. Louis: Mosby-Year Book.

National Institute for Occupational Safety and Health. 1981. *Work practices guide for manual lifting* (DHHS [NIOSH] Publication No. 81:122). Cincinnati: U.S. Department of Health, Education and Welfare.

Neff, C. 1987. He ran a crooked 26 miles, 385 yards. *Sports Illustrated* 67(21), 18.

Neilsen, P.D., and J.W. Lance. 1978. Reflex transmission characteristics during voluntary activity in normal man and patients with movement disorders. In *Cerebral motor control in man: Long loop mechanisms. Progress in neurophysiology* (Vol 4), ed. J.E. Desmedt, 263-299. Basel, Switzerland: S. Kagar AG Medical and Scientific.

Nelson, A.G., I.K. Guillory, A. Cornwell, and J. Kokkonen. 2001. Inhibition of maximal voluntary isokinetic torque production following stretching is velocity-specific. *Journal of Strength Conditioning Research* 15(2), 241-246.

Nelson, J.K., B.L. Johnson, and G.C. Smith. 1983. Physical characteristics, hip, flexibility and arm strength of female gymnasts classified by intensity of training across age. *Journal of Sports Medicine and Physical Fitness* 23(1), 95-100.

Nelson, S.H., and E. Blades-Zeller. 2002. *Singing with your whole self: The Feldenkrais method and voice*. Lanham, MD: Scarecrow Press.

Neu, H.N., and H.R. Dinnel. 1957. The shoulder girdle in the chronic respirator patient. *Physical Therapy Review* 37(6), 373-375.

Neumann, D.A. 2000. Arthrokinesiologic considerations in the aged adult. In *Geriatric physical therapy*. 2nd ed. ed. A.A. Guccione, 56-77. St. Louis: Mosby.

Newham, D.J. 1988. The consequences of eccentric contraction and their relationships to delayed onset muscle pain. *European Journal of Applied Physiology* 57(3), 353-359.

Newham, D.J., D.A. Jones, G. Ghosh, and P. Aurora. 1988. Muscle fatigue and pain after eccentric contractions at long and short length. *Clinical Science (London)* 74(5), 553-557.

Newham, D.J., G. McPhail, K.R. Mills, and R.H.T. Edwards. 1983. Ultrastructural changes after concentric and eccentric contractions of human muscle. *Journal of Neurological Sciences* 61(1), 109-122.

Newham, D.J., K.R. Mills, B.M. Quigley, and R.H.T. Edwards. 1982. Muscle pain and tenderness after exercise. *Australian Journal of Sports Medicine* 14(4), 129-131.

Newham, D.J., K.R. Mills, B.M. Quigley, and R.H.T. Edwards. 1983. Pain and fatigue after concentric and eccentric muscle contractions. *Clinical Science* 64(1), 55-62.

Newton, R. 1985. Effects of vapocoolants on passive hip flexion in healthy subjects. *Physical Therapy* 65(7), 1034-1036.

Ng, G., and J. Walter. 1995. Ageing does not affect flexion relaxation of erector spinae. *Australian Physiotherapy* 41(2), 91-95.

Nicholas, J.A. 1970. Injuries to the knee ligaments: Relationship to looseness and tightness in football players. *Journal of the American Medical Association* 212(13), 2236-2239.

Nicholas, S.J., and T.F. Tyler. 2002. Adductor muscle strains in sport. *Sports Medicine* 32(5), 339-344.

Nielsen, J., C. Crone, and H. Hultborn. 1993. H-reflexes are smaller in dancers from the Royal Danish Ballet than in well-trained athletes. *European Journal of Applied Physiology* 66(2), 116-121.

Nieman, D.C. 1990. *Fitness and sports medicine: An introduction.* Palo Alto, CA: Bull.

Nigg, B.M., and W. Liu. 1999. The effect of muscle stiffness and damping on simulated impact force peaks during running. *Journal of Biomechanics* 32(8), 849-856.

Nikolic, V., and B. Zimmermann. 1968. Functional changes of the tarsal bones of ballet dancers. *Radovi Fakulteta u Zagrebu* 16, 131-146.

Nimmo, M.A., and D.H. Snow. 1982. Time course of ultrastructural changes in skeletal muscle after two types of exercise. *Journal of Applied Physiology* 52(4), 910-913.

Nimmo, R.L. 1958. *The Receptor* 1(3), 1-4.

Nimz, R., U. Radar, K. Wilke, and W. Skipka. 1988. The relationship of anthropometric measures to different types of breaststroke kicks. In *Swimming science V*, ed. B.E. Ungerechts, K. Wilke, and K. Reischle, 115-119. Champaign, IL: Human Kinetics.

Ninos, J. 1996a. Stretching the quadriceps. *Strength and Conditioning* 18(1), 68-69.

Ninos, J. 1996b. Stretch those hamstrings. *Strength and Conditioning* 18(2), 42-43.

Ninos, J. 2001. A chain reaction: The hip rotators. *Strength and Conditioning Journal* 23(2), 26-27.

Nirschl, R.P. 1973. Good tennis-good medicine. *The Physician and Sportsmedicine* 1(1), 26-36.

Noonan, T.J., T.M. Best, A.V. Seaber, and W.E. Garrett. 1993. Thermal effects on skeletal muscle tensile behavior. *American Journal of Sports Medicine* 21(4), 517-522.

Noonan, T.J., T.M. Best, A.V. Seaber, and W.E. Garrett. 1994. Identification of a threshold for skeletal muscle injury. *American Journal of Sports Medicine* 22(2), 257-261.

Noonan, T.J., and W.E. Garrett. 1999. Muscle strain injury: Diagnosis and treatment. *Journal of the American Academy of Orthopaedic Surgeons* 7(4), 262-269.

Nordin, M., and V.H. Frankel. 2001. *Basic biomechanics of the musculoskeletal system.* 3rd ed. Philadelphia: Lippincott, Williams & Wilkins.

Nordschow, M., and W. Bierman. 1962. Influence of manual massage on muscle relaxation. *Journal of the American Physical Therapy Association* 42(10), 653-657.

Norris, F.H., E.L. Gasteiger, and P.O. Chatfield. 1957. An electromyographic study of induced and spontaneous muscle cramps. *Electroencephalography and Clinical Neurophysiology* 9(1), 139-147.

Norris, R. 1993. *The musician's survival manual: A guide to preventing and treating injuries in instrumentalists.* St. Louis, MO: MMB Music.

Northrip, J.W., G.A. Logan, and W.C. McKinney. 1983. *Analysis of sport motion: Anatomic and biomechanic perspectives.* 3rd ed. Dubuque, IA: Brown.

Nosse, L.J. 1978. Inverted spinal traction. *Archives of Physical Medicine and Rehabilitation* 59(8), 367-370.

Noverre, J.G. [1782-1783]. 1978. *The works of Monsieur Noverre* (Vol. II). Reprint, New York: AMS.

Nwuga, V.C. 1982. Relative therapeutic efficiency of vertebral manipulation and conventional treatment in back pain management. *American Journal of Physical Medicine* 61(6), 273-278.

Oakes, B.W. 1981. Acute soft tissue injuries: Nature and management. *Australian Family Physician* 13(Suppl.), 3-16.

Öberg, B. 1993. Evaluation and improvement of strength in competitive athletes. In *Muscle strength*, ed. K. Harms-Ringdahl, 167-185. Edinburgh: Churchill Livingstone.

Ochs, A., Newberry, J., Lenhardt, M., and Harkins, S.W. 1985. Neural and vestibular aging associated with falls. In *Handbook of the psychology of aging.* 2nd ed, ed. J.E. Birren and K.W. Schaie, 378-399. New York: Van Nostrand Reinhold.

O'Driscoll, S.L., and J. Tomenson. 1982. The cervical spine. *Clinical Rheumatic Diseases* 8(3), 617-630.

Ogata, K., and M. Naito. 1986. Blood flow of peripheral nerve effects of dissection, stretching and compression. *Journal of Hand Surgery* 11B(1), 10-14.

Ohshiro, T. 1991. *Low reactive-level laser therapy.* New York: Wiley.

Okada, M. 1970. Electromyographic assessment of muscular load in forward bending postures. *Journal of Faculty Science* (University of Tokyo) 8, 311-336.

Olcott, S. 1980. Partner flexibility exercises. *Coaching Women's Athletics* 6(2), 10-14.

Oliver, J., and A. Middleditch. 1991. *Functional anatomy of the spine.* Oxford: Butterworth Heinemann.

O'Malley, E.F., and R.L. Sprinkle. 1986. Stretching exercises for pretibial periostitis. *Current Podiatric Medicine* 35(7), 22-23.

Oppliger, R., B.A. Clark, J.L. Mayhew, and K.M. Haywood. 1986. Strength, flexibility, and body composition differences between age-group swimmers and non-swimmers. *Australian Journal of Science and Medicine in Sport* 18(2), 14-16.

Ortmann, O. 1962. *The physiological mechanics of piano technique.* New York: E.P. Dutton.

Oseid, S., G. Evjenth, O. Evjenth, H. Gunnari, and D. Meen. 1974. Lower back troubles in young female gymnasts. Frequency, symptoms and possible causes. *Bulletin of Physical Education* 10, 25-28.

Osolin, N.G. 1952. *Das Training des Leichtathleten.* Berlin: Sportverlag.

Osolin, N.G. 1971. *Sovremennaia sistema sportnnoi trenirovky* [Athlete's training system for competitions]. Moscow: Phyzkultura i sport.

Osternig, L.R., R.N. Robertson, R.K. Troxel, and P. Hansen. 1990. Differential responses to proprioceptive neuromuscular facilitation (PNF) stretch techniques. *Medicine and Science in Sports and Exercise* 22(1), 106-111.

Overend, T.J., D.A. Cunningham, D.H. Paterson, and M.S. Lefcoe. 1992. Thigh composition in young and elderly men determined by computed tomography. *Clinical Physiology* 12(6), 629-640.

Owen, E. 1882. Notes on the voluntary dislocations of a contortionist. *British Medical Journal* 1, 650-653.

Özkaya, N., and M. Nordin, M. 1999. *Fundamentals of biomechanics, equilibrium, motion and deformation.* New York: Van Nostrand Reinhold.

Pachter, B.R., and A. Eberstein. 1985. Effects of passive exercise on neurogenic atrophy in rat skeletal muscle. *Experimental Neurology* 90(2), 467-470.

Palmerud, G., H. Sporrong, P. Herberts, and R. Kadefors, 1998. Consequences of trapezius relaxation on the distribution of shoulder muscle forces: An electromyographic study. *Journal of Electromyography and Kinesiology* (3), 185-193.

Panagiotacopulos, N.D., W.G. Knauss, and R. Bloch. 1979. On the mechanical properties of human intervertebral disc material. *Biorheology* 16(4-5), 317-330.

Pang. *See* Barker (1974).

Pappas, A.M., R.M. Zawacki, and C.F. McCarthy. 1985a. Rehabilitation of the pitching shoulder. *American Journal of Sports Medicine* 13(4), 223-235.

Pappas, A.M., R.M. Zawacki, and T.M. Sullivan. 1985. Biomechanics of baseball pitching: A preliminary report. *American Journal of Sports Medicine* 13(4), 216-222.

Pardini, A. 1984. Exercise, vitality and aging. *Aging* 344, 19-29.

Paris, S.V. 1990. Cervical symptoms of forward head posture. *Topics in Geriatric Rehabilitation* 5(4), 11-19.

Parker, M.G., R.O. Ruhling, D. Holt, E. Bauman, and M. Drayna. 1983. Descriptive analysis of quadriceps and hamstrings muscle torque in high school football players. *Journal of Orthopaedic and Sports Physical Therapy* 5(1), 2-6.

Parks, K.A., K.S. Crichton, R.J. Goldford, and S.M. McGill. 2003. A comparison of lumbar range of motion and functional ability scores in patients with low back pain. *Spine* 28(4), 380-384.

Partridge, S.M. 1966. Elastin. In *The physiology and biochemistry of muscle as food*, ed. E.J. Briskey, R.G. Cassens, and J.C. Trautman, 327-337. Madison, WI: University of Wisconsin Press.

Pate, R.R., M. Pratt, S.N. Blair, W.L. Haskell, C.A. Macera, C. Bouchard, D. Buchner, W. Ettinger, G.W. Health, A.C. King, A. Kriska, A.S. Leon, B.H. Marcus, J. Morris, R.S. Paffenbarger, K. Patrick, M.L. Pollock, J.M. Rippe, J. Sallis, and J.H. Wilmore. 1995. Physical activity and public health: A recommendation from the Centers for Disease Control and Prevention and the American College of Sports Medicine. *Journal of the American Medical Association* 273(5), 402-407.

Patel, D.J., and D.L. Fry. 1964. In situ pressure-radius-length measurements in ascending aorta of anesthetized dogs. *Journal of Applied Physiology* 19(3), 413-416.

Patel, D.J., J.C. Greenfield, and D.L. Fry. 1963. In vivo pressure-length-radius relationship of certain blood vessels in man and dog. In *Pulsatile blood flow*, ed. E.O. Attinger, 293-306. Philadelphia: McGraw-Hill.

Patterson, P., D.L. Wiksten, L. Ray, C. Flanders, and D. Sanphy. 1996. The validity and reliability of the back saver-sit-and-reach test in middle school girls and boys. *Research Quarterly for Exercise and Sport* 67(4), 448-451.

Paull, B., and C. Harrison. 1997. *The athlete musician: A guide to playing without pain*. Lanham, MD: Scarecrow Press.

Pauly, J.E. 1966. An electromyographic analysis of certain movements and exercises. I. Some deep muscles of the back. *Anatomical Record* 155(2), 223-234.

Payne, R.A. 1995. *Relaxation techniques, a practical handbook for the health care professional*. Edinburgh: Churchill Livingstone.

Pearcy, M., I. Portek, and J. Shepherd. 1985. The effect of low-back pain on lumbar spinal movements measured by three-dimensional x-ray analysis. *Spine* 10(2), 150-153.

Pearson, K., and J. Gordon. 2000. Spinal reflexes. In *Principles of neural science*. 4th ed, ed. E.R. Kandel, J.H. Schwartz and T.M. Jessell, 713-736. New York: McGraw-Hill.

Pechinski, J.M. 1966. *The effects of interval running and breath-holding on cardiac intervals*. Master's thesis, University of Illinois, Champaign.

Pechtl, V. 1982. Fundamentals and methods for the development of flexibility. In *Principles of sports training*, ed. D. Harre, 146-152. Berlin: Sportverlag.

Peck, C. 1999. Non-compliance and clinical trials: Regulatory perspectives. In *Drug regimen compliance issues in clinical trials and patient management*, ed. J.-M. Métry and U. A. Meyer, 97-102. Chichester: John Wiley & Sons.

Pedersen, M. 2003. Warm up exercises. [Online]. Available: www.pgaprofessional.com/tips10_warmup.html [October 31, 2003].

PennState Sports Medicine Newsletter. 1998. The active isolated stretching controversy. Author: 7(1), 4.

Peres, S., D.O. Draper, K.L. Knight and M.D. Richard. 2001. Pulsed shortwave diathermy and prolonged stretch increases dorsiflexion range of motion more than prolonged stretch alone. *Journal of Athletic Training* 36(2), S49.

Peres, S., D.O. Draper, K.L. Knight and M.D. Richard. 2002. Pulsed shortwave diathermy and prolonged stretching increases dorsiflexion. *Journal of Athletic Training* 37(1), 43-50.

Perez, H.R., and S. Fumasoli. 1984. Benefit of proprioceptive neuromuscular facilitation on the joint mobility of youth-aged female gymnasts with correlations for rehabilitation. *American Corrective Therapy Journal* 38(6), 142-146.

Perkins, K.A., and L.H. Epstein. 1988. Methodology in exercise adherence research. In *Exercise adherence: Its impact on public health*, ed. R.K. Dishman, 399-416. Champaign, IL: Human Kinetics.

Pérusse, L., C. Leblanc and C. Bouchard. 1988. Inter-generation transmission of physical fitness in the Canadian population. *Canadian Journal of Sports Science* 13(1), 8-14.

Peters, J.M., and H.K. Peters. 1983. *The flexibility manual*. Berwyn, PA: Sports Kinetics.

Peterson, D.H., and T.F. Bergmann. 2002. *Chiropractic technique: Principles and procedures*. 2nd ed. St. Louis: Mosby.

Peterson, L., and P. Renstrom. 1986. *Sports injuries: Their prevention and treatment*. Chicago: Year Book Medical.

Pezzullo, D.J., and J.J. Irrgang. 2001. Rehabilitation. In *Sports injuries mechanisms, prevention, treatment*. 2nd ed, ed. F.H. Fu and D.A. Stone, 106-123. Philadelphia: Lippincott Williams & Wilkins.

Pheasant, S. 1991. *Ergonomics, work and health*. Gaithersburg, MD: Aspen.

Pheasant, S. 1996. *Bodyspace-Anthropometry, ergonomics and the design of work*. 2nd ed. London: Taylor and Francis.

Phillips, C.G. 1969. The ferrier lecture, 1968. Motor apparatus of the baboon's hand. *Proceedings of the Royal Society* (Biology) 173(31), 141-174.

Physicians for Human Rights. 2001. General interview considerations. In *Examining asylum seekers—A health professional's guide to medical and psychological evaluations of torture*. 19-35. Boston: Physicians for Human Rights.

Pieper, H-G. 1998. Humeral torsion in the throwing arm of handball players. *American Journal of Sports Medicine* 26(2), 247-253.

Pierce, R. 1983-1984. Doing bodywork as a spiritual discipline. *Somatics* 4(3), 10-27.

Piperek, M. 1971. *Stress und kunst*. Wien-Stuttgart: Wilhelm Braumüller.

Piwowarczyk, L., A. Moreno, and M. Grodin. 2000. Health care of torture survivors. *Journal of the American Medical Association* 284(5), 539-541.

Ploucher, D.W. 1982. Inversion petechiae. *New England Journal of Medicine* 307(22), 1406-1407.

Poggini, L., S. Losasso, and S. Iannone. 1999. Injuries during the dancer's growth spurt: Etiology, prevention, and treatment. *Journal of Dance Medicine & Science* 3(2), 73-79.

Pokorny, M.J., T.D. Smith, S.A. Calus, and E.A. Dennison. 2000. Self-reported oral contraceptive use and peripheral joint laxity. *Journal of Orthopaedic and Sports Physical Therapy* 30(11), 683-692.

Politou, A.S.M., S. Gautel, L. Improta, L. Vanelista, and A. Pastore. 1996. The elastic I-band region of titin is assembled in a "modular" fashion by weakly interacting Ig-like domains. *Molecular Biology* 255 (4), 604-616.

Politou, A.S.M., D.J. Thomas, and A. Pastore. 1995. The folding and stability of titin immunoglobin-like modules, with implications for the mechanism of elasticity. *Biophysical Journal* 69(6), 2601-2610.

Pollack, G.H. 1983. The cross-bridge theory. *Physiological Review* 63(3), 1049-1113.

Pollack, G.H. 1990. *Muscles & molecules: Uncovering the principles of biological motion*. Seattle: Ebner & Sons.

Pollock, M.L., and J.H. Wilmore. 1990. *Exercise in health and disease: Evaluation and prescription for prevention and rehabilitation*. Philadelphia: Saunders.

Poole, D.C., T.I. Musch, and C.A. Kindig. 1997. In vivo microvascular structural and functional consequences of muscle length changes. *American Journal of Physiology* 272 (Heart Circulation Physiology 41), H2107-H2114.

Pope, F.M., and N.P. Burrows. 1997. Ehlers-Danlos syndrome has varied molecular mechanisms. *Journal of Medical Genetics* 34(5), 400-410.

Pope, M.H., G.B.J. Andersson, J.W. Frymoyer, and D.B. Chaffin. 1991. *Occupational low back pain: Assessment, treatment and prevention*. Chicago: Mosby Yearbook.

Pope, M.H., and U. Klingenstierna. 1986. Height changes due to autotraction. *Clinical Biomechanics* 1(4), 191-195.

Pope, R.P., R.D. Herbert, and J.D. Kirwan. 1998. Effects of ankle dorsiflexion range and pre-exercise calf muscle stretching on injury risk in Army recruits. *Australian Physiotherapy* 44(3), 165-172.

Pope, R.P., R.D. Herbert, J.D. Kirwan, and B.J. Graham. 2000. A randomized trial of preexercise stretching for prevention of lower-limb injury. *Medicine and Science in Sports and Exercise* 32(2), 271-277.

Porter, R.W., and I.F. Trailescu. 1990. Diurnal changes in straight leg raising. *Spine* 15(2), 103-106.

Portnoy, H., and F. Morin. 1956. Electromyographic study of postural muscles in various positions and movements. *American Journal of Physiology* 186(1), 122-126.

Poumeau-Deville, G.A., and P. Soulie. 1934. Un cas d'hyperlaxite cutanee et articulaire avec cicatrices atrophiques et pseudo-tumeurs molluscoides (syndrome d'Ehlers-Danlos). *Bulletin de la Societe Medicale des Hopitaux de Paris* 50, 593-595.

Pountain, G. 1992. Musculoskeletal pain in Omanis, and the relationship to joint mobility and body mass index. *British Journal of Rheumatology* 31(2), 81-85.

Pratt, M. 1989. Strength, flexibility, and maturity in adolescent athletes. *American Journal of Diseases of Children* 143(5), 560-563.

Prentice, W.E. 1982. An electromyographic analysis of the effectiveness of heat or cold and stretching for inducing relaxation in injured muscle. *Journal of Orthopaedic and Sports Physical Therapy* 3(3), 133-140.

Prentice, W.E. 1983. A comparison of static stretching and PNF stretching for improving hip joint flexibility. *Athletic Training* 18(1), 56-59.

Prentice, W.E. 1999. *Rehabilitation techniques in sports medicine*. 3rd ed. Boston: McGraw-Hill.

Prentice, W.E. 2001. Impaired mobility: Restoring range of motion and improving flexibility. In *Techniques in musculoskeletal rehabilitation*, ed. W.E. Prentice and M.L. Voight, 83-233. New York: McGraw-Hill.

Prentice, W.E., D.O. Draper, and P.B. Donley. 1999. Shortwave and microwave diathermy. In *Therapeutic modalities in sports medicine*. 4th ed, ed. W.E. Prentice, 148-172. Boston: WCB McGraw-Hill.

Preyde, M. 2000. Effectiveness of massage therapy for subacute low-back pain: A randomized controlled trial. *Canadian Medical Association Journal* 162(13), 1815-1820.

Price, M.G. 1991. In *Advances in structural biology*. Vol. 1, ed. S.K.J. Melhorta, 175-207. New York: JAI Press.

Prichard, B. 1984. *Lower extremity injuries in runners induced by upper body torque (UBT)*. Presented at the Biomechanics and Kinesiology in Sports U.S. Olympic Sports Medicine Conference, Colorado Springs, CO.

Priest, J.D. 1989. A physical phenomenon: Shoulder depression in athletes. *SportCare & Fitness* 2(2), 20-25.

Priest, J.D., H.H. Jones, C.J. Tichenor, and D.A. Nagel. 1977. Arm and elbow changes in expert tennis players. *Minnesota Medicine* 60(5), 399-404.

Priest, J.D., and D.A. Nagel. 1976. Tennis shoulder. *American Journal of Sports Medicine* 4(1), 28-42.

Proske, U., and D.L. Morgan. 1987. Tendon stiffness: Methods of measurement and significance for the control of movement. A review. *Journal of Biomechanics* 20(1), 75-82.

Proske, U., and D.L. Morgan. 1999. Do cross-bridges contribute to the tension during stretch of passive muscle? *Journal of Muscle Research and Cell Motility* 20(5-6), 433-442.

Proske, U., D. Morgan, and J. Gregory. 1992. Muscle history dependence of responses to stretch of primary and secondary endings of cat soleus muscle spindles. *Journal of Physiology (London)* 445(Jan), 81-95.

Proske, U., D. Morgan, and J. Gregory. 1993. Thixotrophy in skeletal muscle and in muscle spindles: A review. *Progress in Neurobiology* 41(6), 705-721.

Proske, U., D. Morgan, and J. Gregory. 1998. The dependence of a muscle's mechanical properties and the sensitivity of its sensory receptors on the previous history of contraction and length changes. Australian Conference of Science and Medicine in Sport 1998 at Adelaide, 13-16 October.

Protas, E.J. 2001. Flexibility and range of motion. In *ACSM's resource manual for guidelines for exercise testing and prescription*. 4th ed, ed. B.A. Franklin, 468-477. Baltimore: Lippincott Williams & Wilkins.

Purslow, P.P. 1989. Strain-induced reorientation of an intramuscular connective tissue network: Implications for passive muscle elasticity. *Journal of Biomechanics* 22(1), 21-31.

Puschel, J. 1930. Der Wassergehalt voraler un degenerieter Zwischenwirbelschiben. *Beitrage zur Pathologischen Anatomie und zur Allgemeinen Pathologie* 84, 123-130.

Pyeritz, R.E. 2000a. Ehlers-Danlos syndromes. In *Cecil textbook of medicine*. 21st ed. Vol. 1, ed. L. Goldman and J.C. Bennett, 1119-1120. Philadelphia: W.B. Saunders.

Pyeritz, R.E. 2000b. Ehlers-Danlos Syndrome. *New England Journal of Medicine* 342(10), 730-732.

Quebec Task Force on Spinal Disorders. 1987. Scientific approach to the assessment and management of activity-related spinal disorders: A monograph for clinicians. *Spine* 12(7), S1-S55.

Quirk, R. 1994. Common foot and ankle injuries in dance. *Orthopaedic Clinics of North America* 25(1), 123-133.

Raab, D.M., J.C. Agre, M. McAdam, and E.L. Smith. 1988. Light resistance and stretching exercise in elderly women: Effect upon flexibility. *Archives of Physical Rehabilitation* 69(4), 268-272.

Radin, E.L. 1989. Role of muscles in protecting athletes from injury. *Acta Medica Scandinavica* 711(Suppl.), 143-147.

Ramacharaka, Y. 1960. *The hindu-yogi science of breath*. London: L.N. Fowler.

Rankin, J., L. Greninger, and C. Ingersoll. 1992. The effects of the power stretch device on flexibility of normal hip joints. *Clinical Kinesiology* 45(4), 23-25.

Rankin, J.M., and C.B. Thompson. 1983. Isokinetic evaluation of quadriceps and hamstrings function: Normative data concerning body weight and sport. *Athletic Training* 18(2), 110-114.

Rao, V. 1965. Reciprocal inhibition: Inapplicability to tendon jerks. *Journal of Postgraduate Medicine* 11(July), 123-125.

Rasch, P.J., and J. Burke. 1989. *Kinesiology and applied anatomy*. 7th ed. Philadelphia: Lea & Febiger.

Rasmussen, G.G. 1979. Manipulation in low back pain: A randomized clinical trial. *Manual Medicine* 1(1), 8-10.

Ray, W.A., and M.R. Griffin. 1990. Prescribed medications and the risk of falling. *Topics in Geriatric Rehabilitation* 5(2), 12-20.

Read, M. 1989. Over stretched. *British Journal of Sports Medicine* 23(4), 257-258.

Rechtien, J.J., M. Andary, T.G. Holmes, and J.M. Wieting. 1998. Manipulation, massage, and traction. In *Rehabilitation medicine: Principles and practice*. 3rd ed, ed. J.A. DeLisa and B.M. Gans, 521-552. Philadelphia: Lippincott-Raven.

Reedy, M.K. 1971. Electron microscope observations concerning the behavior of the cross-bridge in striated muscle. In *Contractility of muscle cells and related processes*, ed. R.J. Podolsky, 229-246. Englewood Cliffs, NJ: Prentice-Hall.

Reich, T.E., S.L. Lindstedt, P.C. LaStayo, and D.J. Pierotti. 2000. Is the spring quality of muscle plastic? *American Journal of Physiology. Regulatory, Integrative and Comparative Physiology* 278(6), R1661-1666.

Reid, D.C. 1992. *Sports injury assessment and rehabilitation*. London: Churchill Livingstone.

Reid, D.C., R.S. Burnham, L.A. Saboe, and S.F. Kushner. 1987. Lower extremity flexibility patterns in classical ballet dancers and their correlation to lateral hip and knee injuries. *American Journal of Sports Medicine* 15(4), 347-352.

Reilly, T. 1998. Circadian rhythms. In *Oxford textbook of sports medicine*. 2nd ed, ed. M. Harries, C. Williams, W.D. Stanish and L.J. Micheli, 281-300. Oxford: Oxford University Press.

Reilly, T., and A. Stirling. 1993. Flexibility, warm-up and injuries in mature games players. In *Kinanthropometry IV*, ed. W. Duquet and J.A.P. Day, 119-123. London: E. & F.N. Spon.

Rennison, C.M. 2001. *Bureau of Justice Statistics National Crime Victimization Survey*. Washington, DC: U.S. Justice Department.

Renstrom, P., and C. Roux. 1988. Clinical implications of youth participation in sports. In *The Olympic book of sports medicine* Vol. 1, ed. A. Dirix, H.G. Knuttgen, and K. Tittel, 469-488. London: Blackwell Scientific.

Requejo, S.M., R. Barnes, K. Kulig, R. Landel, and S. Gonzalez. 2002. The use of a modified classification system in the treatment of low back pain during pregnancy: A case report. *Journal of Orthopaedic and Sports Physical Therapy* 32(7), 318-326.

Rice, C.L., D.A. Cunninham, D.H. Paterson, and M.S. Defcoe. 1989. Arm and leg composition determined by computed tomography in young and elderly men. *Clinical Physiology* 9(3), 207-220.

Richie, D.H., H.A. deVries, and C.K. Endo, C.K. 1993. Shin muscle activity and sports surfaces: An electomyographic study. *Journal of the American Podiatric Medical Association* 83(4), 181-190.

Richardson, A.B., F.W. Jobe, and H.R. Collins. 1980. The shoulder in competitive swimming. *Amercian Journal of Sports Medicine* 8(3), 150-163.

Rider, R., and J. Daly. 1991. Effects of flexibility training on changing spinal mobility in older women. *Journal of Sports Medicine and Physical Fitness* 31(2), 213-217.

Riddle, K.S. 1956. *A comparison of three methods for increasing flexibility of the trunk and hip joints.* PhD diss., University of Oregon, Eugene, Oregon.

Rigby, B. 1964. The effect of mechanical extension under thermal stability of collagen. *Biochimica et Biophysica Acta* 79 (SC 43008), 634-636.

Rigby, B.J., N. Hirai, J.D. Spikes, and J. Eyring. 1959. The mechanical properties of rat tail tendon. *Journal of General Physiology* 43(2), 265-283.

Rikken-Bultman, D.G., L. Wellink, and P.W. van Dongen. 1997. Hypermobility in two Dutch school populations. *European Journal of Obstetrics, Gynecology, and Reproductive Biology* 73(2), 189-192.

Rikkers, R. 1986. *Seniors on the move.* Champaign, IL: Human Kinetics.

Rikli, R., and S. Busch. 1986. Motor performance of women as a function of age and physical activity. *Journal of Gerontology* 41(5), 645-649.

Rippe, J.M. 1990. Staying loose. *Modern Maturity* 33(3), 72-77.

Roaf, R. 1977. *Posture.* New York: Academic Press.

Roberts, J., and K. Wilson. 1999. Effect of stretching duration on active and passive range of motion in the lower extremity. *British Journal of Sports Medicine* 33(4), 259-263.

Roberts, N., D. Hogg, G.H. Whitehouse, and P. Dangerfield. 1998. Quantitative analysis of diurnal variation in volume and water content of lumbar intervertebral discs. *Clinical Anatomy* 11(1), 1-8.

Robertson, D.F. 1960. *Relationship of strength of selected muscle groups and ankle flexibility to flutter kick in swimming.* Master's thesis, Iowa State University, Ames.

Robison, C. 1974. *Modern techniques of track and field.* Philadelphia: Lea & Febiger.

Robison, C., C. Jensen, S. James, and W. Hirschi. 1974. *Prevention, evaluation, management & rehabilitation.* New Jersey: Prentice-Hall.

Rochcongar, P., J. Dassonville, and R. Le Bars. 1979. Modifications of the Hoffmann reflex in function of athletic training. *European Journal of Applied Physiology* 40(3), 165-170.

Rockwood, C.A., and F.A. Matsen. eds. 1998. *The shoulder*, Vol. 2. Philadelphia: WB Saunders.

Rodenburg, J.B., D. Steenbeek, P. Schiereck, and P.R. Bar. 1994. Warm-up, stretching and massage diminish harmful effects of eccentric exercise. *International Journal of Sports Medicine* 15(7), 414-419.

Rodeo, S. 1984. Swimming the breaststroke—A kinesiological analysis and considerations for strength straining. *NSCA Journal* 6(4), 4-6, 74-76, 80.

Rodeo, S. 1985a. The butterfly: A kinesiological analysis and strength training program. *NSCA Journal* 7(4), 4-10, 74.

Rodeo, S. 1985b. The butterfly: Physiologically speaking. *Swimming Technique* 21(4), 14-19.

Roetert, E.P., T.S. Ellenbecker, and S.W. Brown. 2000. Shoulder internal and external rotation range of motion in nationally ranked junior tennis players: A longitudinal analysis. *Journal of Strength and Conditioning Research* 14(2), 140-143.

Roland, P.E., and H. Ladegaard-Pedersen. 1977. A quantitative analysis of sensations of tension and of kinesthesia in man. Evidence for a peripherally originating muscular sense and for a sense of effort. *Brain* 100(4), 671-692.

Rollins, J., J. Puffer, W. Whiting, R. Gregor, and G. Finerman. 1985. Water polo injuries to the upper extremity. In *Injuries to the throwing arm*, ed. B. Zarins, J.R. Andrews and W.G. Carson, 311-317. Philadelphia: W.B. Saunders.

Rondinelli, R.D., and R.T. Katz. 2000. *Impairing rating and disability evaluation.* Philadelphia: W.B. Saunders.

Ronsky, J.L., B.M. Nigg, and V. Fisher. 1995. Correlation between physical activity and the gait characteristics and ankle joint flexibility of the elderly. *Clinical Biomechanics* 10(1), 41-49.

Rose, B.S. 1985. The hypermobility syndrome loose-limbed and liable. *New Zealand Journal of Physiotherapy* 13(2), 18-19.

Rose, D.L., S.F. Radzyminski, and R.R. Beatty. 1957. Effect of brief maximal exercise on strength of the quadriceps femoris. *Archives of Physical Medicine and Rehabilitation* 38(3), 157-164.

Rose, L., R. Örtengren, and M. Ericson, M. 2001. Endurance, pain, and resumption in fully flexed postures. *Applied Ergonomics* 32(5), 501-508.

Rose, S., D.O. Draper, S.S. Schulthies, and E. Durant. 1996. The stretching window part two: Rate of thermal decay in deep muscle following 1-MHz ultrasound. *Journal of Athletic Training* 31(2), 139-143.

Rosenbaum, D., and E.M. Hennig. 1995. The influence of stretching and warm-up exercises on Achilles tendon reflex activity. *Journal of Sports Sciences* 13(6), 481-490.

Rosenberg, B.S., W.L. Cornelius, and A.W. Jackson. 1990. The effects of cryotherapy and PNF stretching techniques on hip extensor flexibility in elderly females. *Journal of Physical Education and Sport Sciences* 2, 31-36.

Rosenberg, B.S., W.L. Cornelius, A.W. Jackson, and S. Czubakowski. 1985. The effects of proprioceptive neuromuscular facilitation (PNF) flexibility techniques with local cold application on hip joint range of motion in 55-84 year old females. In *Abstracts research papers 1977* (p. 110). Washington, DC: AAHPER.

Rosenbloom, J., W.R. Abrams, and R. Mecham. 1993. Extracellular matrix 4: The elastic fiber. *The FASEB Journal* 7(13), 1208-1218.

Roskell, P. 1998. Yoga for pianists. *Piano & Keyboard* 192 (May/June), 44-46.

Roston, J.B., and R.W. Haines. 1947. Cracking in the metacarpophalangeal joint. *Journal of Anatomy* 81(2), 165-173.

Rotés, J. 1983. *Rheumatologia Clinica.* Barcelona, Spain: Espaxs.

Round, J.M., D.A. Jones, and G. Cambridge. 1987. Cellular infiltrates in human skeletal muscle: Exercise induced damage as a model for inflammatory disease? *Journal of the Neurological Sciences* 82(1), 1-11.

Rowe, R.W.D. 1981. Morphology of perimysial and endomysial connective tissue in skeletal muscle. *Tissue & Cell* 13(4), 681-690.

Rowinski, M.J. 1997. Neurobiology for orthopaedic and sports physical therapy. In *Orthopaedic and sports physical therapy.* 3rd ed, ed. T.R. Malone, T.G. McPoil and A.J. Nitz, 47-63. St. Louis: Mosby.

Russek, L.N. 1999. Hypermobility syndrome. *Physical Therapy* 79(6), 591-599.

Russell, B., and D.J. Dix. 1992. Mechanisms for intracellular distribution of mRNA: In situ hybridization studies in muscle. *American Journal of Physiology* 262 (31:1), C1-C8.

Russell, B., D.J. Dix, D.L. Haller, and J. Jacobs-El. 1992. Repair of injured skeletal muscle: A molecular approach. *Medicine and Science in Sports and Exercise* 24(2), 189-196.

Russell, G.S., and T.R. Highland. 1990. *Care of the low back.* Columbia, MO: Spine.

Russell, P., A. Weld, M.J. Pearcy, R. Hogg, and A. Unsworth. 1992. Variation in lumbar spine mobility measured over a 24-hour period. *British Journal of Rheumatology* 31(5), 329-332.

Rydevik, B.L., M.K. Kwan, R.R. Myers, R.A. Brown, K.J. Triggs, S.L-Y. Woo, and S.R. Garfin. 1990. An in vitro mechanical and histological study of acute stretching on rabbit tibial nerve. *Journal of Orthopaedic Research* 8(5), 694-701.

Rydevik, B., G. Lundborg, and R. Skalak. 1989. Biomechanics of peripheral nerves. In *Basic biomechanics of the musculoskeletal system*, ed. M. Nordin and V.H. Frankel, 76-87. Philadelphia: Lea & Febiger.

Rymer, W.Z., J.C. Houk, and P.E. Crago. 1979. Mechanisms of the clasp-knife reflex studied in an animal model. *Experimental Brain Research* 37(1), 93-113.

Saal, J.S. 1998. Flexibility training. In *Functional rehabilitation of sports and musculoskeletal injuries*, eds. W.B. Kibler, S.A. Herring, and J.M. Press, 85-97. Gaithersburg, Maryland: Aspen.

Sachse, J., and M. Berger. 1989. Cervical mobilization induced by eye movement. *Journal of Manual Medicine* 4(4), 154-156.

Sackett, D.L., and J.C. Snow. 1979. The magnitude of compliance and noncompliance. In *Compliance in health care*, ed. R.B. Haynes, D.W. Taylor, and D.L. Sackett, 11-22. Baltimore: Johns Hopkins Press.

Sacks, R.D., and R.R. Roy. 1982. Architecture of the hindlimb muscles of cats: Functional significance. *Journal of Morphology* 173(2), 185-195.

Sadoshima, J., and S. Izumo. 1993. Mechanical stretch rapidly activates multiple signal transduction pathways in cardiac myocytes: Potential involvement of an autocrine/paracrine mechanism. *EMBO Journal* 12(4), 1681-1993.

Sady, S.P., M. Wortman, and D. Blanke. 1982. Flexibility training: Ballistic, static or proprioceptive neuromuscular facilitation. *Archives of Physical Medicine and Rehabilitation* 63(6), 261-263.

Safran, M.R., W.E. Garrett, A.V. Seaber, R.R. Glisson, and B.M. Ribbeck. 1998. The role of warm-up in muscular injury prevention. *American Journal of Sports Medicine* 16(2), 123-129.

Sage, G.H. 1984. *Motor learning and control: A neuropsychological approach*. Dubuque, IA: Wm. C. Brown.

Sah, R.L., J.Y.H. Doong, A.J. Grodzinsky, A.H.K. Plaas, and J.D. Sandy. 1991. Effects of compression on the loss of newly synthesized proteoglycans and proteins from cartilage explants. *Archives of Biochemistry and Biophysics* 286(1), 20-29.

Sah, R.L., A.J. Grodzinsky, A.H.K. Plaas, and J.D. Sandy. 1992. Effects of static and dynamic compression on matrix metabolism in cartilage explants. In *Articular cartilage and osteoarthritis*, ed. K.E. Kuettner, R. Schleyerbach and J.G. Peyron, 373-391. New York: Raven Press.

Sahrmann, S. 2002. *Diagnosis and treatment of movement impairment syndromes*. St. Louis: Mosby.

Sale, D.G. 1986. Neural adaptation in strength and power training. In *Human muscle power*, ed. N.L. Jones, N. McCartney, and A.J. McComas, 289-307. Champaign, IL: Human Kinetics.

Sale, D.G., A.J. McComas, J.D. MacDougall, and A.R.M. Upton. 1982. Neuromuscular adaptation in human thenar muscles following strength training and immobilization. *Journal of Applied Physiology* 53(2), 419-424.

Sale, D.G., J.D. MacDougall, A.R.M. Upton, and A.J. McComas. 1983. Effect of strength training upon motorneuron excitability in man. *Medicine and Science in Sports and Exercise* 15(1), 57-62.

Sale, D.G., A.R.M. Upton, A.J. McComas, and J.D. MacDougall. 1983. Neuromuscular function in weight-trainers. *Experimental Neurology* 82(3), 521-531.

Sallay, P.I., R.L. Friedman, P.G. Coogan, and W.E. Garrett. 1996. Hamstring muscle injuries among water skiers: Functional outcome and prevention. *American Journal of Sports Medicine* 24(2), 130-136.

Salminen, J.J. 1984. The adolescent back. A field survey of 370 Finnish schoolchildren *Acta Pædiatrica Scandinavica* 315 (Suppl.), 1-122.

Salminen, J.J., A. Oksanen, P. Maki, J. Pentti, and U.M. Kujala. 1993. Leisure time physical activity in the young. Correlation with low-back pain, spinal mobility and trunk muscle strength in 15-year-old school children. *International Journal of Sports Medicine* 14(7), 406-410.

Sammarco GJ. 1983. The dancer's hip. *Clinics in Sports Medicine* 2(3), 485-498.

Sams, E. 1971. Schumann's hand injury. *Musical Times* 112(1546), 1156-1159.

Samuel, C.S., A. Butkus, J.P. Coghlan, and J. Bateman. 1996. The effect of relaxin on collagen metabolism in the non-pregnant rat pubic symphysis: The influence of estrogen and progesterone in regulating relaxin activity. *Endocrinology* 137(9), 3884-3890.

Sanders, G.E., O. Reinert, R. Tepe, and P. Maloney. 1990. Chiropractic adjustive manipulation on subjects with acute lowback pain: Visual analog pain scores and plasma endorphin levels. *Journal of Manipulative and Physiological Therapeutics* 13(7), 391-395.

Sandoz, R. 1969. The significance of the manipulative crack and of other articular noises. *Annals of the Swiss Chiropractic Association* 4, 47-68.

Sandoz, R. 1976. Some physical mechanisms and effects of spinal adjustments. *Annals of the Swiss Chiropractic Association* 6, 91-141.

Sandstead, H.L. 1968. The relationship of outward rotation of the humerus to baseball throwing velocity. Master's thesis, Eastern Illinois University, Charleston.

Sandyk, R. 1998. Yawning and stretching—A behavioral syndrome associated with transcranial application of electromagnetic fields in multiple sclerosis. *International Journal of Neuroscience* 95(1-2), 107-113.

Sanes, J.N., J.P. Donoghue, V. Thangaraj, R.R. Edelman, and S. Warach. 1995. Shared neural substrates controlling hand movements in human motor cortex. *Science* 268 (5218), 1775-1777.

Sapega, A.A., T.C. Quedenfeld, R.A. Moyer, and R.A. Butler. 1981. Biophysical factors in range-of-motion exercise. *The Physician and Sportsmedicine* 9(12), 57-65.

Sarti, M.A., J.F. Lisón, M. Monfort, and M.A. Fuster. 2001. Response of flexion-relaxation phenomenon relative to the lumbar motion to load and speed. *Spine* 26(18), E416-E420.

Sato-Suzuki, I., I. Kita, M. Oguri, and H. Arita. 1998. Stereotyped yawning responses induced by electrical and chemical stimulation of paraventricular nucleus of the rat. *Journal of Neurophysiology* 80(5), 2765-2775.

Saunders, H.D. 1986. Lumbar traction. In *Modern manual therapy of the vertebral column*, ed. G.P. Grieve, 787-795. Edinburgh: Churchill Livingstone.

Saunders, H.D. 1998. The controversy over traction for neck and low back pain. *Physiotherapy* 84(6), 285-288.

Sawyer, P.C., T.L. Uhl, C.G. Mattacola, D.L. Johnson, and J.W. Yates. 2003. Effects of moist heat on hamstring flexibility and muscle temperature. *Journal of Strength and Conditioning Research* 17(2), 285-290.

Scala, A. 2001. Rehabilitation of the foot following sports-related injuries and surgical treatment. In *Rehabilitation of sports injuries*, ed. G. Puddu, A. Giombini, and A. Selvanetti, 167-184. New York: Springer-Verlag.

Schache, A.G., P.D. Blanch, and A.T. Murphy. 2000. Relation of anterior pelvic tilt during running to clinical and kinematic measures of hip extension. *British Journal of Sports Medicine* 34(4), 279-283.

Schenk, R., K. Adelman, and J. Rousselle. 1994. The effects of muscle energy technique on cervical range of motion. *Journal of Manual & Manipulative Therapy* 2(4), 149-155.

Schiaffino, S. 1974. Hypertrophy of skeletal muscle induced by tendon shortening. *Experimentia* 30(10), 1163-1164.

Schiaffino, S., and V. Hanzlíková. 1970. On the mechanisms of compensatory hypertrophy in skeletal muscle. *Experimentia* 26(2), 152-153.

Schieber, M.H. 1995. Muscular production of individual finger movements: The role of extrinsic finger muscles. *Journal of Neuroscience* 15(1), 284-297.

Schmitt, G.D., T.W. Pelham, and L.E. Holt. 1998. Changes in flexibility of elite female soccer players resulting from a flexibility program or combined flexibility and strength program: A pilot study. *Clinical Kinesiology* 52(3), 64-67.

Schneider, H.J., A.Y. King, J.L. Bronson, and E.H. Miller. 1974. Stress injuries and developmental change of lower extremities in ballet dancers. *Radiology* 113(3), 627-632.

Schneiderman, R., D. Kevet, and A. Maroudas. 1986. Effects of mechanical and osmotic pressure on the rate of glycosaminoglycan synthesis in the human adult femoral head cartilage: An in vivo study. *Journal of Orthopaedic Research* 4, 393-408.

Schnitt, J.M., and D. Schnitt. 1987. Psychological issues in a dancer's career. In *Dance medicine: A comprehensive guide*, ed. A.J. Ryan and R.E. Stephens, 334-349. Chicago: Pluribus.

Schoenfeld, M.R. 1978. Nicolo Paganini: Musical magician and Marfan mutant? *Journal of the American Medical Association* 239(1), 40-42.

Schottelius, B.A., and L.C. Senay. 1956. Effect of stimulation-length sequence on shape of length-tension diagram. *American Journal of Physiology* 186(1), 127-130.

Schultz, A.B., G.B. Andersson, K. Haderspeck, R. Ortengren, M. Nordin, and R. Bjork. 1982. Analysis and measurement of lumbar trunk loads in tasks involving bends and twists. *Journal of Biomechanics* 15(9), 669-675.

Schultz, A.B., K. Haderspeck-Grib, G. Sinkora, and D.N. Warwick. 1985. Quantitative studies of the flexion-relaxation phenomenon in the back muscles. *Journal of Orthopaedic Research* 3(2), 189-197.

Schultz, J.S., and J.A. Leonard. 1992. Long thoracic neuropathy from athletic activity. *Achives of Physical Medicine and Rehabilitation* 73(1), 87-90.

Schultz, P. 1979. Flexibility: Day of the static stretch. *The Physician and Sportsmedicine* 7(11), 109-117.

Schuppert, M., and C. Wagner. 1996. Wrist symptoms in instrumental musicians: Due to biomechanical restrictions? *Medical Problems of Performing Artists* 11(2), 37-42.

Schur, P.E. 2001a. Effectiveness of stretching to reduce injury. *British Journal of Sports Medicine* 35(2), 138.

Schur, P.E. 2001b. Author's reply. *British Journal of Sports Medicine* 35(5), 364.

Schuster, D.F. 1988. Exploring backbends. *Yoga Journal* 80(May-June), 55-60.

Schwane, J.A., and R.B. Armstrong. 1983. Effect of training on skeletal muscle injury from downhill running in rats. *Journal of Applied Physiology* 55(3) 969-975.

Schwane, J.A., J.S. Williams, and J.H. Sloan. 1987. Effects of training on delayed muscle soreness and serum creatine kinase activity after running. *Medicine and Science in Sports and Exercise* 19(6), 584-590.

Schweitzer, G. 1970. Laxity of the metacarpo-phalangeal joints of the finger and interphalangeal joint of the thumb in comparative interracial studies. *South African Medical Journal* 44(9), 246-249.

Scott, A.B. 1994. Change of eye muscle sarcomeres according to eye position. *Journal of Pediatric Ophthalmology and Strabismus* 31(2), 85-88.

Scott, D., H.A. Bird, and V. Wright. 1979. Joint laxity leading to osteoarthrosis. *Rheumatology and Rehabilitation* 18(3), 167-169.

Sechrist, W.C., and G.A. Stull. 1969. Effects of mild activity, heat applications, and cold applications on range of joint movement. *American Corrective Therapy Journal* 23(4), 120-123.

Sédat, J., M. Dib, H. Mahagne, M. Lonjon, and P. Paquis. 2002. Stroke after chiropractic manipulation as a result of extracranial postero-inferior cerebellar artery dissection. *Journal of Manipulative and Physiological Therapeutics* 25(9), 588-590.

Segal, D.D. 1983. An anatomic and biomechanical approach to low back health: A preventive approach. *Journal of Sports Medicine and Physical Fitness* 23(4), 411-421.

Segal, R.L., and S.L. Wolf. 1994. Operant conditions of spinal stretch reflexes in patients with spinal cord injuries. *Experimental Neurology* 130(2), 202-213.

Seimon, L.P. 1983. *Low back pain: Clinical diagnosis and management.* Norwalk, CT: Appleton-Century-Crofts.

Seliger, V., L. Dolejs, and V. Karas. 1980. A dynamometric comparison of maximum eccentric, concentric and isometric contraction using EMG and energy expenditure measurements. *European Journal of Applied Physiology* 45(2-3), 235-244.

Seno, S. 1968. The motion of the spine and the related electromyogram of the patient suffering from lumbago. *Electromyography* 8(2), 185-186.

Sereika, S.M., and C.E. Davis. 2001. Analysis of clinical trials and treatment nonadherence. In *Compliance in healthcare and research*, ed. L.E. Burhe and I.S. Ockene, 263-284. Armonk, NY: Futura Publishing Company.

Sermeev, B.V. 1966. Development of mobility in the hip joint in sportsmen. *Yessis Review* 2(1), 16-17.

Shambaugh, J.P., A. Klein, and J.P. Herbert. 1991. Structural measures as predictors of injury in basketball players. *Medicine and Science in Sports and Exercise* 23(5), 522-527.

Shambaugh, P. 1987. Changes in electrical activity in muscles resulting from chiropractic adjustment: A pilot study. *Journal of Manipulative and Physiological Therapeutics* 10(6), 300-304.

Shamos, M.H., and L.S. Lavine. 1967. Piezoelectricity as a fundamental property of biological tissues. *Nature* 213(5073), 267-269.

Sharratt, M.T. 1984. Wrestling profile. *Clinics in Sports Medicine* 3(1), 273-289.

Shellock, F.G., and W.E. Prentice. 1985. Warming-up and stretching for improved physical performance and prevention of sports-related injuries. *Sports Medicine* 2(4), 267-278.

Shephard, R.J. 1978. *The fit athlete.* Oxford: Oxford University Press.

Shephard, R.J. 1982. *Physiology and biochemistry of exercise.* New York: Praeger.

Shepard, R.J. 1997. *Aging, physica activity, and health.* Champaign, IL: Human Kinetics.

Shephard, R.J., M. Berridge, and W. Montelpare. 1990. On the generality of the "sit and reach" test: An analysis of flexibility data for an aging population. *Research Quarterly for Exercise and Sport* 61(4), 326-330.

Shirado, O., T. Ito, K. Kaneda, and T.E. Strax. 1995. Flexion-relaxation phenomenon in the back muscles. *American Journal of Physical Medicine and Rehabilitation* 74(2), 139-144.

Shrier, I. 1999. Stretching before exercise does not reduce the risk of local muscle injury: A critical review of the clinical and basic science literature. *Clinical Journal of Sports Medicine* 9(4), 221-227.

Shrier, I. 2000. Stretching before exercise: An evidence based approach. *British Journal of Sports Medicine* 34(5), 324-325.

Shrier, I. 2001. Flexibility versus stretching. *British Journal of Sports Medicine* 35(5), 364.

Shrier, I. 2002. Does stretching help prevent injuries? In *Evidence-based sports medicine*, ed. D. MacAuley and T.M. Best, 97-116. London: BMJ Books.

Shrier, I., and K. Gossal. 2000. Myths and truths of stretching. *The Physician and Sportsmedicine* 28(8), 57-63.

Shustova, N.Y., N.A. Maltsev, Y.I. Levkovich, and V.A. Levtov. 1985. Postelongation hyperemia in gastrocnemius muscle capillaries. *Fiziologicheskii Zhurnal SSR Imeni I.M. Sechenova* 71(5), 599-608. (In *Biological Abstract* 81(4), p. 169. No. 30857, Feb. 1986.)

Shustova, N.Y., A.T. Matchanov, and V.A. Levtov. 1985. Effect of the compression of gastrocnemius muscle vessels on the muscle blood supply in stretching. *Fiziologicheskii Zhurnal SSSR Imeni I.M. Sechenova* 71(9), 1105-1111. (In *Biological Abstract* 81(9), p. 164. No. 79766, May 1986.)

Shyne, K. 1982. Richard H. Dominguez, M.D.: To stretch or not to stretch? *The Physician and Sportsmedicine* 10(9), 137-140.

Siff, M.C. 1992. A flat back. *Fitness and Sports Review International* 27(3), 88.

Siff, M.C. 1993a. Exercise and the soft tissues. *Fitness and Sports Review International* 28(1), 32.

Siff, M.C. 1993b. Soft tissue biomechanics and flexibility. *Fitness and Sports Review International* 28(4), 127-128.

Siff, M.C., and Y.V. Verkhoshansky. 1999. *Supertraining.* 4th ed. Denver, Colorado: Supertraining International.

Sihvonen, T. 1997. Flexion relaxation of the hamstring muscles during lumbar-pelvic rhythm. *Archives of Physical Medicine and Rehabilitation* 78(5), 486-490.

Sihvonen, T., J. Partanen, O. Hänninen, and S. Soimakallio. 1991. Electric behavior of low back muscles during lumbar pelvic rhythm in low back pain patients and healthy controls. *Archives of Physical Medicine and Rehabilitation* 72(13), 1080-1087.

Silman, A.J., D. Haskard, and S. Day. 1986. Distribution of joint mobility in a normal population: Results of the use of fixed torque measuring devices. *Annals of the Rheumatic Diseases* 45(1), 27-30.

Simard, T.G., and J.V. Basmajian. 1967. Methods in training conscious control of motor units. *Archives of Physical Medicine and Rehabilitation* 48(1), 12-19.

Simon, R.W. 1992. *Stretching and warm-up habits of selected college students.* Master's thesis. University of Florida, Gainesville, Florida.

Simons, D.G., J.G. Travell, and L.S. Simons. 1999. *Travel & Simons' myofascial pain and dysfunction: The trigger point manual, Volume 1. Upper half of the body.* 2nd ed. Philadelphia: Williams & Wilkins.

Simpson, D.G., W. Carver, T.K. Borg, and L. Terracio. 1994. Role of mechanical stimulation in the establishment and maintenance of muscle cell differentiation. *International Review of Cytology* 150, 69-94.

Sing, R.F. 1984. *The dynamics of the javelin throw*. Cherry Hill, NJ: Reynolds.

Singer, K.P. 1997. Contradictions to spinal manipulation. In *Clinical anatomy and management of low back pain*, ed. L.G.F. Giles and K.P. Singer, 387-391. Oxford: Butterworth Heinmann.

Singh, M., and P.V. Karpovich. 1966. Isotonic and isometric forces of forearm flexors and extensors. *Journal of Applied Physiology* 21(4), 1435-1437.

Sirbaugh, N. 1995. Pedagogical opinion: The effects of exercise on singing. *The NATS Journal* 51(5), 27-29.

Slocum, D.B., and S.L. James. 1968. Biomechanics of running. *Journal of the American Medical Association* 205(11), 97-104.

Sluijs, E.M., J.J. Kerssens, J. van der Zee, and L.B. Myers. 1998. Adherence to physiotherapy. In *Adherence to treatment in medical conditions*, ed. L.B. Myers and K. Midence, 363-382. Amsterdam: Hardwood Academic Publishers.

Sluijs, E.M., G.J. Kok, and J. van der Zee. 1993. Correlates of exercise compliance in physical therapy. *Physical Therapy* 73(11), 771-786.

Smith, C.A. 1994. The warm-up procedure: To stretch or not to stretch. A brief review. *Journal of Orthopaedic and Sports Physical Therapy* 19(1), 12-17.

Smith, C.F. 1977. Physical management of muscular low back pain in the athlete. *Canadian Medical Association Journal* 117(September 17), 632-635.

Smith, J.L., R.S. Hutton, and E. Eldred. 1974. Post contraction changes in sensitivity of muscle afferents to static and dynamic stretch. *Brain Research* 78(September-October), 193-202.

Smith, J.W. 1966. Factors influencing nerve repair. I. Blood supply of peripheral nerves. *Archives of Surgery* 93(2), 335-341.

Smith, R.E. 1986. Toward a cognitive-affective model of athletic burnout. *Journal of Sport Psychology* 8(1), 36-50.

Solomonow, M., and R. D'Ambrosia. 1991. Neural reflex arcs and muscle control of knee stability and motion. In *Ligament and extensor mechanism injuries of the knee*, ed. W.N. Scott, 389-400. St. Louis: Mosby-Year Book.

Song, T.M.K. 1979. Flexibility of ice hockey players and comparison with other groups. In *Science in skiing, skating and hockey*, ed. J. Terauds and H.J. Gros, 117-125. Del Mar, CA: Academic.

Song, T.M., and G.T. Garvie. 1976. Wrestling with flexibility. *Canadian Journal for Health, Physical Education and Recreation* 43(1), 18-26.

Song, T.M.K., and G.T. Garvie. 1980. Anthropometric, flexibility, strength, and physiological measures of Canadian and Japanese Olympic wrestlers. *Canadian Journal of Applied Sport Science* 5(1), 1-8.

Sontag, S., and J.N. Wanner. 1988. The cause of leg cramps and knee pains: A hypothesis and effective treatment. *Medical Hypotheses* 25(1), 35-41.

Sorimachi, H., Y. Ono, and K. Suzuki. 2000. Skeletal muscle-specific calpain, p94, and connectin/titin: Their physiological functions and relationship to limb-girdle muscular dystrophy type 2a. In *Advances in experimental medicine and biology. Elastic filaments of the cell*, 481, ed. H.L. Granzier and G.H. Pollack, 383-397. New York: Kluwer Academic/Plenum Publishers.

Soussi-Yanicostas, N., C.B. Hamida, G.S. Butler-Browne, F. Hentati, K. Bejaoui, and M.B. Hamida. 1991. Modification in the expression and location of contractile and cytoskeletal proteins in Schwartz-Jampel syndrome. *Journal of the Neurological Sciences* 104(1), 64-73.

Souza, T.A. 1994. General treatment approaches for shoulder disorder. In *Sports injuries of the shoulder: Conservative management*, ed. T.A. Souza, 107-124. Edinburgh: Churchill Livingstone.

Sovik, R. 2000. The science of breathing—The yogic view. *Progress in Brain Research* 122, 491-505.

Speaight, G. 1980. *A history of the circus*. New York: A.S. Barnes and Company.

Spernoga, S.G., T.L. Uhl, B.L. Arnold, and B.M. Gansneder. 2001. Duration of maintained hamstring flexibility after a one-time, modified hold-relax stretching protocol. *Journal of Athletic Training* 36(1), 44-48.

Spielholz, N.I. 1990. Scientific basis of exercise. In *Therapeutic exercise*. 5th ed. eds. J.V. Basmajian and S.L. Wolf, 49-76. Baltimore: Williams & Wilkins.

Spindler, K.P., and E.M. Benson. 1994. Natural history of posterior cruciate ligament injury. *Sports Medicine and Arthroscopy Review* 2(2), 73-79.

Spoerl, J., M. Mottice, and E.K. Benner. 1994. *Soft tissue mobilization-techniques*. 2nd ed. Canton, Ohio: JEMD.

Stafford, M., and W. Grana. 1984. Hamstring/quadriceps ratios in college football players: A high velocity evaluation. *American Journal of Sports Medicine* 12(3), 209-211.

Stainsby, W.N., J.T. Fales, and J.L. Lilienthal. 1956. Effect of stretch on oxygen consumption of dog skeletal muscle in situ. *Bulletin of the Johns Hopkins Hospital* 99(5), 249-261.

Stamford, B. 1981. Flexibility and stretching. *The Physician and Sportsmedicine* 12(2), 171.

Stanitski, C.L. 1995. Articular hypermobility and chondral injury in patients with acute patellar dislocation. *American Journal of Sports Medicine* 23(2), 146-150.

Starring, D.T., M.R. Gossman, G.G. Nicholson, Jr., and J. Lemons. 1988. Comparison of cyclic and sustained passive stretching using a mechanical device to increase resting length of hamstring muscles. *Physical Therapy* 68(3), 314-320.

Stauber, W.T. 1989. Eccentric action of muscles: Physiology, injury, and adaptation. In *Exercise and sports sciences reviews*, ed. K. Pandolf, 157-185. Baltimore: Williams & Wilkins.

Steban, R.E., and S. Bell. 1978. *Track & field: An administrative approach to the science of coaching*. New York: Wiley & Sons.

Steele, V.A., and J.A. White. 1986. Injury prevention in female gymnasts. *British Journal of Sports Medicine* 20(1), 31-33.

Steinacker, J.M., M. Both, and B.J. Whipp. 1993. Pulmonary mechanics and entrainment of respiration and stroke rate during rowing. *International Journal of Sports Medicine* 14(Suppl. 1), S15-S19.

Steindler, A. 1977. *Kinesiology of the human body*. Springfield, IL: Charles C Thomas.

Steinmann, B., P.M. Royce, and A. Superti-Furga. 1993. The Ehlers-Danlos syndrome. In *Connective tissue and its heritable disorders: Molecular, genetic and medical aspects*, eds., P.M. Royce and B. Steinmann, 351-407. New York: Wiley-Liss.

Stevens, A., H. Stijns, N. Rosselle, and F. Decock. 1977. Litheness and hamstring muscles. *Electromyography and Clinical Neurophysiology* 17(6), 507-511.

Stevens, A., H. Stijns, N. Rosselle, K. Stappaerts, and A. Michels. 1974. Slowly stretching the hamstrings and compliance. *Electromyography and Clinical Neurophysiology* 14(5-6), 495-496.

Steventon, C., and G. Ng. 1995. Effect of trunk flexion speed on flexion relaxation or erector spinae. *Australian Journal of Physiotherapy* 41(4), 239-241.

Stewart, I.B. and G.G. Sleivert. 1998. The effect of warm-up intensity on range of motion and anaerobic performance. *Journal of Orthopaedic and Sports Physical Therapy* 27(2), 154-161.

Stewart, R.B. 1987. Drug use and adverse drug reactions in the elderly: An epidemiological perspective. *Topics in Geriatric Rehabilitation* 2(3), 1-11.

Stiles, E.G. 1984. Manipulation: A tool for your practice? *Patient Care* 18(9), 16-42.

Stockton, I.D., T. Reilly, F.H. Sanderson, and T.J. Walsh. 1980. Investigations of circadian rhythm in selected components of sports performance. *Bulletin of the Society of Sports Sciences* 1(1), 14-15.

Stoddard, A. 1979. *The back, relief from pain*. New York: Arco.

Stokes, I.A., D.G. Wilder, J.W. Frymoyer, and M.H. Pope. 1981. Assessment of patients with low back pain by biplanar radiographic measurement of intervertebral motion. *Spine* 6(3), 233-238.

Stone, D.A., R. Kamenski, J. Shaw, K.M.J. Nachazel, S.F. Conti, and F.H. Fu. 2001. Dance. In *Sports injuries: Mechanisms, prevention, treatment*. 2nd ed, ed. F.H. Fu and D.A. Stone, 380-397. Philadelphia: Lippincott Williams & Wilkins.

Stone, W.J., and W.A. Kroll. 1991. *Sports conditioning and weight training: Programs for athletic competition*. 3rd ed. Dubuque, Iowa: Wm. C. Brown.

Stopka, C., K. Morley, R. Siders, J. Schuette, A. Houck, and Y. Gilmet. 2002. Stretching techniques to improve flexibility in Special Olympics athletes and their coaches. *Journal of Sport Rehabilitation* 11(1), 22-34.

Stover, C.N., G. Wiren, and S.R. Topaz. 1976. The modern golf swing and stress syndromes. *The Physician and Sportsmedicine* 4(9), 43-47.

Strauhal, M.J. 1999. Therapeutic exercise in obstetrics. In *Therapeutic exercise: Moving toward function.* eds. C. Hall and L.T. Brody, 211-232. Philadelphia: Lippincott, Williams & Wilkins.

Strauss, J.B. 1993. *Chiropractic philosophy.* Levittown, PA: Foundation for the Advancement of Chiropractic Education.

Strickler, T., T. Malone, and W.E. Garrett. 1990. The effects of passive warming on muscle injury. *American Journal of Sports Medicine* 18(2), 141-145.

Strocchi, R., L. Leonardi, S. Guizzardi, M. Marchini, and A. Ruggeri. 1985. Ultrastructural aspects of rat tail tendon sheaths. *Journal of Anatomy* 140(1), 57-67.

Stroebel, C.F. 1979. Non-specific effects and psychodynamic issues in self-regulatory techniques. Paper presented at the Johns Hopkins Conference on Clinical Biofeedback. Baltimore, MD.

Sturkie, P.D. 1941. Hypermobile joints in all descendants for two generations. *Journal of Heredity* 32(7), 232-234.

Sugamoto, K., T. Harada, A. Machida, H. Inui, T. Miyamoto, E. Takeuchi, H. Yoshikawa, and T. Ochi. 2002. Scapulohemeral rhythm: Relationship between motion velocity and rhythm. *Clinical Orthopaedics and Related Research* Aug(401), 119-124.

Sugaya, H., A. Tsuchiya, H. Moriya, D. Morgan, and S.A. Banks. 1999. Low back injury in elite and professional golfers: An epdemiologic and radiographic study. In *Science and golf III: Proceedings of the 1998 World Scientific Congress of Golf,* eds. M.R. Farrally and A.J. Cochran, 38-91. Champaign, IL: Human Kinetics.

Sullivan, M.K., J.J. Dejulia, and T.W. Worrell. 1992. Effect of pelvic position and stretching method on hamstring muscle flexibility. *Medicine and Science in Sports and Exercise* 24(12), 1383-1389.

Sullivan, P.D., P.E. Markos, and M.D. Minor. 1982. *An integrated approach to therapeutic exercise theory and clinical application.* Reston, VA: Reston.

Suminski, R.R., C.O. Mattern, and S.T. Devor. 2002. Influence of racial origin and skeletal muscle properties on disease prevalence and physical performance. *Sports Medicine* 32(11), 667-673.

Sun, J-S., Y-H. Tsuang, T-K. Liu, Y-S. Hang, C-K. Cheng, and W.W-L. Lee. 1995. Viscoplasticity of rabbit skeletal muscle under dynamic cyclic loading. *Clinical Biomechanics* 10(5), 258-262.

Sundberg, J. 1983. Chest wall vibrations in singers. *Journal of Speech and Hearing Research* 26(3), 329-340.

Sunderland, S. 1978. Traumatized nerves, roots and ganglia: Musculoskeletal factors and neuropathological consequences. In *The neurobiologic mechanism in manipulative therapy,* ed. I.M. Korr, 137-166. New York: Plenum Press.

Sunderland, S. 1991. *Nerve injuries and their repair: A critical appraisal.* 3rd ed. London: Churchill Livingstone.

Sunderland, S., and K.C. Bradley. 1961. Stress-strain phenomena in human spinal nerve roots. *Brain* 84(1), 102-119.

Surburg, P.R. 1981. Neuromuscular facilitation techniques in sportsmedicine. *The Physician and Sportsmedicine* 18(1), 114-127.

Surburg, P.R. 1983. Flexibility exercise re-examined. *Athletic Training* 18(1), 37-40.

Sutcliffe, M.C., and J.M. Davidson. 1990. Effect of static stretching on elastin production by porchine aortic smooth muscle cells. *Matrix* 10(3), 148-153.

Sutro, C.J. 1947. Hypermobility of bones due to "overlengthened" capsular and ligamentous tissues. *Surgery* 21(1), 67-76.

Sutton, G. 1984. Hamstrung by hamstring strains: A review of the literature. *Journal of Orthopaedic and Sports Physical Therapy* 5(4), 184-195.

Suzuki, S., and R.S. Hutton. 1976. Postcontractile motorneuron discharge produced by muscle afferent activation. *Medicine and Science in Sports* 8(4), 258-264.

Suzuki, S., and G.H. Pollack. 1986. Bridge-like interconnections between thick filaments in stretched skeletal muscle fibers observed by the freeze-fractured method. *Journal of Cell Biology* 102(3), 1093-1098.

Sward, L., B. Eriksson, and L. Peterson. 1990. Anthropometric characteristics, passive hip flexion, and spinal mobility in relation to back pain in athletes. *Spine* 15(5), 376-382.

Sweet, S. 2001. Warm-up or no warm-up *Strength and Conditioning Journal* 23(6), 36.

Tabary, J.C., C. Tabary, C. Tardieu, G. Tardieu, and G. Goldspink. 1972. Physiological and structural changes in the cat's soleus muscle due to immobilization at different lengths by plaster casts. *Journal of Physiology (London)* 224(1), 231-244.

Talag, T. 1973. Residual muscle soreness as influenced by concentric, eccentric, and static contractions. *Research Quarterly* 44(4), 458-469.

Talbot, J.A., and D.L. Morgan. 1996. Quantitative analysis of sarcomere non-uniformities in active muscle following a stretch. *Journal of Muscle Research and Cell Motility* 17(2), 261-268.

Talbot, J.A., and D.L. Morgan. 1998. The effects of stretch parameters on eccentric exercise-induced damage to toad skeletal muscle. *Journal of Muscle Research and Cell Motility* 19(3), 237-245.

Tamkun, J.W., D.W. DeSimone, D. Fonda, R.S. Patel, C. Buck, A.F. Horwitz, and R.O. Hynes. 1986. Structure of integrin, a glycoprotein involved in the transmembrane linkage between fibronectin and actin. *Cell* 46(2), 271-282.

Tanigawa, M.C. 1972. Comparison of the hold-relax procedure and passive mobilization on increasing muscle length. *Physical Therapy* 52(7), 725-735.

Tanii, K., and T. Masuda. 1985. A kinesiologic study of erectores spinae during trunk flexion and extension. *Ergonomics* 28(6), 883-893.

Tatsumi, R., K. Maeda, A. Hattori, and K. Takahashi. 2001. Calcium binding to an elastic portion of connectin/titin filaments. *Journal of Muscle Research and Cell Motility,* 22(2), 149-162.

Taunton, J.E. 1982. Pre-game warm-up and flexibility. *New Zealand Journal of Sports Medicine* 10(1), 14-18.

Taylor, D.C., J.D. Dalton, A.V. Seaber, and W.E. Garrett. 1990. Viscoelastic properties of muscle-tendon units: The biomechanical effects of stretching. *American Journal of Sports Medicine* 18(3), 300-309.

Taylor, J., and S. Taylor. 1997. *Psychological approaches to sports injury rehabilitation.* Gaithersburg, MD: Aspen.

Teaching Music. 2001. Music and medicine: Preventing performance injuries. *Teaching Music* 9(2), 23-30.

Teeter Hang Ups. 2002, Oct. 12. Inversion benefits. [Online]. Available: www.teeterhangups.com/about/benefits.html [October 31, 2003].

Teitz, C.C. 1982. Sports medicine concerns in dance and gymnastics. *Pediatric Clinics of North America* 29(6), 1399-1421.

Terracio, L., D. Gullberg, K. Rubin, S. Craig, and T.K. Borg. 1989. Expression of collagen adhesion proteins and their association with the cytoskeleton in cardiac myocytes. *Anatomical Record* 223(1), 62-71.

Terrett, A.G.J., and H. Vernon. 1984. Manipulation and pain tolerance. *American Journal of Physical Medicine* 63(5), 217-225.

Tesch, P.A., H. Hjort, and U.I. Balldin. 1983. Effects of strength training on G tolerance. *Aviation Space and Environmental Medicine* 54(8), 691-695.

Tesh, K.M., J.H. Evans, J.S. Dunn, and J.P. O'Brien. 1985. The contribution of skin, fascia, and ligaments to resisting flexion of the lumbar spine. In *Biomechanical measurement in orthopaedic practice,* ed. W. Whittle and D. Harris, 179-187. Oxford: Clarendon Press.

Tessman, J.R. 1980. *My back doesn't hurt anymore.* New York: Quickfox.

Thacker, S.B., J. Gilchrist, D.F. Stroup, and C.D. Kimsey. 2002. The prevention of shin splints in sports: A systematic review of literature. *Medicine and Science in Sports and Exercise* 34(1), 32-40.

Thieme, W.T., R. Wynne-Davis, H.A.F. Blair, E.T. Bell, and J.A. Joraine. 1968. Clinical examination and urinary oestrogen assays in newborn children with congenital dislocation of the hip. *The Journal of Bone and Joint Surgery* 50B(3), 546-550.

Thigpen, L.K. 1984. Neuromuscular variation in association with static stretching (Abstract). In *Abstracts of research papers 1984,* ed. W. Kroll, 28. American Alliance for Health, Physical Education and Recreation. Washington, DC.

Thigpen, L.K., T. Moritani, R. Thiebaud, and J.L. Hargis. 1985. The acute effects of static stretching on alpha motoneuron excitability. In *Biomechanics IX-A. International series on biomechanics* Vol. 5A, ed. D.A. Winter, R.W. Norman, R.P. Wells, K.C. Hayes, and A.E. Patla, 352-357. Champaign, IL: Human Kinetics.

Thomas, D.Q., and J.C. Quindry. 1997. Exercise consumerism—Let the buyer beware! *Journal of Physical Education, Recreation & Dance* 68(3), 56-60.

Thomas, E., A. Silman, A. Papageorgiou, G. Macfarlane, and P. Croft. 1998. Association between measures of spinal mobility and low back pain. An analysis of new attenders in primary care. *Spine* 23(3), 343-347.

Thomeé, R., and J. Karlsson. 1995. Muscle and tendon injuries of the groin. *Critical Reviews in Physical and Rehabilitation Medicine* 7(4), 299-313.

Thomsen, P., and J.V. Luco. 1944. Changes of weight and neuromuscular transmission in muscles of immobilized joints. *Journal of Neurophysiology* 7(4), 245-251.

Thurston, A.J. 1985. Spinal and pelvic kinematics in osteoarthritis of the hip joint. *Spine* 10(5), 46-471.

Tideiksaar, R. 1986. Preventing falls: Home hazard checklists to help older patients protect themselves. *Geriatrics* 41(5), 26-28.

Tiidus, P., and J. Shoemaker. 1995. Effleurage massage, muscle blood flow and long-term post-exercise strength recovery. *International Journal of Sports Medicine* 16(7), 478-483.

Tillman, L.J., and G.S. Cummings. 1992. Biologic mechanisms of connective tissue mutability. In *Dynamics of human biologic tissues*, ed. D.P. Currier and R.M. Nelson, 1-44. Philadelphia: F.A. Davis.

Tilney, F., and F.H. Pike. 1925. Muscular coordination experimentally studied in its relation to the cerebellum. *Archives of Neurology and Psychiatry* 13(3), 289-334.

Tinker, D., and R.B. Rucker. 1985. Role of selected nutrients in synthesis, accumulation, and chemical modification of connective tissue proteins. *Physiological Reviews* 65(3), 607-657.

Tippett, S.R. 1986. Lower extremity strength and active range of motion in college baseball pitchers: A comparison between stance leg and kick leg. *Journal of Orthopaedic and Sports Physical Therapy* 8(1), 10-14.

Tobias, M., and M. Stewart. 1985. *Stretch and relax*. Tucson, AZ: Body Press.

Todd, T. 1985. The myth of the muscle-bound lifter. *NSCA Journal* 7(3), 37-41.

Toepfer, K. 1999. Twisted bodies: Aspects of female contortionism in the letters of a connoisseur. *The Drama Review* 43(1), 104-136.

Toft, E., G.T. Espersen, S. Kålund, T. Sinkjær, and B.C. Hornemann. 1989. Passive tension of the ankle before and after stretching. *American Journal of Sports Medicine* 17(4), 489-494.

Tolsma, B. 1985. Flexibility and velocity. *Track & Field Quarterly Review* 84(3), 44-47.

Toppenberg, R., and M. Bullock. 1986. The interrelation of spinal curves, pelvic tilt and muscle length in the adolescent female. *Australian Journal of Physiotherapy* 32, 6-12.

Toppenberg, R., and M. Bullock. 1990. Normal lumbo-pelvic muscle length and their interrelationships in adolescent females. *Australian Journal of Physiotherapy* 36, 105-109.

Torg, J.S., J.J. Vegso, and E. Torg. 1987. *Rehabilitation of athletic injuries: An atlas of therapeutic exercise*. Chicago: Year Book Medical.

Torgan, C.J. 1985. *The effects of static stretching upon muscular distress*. Master's thesis, University of Massachusetts.

Toufexis, A. 1974. The price of an art. *Physician's World* 2(4), 44-50.

Tovin, B., and M. Neyer. 2001. Diving. In *Sports injury prevention & rehabilitation*, ed. E. Shamus and J. Shamus, 155-184. New York: McGraw-Hill.

TRECO. 1987. *Power stretch*. Newport News, VA: TRECO Products.

Trendelenburg, W. 1923. *Zur physiologie de spielbewegung in der musikausübung*. *Pflüger's Archiv für die gesamie Physiologie des Menschen der Tiere* 210, 198-201.

Trendelenburg, W. 1925. *Die natürlichen grundlagen der kunst des streichinstrumentenspiels*. Berlin: Springer.

Trinick, J., P. Knight, and A. Whiting. 1984. Purification and properties of native titin. *Journal of Molecular Biology* 180(2), 331-356.

Troels, B. 1973. Achilles tendon rupture. *Acta Orthopaedica Scandinavica* 152(Suppl.), 1-126.

Trombitás, K., M. Greaser, S. Labeit, J.P. Jin, M. Kellermayer, M. Helmes, and H. Granzier. 1998. Titin extensibility in situ: Entropic elasticity of permanently folded and permanently unfolded molecular segments. *Journal of Cell Biology* 140(4), 853-859.

Trombitás, K., G.H. Pollack, J. Wright, and K. Wang. 1993. Elastic properties of titin filaments demonstrated using a "freeze-break" technique. *Cell Motility and the Cytoskeleton* 24(4), 274-283.

Troup, J.D.G., C.A. Hood, and A.E. Chapman. 1968. Measurement of the sagittal mobility of the lumbar spine and hips. *Annals of Physical Medicine* 9(8), 308-321.

Tsai, L., and T. Wredmark. 1993. Spinal posture, sagittal mobility, and subjective rating of back problems in former elite gymnasts. *Spine* 18(7), 872-875.

Tsatsouline, P. 2001a. *Relax into stretch*. St. Paul, MN: Dragon Door.

Tsatsouline, P. 2001b. *Super joints*. St. Paul, MN: Dragon Door.

Tschernogubow, A. 1892. Cutis laxa. *Monatshefte für Praktische Dermatologie* 14(2), 76.

Tskhovrebova, L., and J. Trinick. 2000. Extensibility in the titin molecule and its relation to muscle elasticity. In *Advances in experimental medicine and biology. Elastic filaments of the cell*, Vol. 481, ed. H.L. Granzier and G.H. Pollack, 163-173. New York: Kluwer Academic/Plenum Publishers.

Tskhovrebova, L., and J. Trinick. 2001. Flexibility and extensibility in the titin molecule: Analysis of electron microscope data. *Journal of Molecular Biology* 310(4), 755-771.

Tucker, C. 1990. *The mechanics of sports injuries: An osteopathic approach*. Oxford: Blackwell Scientific.

Tullos, H.S., and J.W. King. 1973. Throwing mechanism in sport. *Orthopedic Clinics of North America* 4(3), 709-720.

Tullson, P., and R.B. Armstrong. 1968. Exercise induced muscle inflammation. *Federation Proceeding* 37(3), 663.

Tullson, P., and R.B. Armstrong. 1981. Muscle hexose monophosphate shunt activity following exercise. *Experimentia* 37(12), 1311-1312.

Tumanyan, G.S., and S.M. Dzhanyan. 1984. Strength exercises as a means of improving active flexibility of wrestlers. *Soviet Sports Review* 19(3), 146-150.

Turek, S.L. 1984. *Orthopaedics principles and their application*. 4th ed. Philadelphia: Lippincott.

Turk, D.C. 1993. Commentaries. *Physical Therapy* 73(11), 771-786.

Turl, S.E., and K.P. George. 1998. Adverse neural tension: A factor in repetitive hamstring strain? *Journal of Orthopaedic and Sports Physical Therapy* 27(1), 16-21.

Turner, A.A. 1977. *The effects of two training methods on flexibility*. Master's thesis, Lakehead University.

Turner, A.A., and R. Frey. 1984. Active-static flexibility conditioning: A research proposal submitted to the UAA Rights of Human Subjects Committee (Proposal II), School of Education, Department of Physical Education. University of Alaska, Anchorage.

Tuttle, W.W. 1924. The effect of sleep upon the patellar tendon reflex. *American Journal of Physiology* 68(2), 345-348.

Tweitmeyer, T.A. 1974. *A comparison of two stretching techniques for increasing and retaining flexibility*. Master's thesis, University of Iowa.

Twellaar, F.T., F.T.J. Verstappen, A. Huson, and W. van Mechelen. 1997. Physical characteristics as risk factors for sports injuries: A four year prospective study. *International Journal of Sports Medicine* 18(1), 66-71.

Tyne, P.J., and M. Mitchell. 1983. *Total stretching*. Chicago: Contemporary Books.

Tyrance, H.J. 1958. Relationships of extreme body types to ranges of flexibility. *Research Quarterly* 29(3), 349-359.

Tyrer, P.J., and A.J. Bond. 1974. Diurnal variation in physiological tremor. *Electroencephalography and Clinical Neurophysiology* 37(1), 35-40.

Ulmer, R.A. 1989. The past, present, and predicted future of the patient compliance field. [Editorial] *Journal of Compliance in Health Care* 4(2), 89-93.

Unsworth, A., D. Dowson, and V. Wright. 1971. Cracking joints: A bioengineering study of cavitation in the metacarpophalangeal joint. *Annals of the Rheumatic Diseases* 30(4), 348-358.

Upton, A.R.M., and P.F. Radford. 1975. Motoneuron excitability in elite sprinters. In *Biomechanics*, ed. P.V. Komi, 82-87. Baltimore, MD: University Park.

Uram, P. 1980. *The complete stretching book*. Mountain View, CA: Anderson World.

Urban, J.P.G., and M.T. Bayliss. 1989. Regulation of proteoglycan synthesis rate in cartilage in vitro: Influence of extracellular ionic composition. *Biochemica et Biophysica Acta* 992, 59-65.

Urban, J., A. Maroudas, M. Bayliss, and J. Dillon. 1979. Swelling pressures of proteoglycans at the concentration found in cartilagenous tissues. *Biorheology* 16(6), 447-464.

Urban, L.M. 1981. The straight-leg-raising test: A review. *The Journal of Orthopaedic and Sports Physical Therapy* 2(3), 117-134.

Urry, D.W. 1984. Protein elasticity based on conformations of sequential polypeptides: The biological elastic fiber. *Journal of Protein Chemistry* 3(5-6), 403-436.

US Department of Commerce, Bureau of the Census 1998. *Statistical abstract of the United States: The national data book.* 118th ed. Washington, DC: US Government Printing Office.

Ushijama, I., K. Yamada, T. Inoue, T. Tokunaga, T. Furukawa, and Y. Noda. 1984. Muscarinic and nicotinic effects on yawning and tongue protruding in the rat. *Pharmacology Biochemistry and Behavior* 21(2), 297-300.

Vallbo, A.B. 1974a. Afferent discharge from human muscle spindles in non-contracting muscles. Steady state impulse frequency as a function of the joint angle. *Acta Physiologica Scandinavica* 90(2), 303-318.

Vallbo, A.B. 1974b. Human muscle spindle discharge during isometric voluntary contractions. Amplitude relations between spindle frequency and torque. *Acta Physiologica Scandinavica* 90(2), 319-336.

Van Beveren, P.J. 1979. Effects of muscle stretching program on muscle strength. *Empire State Physical Therapy* 20, 9.

Vandenburgh, H.H. 1987. Motion into mass: How does tension stimulate muscle growth? *Medicine and Science in Sports and Exercise* 19(5), S142-S149.

Vandenburgh, H.H. 1992. Mechanical forces and their second messengers in stimulating cell growth in vitro. *American Journal of Physiology* 31(3), R350-R355.

Vandenburgh, H.H., S. Hatfaludy, P. Karlisch, and J. Shansky. 1991. Mechanically induced alterations in cultured skeletal muscle growth. *Journal of Biomechanics* 24 (Suppl. 1), 91-99.

Vandenburgh, H.H., and S. Kaufman. 1979. In vitro model for stretch-induced hypertrophy of skeletal muscle. *Science* 203(4377), 265-268.

Vandenburgh, H.H., and S. Kaufman. 1983. Stretch and skeletal myotube growth: What is the physical to biochemical linkage? *Frontiers of exercise biology*, eds. K.T. Borer, D.W. Edington and T.P. White, 71-84. Champaign, IL: Human Kinetics.

Vander, A.J., J.H. Sherman, and D.S. Luciano. 1975. *Human physiology: The mechanics of body function.* 2nd ed. New York: McGrw-Hill.

van der Heijden, G.J.M.G., A.J.H.M. Beurskens, B.W. Koes, W.J.J. Assendelft, H.C.W. de Vet, and L.M. Bouter. 1995. The efficacy of traction for back and neck pain: A systematic, blinded review of randomized clinical trial methods. *Physical Therapy* 75(2), 93-104.

Van der Meulin, J.H.C. 1982. Present state of knowledge on processes of healing in collagen structures. *International Journal of Sports Medicine* 3(Suppl. 1), 4-8.

van der Ven, P.F.M., S. Wiesner, P. Salmikangas, D. Aurbach, M. Himmel, S. Kempa, K. Hayess, D. Pacholosky, A. Taivainen, R. Schröder, O. Carpén, and D.O. Fürst. 2000. Indications for a novel muscular dystrophy pathway: Gamma-filamin, the muscle-specific filamin isoform, interacts with myotilin, *Journal of Cell Biology* 151(2), 235-247.

Vandervoort, A.A., B.M. Chesworth, D.A. Cunningham, D.H. Patterson, P.A. Rechnitzer, and J.J. Koval. 1992. Age and sex effects on mobility of the human ankle. *Journal of Gerontology* 47(1), M17-M21.

Vandervoort, A.A., K.C. Hayes, and Y. Bélanger. 1986. Strength and endurance of skeletal muscle in the elderly. *Physiotherapy Canada* 38(3), 167-173.

Vandervoort, A.A., and A.J. McComas. 1986. Contractile changes in opposing muscles of the human ankle joint with aging. *Journal of Applied Physiology* 61(1), 361-367.

Van Deusen, J., and D. Harlowe. 1987. A comparison of the ROM dance home exercise rest program with traditional routines. *Occupational Therapy Journal of Research* 7(6), 349-361.

van Dieën, J.H., and H.M. Toussaint. 1993. Spinal shrinkage as a parameter of functional load. *Spine* 18(11), 1504-1514.

van Mechelen, W., H. Hlobil, H.C.C. Kemper, W.J. Voorn, and R. de Jongh. 1993. Prevention of running injuries by warm-up, cool-down, and stretching exercises. *American Journal of Sports Medicine* 21(5), 711-719.

Van Wjimen, P.M. 1986. The management of recurrent low back pain. In *Modern manual therapy of the vertebral column*, ed. G.P. Grieve, 756-776. Edinburgh: Churchill Livingstone.

Vasu, S.C. 1933. *The Gheranda Samhita: A treatise on hatha yoga.* Adyar, Madras, India: Theosophical.

Verkhoshansky, Y., and M.C. Siff. 1993. Some facts on warming up. *Fitness and Sports Review International* 28(2), 64-65.

Vernon, H.T., M.S.I. Dhami, T.P. Howley, and R. Annett. 1986. Spinal manipulation and beta-endorphin: A controlled study of the effect of a spinal manipulation on plasma beta-endorphin levels in normal males. *Journal of Manipulative and Physiological Therapeutics* 9(2), 115-123.

Vernon, H., J. Meschino, and J. Naiman. 1985. Inversion therapy: A study of physiological effects. *Journal of the Canadian Chiropractic Association* 29(3), 135-140.

Verrall, G.M., J.P. Slavotinek, P.G. Barnes, G.T. Fon, and A.J. Spriggins. 2001. Clinical risk factors for hamstring muscle strain injury: A prospective study with correlation of injury by magnetic resonance imaging. *British Journal of Sports Medicine* 35(6), 435-440.

Verzar, F. 1963. Aging of collagen. *Scientific American* 208(4), 104-117.

Verzar, F. 1964. Aging of collagen fiber. In *International review of connective tissue research* Vol. 2, ed. D.A. Hall, 244-300. New York: Academic Press.

Viidik, A. 1973. Functional properties of collagenous tissue. *International Review of Connective Tissue Research* 6, 127-217.

Viidik, A. 1980. Interdependence between structure and function in collagenous tissues. In *Biology of collagen*, ed. A. Viidik, and J. Vuust, 257-280. London: Academic Press.

Viidik, A., C.C. Danielson, and H. Oxlund. 1982. On fundamental and phenomenological models, structure and mechanical properties of collagen, elastin and glycosaminoglycan complexes. *Biorheology* 19(3), 437-451.

Volkov, V.M., and E.G. Milner. 1990. Running and injuries. *Soviet Sports Review* 25(2), 95-98.

Voluntary power of dislocation. 1882. *The British Medical Journal* 1, 515.

Volz, R.G., M. Lieb, and J. Benjamin. 1980. Biomechanics of the wrist. *Clinical Orthopaedics and Related Research* 149(June), 112-117.

von Wasielewski, J.W. 1975. *Life of Robert Schumann.* Translated by A.L. Alger. Detroit, MI: Information Coordinators.

Vorobiev, A.N. 1987. Weightlifting: Development of physical qualities. *Soviet Sports Review* 22(2), 62-68.

Voss, D.E., M.J. Ionta, B.J. Myers, and M. Knott. 1985. *Proprioceptive neuromuscular facilitation.* 3rd ed. New York: Harper & Row.

Vujnovich, A.L. 1995. Neural plasticity, muscle spasm and tissue manipulation: A review of the literature. *Journal of Manual & Manipulative Therapy* 3(4), 152-156.

Vujnovich, A.L., and N.J. Dawson. 1994. The effect of therapeutic muscle stretch on neural processing. *Journal of Orthopaedic and Sports Physical Therapy* 20(3), 145-153.

Waddell, G., G. Feder, A. McIntosh, M. Lewis, and A. Hutchinson. 1996. *Low back pain evidence review.* London: Royal College of General Practitioners.

Waddell, G., D. Somerville, I. Henderson, and M. Newton. 1992. Objective clinical evaluation of physical impairment in chronic low back pain. *Spine* 17(6), 617-628.

Waddington, P.J. 1976. Proprioceptive neuromuscular facilitation techniques. In *Practical exercise therapy*, ed. M. Hollis 207-213, Oxford: Blackwell Scientific.

Wagner, Ch. 1974. Determination of finger flexibility. *European Journal of Applied Physiology* 32(3), 259-278.

Wagner, Ch. 1988. The pianist's hand: Anthropometry and biomechanics. *Ergonomics* 31(1), 97-131.

Walcott, B., and E.B. Ridgeway. 1967. The ultrastructure of myosin-extracted striated muscle fibers. *American Zoologist* 7(3), 499-503.

Walker, J.M. 1981. Development, maturation and aging of human joints: A review. *Physiotherapy Canada* 33(3), 153-160.

Walker, S.M. 1961. Delay of twitch relaxation induced by stress and stress-relaxation. *Journal of Applied Physiology* 16(5), 801-806.

Wall, E.J., J.B. Massie, M.K. Kwan, B.J. Rydevik, R.R. Myers, and S.R. Garfin. 1992. Experimental stretch neuropathy: Changes in nerve conduction under tension. *Journal of Bone and Joint Surgery* 74B(1), 126-129.

Wallensten, R., and B. Eklund. 1983. Intramuscular pressures and muscle metabolism after short-term and long-term exercise. *International Journal of Sports Medicine* 4(4), 231-235.

Wallin, D., B. Ekblom, R. Grahn, and T. Nordenborg. 1985. Improvement of muscle flexibility: A comparison between two techniques. *American Journal of Sports Medicine* 13(4), 263-268.

Wallis, E.L., and G.A. Logan. 1964. *Figure improvement and body conditioning through exercise.* Englewood Cliffs, NJ: Prentice-Hall.

Walro, J.M., and J. Kucera. 1999. Why adult mammalian intrafusal and extrafusal fibers contain different myosin heavy-chain isoforms. *Trends in Neuroscience* 22(4), 180-184.

Walsh, M. 1985. Review. In F.J. Novakovski, *Trainer-assisted isolated stretching (TAIS)* (pp. ii). Lorton, VA: American Canoe Association.

Walshe, A.D., and G.J. Wilson. 1997. The influence of musculotendinous stiffness on drop jump performance. *Canadian Journal of Applied Physiology* 22(2), 117-132.

Walshe, A.D., G.J. Wilson, and A.J. Murphy. 1996. The validity and reliability of a test of lower body musculotendinous stiffness. *European Journal of Applied Physiology* 73(3-4), 332-339.

Walter, J., S.F. Figoni, F.F. Andres, and E. Brown. 1996. Training intensity and duration in flexibility. *Clinical Kinesiology* 50(2), 40-45.

Walter, S.D., L.E. Hart, J.M. McIntosh, and J.R. Sutton. 1989. The Ontario cohort study of running-related injuries. *Archives of Internal Medicine* 149(11), 2561-2564.

Walter, S.D., L.E. Hart, J.R. Sutton, J.M. McIntosh, and M. Gauld. 1988. Training habits and injury experience in distance runners: Age- and sex-related factors. *The Physician and Sportsmedicine* 16(6), 101-113.

Wang, H-K., and T. Cochrane. 2001. Mobility impairment, muscle imbalance, muscle weakness, scapular asymmetry and shoulder injury in elite volleyball athletes. *Journal of Sports Medicine and Physical Fitness* 41(3), 403-410.

Wang, H-K., A. Macfarlane, and T. Cochrane. 2000. Isokinetic performance and shoulder mobility in elite volleyball athletes from the United Kingdom. *British Journal of Sports Medicine* 34(1), 39-43.

Wang, K. 1984. Cytoskeletal matrix in striated muscle: The role of titin, nebulin and intermediate filaments. In *Contractile mechanisms in muscle*, ed. G.H. Pollack and H. Sugi, 285-306. New York: Plenum Press.

Wang, K. 1985. Sarcomere-associated cytoskeletal lattices in striated muscle. In *Cell and muscle motility* Vol. 6, ed. J.W. Shay, 315-369. New York: Plenum.

Wang, K., J.G. Forbes, and A.J. Jin. 2001. Single molecule measurements of titin elasticity. *Progress in Biophysics & Molecular Biology* 77, 1-44.

Wang, K., R. McCarter, J. Wright, J. Beverly, and R. Ramirez-Mitchell. 1991. Regulation of skeletal muscle stiffness and elasticity by titin isoforms: A test of the segmental extension model of resting tension. *Proceedings of the National Academy of Science* (USA) 88(6), 7101-7105.

Wang, K., R. Ramirez-Mitchell, and D. Palter. 1984. Titin is an extraordinarily long, flexible, and slender myofibrillar protein. *Proceedings of the National Academy of Science* (USA) 81(12), 3685-3689.

Wang, K., and J. Wright. 1988. Architecture of the sarcomere matrix of skeletal muscle: Immunoelectron microscopic evidence that suggests a set of parallel inextensible nebulin filaments anchored at the Z-line. *Journal of Cell Biology* 107(6, Pt. 1), 2199-2212.

Wang, K., and R. Ramirez-Mitchell. 1983. A network of transverse and longitudinal intermediate filaments is associated with sarcomeres of adult vertebrate skeletal muscle. *Journal of Cell Biology*, 96 (2), 562-570.

Wang, K., J. Wright, and R. Ramirez-Mitchell. 1985. Architecture of the titin/nebulin containing cytoskeletal lattice of the striated muscle sarcomere: Evidence of elastic and inelastic domains of the bipolar filaments (Abstract). *Biophysical Journal* 47, 349a.

Wang, N., J.P. Butler, and D.E. Ingber. 1993. Mechanotransduction across the cell surface and through the cytoskeleton. *Science* 260(5111), 1124-1127.

Wang, N., K. Naruse, D. Stamenovi, J.J. Fredberg, S.M. Mijailovich, I.M. Toli-Nørrelykke, T. Polte, R. Mannix, and D.E. Ingber. 2001. Mechanical behavior in living cells consistent with the tensegrity model. *Proceedings of the National Academy of Sciences of the United States of America* 98(14),7765-7770.

Warburton, D.E.R., N. Gledhill, and A. Quinney. 2001a. The effects of changes in musculoskeletal fitness on health. *Canadian Journal of Applied Physiology* 26(2), 161-216.

Warburton, D.E.R., N. Gledhill, and A. Quinney. 2001b. Musculoskeletal fitness and health. *Canadian Journal of Applied Physiology* 26(2), 217-237.

Ward, L. 1970. *The effects of the squat jump exercise on the lateral stability of the knee.* Ph.D. diss., Pennsylvania State University, University Park, PA.

Ward, R.C. 1993. Myofascial release concepts. In *Rational manual therapies*, ed. J.V. Basmajian and R. Nyberg, 223-241. Baltimore: Williams & Wilkins.

Ward, R.C. 2001. Myofascial release: A brief history. In *The myofascial release manual.* 3rd ed, ed. C. Manheim, 6-15. Thorofare, New Jersey: Slack.

Warren, A. 1968. Mobilization of the chest wall. *Physical Therapy* 48(6), 582-585.

Warren, C.G., J.F. Lehmann, and J.N. Koblanski. 1971. Elongation of rat tail tendon: Effect of load and temperature. *Archives of Physical Medicine and Rehabilitation* 57(3), 122-126.

Warren, C.G., J.F. Lehmann, and J.N. Koblanski. 1976. Heat and stretch procedures: An evaluation using rat tail tendon. *Archives of Physical Medicine and Rehabilitation* 57(3), 122-126.

Warren, G.L., D.A. Hayes, D.A. Lowe, and R.B. Armstrong 1993. Mechanical factors in the initiation of eccentric contraction-induced injury in rat soleus muscle. *Journal of Physiology* 464(May), 457-475.

Warren, G.W. 1989. *Classical ballet technique.* Tampa, FL: University of South Florida Press.

Waterman-Storer, C.M. 1991. The cytoskeleton of skeletal muscle: Is it affected by exercise? A brief review. *Medicine and Science in Sports and Exercise* 23(11), 1240-1249.

Watkins, A., A.P. Woodhull-McNeal, P.M. Clarkson, and C. Ebbeling. 1989. Lower extremity alignment and injury in young, preprofessional, college, and professional ballet dancers. *Medical Problems of Performing Artists* 4(4), 148-153.

Watson, A.W.S. 2001. Sports injuries related to flexibility, posture, acceleration, clinical defects, and previous injury in high-level players of body contact sports. *International Journal of Sports Medicine* 22(3), 222-225.

Watts, N. 1968. Improvement of breathing patterns. *Physical Therapy* 48(6), 563-581.

Wear, C.R. 1963. Relationship of flexibility measurements to length of body segments. *Research Quarterly* 34(3), 234-238.

Weaver, D. 1979. Weight-lifting advice: Flexibility the key to better lifting. *Strength Health* 47(4), 50-53.

Webber, C.E., and E.S. Garnett. 1976. Density of os calcis and limb dominance. *Journal of Anatomy* 121(1), 203-205.

Weber, F.P. 1936. The Ehlers-Danlos syndrome. *British Journal of Dermatology* 48(December), 609-617.

Webster, A.L., D.G. Syrotuik, G.L. Bell, R.L. Jones, and C.C. Hanstock. 2002. Effects of hyperbaric oxygen on recovery from exercise-induced muscle damage in humans. *Clinical Journal of Sports Medicine* 12(3), 139-150.

Webster, D. 1986. *Preparing for competition weightlifting.* Huddersfield, England: Springfield Books.

Weider, J. 1995. The case for flexibility: Unlock your massive back & shoulder muscles. *Muscle & Fitness* 56(5), 134-139.

Weiner, I.H., and H.L.Weiner. 1980. Nocturnal leg muscle cramps. *Journal of the American Medical Association* 244(20), 2332-2333.

Weinreb, R.N., J. Cook, and T.R. Friberg. 1984. Effect of inverted body position on intraocular pressure. *American Journal of Ophthalmology* 98(6), 784-787.

Weinstein, H., L. Dansky, and V. Iacopino. 1996. Torture and war trauma survivors in primary care. *Western Journal of Medicine* 165(3), 112-118.

Weis-Fogh, T., and S.O. Anderson. 1970a. In *Chemistry and molecular biology of the intracellular matrix* Vol. 1, ed. E.A. Balazs, 671-684. London: Academic Press.

Weis-Fogh, T., and S.O. Anderson. 1970b. New molecular model for the long-range elasticity of elastin. *Nature* 213(5259), 718-721.

Weisler, R.R., M. Hunter, D.F. Martin, W.W. Curl, and H. Hoen. 1996. Ankle flexibility and injury patterns in dancers. *American Journal of Sports Medicine* 24(6), 754-757.

Weldon, E.J., and A.B. Richardson. 2001. Upper extremity overuse injuries in swimming: A discussion of swimmer's shoulder. *Clinics in Sports Medicine* 20(3), 423-438.

Wells, K.B., J.M. Golding, and M.A. Burnam. 1988. Psychiatric disorder in a sample of the general population with and without chronic medical conditions. *American Journal of Psychiatry* 145(8), 976-981.

Welsh, D.G., and S.S. Segal. 1996. Muscle length directs sympathetic nerve activity and vasomotor tone in resistance vessels of hampster retractor. *Circulation Research* 79(3), 551-559.

Werner, S.L., G.S. Fleisig, C.J. Dillman, and J.R. Andrews. 1993. Biomechanics of the elbow during baseball pitching. *Journal of Orthopaedic and Sports Physical Therapy* 17(6), 274-278.

Wessel, J., and A. Wan. 1994. Effect of stretching on the intensity of delayed-onset muscle soreness. *Clinical Journal of Sport Medicine* 4(2), 83-87.

Wessling, K.C., D.A. DeVane, and C.R. Hylton. 1987. Effects of static stretch versus static stretch and ultrasound combined on triceps surae muscle extensibility in healthy women. *Physical Therapy* 67(5), 674-679.

Westgaard, R.H., and R. Björklund. 1987. Generation of muscle tension additional to postural muscle load. *Ergonomics* 30(6), 911-923.

Westling, L., S. Holm, and I. Wallentin. 1992. Temporomandibular joint dysfunction: Connective tissue variations in skin biopsy and mitral valve function. *Oral Surgery, Oral Medicine, and Oral Pathology* 74(6), 709-718.

Westling, L., and A. Mattiasson. 1992. General joint hypermobility and temporomandibular joint derangement in adolescents. *Annals of the Rheumatic Diseases* 51(1), 87-90.

Wharton, J., and P. Wharton. 1996. *The Wharton's stretch book.* New York: Three River Press.

Whelan, K.M., E.M. Gass, and C.C. Morgan. 1999. Warm-up: Efficacy of a program designed for downhill skiiing. *Australiam Journal of Physiotherapy* 45(4), 279-288.

Whipple, R.H., L.I. Wolfson, and P.M. Amerman. 1987. The relationship of knee and ankle weakness to falls in nursing home residents: An isokinetic study. *Journal of the American Geriatric Society* 35(1), 13-20.

White, A.A., and M.M. Panjabi. 1978. *Clinical biomechanics of the spine.* Philadelphia: Lippincott.

White, A.H. 1983. *Back school and other conservative approaches to low back pain.* St. Louis: Mosby.

Whiting, A., J. Wardale, and J. Trinick. 1989. Does titin regulate the length of muscle thick filaments? *Journal of Molecular Biology* 205(1), 263-268.

Whiting, W.C., and R.F. Zernicke. 1998. *Biomechanics of musculoskeletal injury.* Champaign, IL: Human Kinetics.

Wickstrom, R.L. 1963. Weight training and flexibility. *Journal of Health, Physical Education and Recreation,* 34(2), 61-62.

Wiegner, A.W. 1987. Mechanism of thixotropic behavior at relaxed joints in the rat. *Journal of Applied Physiology* 62(4), 1615-1621.

Wieman, H.M., and E. Calkins. 1986. Falls. In *The practice of geriatrics,* ed. E. Calkins, P.J. Davis, and A.B. Ford, 272-280. Philadelphia: Saunders.

Wiemann, K., and K. Hahn. 1997. Influences of strength, stretching and circulatory exercises on flexibility parameters of the human hamstrings. *International Journal of Sports Medicine* 18(5), 340-346.

Wiemann, K., A. Klee, and M. Stratmann. 1998. Filamentäre quellen der muskelruhespannung und die behandlung muskulärer dysbalancen. *Deutsche Zeitschrift für Sportmedizin* 44(4), 111-118.

Wigley, F.M. 1984. Osteoarthritis: Practical management in older patients. *Geriatrics* 39(3), 101-120.

Wiktorssohn-Möller, M., B. Öberg, J. Ekstrand, and J. Gillquist. 1983. Effects of warming up, massage, and stretching on range of motion and muscle strength in the lower extremity. *American Journal of Sports Medicine* 11(4), 249-252.

Wilby, J., K. Linge, T. Reilly, and J.D.G.Troup. 1987. Spinal shrinkage in females: Circadian variation and the effects of circuit weight-training. *Ergonomics* 30(1), 47-54.

Wiles, P. 1935. Movements of the lumbar vertebrae during flexion and extension. *Proceedings of the Royal Society of London* 28(5), 647-651.

Wilkinson, H.A. 1983. *The failed back syndrome: Etiology and therapy.* New York: Harper & Row.

Williams, J.C.P., and G. Sperryn. 1976. *Sports medicine.* 2nd ed. Baltimore: Williams & Wilkins.

Williams, P.C. 1977. *Low back and neck pain: Causes and conservative treatments.* Springfield, IL: Charles C Thomas.

Williams, P.E. 1988. Effect of intermittent stretch on immobilized muscle. *Annals of the Rheumatic Diseases* 47(12), 1014-1016.

Williams, P.E., T. Catanese, E.G. Lucey, and G. Goldspink. 1988. The importance of stretch and contractile activity in the prevention of connective tissue accumulation in muscle. *Journal of Anatomy* 158(June), 109-114.

Williams, P.E., and G. Goldspink. 1971. Longitudinal growth of striated muscle fibres. *Journal of Cell Science* 9(3), 751-767.

Williams, P.E., and G. Goldspink. 1973. The effect of immobilization on the longitudinal growth of striated muscle fibres. *Journal of Anatomy* 116(1), 45-55.

Williams, P.E., and G. Goldspink. 1976. The effect of denervation and dystrophy on the adaptation of sarcomere number to the functional length of the muscle in young and adult mice. *Journal of Anatomy* 122(2), 455-465.

Williams, P.E., and G. Goldspink. 1984. Connective tissue changes in immobilised muscle. *Journal of Anatomy* 138(2), 343-350.

Williams, P.L., L.H. Bannister, M.M. Berry, P. Collins, M. Dyson, J.E. Dussek, and M.W.J. Ferguson. eds. 1995. *Gray's anatomy.* 38th ed. Edinburgh London: Churchill Livingstone.

Williford, H.N., J.B. East, F.H. Smith, and L.A. Burry. 1986. Evaluation of warm-up for improvement in flexibility. *American Journal of Sports Medicine* 14(4), 316-319.

Willy, R.W., B.A. Kyle, S.A. Moore, and G.S. Chlebourn. 2001. Effect of cessation and resumption of static hamstring muscle stretching on joint range of motion. *Journal of Orthopaedic and Sports Physical Therapy* 31(3), 138-144.

Wilmore, J.H. 1991. The aging of bone and muscle. *Clinics in Sports Medicine* 10(2), 231-244.

Wilmore, J., and D. Costill. 1999. *Physiology of sports and exercise.* 2nd ed. Champaign, IL: Human Kinetics.

Wilmore, J., R.B. Parr, R.N. Girandola, P. Ward, P.A. Vodak, T.V. Pipes, G.T. Romerom, and P. Leslie. 1978. Physiological alterations consequent to circuit weight training. *Medicine and Science in Sports* 10(2), 79-84.

Wilson, G.J., A.J. Murphy, and J.F. Pryor. 1994. Musculotendinous stiffness: Its relationship to eccentric, isometric, and concentric performance. *Journal of Applied Physiology* 76(6), 2714-2719.

Wilson, G.J., G.A. Wood, and B.C. Elliott. 1991. The relationship between stiffness of the musculature and static flexibility: An alternative explanation for the occurrence of muscular injury. *International Journal of Sports Medicine* 12(4), 403-407.

Wilson, L.R., S.C. Gandevia, and D. Burke. 1995. Increased resting discharge of human spindle afferents following voluntary contractions. *Journal of Physiology (London)* 488(3), 833-840.

Wilson, V.E., and E.I. Bird. 1981. Effects of relation and/or biofeedback training upon hip flexion in gymnasts. *Biofeedback and Self-Regulation* 6(1), 25-34.

Wing, P., I. Tsang, F. Gagnon, L. Susak, and R. Gagnon. 1992. Diurnal changes in the profile shape and range of motion of the back. *Spine* 17(7), 761-766.

Winget, C.M., C.W. DeRoshia, and D.C. Holley. 1985. Circadian rhythms and athletic performance. *Medicine and Science in Sports and Exercise* 17(5), 498-516.

Winkenwerder, E.H., and K. Shankar. 2002. Spinal traction. In *Therapeutic physical modalities*, ed. K. Shankar and K.D. Randall, 161-176. Philadelphia: Hanley & Belfus.

Winterstein, J.F. 1989. In what way would a graduate of a SCASA college practice differently from a graduate of a CCE college? *Dynamic Chiropractic* 7(15), 1.

Wirhed, R. 1984. *Athletic ability: The anatomy of winning*. New York: Harmony Books.

Wisnes, A., and A. Kirkebø. 1976. Regional distribution of blood flow in calf muscles of rat during passive stretch and sustained contraction. *Acta Physiologica Scandinavica* 96(2), 256-266.

Witvrouw, E., L. Danneels, P. Asselman, T. D'Have, and D. Cambier. 2003. Muscle flexibility as a risk factor for developing muscle injuries in male professional soccer players: A prospective study. *American Journal of Sports Medicine* 31(1), 41-46.

Wolf, L.B., R.L. Segal, S.L. Wolf, and N. Nyberg. 1991. Quantitative analysis of surface and percutaneous electromyographic activity in lumbar erector spinae of normal young women. *Spine* 16(2), 155-161.

Wolf, M.D. 1983. Stretching a point. *Women's Sports* 5(8), 53.

Wolf, P. 2001. Creativity and chronic disease: Nicolo Paganini (1782-1840). *Western Journal of Medicine* 175(5), 345.

Wolf, S.L. 1994. Biofeedback. In *The physiological basis of rehabilitation medicine*. 2nd ed, ed. J.A. Downey, S.J. Myers, E.G. Gonzalez and J.S. Lieberman, 563-571. Boston: Butterworth-Heinmann.

Wolf, S.L., and R.L. Segal. 1990. Conditioning of the spinal stretch reflex: Implication for rehabilitation. *Physical Therapy* 70(10), 652-656.

Wolfson, M.D. 1991. The effect of muscle energy technique for increasing flexion of the lumbar spine. Master's thesis, D'Youville College, Buffalo, New York.

Wolpaw, J.R. 1983. Adaptive plasticity in the primate spinal stretch reflex: Reversal and redevelopment. *Brain Research* 278(1-2), 299-304.

Wolpaw, J.R., D.J. Braitman, and R.F. Seegal. 1983. Adaptive plasticity in the primate spinal stretch reflex: Initial development. *Journal of Neurophysiology* 50(6), 1296-1311.

Wolpaw, J.R., and J.S. Carp. 1990. Memory traces in spinal cord. *Trends in Neuroscience* 13(4), 137-142.

Wolpaw, J.R., and C.L. Lee. 1989. Memory traces in primate spinal cord produced by operant conditioning of H-reflex. *Journal of Neurophysiology* 61(3), 563-572.

Wolpaw, J.R., C.L. Lee, and J.S. Carp. 1991. Operantly conditioned plasticity in spinal cord. *Annals of the New York Academy of Sciences* 627, 338-348.

Wolpaw, J.R., P.A. Noonan, and J.A. O'Keefe. 1984. Adaptive plasticity and diurnal rhythm in the primate spinal stretch reflex are independent phenomenon. *Brain Research* 33(2), 385-391.

Wolpaw, J.R., and R.F. Seegal. 1982. Diurnal rhythm in the spinal stretch reflex. *Brain Research* 244(2), 365-369.

Wolpaw, J.R., and A.N. Tennissen. 2001. Activity-dependent spinal cord plasticity in health and disease. *Annual Review of Neuroscience* 24, 807-843.

Wolpe, J. 1958. *Psychotherapy by reciprocal inhibition*. Stanford: Stanford University Press.

Woo, S.L.-Y. 1982. Mechanical properties of tendon and ligament: I. Quasi-static and nonlinear viscoelastic properties. *Biorheology* 19(3), 385-396.

Woo, S.L.-Y., M.A. Gomez, and W.H. Akeson. 1985. Mechanical behaviors of soft tissues: Measurements, modifications, injuries, and treatments. In *The biomechanics of trauma*, ed. A.M. Nahum and J. Melvin. Norwalk, CT: Appleton-Century-Crofts.

Woo, S., J.V. Matthews, W.H. Akeson, D. Amiel, and R. Convery. 1975. Connective tissue response to immobility: Correlative study of bio-mechanical and biologic measurements of normal and immobilized rabbit knees. *Arthritis Rheumatology* 18(3), 257-264.

Wood, P.H.N. 1971. Is hypermobility a discrete entity? *Proceedings of the Royal Society of Medicine* 64(6), 690-692.

Wood, P.L., D. Cheney, and E. Costa. 1978b. Modulation of the turn-over rate of hippocampal acetylcholine by neuropeptides: Possible site of action of alpha-melanocyte stimulating hormone, adreno-corticotrophic hormone, and somatostatin. *Journal of Pharmacology and Experimental Therapeutics* 209(1), 97-103.

Wood, P.L., D. Malthe-Sørenssen, D.L. Cheney, and E. Costa. 1978a. Increase of hippocampal acetylcholine turnover rate and the stretch-ing-yawning syndromes elicited by alpha-MSH and ACTH. *Life Sciences* 22(8), 673-678.

Woods, M.J. 2002. Shin splints. In *Essentials of physical medicine and rehabilitation*, ed. W.R. Frontera and J.K. Silver, 375-378. Philadelphia: Hanley & Belfus.

Wordsworth, P., D. Ogilvie, R. Smith, and B. Sykes. 1987. Joint mobility with particular reference to racial variation and inherited connective tissue disorders. *British Journal of Rheumatology* 26(1), 9-12.

Workman, D. 1999. Injury prevention: The teacher's responsibility. *Percussive Notes* 37(3), 57, 59-60.

Workman, D. 2002. Preparing for performance. Part 3: Physical preparation. *Percussive Notes* 40(3), 54-59.

World Chiropractic Alliance. 1993. *Practice guidelines for straight chiropractic*. Chandler, AZ: Author.

World Chiropractic Alliance. 1998. *Clinical practice guideline: Vertebral subluxation in chiropractic practice*. Council on Chiropractic Practice.

Worrell, T.W., and D.H. Perrin. 1992. Hamstring muscle injury: The influence of strength, flexibility, warm-up, and fatigue. *Journal of Orthopaedic and Sports Physical Therapy* 16(1), 12-18.

Worrell, T.W., D.H. Perrin, B.M. Gansneder, and J.H. Gieck. 1991. Comparison of isokinetic strength and flexibility measures between hamstring injured and noninjured athletes. *Journal of Orthopaedic and Sports Physical Therapy* 13(3), 118-125.

Worrell, T.W., T.L. Smith, and J. Winegardner. 1994. Effect of hamstring stretching on hamstring muscle performance. *Journal of Orthopaedic and Sports Physical Therapy* 20(3), 154-159.

Worrell, T.W., M.K. Sullivan, and J.J. DeJulia. 1992. Reliability of an active-knee-extension test for determining hamstring muscle flexibility. *Journal of Sport Rehabilitation* 1(3), 181-187.

Wreje, U., P. Kristiansson, H. Åberg, B. Byström, and B-V. Schoultz. 1995. Serum levels of relaxin during the menstrual cycle and oral contraceptive use. *Gynecologic and Obstetric Investigation* 39(3), 197-200.

Wright, V., and R.J. Johns. 1960. Physical factors concerned with the stiffness of normal and diseased joints. *Bulletin of the Johns Hopkins Hospital* 106(4), 215-231.

Wristen, B.G. 2000. Avoiding piano-related injury: A proposed theoretical procedure for biomechanical analysis of piano technique. *Medical Problems of Performing Artists* 15(2), 55-64.

Wyke, B. 1967. The neurology of joints. *Annals of the Royal College of Surgeons of England* 41(1), 25-50.

Wyke, B. 1972. Articular neurology—A review. *Physiotherapy* 58(3), 94-99.

Wyke, B. 1979. Neurology of the cervical spinal joints. *Physiotherapy* 65(3), 72-76.

Wyke, B. 1985. Articular neurology and manipulative theray. In *Aspects of manipulative therapy*. 2nd ed. ed. E.F. Glasgow, L.T. Twomey, E.R. Scull, and A.M. Kleynhans, 72-77. London: Churchill Livingstone.

Wynne-Davies, R. 1971. Familial joint laxity. *Proceedings of the Royal Society of Medicine* 64(6), 689-690.

Yaggie, J.A., and W.J. Armstrong. 2002. Flexibility outcomes of children with spastic cerebral palsy during a semester of play-based therapy. *Clinical Kinesiology* 56(2), 19-24.

Yagi, N., and I. Matsubara. 1984. Cross-bridge movements during a slow length change of active muscle. *Biophysical Journal* 45(3), 611-614.

Yamada, K., and T. Furukawa. 1980. Direct evidence for involvement of dopiminergic inhibition and cholinergic activation of yawning. *Psychopharmacology* 67(1), 39-43.

Yamamoto, T. 1993. Relationship between hamstring strains and leg muscle strength. *Journal of Sports Medicine and Physical Fitness* 33(2), 194-199.

Yanicostas, N.S., C.B. Hamida, G.S. Butler-Browne, F. Hentati, K. Bejaoui, and M.B. Hamida. 1991. Modification in the expression and localization of contractile and cytoskeletal proteins in Schwartz-Jampel syndrome. *Journal of the Neurological Sciences* 104(1), 64-73.

Yates, J. 1990. *A physician's guide to therapeutic massage: Its physiological effects and their application to treatment.* Vancouver: Massage Therapists' Association of British Columbia.

Yazici, Y., D. Erkan, M.G.E. Peterson, and L.J. Kagen. 2001. Morning stiffness: How common is it and does it correlate with physician and patient global assessment of disease activity? *Journal of Rheumatology* 28(6), 1468-1469.

Yeomans, S.G. 1992. The assessment of cervical intersegmental mobility before and after spinal manipulative therapy. *Journal of Manipulative and Physiological Therapeutics* 15(2), 106-114.

Yeung, E.W., and S.S. Yeung. 2001. A systematic review of interventions to prevent lower limb soft tissue running injuries. *British Journal of Sports Medicine* 35(6), 383-389.

Yessis, M. 1986. A flexible spine: How you can develop one. *Muscle & Fitness* 47(5), 60-63, 203-204.

Yingling, V.R. 1997. *Shear loading of the lumbar spine: Modulators of motion segment tolerance and the resulting injuries.* Ph.D. diss. Waterloo, Ontario, Canada: University of Waterloo.

Yoshioka, T., H. Higuchi, S. Kimura, K. Ohashi, Y. Umazume, and K. Maruyama. 1986. Effects of mild trypsin treatment on the passive tension genereation and connectin splitting in stretched skinned fibers from frog skeletal muscle. *Biomedical Research* 7, 181-186.

Young, T. (Interview Wednesday 12/04/02).

Young, W., and S. Elliott. 2001. Acute effects of static stretching, proprioceptive neuromuscular facilitation stretching, and maximum voluntary contractions on explosive force production and jumping performance. *Research Quarterly for Exercise and Sport* 72(3), 273-279.

Young, W.B., and D.G. Behm. 2003. Effects of running, static stretching and practice jumps on explosive force production and jumping performance. *Journal of Sports Medicine and Physical Fitness* 43(1), 21-27.

Zacharkow, D. 1984. *The healthy lower back.* Springfield, IL: Charles C Thomas.

Zachazewski, J.E. 1990. Flexibility for sports. In *Sports physical therapy,* ed. B. Sanders, 201-238. Norwalk, CT: Appleton & Lange.

Zahourek, R.P., ed. 1988. *Relaxation and imagery: Tools for therapeutic communication and intervention.* Philadelphia: W.B. Saunders.

Zajonc, R.B. 1965. Social facilitation. *Science* 149(3681), 269-274.

Zarins, B., J.R. Andrews, and W.G. Carson. eds. 1985. *Injuries to the throwing arm.* Philadelphia: Saunders.

Zebas, C.J., and M.L. Rivera. 1985. Retention of flexibility in selected joints after cessation of a stretching exercise program. In *Exercise physiology. Current selected research I,* ed. C.O. Dotson and J.H. Humphrey, 181-191. New York: AMS Press.

Zehr, E.P., and D.G. Sale. 1994. Ballistic movement: Muscle activation and neuromuscular adaptation. *Canadian Journal of Applied Physiology* 19(4), 363-378.

Zemek, M.J., and D.J. Magee. 1996. Comparison of glenohumeral joint laxity in elite and recreational swimmers. *Clinical Journal of Sports Medicine* 6(1), 40-47.

Zernicke, R.F., and G.J. Salem. 1996. Flexibility training. In. *Sports medicine: The school-age athlete.* 2nd ed. 41-52. Philadelphia: W.B. Saunders.

Zito, M., D. Driver, C. Parker, and R. Bohannon. 1997. Lasting effects of one bout of two 15-second passive stretches on ankle dorsiflexion range of motion. *Journal of Orthopaedic and Sports Physical Therapy* 26(4), 214-221.

Zuberbier, O.A., Kozowski, A.J., Hunt, D.G., Berkowitz, J., Schultz, I.Z., Crook, J.M., and Milner, R.A. 2001. Analysis of the convergent and discriminant validity of published lumbar flexion, extension, and lateral flexion scores. *Spine* 26(20), E472-E478.

Zulak, G. 1991. Fascial stretching: The ignored exercise technique. *Flex* 9(1), 94, 107-108.

Author Index

A

Aarskog, D., 120
Aberdeen, D.L., 267
Abraham, W.M., 110, 111, 10
Abrahams, M., 45
Abramson, D., 120
Adair, S.M., 90
Adams, M.A., 132, 133, 155, 196, 197, 198
Adams, P., 234
Adler, S.S., 165, 166, 167, 168
Agre, J.C., 5
Ahmed, I.M., 218
Ahtikoski, A.M., 32, 50
Akagawa, M., 43
Akeson, W.H., 50, 51
Akster, H.A., 23
Alabin, V.G., 202
Alexander, M.J.L., 119
Alexander, R.M., 39, 55, 60
Allander, E., 120
Allander, E., 125, 204
Allen, C.E.L., 194, 195
Allen, D.G., 111
Allen, D.G., 112, 113
Almeida-Silveira, M-I., 29
Almekinders, L.C., 91
Alnaqeeb, M.A., 31
Al-Rawi, Z.S., 90
Alter, J., 192, 193, 202, 216
Alter, M., 37, 59, 153, 161, 164, 187, 188, 189, 190, 191, 192, 193, 198, 199, 201, 215, 226, 237, 272
Alvarez, R., 121
American Academy of Orthopaedic Surgeons, 189, 216
American Alliance for Health, Physical Education, and Recreation, 149
American Chiropractic Association (ACA), 175
American College of Obstetricians and Gynecologists (ACOG), 209, 210
American College of Sports Medicine (ACSM), 4, 8, 121, 154, 207
American College of Sports Medicine Position [1998], 12, 13, 154
American Medical Association, 150, 228
American Orthopaedic Association. 248
Amis, A.A., 5, 120, 124, 253
Amnesty International, 142
Anderson, B., 154, 187, 188, 189, 190, 191, 192, 193, 198, 202
Anderson, M.B., 266
Anderson, O., 155, 217
Andersson, G.B.J., 195, 196
Andren, L., 120
Andrish, J.T., 219
Ansell, B.A., 88, 90

AOSSM [American Orthopaedic Society for Sports Medicine] Research Committee, 116
Apostolopoulos, N., 154, 155
Arampatzis, A., 54, 260
Araujo, D., 211
Argiolas, A., 183
Armstrong, C.G., 47
Armstrong, R.B., 11, 108, 110, 112, 114
Arner, O., 218
Arnheim, D.D., 115, 185, 222, 223
Arskey, M., 280
Ashmen, K.J., 8, 9
Ashmore, C.R., 272
Askensay, J.J.M., 183
Asmussen, E., 110, 112, 257
Aspden, R.M., 196
Asterita, M.F., 138
Aten, D.W., 5, 11
Athenstaedt, H., 39
Atwater, A.A., 266
Aura, O., 112
Avela, J., 23, 86
Axelson, H.W., 166

B

Baatsen, P.H., 25
Bachrach, R.M., 17, 119
Baddeley, S., 210
Badtke, G., 131
Baenninger, R., 183
Bak, K., 265
Baker, M.M., 121
Balaftsalis, H., 88, 184
Baldissera, F., 83
Ballantyne, B.T., 200
Baltaci, G., 266
Bandy, W.D., 153, 157, 159, 160
Banker, I.A., 76
Baratta, R., 82
Barbizet, J., 183
Barbosa, A.R., 130
Barker, D., 78, 79
Barlow, J.C., 128
Barnard, R.J., 127
Barnes, J., 50
Barnett, C.H., 89
Barnett, J.G., 272
Barone, J.N., 107
Barrack, R.L., 88, 90, 182, 183
Barrett, C., 119, 207
Barrett, J., 131, 132
Barry, W., 273
Bartelink, D.L., 196
Basmajian, J.V., 97, 106
Bassey, E.J., 119
Bates, R.A., 135, 136, 154
Batson, G., 136, 137
Battié, M.C., 8, 9, 10, 204
Bauman, P.A., 231, 278
Baxter, C., 130
Baxter, D.E., 216
Baxter, M.P., 17
Beach, M.L., 265

Beaulieu, J.E., 166, 167, 187, 202
Bechbache, R.R., 98
Beekman, S., 224
Beel, J.A., 68
Behm, D.G., 258
Beighton, P., 88, 89, 90, 91, 92, 93, 184, 220, 279, 280
Bell, G.W., 104
Bell, R.D., 119, 204
Benjamin, B.E., 191
Benjamin, M., 36, 192
Bennell, K., 121, 233
Bennell, K.L., 185
Benson, H., 105
Bentivoglio, M., 78
Berland, T., 192, 202
Bernstein, D.A., 105
Berque, P., 106
Bertolasi, L., 10
Best, T.M., 108, 114, 116
Bestcourses.com, 274
Beynon, C., 131
Bick, E.M., 43
Biering-Sørensen, F., 8, 9
Biesterfeldt, H.J., 225
Bigland-Ritchie, B., 110, 112
Bigliani, L.U., 266
Bilkey, W.J., 50
Billig, H.E., 10
Bird, H., 88, 89, 90, 120, 182, 184, 185
Biro, F., 90, 91, 280
Birrell, F.N., 90
Bischoff, C., 156
Bishop, D., 127
Bissell, M.J., 33
Bixler, B., 185
Björklund, K., 120
Black, J.D.J., 62, 112, 161, 182
Blau, H., 34
Blecher, A.M., 120
Bledsoe, J., 155
Block, R.A., 121
Bloom, W., 43
Bloomfield, J., 5, 263, 264, 268, 273
Blumenthal, J.A., 206, 207
Bobbert, M.F., 11, 110, 111
Bogduk, N., 196
Bohannon, R., 32, 223, 228, 229
Boland, R.A., 229
Bompa, T., 130
Bonci, C.M., 126
Boocock, M.G., 131
Boone, D.C., 204
Borg, G., 59, 142
Borg, T.K., 34, 48
Borkovec, T.D., 105
Borms, J., 153
Boscardin, J.B., 268
Boscoe, C., 258
Bosien, W.R., 85
Botsford, D.J., 132
Bouchard, C., 124
Boulgarides, L.K., 207

Bovens, A.M.P.M., 150
Bowen, W.P., 272
Bowker, J.H., 88
Bowman, M.W., 216
Bozeman, M., 222
Brainum, J., 128, 180
Brand, R.A., 47
Brandfonbrener, A.G., 280
Brandon, R., 217
Brant, J., 261, 263
Breig, A., 228, 229
Brendstrup, P., 110
Bressel, E., 30, 159
Brewer, B., 251
Brewer, V., 120
Brill, P.A., 185
Brodelius, A., 217
Brodie, D.A., 88, 89
Brodowicz, G.R., 103, 104
Brody, D.M., 216
Brody, L.T., 4, 152, 153, 154, 182, 260
Broer, M.R., 121
Brooks, G.A., 79
Brown, L.E., 11
Brown, L.P., 266
Brown, M., 206
Browne, A.O., 250
Browse, N.L., 66
Brukner, P., 188, 223
Bruser, M., 279, 281
Bryant, S., 4, 11
Buckingham, R.B., 88
Bulbena, A., 90
Bunch, M., 279
Bunn, J.W., 263, 265
Burgener, M., 270
Burke, D., 172
Burke, D.G., 103, 104
Burke, R.E., 83
Burkett, L.N., 180, 222, 223
Burley, L.R., 118
Buroker, K.C., 160
Burrows, N.P., 92
Burton, A.K., 8, 9
Butler, D.S., 229
Buxton, D., 118
Byers, P.H., 92
Byrd, R.J., 86
Byrd, S.K., 108
Byrnes, W.C., 113, 114

C

Cailliet, R., 8, 122, 167, 187, 188, 189, 190, 191, 192, 193, 198, 200, 202, 215, 224, 226, 234, 236, 237, 239, 248, 249, 250, 261
Calais-Germain, B., 230, 231
Caldwell, R., 278, 279
Caldwell, W.E., 120
Calguneri, M., 121, 210
Campbell, E.J.M., 98
Campbell, K.S., 56
Campbell, R., 139

Cantu, R.I., 50
Cao, X., 104
Capaday, C., 83
Carborn, D.N.M., 154
Carlson, F.D., 63
Carp, J.S., 84
Carr, G., 260, 261, 274
Carranza, J., 274
Carrico, M., 192, 193
Carson, J.A., 272
Carter, C., 88, 89, 92, 220, 253
Carter, R.L., 274
Cassidy, J.D., 175
Cassidy, S.S., 273
Cavagna, G.A., 258
Cerretelli, P., 183
Chaitow, L., 173, 174
Chan, S.P., 166
Chandler, T.J., 3, 5, 125, 184, 266, 267, 268
Chang, D.E., 5
Chapman, E.A., 206
Chapron, D.J., 208
Chatfield, S.J., 119, 277
Chatterjee, S., 124
Chen, C-Y., 138
Cheng, J.C.Y., 88, 90
Cherry, D.B., 162, 166, 167
Chiarello, C.M., 8
Child, A.H., 88, 89, 90, 91
Chinn, C.J., 125, 266, 267
Chissell, J., 281
Cholewicki, J., 82, 193, 194
Christian, G.F., 102
Chujoy, A., 231
Church, J.B., 259
Cipriani, D., 153
Ciullo, J.V., 117, 257, 258, 266
Clanton, T.O., 220, 222, 224
Clark, J.M., 98
Clarke, H.H., 118
Clarkson, P.M., 11, 114
Cleak, M.J., 113
Clemente, C.D., 48
Cleveland, T.F., 98
Clippinger-Roberson, K., 4, 187, 188, 191, 202
Cohen, D.B., 267
Colachis, S.C., 178
Comeau, M.J., 11
Comwell, D.B., 128
Concu, A., 183
Condon, S.A., 167, 172, 173
Conroy, R.T.W.L., 13
Contortionist, A., 88
Cook, E.E., 266
Cooper Fitness Center, 13
Corbett, M., 102
Corbin, C.B., 4, 5, 8, 11, 13, 119, 157, 183, 184, 185
Cornbleet, S.L., 122
Cornelius, W.L., 103, 155, 164, 166, 167, 187, 189
Cottrell, N.B., 134
Couch, J., 192, 193
Coulter, H.D., 101
Counsilman, J.E., 135, 263, 264, 265
Coville, C.A., 97
Coyle, E.F., 172
Craib, M.W., 161, 259, 260
Craig, E.J., 178

Cramer, L.M., 216
Crawford, H.J., 7
Crisp, J., 45
Crosman, L.J., 101
Cross, K.M., 62, 186
Cummings, G.S., 39, 117, 253
Cummings, M.S., 106
Cureton, T.K., 263

D
Dahm, D.L., 267
Daleiden, S., 192
Danforth, D.W., 121
Daniell, H.W., 10
Danlos, P.M., 92
Davies, A., 258
Davies, C., 280
Davies, C.T.M., 86, 110
Davies, G.J., 221
Davis, E.C., 11
Davis, L., 182
Davison, S., 10
Davson, H., 63
Dawson, W.J., 280
Day, R.K., 272
Day, R.W., 85
Dean, E., 112
Debevoise, N.T., 251
Debreceni, L., 104
Decoster, L.C., 90
Delforge, G., 39
de Jong, R.H., 58
de Koninick, J., 13
de Lateur, B.J., 30
Delitto, R.S., 196
DeLuca, C., 82
Denny-Brown, D., 68
DePino, G.M., 146, 147, 160
DePriest, S.M., 180
De Smet, A.A., 45
De Troyer, A., 99
Devor, E.J., 124, 125
de Vries, H.A., 3, 6, 7, 10, 11, 108, 111, 114, 159, 160, 200, 262, 263
Deyo, R.A, 8
Dick, F.W., 130, 160
Dick, R.W., 110
Dickenson, R.V., 121
Dickerson, R.V., 121
Dillman, C.J., 266
DiMatteo, M.R., 138
Dintiman, G., 260, 261
DiRaimondo, 216
Dishman, R.K., 139
DiTullio, M., 5, 277
Dix, D.J., 33
Dobeln, K.J.W., 125
Dobrin, P.B., 65, 66
Docherty, D., 118
Doherty, K., 145
Dolan, F., 8, 9
Dominguez, R.H., 164, 192, 265
Donatelli, R., 51
Donisch, E.W., 195
Donison, C., 280
DonTigny, R.L., 121
Doran, D.M.L., 175
Dorland's Illustrated Medical Dictionary, 174
Doss, W.S., 112
Douglas, S., 265
Downer, A.H., 178
Dowsing, G.S., 158, 162

Draper, D.O., 103, 127
Drezner, J.A., 116, 223
Dubrovskii, V.I., 101
Dummer, G.M., 119
Dvorkin, L.S., 269, 270
Dyson, G.H.G., 260, 261

E
Ebbeling, C.B., 114
Ecker, T., 261
Edworthy, S.M., 132
Ehlers, E., 92
Ehrhart, B., 189
Einkauf, D.K., 204
Eklund, J.A.E., 131
Ekman, B., 125
Ekstrand, J., 12, 160
Eldred, E., 167
Eldren, H.R., 44
Ellenbecker, T.S., 267, 268
Elliott, D.H., 41
Elliott, J., 265
Ellis, C.G., 65
Ellis, J., 219
Elnaggar, I.M., 8, 9
el-Shahaly, H.A., 90
Emery, C.A., 225
Emmons, M., 105
Ende, L.S., 217, 278
Engesvik, F., 264
Enoka, R.M., 56, 82, 86
Ensink, F-B., 131, 239
Eppel, W., 120
Ernst, E., 11
Esola, M.A., 8
Etnyre, B., 101, 167, 168, 172, 173
Evans, D.P., 175
Evans, G.A., 85
Evans, S.A., 268
Evans, W.J., 112
Evatt, M.L., 84, 160
Everly, G.S., 105
Evjenth, O., 5, 152

F
Fairbank, J.C.T., 198
Falkel, J.E., 265
Falls, H.B., 192, 203
Fardy, P.S., 167
Farfan, H.F., 8, 195, 237
Farley, C.T., 54, 261
Farrell, J., 175
Fatouros, I.G., 130
Faulkner, J.A., 112
Federation of Straight Chiropractic Organizations (FSCO), 175
Feinberg, J., 139
Feit, E.M., 219
Feland, J.B., 153, 206
Feldman, D., 17, 18, 119
Fellabaum, J., 199
Feltner, M., 266
Ferlic, D., 204
Ferrari, W., 183
Fick, R., 194
Fick, S., 219
Finkelstein, H., (1916) 88, 92
Finkelstein, H., (1990) 127
Finneson, B.E., 192
Fisher, A.C., 138

Fisk, J.W., 175, 191, 236, 237
Fitness and Sports Review International, 167
Fitt, S.S., 202
Fixx, J., 182, 184, 263
Fleckenstein, J.L., 45
Fleischman, E.A., 4
Fleisg, G.S., 5, 266
Flint, M.M., 198, 232
Flintney, F.W., 65
Flood, J., 219
Floyd, W.F., 194, 195
Follan, L.M., 220
Found, E., 219
Fowler, A.W., 10
Fowler, P.J., 190
Fowles, J.R., 258, 259, 272
Fradkin, A.J., 127
Francis, K.T., 111
Frankeny, J.R., 272
Franzblau, C., 43
Franzini-Armstrong, C., 25
Frederick, E.C., 182, 263
Frederickson, K.B., 280
Fredette, D.M., 11, 149
Freed, D.C., 98
Freeman, M.A.R., 85
Freivalds, A., 131
Frekany, G.A., 119, 206
Frey, C., 216
Friberg, T.R., 200
Fridén, J., 29, 32, 108, 110, 112, 113, 114
Fried, R., 105
Friedman, L.M., 138
Friedmann, L.W., 192
Fry, A.C., 23
Fujiwara, M., 220
Fukashiro, S., 47, 124
Fulton, A.B., 24
Funatsu, T., 63
Furst, D.O., 20

G
Gabbard, C., 119, 120, 124
Gajda, R., 160
Gajdosik, R., 3, 5, 8, 24, 31, 32, 48, 53, 55, 124, 150, 228
Gál, J., 175
Galin, M.A., 200
Galley, P.M., 3
Galloway, M.T., 208
Gallup Organization 2000, 278
Garamvölgyi, N., 63
Garde, R.E., 57, 58
Garfin, S.R., 49
Garhammer, J., 257, 269
Garrett, W.E., 11, 29, 45, 56, 62, 114, 116, 221, 222, 223, 224
Garu, J., 241
Gaskell, W.H., 66
Gatton, M.L., 122
Gaughran, J.A., 263
Gaymans, F., 100
Gedalia, A., 91
Geisler, P.R., 276, 277
Gelabert, 277
George, G.S., 257
Germain, N.W., 118, 119, 204
Gibala, M.J., 110
Giel, D., 270
Gifford, L.S., 55, 130, 150
Gilad, G.M., 183

Gilhodges, J.C., 166
Gillberg, M., 131
Gillette, P.D., 29, 32
Gilliam, T.B., 222
Girouard, C.K., 129
Glazer, R.M., 60
Gleim, G.W., 11, 259
Goats, G.C., 127
Godges, J.J., 161, 259
Goebel, H.H., 24
Göeken, L.N., 228, 229
Gold, R., 199
Goldberg, B., 41, 43
Goldspink, G., 31, 32, 34, 49, 272
Goldstein, J.D., 198
Goldthwait, J.E., 3
Golub, L.J., 10
Goode, D.J., 85, 86
Goode, J.D., 131
Goodridge, J.P., 173, 174
Gordon, A.M., 26, 112
Gordon, G.M., 223
Gordon, S.J., 13, 14
Gosline, J.M., 43, 44
Gosselin, L.E., 29, 39
Gould, D., 134, 135
Gould, G.M., 88
Goulding, D., 24
Gowitzke, B.A., 64
Grace, T.G., 223
Gracovetsky, S., 195, 196, 197
Grady, J.F., 153
Graham, C.E., 216
Graham, G., 10
Grahame, R., 88, 89, 90, 91, 220, 277
Grana, W.A., 88, 127, 184
Granit, R., 158
Grant, M.E., 39
Granzier, H., 23
Grassino, A., 273
Gray, M.L., 41
Gray, S.D., 66
Green, J.D., 183
Greenberg, D., 140, 142
Greene, W.B., 217, 220, 238, 248, 250, 252, 254
Greey, G.W., 206
Gregory, J.E., 166
Greipp, J.F., 264, 265
Grewal, R., 68, 69
Gribble, P.A., 180
Grieve, D.W., 258
Grieve, G.P., 192
Grodzinsky, A.J., 40
Groth, G.N., 139
Guissard, N., 259
Gulick, D.T., 11
Gurewitsch, A.D., 17, 118
Gurry, M., 5, 125
Gustavsen, R., 88
Gutman, G.M., 206
Gutmann, E., 31, 272
Guyton, A.C., 196

H
Haftek, J., 68
Hagbarth, K.-E., 56, 166
Hagerman, P., 126
Halbertsma, J.P.K., 3, 12, 87, 166
Hald, R.D., 142, 278
Haley, T.L., 120, 281

Hall, A.C., 41
Hall, T., 228
Halvorson, G.A., 3, 102, 104
Hamberg, J., 226
Hamill, J., 253
Hamilton, W.G., 5, 215, 217, 227, 228, 231
Hammer, W.I., 30, 173
Han, J-S., 105
Handel, M., 166
Hansson, L., 139
Hanus, S.H., 198
Haravuori, H., 23
Hardakler, W.T., 277, 278
Hardy, L., 126, 163, 168
Hardy, M., 61, 102, 103, 104, 149
Harmer, P., 126
Harris, F.A., 165, 178
Harris, H., 89, 90
Harris, M.L., 4, 119, 121, 204
Harris, P.M., 174
Harryman, D.T., 267
Hartig, D.E., 186
Hartley-O'Brien, S.J., 148, 164, 166
Harvey, C., 104
Harvey, L., 146
Harvey, L.A., 29
Harvey, V.P., 121, 122
Hasselman, C.T., 114
Hatfield, F.C., 166
Hay, J.G., 263, 264
Haynes, R.B., 139
Haynes, S.C., 107, 139
Haywood, K.M., 125
Hebbelinck, M., 3, 128, 257
Hedrick, A., 145
Heil, J., 142
Heil, J.O., 140, 142
Heino, J.G., 232
Heiser, T.M., 223
Helin, P., 10
Hellig, D., 100
Helliwell, P.S., 55, 150
Hemmings, B., 101, 127
Heng, M.K., 200
Hennessy, L., 12, 224
Henricson, A.S., 102, 127
Henry, J.H., 126
Henry, J.P., 200
Henry, K.D., 204
Herbert, R.D., 11
Herbison, G.J., 208
Herrington, L., 267
Hertling, D.M., 98, 105
Hesselink, M.K.C., 113
Heusner, A.P., 183
Hewett, T.E., 121
High, D.M., 11
Highet, W.B., 68
Hill, A.R., 98
Hill, A.V., 110, 258
Hill, C., 23
Hill, D.K., 56
Hilyer, J.C., 11, 138
Hinrichs, R.N., 261
Hinterbuchner, C., 178, 179
Hirche, H., 66
Hoeger, W.W.K., 122, 123
Hoehler, F.K., 175
Hoen, T.I., 68
Hoeve, C.A.J., 43
Holcomb, W.R., 129

Holland, G.W., 4
Holly, R.G., 272
Holmer, I., 98
Hölmich, P., 225
Holt, L.E., 164, 165, 166
Hong, Y., 119, 206
Hooker, D.N., 178
Hooper, A.C.B., 31
Hoover, H.V., 174
Hopkins, D.R., 119, 122, 206
Horowits, R., 23, 24, 63
Hosea, T.M., 276
Hossler, P., 193
Hough, T., 108
Houglum, P.A., 117, 168, 169, 228
Houk, J.C., 79, 172
Howard, B.K., 210
Howell, J.N., 110
Howes, R.G., 8, 9
Howse, A.J., 17, 217
Hsieh, C., 228
Hu, D.H., 23
Huang, Q-M., 239
Hubley-Kozey, C.L., 3, 11, 13, 146, 150, 262, 263
Huijing, P.A., 49
Hull, M., 263
Hulliger, J., 39
Hunt, D.G., 10, 228
Hunter, D.G., 11, 12, 161
Hunter, G., 59
Hunter, J.P., 259
Hunter, S.C., 149
Hupprich, F.L., 118
Hussain, S.N.A., 273
Hutson, M.A., 260
Hutton, R.S., 166, 167
Huwyler, J., 277
Huxley, H.E., 63
Hyman, J., 45

I
Iashvili, A.V., 160, 162, 163, 164
Ice, R., 138
Ichiyama, R.M., 107
Ikai, M., 86
Ingber, D.E., 33, 34, 49
Inman, V.T., 249
Inoue, S., 36, 37
International Chiropractors Association, 175
International Dance-Exercise Association, 193
Irvin, R., 218
Itay, S., 85
Itoh, Y., 20
Iyengar, B.K.S., 6, 188, 189, 201

J
Jackman, R.V., 60
Jackson, A.W., 8, 122
Jackson, C.P., 10
Jackson, D.W., 198
Jackson, M., 193
Jacobs, M., 162
Jacobs, S.J., 185
Jacobson, E., 105
Jahnke, M.T., 166
Jahss, S.A., 88
Jami, L., 78, 79, 83
Jamieson, A.H., 13, 14
Japan Information Network, 274
Järvinen, T.A.H., 37, 116

Javurek, I., 184, 185
Jay, I., 200
Jayson, M., 175
Jenkins, R., 43
Jerome, J., 279
Jervey, A.A., 206
Jesse, E.F., 89, 90
Jette, A.M., 139, 204
Jobbins, B., 89
Johansson, P.H., 11
Johns, R.J., 47, 49
Johnson, J.E., 264, 265
Johnson, J.N., 265
Johnson, R.J., 138
Jones, A., 128, 145
Jones, A.M., 259, 260
Jones, B.H., 12, 182
Jones, C.J., 122
Jones, D., 276
Jones, D.A., 86, 110, 111, 114
Jones, H.H., 167
Jones, L.H., 173, 174
Jones, M.A., 120, 124
Jones, R.E., 220
Józsa, L.G., 45
Jungueira, L.C., 36

K
Kabat, H., 168
Kadi, F., 272
Kadler, K., 90
Kaigle, A.M., 195
Kalenak, A., 184, 185
Kanamaru, A., 273
Kane, M.D., 131, 200
Kannus, P., 37, 44
Kapandji, I.A., 192, 215, 216, 226, 229, 233, 234, 235, 243, 247, 249, 250, 252, 254
Karmenov, B., 164
Karpovich, P.V., 184
Karvonen, J., 126, 127, 128
Kasteler, J., 138
Kastelic, J., 36
Kattenberg, B., 93, 96
Kauffman, T., 192, 202
Kawashima, K., 98
Kegerris, S., 49
Keirns, M., 50
Kellett, J., 116
Kellermayer, M.S.Z., 22
Kendall, F.P., 122, 232,
Kendall, H.O., 17, 118, 119, 122, 229, 239
Kent, M., 3
Kerner, J.A., 185
Kerr, K., 97, 98
Keskinen, K.L., 98
Kettunen, J.A., 124
Key, J.A., 88, 92
Khalil, T.M., 8
Khan, K.M., 277, 278
Kibler, W.B., 268
Kihira, M., 280
Kim, P.S., 175
Kim, Y.-J., 41
Kindig, C.A., 67
King, J.W., 267
King, N.J., 105
Kippers, V., 195
Kirk, J.A., 88, 89, 91
Kirkebø A., 66
Kirkendall, D.T., 223

Kirstein, L., 179
Kirwan, T., 138, 139
Kisner, C., 3, 5, 149, 178, 202, 207
Klatz, R.M., 200
Klee, A., 8, 24, 30
Klein, K.K., 184, 223
Klemp, P., 88, 89, 90, 119, 277
Klinge, K., 91, 128
Kloeppel, R., 280, 281
Knapik, J.J., 12, 182, 184
Knapp, M.E., 101
Knight, E.L., 194
Knight, K.L., 103, 104
Knott, M., 165, 167, 168
Knudson, D., 4, 11, 153, 155
Knuttgen, H.G., 110, 114
Kobet, K.A., 200
Koceja, D.M., 86
Kokjohn, K., 102
Kokkonen, J., 258, 259
Komi, P.V., 29, 86, 114, 258
Kopell, H.P., 127
Kornberg, L., 34
Kornecki, S., 82
Korr, I.M., 174
Koslow, R.E., 118, 126
Kotoulas, M., 53
Kottke, F.J., 60
Koutedakis, Y., 278
Kovanen, V., 29
Kovar, R., 124
Krabak, B.J., 12, 187
Kraeger, D.R., 216
Kraemer, W.J., 266
Krahenbuhl, G.S., 118, 124
Kramer, A.M., 204
Kranz, K.C., 174, 177
Kraus, H., 192
Kreighbaum, E., 268, 269
Krejci, V., 202
Krieglstein, G.K., 200
Krivickas, L.S., 3, 12, 154
Kroll, P.G., 224, 257
Kronberg, M., 125, 251
Krugman, M., 281
Kubo, K., 41, 47, 54, 58, 63, 124
Kuchera, W.A., 49
Kudina, L., 82
Kuipers, H.J., 108
Kulakov, V., 263
Kulkarni, J., 208
Kulund, D.N., 126, 189, 270
Kunz, H., 261
Kuo, P-L., 45
Kurzban, G.P., 20
Kushner, S., 231, 277
Kuukkanen, T., 9

L
Laban, M.M., 39, 41, 59, 61, 158, 159
Labeit, S., 20
LaFreniere, J.G., 192, 193
Lakie, M., 56
Lan, C., 119, 206
Langeland, R.H., 224
Lankhorst, G.J., 9
Larsson, L.-G., 90, 280
Larsson, R., 7
Larsson, S.-E., 6, 106
Lasater, J., 188, 189, 190, 191, 192, 193
Laskowski, E.R., 211
Laubach, L.C., 124

Laughlin, K., 13, 182
Lavender, S.A., 82
Lawton, R.W., 65
Laxton, A.H., 174
Leard, J.S., 17, 119
Leardini, A., 216
Leboeuf, C., 200
Lebrun, C.M., 121
Lederman, E., 40, 45, 53, 58, 162
Lee, D., 194
Lee, G.C., 53, 71
Lee, J., 65
Lee, M.A., 131
Lee, R.Y.W., 228, 229
Lehmann, J.F., 59, 61, 103, 127
Lehrer, P.M., 105
Leighton, J.R., 118, 128
Le Marr, J.D., 200
Lentell, G., 61, 102, 104
Leonard, T.J.K., 200
Lerda, R., 98
Levin, R.M., 106
Levine, M., 185
Levine, M.G., 82
Levtov, V.A., 67
Lew, P.C., 243
Lewin, G., 264, 265
Lewit, K., 98, 99, 100
Ley, P., 139, 140
Li, B., 44
Li, Y., 8, 232
Liberson, W.T., 86
Lichtor, J., 88, 182
Lieber, R.L., 32, 111, 113
Liemohn, W., 3, 122, 222
Light, K.E., 48, 158
Lin, D.C., 82
Lindner, E., 266
Lindsay, D., 276
Linke, W.A., 23, 24
Lineker, S., 132
Linz, J.C., 216
Litchfield, R., 265
Liu, J.X., 76
Liu, S.H., 121
Liu, W., 184
Liversage, A.D., 24
Locke, J.C., 8, 138
Logan, G.A., 157
Long, P.A., 147
Longworth, J.C., 101
Loughna, P.T., 272
Louttit, C.M., 272
Louis, M., 93, 94, 95
Low, F.N., 36
Lowe, D.A., 272
Lubell, A., 187, 202, 203
Luby, S., 190, 191, 192, 193, 202
Lucas, G.L., 45, 47
Lucas, R.C., 168
Lund, H., 11
Lund, J.P., 111
Lundberg, U., 6
Lundborg, G., 8, 69
Lunde, B.K., 125
Lung, M.W., 150
Lustig, S.A., 166, 173
Luthe, W., 105
Lysens, R.J., 182, 184, 217

M
MacAuley, D., 116
MacDonald, J., 208
MacDonald, J.B., 208
Macera, C.A., 185

Macintosh, J.E., 195
Maclennan, S.E., 98
Maddalozzo, G.F.J., 274, 275, 276
Madding, S.W., 153
Magder, R., 133
Magee, D.J., 7, 18
Magid, A., 25
Magnusson, M., 131
Magnusson, S.P., 3, 4, 5, 12, 88, 90, 91, 124, 146, 153, 160, 166, 266, 267
Maher, C., 55
Mahler, D.A., 98
Mair, S.D., 222
Maitland, G.D., 55, 174
Malina, R.M., 124
Mallac, C., 5
Mallik, A.K., 90
Malm, C., 109
Maltz, M., 135, 136
Manheim, C.J., 49, 50
Mann, R.A., 231
Mantel, G., 280
Mao, J-R., 92, 93
Marino, M., 265
Markee, J.E., 220
Marras, W.S., 8, 9, 10, 82
Marshall, J.L., 88
Martin, D., 261, 262, 263
Martin, P.E., 207
Martin, R.B., 152
Martin, R.M., 200
Martín-Santos, R., 93
Maruyama, K., 20
Marvey, D., 31
Marx, R.G., 268
Mason, T., 61, 127
Massey, B.A., 128
Massie, W.K., 88
Matchanov, A.T., 66
Mathews, D.K., 54, 121
Mathieu-Costello, O., 65
Matsumura, K., 23
Mattes, A.L., 154, 163
Matveyev, L., 5, 163
Matvienko, L.A., 10
Maud, P.J., 150
May, B.J., 207
Mayer, T.G., 8, 9
Mayhew, T.P., 223, 229
McAtee, R.E., 166, 169
McBride, J.M., 23
McCarroll, J.R., 275, 276
McCue, B.F., 122, 147
McCully, K.K., 111
McComas, A.J., 34
McCune, D.A., 39
McCutcheon, L.J., 108
McDonagh, M.J.N., 86
McDonough, A.L., 51
McEwen, B.S., 183
McFarlane, A.C., 139
McFarlane, B., 138, 261, 262
McGee, S.R., 10
McGill, S.M., 9, 57, 158, 194
McGlynn, G.H., 11, 106, 160
McGonigle, T., 117
McGorry, R.W., 195
McHugh, M.P., 3, 12, 55, 63, 120, 161
McKenzie, R., 177
McKusick, V.A., 92
McLaughlin, P.A., 275
McMaster, W., 265
McMaster, W.C., 265

McNair, P.J., 62
McNeal, J.R., 258
McNitt-Gray, J.L., 120, 210
McPoil, T.G., 216
McTeigue, M., 274, 276
Mead, N., 52
Medoff, L.E., 280
Meichenbaum, D., 139
Mellin, G., 8, 9, 119
Mens, J.M.A., 229
Merletti, R., 125
Merni, F., 4
Merskey, H., 58
Metheny, E., 3
Mewis, J., 56
Meyer, J.J., 195
Meyers, E.J., 185
Michael, R.H., 219
Michaud, T., 267
Micheli, L.J., 17, 18, 119, 277
Michelson, L., 105
Mikawa, Y., 121
Mikula, P.J., 281
Milberg, S., 139
Miller, E.H., 278
Miller, G., 139
Miller, G., 114
Miller, J., 126
Miller, M.D., 190
Miller, W.A., 218
Milne, C., 118, 119
Milne, R.A., 119
Milner-Brown, H.S., 86
Minton, J., 103
Mironov, V.M., 98
Mishra, M.B., 88
Mitchell, F.L., 99
Mittelmark, R.A., 209, 210
Modis, L., 43
Mohan, S., 42
Mohr, K.J., 29, 97, 160
Moll, J.M.H., 119
Möller, M.H.L., 146
Möller-Nielsen, J., 121
Montgomery, L.C., 219
Moore, J.C., 79, 83
Moore, M.A., 97, 164, 166, 167, 172, 173
Mora, J., 160
Moran, H.M., 119
Morelli, M., 101
Moreno, A., 142
Moretz, A.J., 184, 185
Morey, M.C., 119, 206
Morgan, D., [1994] 50
Morgan, D., [1997] 277
Morgan, D.L., 27, 64, 112, 113
Morgan-Jones, R.L., 220, 222, 223, 224
Moritani, T., 86
Morris, J.M., 195
Morrissey, M., 225
Mortimer, J.A., 158
Moseley, A.M., 125
Moss, F.P., 33
Moulton, B., 7
Mow, V.C., 45
Muckle, D.S., 224
Mühlemann, D., 5, 149
Muir, H., 40
Muir, L.W., 40, 263
Muller, G.E., 166
Munns, K., 206
Munroe, R.A., 4
Murphy, D.R., 160

Murphy, P., 128
Murray, M.P., 125
Murray, P.M., 276
Mutungi, G., 23, 29
Myers, E.J., 184
Myers, M., 188
Myklebust, B.M., 85
Myllyharju, J., 92
Mysorekar, V.R., 125

N

Nadler, S.F., 8, 9
Nagler, W., 198
Naish, J.M., 17
Nakazawa, K., 82
Nako, M., 65
Nansel, D., 176, 177
National Institute for Occupational Safety and Health, 196
Neff, C., 261
Neilson, P.D., 84
Nelson, A.G., 258
Nelson, J.K., 119
Nelson, S.H., 279
Neu, H.N., 273
Neumann, D.A., 15
Newham, D.J., 108, 110, 111
Newton, R., 103
Ng, G., 194
Nicholas, J.A., 182, 183, 184
Nicholas, S.J., 225
Nielsen, J., 85, 86
Nieman, D.C., 193
Nigg, B.M., 54
Nikolic, V., 217
Nimmo, M.A., 108
Nimmo, R.L., 105
Nimz, R., 263
Ninos, J., 187, 226, 277
Nirschl, R.P., 267
Noonan, T.J., 61, 114, 155
Nordin, M., 44, 47
Nordschow, M., 101
Norris, F.H., 10
Norris, R., 281
Northrip, J.W., 266
Nosse, L.J., 131, 200
Noverre, J.G., 179
Nwuga, V.C., 175

O

Oakes, B.W., 116
Öberg, B., 258
Ochs, A., 192
O'Driscoll, S.L., 130
Ogata, K., 69
Ohshiro, T., 105
Okada, M., 194, 195, 196
Olcott, S., 158, 162
Oliver, J., 229
O'Malley, E.F., 189, 219
Oppliger, R., 5, 263
Ortmann, O., 281
Oseid, S., 198
Osolin, N.G., 130
Osternig, L.R., 164, 173
Overend, T.J., 31
Owen, E., 88
Özkaya, N., 37

P

Pachter, B.R., 272
Palmerud, G., 106
Panagiotacopulos, N.D., 236
Pang., *See* Barker, D., (1974)
Pappas, A.M., 266, 268

Pardini, A., 207
Paris, S.V., 202
Parker, M.G., 221, 222
Parks, K.A., 9
Partridge, S.M., 43
Pate, R.R., 207
Patel, D.J., 65
Patterson, P., 122
Paull, B., 279
Pauly, J.E., 194
Payne, R.A., 98
Pearcy, M., 9
Pearson, K., 77, 79
Pechinski, J.M., 98
Pechtl, V., 163
Peck, C., 138
Pedersen, M., 274
PennState Sports Medicine Newsletter, 163
Peres, S., 61, 103
Perez, H.R., 166
Perkins, K.A., 139
Pérusse, L., 124, 125
Peters, J.M., 187, 193, 202
Peterson, D.H., 4
Peterson, L., 202
Pezzullo, D.J., 5, 55, 161, 162
Pheasant, S., 119
Phillips, C.G., 172
Physicians for Human Rights, 142
Pieper, H-G., 268
Pierce, R., 136
Piperek, M., 281
Piwowarczyk, L., 142
Ploucher, D.W., 200
Poggini, L.S., 17
Pokorny, M.J., 121
Politou, A.S.M., 22, 23
Pollack, G.H., 20, 21, 22, 24, 25, 63, 64
Pollock, M.L., 202
Poole, D.C., 65, 67
Pope, F.M., 92
Pope, M.H., 131, 195
Pope, R.P., 11, 186, 219
Porter, R.W., 229
Portnoy, H., 194, 195
Poumeau-Deville, G.A., 92
Pountain, G., 90
Pratt, M., 17, 119
Prentice, W.E., 103, 104, 127, 128, 153, 159, 165, 167
Preyde, M., 101
Price, M.G., 34
Prichard, B., 261, 263
Priest, J.D., 267, 268
Proske, U., 56, 154, 166
Protas, E.J., 150, 152
Purslow, P.P., 48
Pushel, J., 202, 234
Pyeritz, R.E., 92

Q

Quebec Task Force on Spinal Disorders, 177
Quirk, R., 277

R

Raab, D.M., 206
Radin, E.L., 160
Ramacharaka, Y., 6
Rankin, J., 180
Rankin, J.M., 222
Rao, V., 82
Rasch, P.J., 8, 10, 154
Rasmussen, G.G., 175

Ray, W.A., 208
Read, M., 182, 184
Rechtien, J.J., 178
Reedy, M.K., 25
Reich, T.E., 91, 179
Reid, D.C., 188, 189, 278
Reilly, T., 130
Rennison, C.M., 142
Renstrom, P., 267
Requejo, S.M., 210
Rice, C.L., 31
Richardson, A.B., 265
Richie, D.H., 219
Rider, R., 119, 206
Riddle, K.S., 147
Rigby, B.J., 45, 61, 127
Rikken-Bultman, D.G., 90
Rikkers, R., 208, 209
Rikli, R., 119
Rippe, J.M., 200
Roaf, R., 98
Roberts, J., 154, 163
Robertson, D.F., 263
Robison, C., 261
Rochcongar, P., 85
Rockwood, C.A., 265
Rodenburg, J.B., 11
Rodeo, S., 263, 264
Roetert, E.P., 267, 268
Roland, P.E., 79
Rollins, J., 265
Rondinelli, R.D., 150
Ronsky, J.L., 206
Rose, B.S., 88, 89, 91
Rose, D.L., 86
Rose, L., 192, 193, 197
Rose, S., 127
Rosenbaum, D., 258
Rosenberg, B.S., 103, 206
Rosenbloom, J., 44
Roskell, P., 281
Rotés, J., 89
Round, J.M., 114
Rowe, R.W.D., 49
Rowinski, M.J., 47
Russek, L.N., 89, 90, 91, 184
Russell, B., 33, 34
Russell, G.S., 8
Russell, P., 130
Rydevik, B., 61, 68, 69
Rymer, W.Z., 172

S

Saal, J.S., 3, 4, 12, 184
Sachse, J., 199, 262
Sackett, D.L., 138
Sacks, R.D., 29
Sadoshima, J., 33, 34
Sady, S.P., 157, 168
Safran, M.R., 11, 45, 165
Sage, G.H., 134
Sah, R.L., 41
Sahrmann, S., 5, 252
Sale, D.G., 86
Sallay, P.I., 222
Salminen, J.J., 119
Sams, E., 281
Samuel, C.S., 120
Sanders, G.E., 102
Sandoz, R., 174, 175, 176
Sandstead, H.L., 266, 267
Sandyk, R., 183
Sanes, J.N., 82
Sapega, A.A., 39, 61, 104, 127, 128, 155, 159, 165

Sarti, M.A., 194
Sato-Suzuki, I., 183
Saunders, H.D., 177, 178
Sawyer, P.C., 102
Scala, A., 216
Schache, A.G., 262
Schenk, R., 173, 174
Schiaffino, S., 272
Schieber, M.H., 82
Schmitt, G.D., 128
Schneider, H.J., 217
Schneiderman, R., 41
Schnitt, J.M., 133
Schoenfeld, M.R., 280
Schultz, A.B., 194, 241
Schultz, J.S., 276
Schultz, P., 160
Schuppert, M., 280
Schur, P.E., 13
Schuster, D.F., 189
Schwane, J.A., 114
Schweitzer, G., 90
Scott, A.B., 32
Scott, D., 89, 90
Sechrist, W.C., 102, 103
Segal, D.D., 241
Seimon, L.P., 192
Seliger, V., 110, 112
Seno, S., 9
Sereika, S.M., 138
Sermeev, B.V., 119
Shambaugh, J.P., 12
Shambaugh, P., 102
Shamos, M.H., 39
Sharratt, M.T., 268
Shellock, F.G., 126
Shephard, R.J., 204, 206
Shirado, O., 194, 195
Shrier, I., 12, 13, 62, 127, 153, 158, 182, 187
Shustova, N.Y., 66
Shyne, K., 182, 192, 202, 263
Siff, M.C., 4, 129, 151, 152, 157, 158, 160, 162, 164, 170, 192, 196, 203, 222, 258
Sihvonen, T., 194, 195
Silman, A.J., 89
Simard, T.G., 106
Simon, R.W., 127
Simons, D.G., 7
Simpson, D.G., 33, 34
Sing, R.F., 189
Singh, M., 112
Sirbaugh, N., 279, 281
Slocum, D.B., 260, 261
Sluijs, E.M., 139
Smith, C.A., 11, 154
Smith, C.F., 189
Smith, J.L., 167
Smith, J.W., 69
Smith, R.E., 134
Solomonow, M., 82
Song, T.M.K., 5, 268, 269
Sontag, S., 10
Sorimachi, H., 23
Soussi-Yanicostas, N., 23
Souza, T.A., 50, 264
Sovik, R., 101
Speaight, G., 93
Spernoga, S.G., 146, 147
Spielholz, N.I., 39
Spindler, K.P., 190
Spoerl, J., 50
Stafford, M.C., 160, 222
Stainsby, W.N., 66

Stamford, B., 157
Stanitski, C.L., 90
Starring, D.T., 44, 147, 163, 180
Stauber, W.T., 108, 110
Steban, R.E., 260, 261
Steele, V.A., 184
Steinacker, J.M., 98
Steindler, A., 227
Steinmann, B., 92
Stevens, A., 86, 87
Steventon, C., 194
Stewart, R.B., 126, 208
Stiles, E.G., 174
Stockton, I.D., 130
Stoddart, A., 192
Stokes, I.A., 9
Stone, D.A., 278
Stone, W.J., 3, 257
Stopka, 160, 167
Stover, C.N., 276
Strauhal, M.J., 210
Strickler, T., 128
Strocchi, R., 36
Stroebel, C.F., 105
Sturkie, P.D., 92
Sugamato, K., 248
Sugaya, H., 276
Sullivan, M.K., 152, 224, 225
Sullivan, P.D., 136, 166, 167, 168
Suminski, R.R., 124
Sun, J-S., 158
Sundberg, J., 279
Sunderland, S., 68, 69, 70
Surburg, P.R., 165, 166, 167, 168, 182
Sutcliffe, M.C., 33, 40
Sutro, C.J., 17, 183
Sutton, G., 110, 222, 224, 229
Suzuki, S., 25, 129, 167
Sward, L., 198
Sweet, S., 126

T
Tabary, J.C., 31, 32,
Talag, T., 111
Talbot, J.A., 111, 112
Tamkun, J.W., 33
Tanigawa, M.C., 167
Tanii, K., 194
Tatsumi, R., 24
Taylor, D.C., 45, 46, 47, 61, 62, 154, 155, 158, 160
Taylor, J., 142
Teaching Music 2001, 279, 280, 281
Teeter Hang Ups, 201
Teitz, C.C., 278
Terracio, L., 33
Terrett, A.G.J., 102
Tesch, P.A., 86
Tesh, K.M., 195
Tessman, J.R., 192
Thacker, S.B., 219
Thieme, W.T., 120
Thigpen, L.K., 11, 101, 159
Thomas, D.Q., 180
Thomeé, R., 225
Thomsen, P., 272
Thurston, A.J., 224
Tideiksaar, R., 192

Tiidus, P., 126
Tillman, L.J., 39, 117
Tilney, F., 82
Tinker, D., 51, 52
Tippett, S.R., 5, 125, 268
Tobias, M., 210
Todd, T., 128
Toepfer, K., 93
Toft, E., 4, 146, 263
Tolsma, B., 261, 262, 263
Toppenberg, R., 8, 232
Torg, J.S., 192
Torgan, C.J., 111
Toufexis, A., 134
Tovin, B., 273
TRECO, 260
Trendelenburg, W., 281
Trinick, J., 20, 22
Troels, B., 127
Trombitas, K., 21, 24, 27
Troup, J.D.G., 89
Tsai, L., 198
Tsatsouline, P., 137, 164, 182
Tschernogubow, A., 92
Tskhovrebova, L., 22, 23
Tucker, C., 187, 202
Tullos, H.S., 266
Tullson, P., 110
Tumanyan, G.S., 163
Turek, S.L., 248, 249, 252
Turk, D.C., 139
Turl, S.E., 223, 248, 249, 252
Turner, A.A., 147, 164
Tuttle, W.W., 131
Twellaar, F.T., 12
Tweitmeyer, T.A., 147
Tyne, P.J., 187, 188, 192, 193, 202
Tyrance, H.J., 124
Tyrer, P.J., 131

U
Ulmer, R.A., 138
Upton, A.R.M., 86
Uram, P., 193
Urban, J., 40, 41
Urban, L.M., 228
Urry, D.W., 43
U.S. Department of Commerce, Bureau of the Census, 205
Ushijima, I., 183

V
Vallbo, A.B., 172
Van Beveren, P.J., 258
Vandenburgh, H.H., 33, 34, 155, 272
Vander, A.J., 19
van der Heijden, G.J.M.G., 177
van der Ven, P.F.M., 23
Vandervoot, A.A., 31, 204
Van Deusen, J., 119
van Mechelen, W., 12, 128, 185
van Wijmen, P.M., 192
Vasu, S.C., 6
Verkhoshansky, Y., 127
Vernon, H., 200
Vernon, H.T., 102
Verrall, G.M., 224
Verzar, F., 41, 44
Viidik, A., 39, 45, 86
Volkov, V.M., 261

Voluntary power of dislocation, 88
Volz, R.G., 254
von Wasielewski, J.W., 281
Vorobiev, A.N., 270
Voss, D.E., 165, 168
Vujnovich, A.L., 87, 115, 158

W
Waddell, G., 8, 177
Waddington, P.J., 164
Wagner, Ch., 281
Walker, J.M., 236
Walker, S.M., 158
Wall, E.J., 68, 69
Wallensten, R., 110
Wallin, D., 147, 157, 158
Wallis, E.L., 153
Walro, J.M., 75, 77, 86
Walsh, M., 54, 182
Walshe, A.D., 63, 64, 258, 259
Walter, J., 127, 153, 155
Walter, S.D., 184, 185
Wang, H-K., 267
Wang, K., 20, 23, 24, 27, 28, 34, 63
Wang, N., 33, 49
Warburton, D.E.R., 208
Ward, L., 184
Ward, R.C., 50
Warren, A., 273
Warren, C.G., 61, 158, 159
Warren, G.I., 111
Warren, G.W., 216, 278
Waterman-Storer, C., M., 108
Watkins, A., 231
Watson, A.W.S., 12
Watts, N., 273
Wear, C.R., 121, 122
Weaver, D., 189
Webber, C.E., 125
Weber, F.P., 92
Webster, A.L., 116
Webster, D., 270
Weider, J., 154, 272
Weiner, I.H., 10
Weinreb, R.N., 200
Weinstein, H.M., 142
Weis-Fogh, T., 43
Weisler, R.R., 151, 277
Weldon, E.J., 265
Wells, K.B., 90
Welsh, D.G., 67
Werner, S.L., 266
Wessel, J., 11
Wessling, K.C., 103
Westgaard, R.H., 106
Westling, L., 90
Wharton, J., 154, 163, 164
Whelan, K.M., 126, 127
Whipple, R.H., 192
White, A.H., 193, 238, 241
Whiting, A., 20
Whiting, W.C., 45
Wickstrom, R.L., 128
Wiegner, A.W., 56
Wieman, H.M., 8, 208
Wiemann, K., 128
Wigley, F.M., 207
Wiktorsson-Möller, M., 11, 101
Wilby, J., 131

Wiles, P., 88
Wilkinson, H.A., 192
Williams, J.C.P., 113
Williams, P.C., 192
Williams, P.E., 31, 32, 33
Williams, P.L., 15, 18, 121, 254
Williford, H.N., 127
Willy, R.W., 146, 147
Wilmore, J.H., 29, 31, 76, 99, 109, 128
Wilson, G.J., 12, 54, 55, 63, 112, 223, 259
Wilson, L.R., 166
Wilson, V.E., 106
Wing, P., 229
Winget, C.M., 130, 131
Winkenwerder, E.H., 178
Wirhed, R., 226
Wisnes, A., 66
Witvrouw, E., 12
Wolf, L.B., 194
Wolf, M.D., 182, 263
Wolf, P., 280
Wolf, S.L., 84, 106
Wolfson, M.D., 174
Wolpaw, J.R., 77, 83, 84, 85, 131, 160
Wolpe, J., 105
Woo, S.L.-Y., 45, 50
Wood, P.H.N., 90
Wood, P.L., 183
Woods, M.J., 219
Wordsworth, P., 90
Workman, D., 281
World Chiropractic Alliance, 175
Worrell, T.W., 223, 224
Wright, V., 54, 56, 57, 133, 150
Wristen, B.G., 281
Wyke, B., 80, 81
Wynne-Davies, R., 220

Y
Yaggie, J.A., 211
Yagi, N., 64
Yamada, K., 183
Yamamato, T., 222
Yates, J., 101
Yazici, Y., 132
Yeomans, S.G., 175
Yessis, M., 200
Yeung, E.W., 186
Yingling, V.R., 57, 158
Yoshioka, T., 63
Young, T., 93, 95
Young, W., 258, 259
Young, W.B., 259

Z
Zacharkow, D., 192
Zachazewski, J.E., 45, 158, 159
Zahourek, R.P., 97
Zajonc, R.B., 134
Zarins, B., 267
Zebas, C.J., 5, 146, 147
Zehr, E.P., 157
Zemek, M.J., 265
Zernicke, R.F., 5
Zito, M., 146
Zuberbier, O.A., 9
Zulak, G., 270, 271

Subject Index

A

A-band, 20, 21, 25
A-bridge, 24, 25
Acetabulum, 120, 227, 231, 239
Achilles tendon, 190, 215, 217, 218, 219, 258, 270, 275
Actin (thin filaments), 19, 20, 21, 22, 24, 25, 26, 27, 31, 32, 35, 37, 56, 62, 63, 64, 65, 97, 109, 112
Active-assisted flexibility/stretching, 162
Active flexibility/stretching, 3, 34, 152, 162, 163, 181, 281
Active Isolated Stretching, 154, 163, 164, 165
Activities of daily living (ADLs), 207
Acupressure, 98
Acupuncture, 49, 91, 104
Adaptation, 145
Adenosine triphosphate (ATP), 25
Adhesion(s), 70, 101, 102, 104, 176, 177, 178
Adhesive capsulitis, 47
Adipose tissue, 147
Adjustment, chiropractic, 47, 85, 98, 102, 174, 175, 176
    cracking noise, 175, 176
    elastic barrier of resistance, 175, 176
    limit of anatomical integrity, 175, 176
    paraphysiological space/zone, 176
Aerobic/Aerobic training, 5, 27
Aesthetics, 273
Age/Aging
    and sleep, 13, 14
    effects on annulus fibrosus, 234, 235, 236
    effects on collagen, 41, 49
    effects on elastin, 43 , 207
    effects on muscle, 17, 18, 31, 208
    effects on nucleus pulposus, 234
    effects on shoulder flexion and extension, 118
    effects on modified sit-and-reach test, 118
    flexibility changes in young children, 17, 18, 118
    geriatric (elderly/older/senior) population, 119, 129, 130, 193, 194, 197, 205
    growing pains, 17
Agonistic reversal (AR), 170, 171, 173
Altered reflex sensitivity, 23, 86, 166
Amino acids, 19, 22, 36, 38, 39, 43, 155
Amplitude, 257
Analgesic effect, 62, 107
Analgesics, 106, 107
Angle of declination, 227, 228
Angle of inclination, 227, 228
Ankle(s), 159, 178, 186, 204
    dorsiflexion, 17, 18, 89, 125, 126, 146, 186, 187, 217, 218, 219, 261, 262, 263
    eversion, 89, 217, 224, 277
    inversion, 216, 217, 229, 277
    plantar flexion, 17, 125, 180, 206, 217, 218, 219, 224, 229, 261, 263, 268, 273
Ankylosis, 182
Annulus fibrosus. See Vertebral disk
Anteversion, 231, 277, 268
Arabesque, 7, 31
Arch, the, 187, 199, 200, 203
Artery, 65, 66
Arthritis, 207, 209

Arthrokinematics, 15, 182, 268
Articular mechanoreceptors. See Mechano-receptors
Articular noise. See Crack
Asanas, 6, 7, 187
Asymmetrical arm action, 261
Asymmetrical leg action, 261
Athletic trainer(s), 13, 103, 139, 151, 187, 192
Athletic training, 23
Atrophy, 31, 208
Audience, 134, 135

B

Ballet (ballerinas), 23, 29, 31, 77, 86, 89, 95, 151, 152, 179, 182, 191, 215, 216, 228, 231, 257, 277, 278
    foot and ankle flexibility, 215, 216, 277, 278
    low back injury and pain, 17
    muscle control, 4, 31, 277
    neural plasticity, 86
    specificity, 5
    turnout, 151, 228, 231, 277, 278
    and use of non-traditional stretching devices, 179
Ballistic flexibility 14, 34
    defined, 4
    classification, 4
Ballistic movements/stretching
    advantages of, 156, 157, 158, 163
    applied force, 8, 61, 71, 87
    arguments against, 41, 61, 64, 156, 157, 158, 192, 193, 196, 209, 210, 219, 241
    defined, 4, 157
    injury, 41, 61, 157, 158, 194, 210, 219, 241
    neural plasticity, 85
    safety of, 41, 157, 158, 193
Baseball, 5, 125, 126, 158, 190, 198, 253, 266
Biarticular muscles, 31, 218, 220
Bicycling, 98, 146
Biofeedback, 83, 98, 106, 107, 135, 148
Biomechanics, 257, 273
Biophysics, 53, 55, 60
Blood
    flow/supply, 6, 7, 65, 66, 67, 68, 69, 71, 98, 101, 102, 103, 104, 107, 110, 111, 115, 121, 127, 160, 163, 167, 177, 178, 200, 218
    pressure, 6, 65, 66, 97, 98, 99, 106, 130, 167, 189, 200, 208
    pressure changes, 66, 97, 130, 167, 200, 208
    vessels, 49, 65, 66, 67, 71, 103, 107, 114, 142, 200, 202, 218
Body
    build, 118, 124, 195
    proportions (segment lengths) and symmetry, 7, 121, 122, 123, 124, 133
    surface area, 121, 122, 124
    weight, 91, 121, 122, 124, 133
Bodybuilders/building, 129, 135, 196, 269, 270, 271, 272
Body temperature, 130, 131, 132, 160
Bone(s)
    as limiting factor of flexibility, 17, 147
    growth, 17, 18, 119
    individual/specific
        atlas, 15, 243
        axis, 15, 243

calcaneus, 215, 217
capitate, 253
Carpal, 15
clavicle, 17, 247, 248, 249
coccyx, 232
cuboid, 215
femur, 136, 137, 187, 220, 221, 225, 227, 231, 239
fibula, 216, 217, 218, 220
hamate, 253
humerus, 125, 129, 247, 248, 249, 250, 251, 252, 253, 265, 267
hyoid, 15
ilium, 227
ischium, 187, 227, 240
lunate, 253
metatarsals, 215
navicular, 215
phalanges, 215
pisiform, 253
pubis, 119, 227
radius, 15, 125, 252, 254
ribs, 99, 237, 238, 247, 279
sacrum, 120, 194, 224, 232
scaphoid, 253
scapula, 17, 129, 243, 247, 248, 249, 250, 251, 252
sternum, 99, 238, 247, 279
talus, 18, 216, 217, 218
tarsal, 215, 216, 217
tibia, 18, 136, 137, 189, 215, 216, 217, 218, 219, 220, 231, 278
trapezoid, 253
trapezium, 253
triquetrum, 253
ulna, 15, 252, 253, 254
Bone growth, 17
Bowling, 250
Breath-holding, 151, 152, 167, 209
Breathing, 14, 98, 99, 100, 101, 151, 152, 210, 279
Bridge, the, 41, 187, 199, 203

C

Calcium ions, 24, 25, 27
Calcium deposit(s), 129, 207
Capillary, 65, 66, 67, 69, 115
Cardiorespiratory endurance, 4
Cartilage, 40, 41, 55, 226, 232
Cats, 182, 183
Central nervous system (CNS), 75, 76, 83, 85, 130, 165
    defined, 75
    diurnal rhythm, 130
    neural plasticity, 83, 84, 85
Cervical, 14, 100, 177, 201, 232, 243, 244, 246, 273
    extension, 118, 243, 244
    flexion, 229, 243, 273
    hyperextension, 198, 243
    lateral bend/flexion, 243, 244
    rotation, 206, 243, 246
Cheerleader/Cheerleading, 134, 221
Chiropractic, 85
Chiropractor, 47, 49, 81, 91, 120, 142, 174
    importance of type IV mechanoreceptors, 81

Chromosomes, 19
Circadian/diurnal cycles/rhythms/variations, 118, 130, 131, 132, 133, 148, 150, 229
Circumduction, 17
Circus, 93, 95
Close-packing, 18
Clowns, 95, 96
Coaction, 135
Coactivation, 82, 86, 87
Cocontraction, 82, 86, 87, 173
Cold, 103, 104, 206
Collagen, 29, 36, 38, 39, 49, 50, 51, 61, 66, 67, 71, 79, 86, 90, 92, 93, 102, 115, 117, 120, 124, 153, 184, 236
  composition and structure, 36, 37
  concentration related to stiffness, 66
  cross-linking, 29, 37, 41, 42, 51, 115, 117
  effects of aging on, 31, 41, 42, 153, 202, 236
  electromechanical properties, 39, 40
  fiber orientations, 29, 32, 51, 71
  gender differences, 44, 124
  genetic and biomechanical defects, 92, 93
  mechanical properties, 41, 71, 236
  nerves, 67, 68, 71
  remodeling, 116, 117
  synthesis, 117
  thermal transition, 61
  turnover, 39, 117
Competing, 150
Compliance
  athlete/patient, 127, 134, 138, 139, 140, 141, 142, 149, 160, 208
  biomechamical, 3, 11, 12, 23, 31, 32, 41, 47, 53, 54, 55, 62, 86, 150, 187, 258, 259, 272
Compression, 53
Concentric contraction. *See* Contraction
Connectin. *See* Titin
Connective tissue(s), 10, 13, 15, 17, 25, 27, 32, 33, 51, 52, 60, 61, 87, 92, 93, 102, 105, 112, 113, 136, 148, 158, 159, 176, 177, 196, 226, 262, 278
  effects of immobilization, 32
  gender differences, 44, 124
  research regarding stretching, 33
  uterus, 10
Consumerism, 181
Contortionism/Contortionist(s), 47, 88, 90, 93, 94, 95, 96, 148
Contraceptives, 121
Contractile component/element (CC), 62, 63, 64, 65, 97, 114, 158, 259
Contractility, 58
Contraction, 25
  concentric, 110, 111, 148, 162, 165, 168, 170, 172, 173, 195, 258
  eccentric, 11, 12, 62, 106, 108, 110, 111, 112, 129, 130, 148, 162, 165, 168, 170, 171, 187, 195, 219, 221, 222, 238, 252, 253, 258
  isometric (static), 24, 47, 101, 110, 111, 112, 148, 163, 164, 165, 166, 167, 168, 169, 170, 171, 172, 183, 196
  isotonic, 101, 111, 164, 165, 168, 169, 170, 171
  negative work, 112, 113, 130
  positive work, 111
Contract-relax (CR), 146, 164, 170, 171, 173, 225, 262
Contract-relax agonist-contract (CRAC), 165, 172, 173
Contracture, 7, 29, 30, 147, 149, 215, 229

Cool-down, 5, 110, 117, 126, 128, 133, 156, 160, 185
Counterirritants (topical ointments), 11, 106, 107
Coxa valga, 227, 228
Coxa vara, 227, 228
Crack, 174, 175, 176
Cramp, 10, 13, 14, 226
Creatine kinase (CK), 11, 109, 113
Creep, 56, 59, 61, 101, 158, 160
Crimp, 38, 41, 45
Critical periods, 23, 119
Critical point, 194, 195
Cross-bridge(s), 23, 25, 27, 62, 64, 65, 86, 112
Cross-links, 38, 39, 41, 43, 45, 55, 59, 60, 93
Crossover, 261
Cryotherapy, 103, 104
Cybernetic stretch, 135, 136
Cyclic loading, 41, 45, 46, 62, 71, 159, 163, 164
Cycling. *See* Bicycle/Bicycling
Cytoskeleton, 33, 34

D

Damping, 4, 146, 258
Dance/Dancing, 5, 61, 70, 93, 106, 119, 134, 142, 147, 148, 180, 181, 187, 190, 193, 203, 277
Dancer(s), 3, 4, 18, 47, 67, 86, 90, 137, 179, 216, 217, 221, 277, 278, 279
  GAG, 47
  modified reflexes, 86
  non-traditional stretching devices, 180
  social facilitation. *See also* Ballet
  turnout, 180
Deep knee bends, 187, 190, 191, 203
Deformation, 53
Dehydration, 13, 41, 52, 207, 224
Delayed muscle soreness (DMS, DOMS), 10, 11, 55, 108, 109, 110, 111, 113, 114, 117, 160
Denervation, 32
Deoxyribonucleic acid (DNA), 34, 90, 271
Desmin, 24, 34
Desmosine, 43
Diagonal pattern, 168, 169
Diathermy, 7, 103, 127
  stretching window, 103
Discus, 198
Disk. *See* Vertebral disk
Dislocation, 12, 91, 92, 93, 120, 182, 252, 265
Distensibility, 58
Divers/Diving, 197, 257, 272, 273
Dominant side. *See* Laterality
Dorsiflexion. *See* Ankle(s)
Double jointed, 88, 95
Downtrain, 83, 84, 106, 160
Drugs, 98, 106, 107, 130, 150, 208
Duchenne muscular dystrophy (DMD), 23
Dynamic flexibility. *See* Flexibility
Dynamic sensitivity, 79
Dynamometers, 5
Dysmenorrhea, 10

E

Eccentric contraction. *See* Contraction
Edema, 178, 209
Ehlers-Danlos syndrome (EDS), 4, 88, 89, 91, 92, 93, 96, 124
Elastic
  deformation, 71
  energy, 23, 158, 257, 258
  limit, 23, 56, 59, 68, 197
  tissues, 41, 43, 65, 67, 207

region, 45
Elasticity
  of connective tissue, 25, 39, 44, 59, 71, 117, 147
  defined, 23, 53, 54, 70, 258
  elastin, 44
  modulus of elasticity, 60
  of muscle, 20, 22, 63, 124, 147
  of nerves, 67, 68, 69, 70
  relation to cross-links, 39, 59, 60
  relation to injury, 54, 62, 70
  relation to nebulin, 63
  relation to race, 124
  relation to titin, 22, 23, 24, 63
  terminology, 53
Elastin, 43, 44, 66, 71
Elbow, 88, 89, 120, 124, 252, 253
  extension, 112, 152, 252, 253, 270
  flexion, 70, 152, 252
  hyperextension, 89, 120, 124, 253
  pronation, 15, 152, 252, 253
  supination, 15, 152, 252, 253
Electroencephalography (EEG), 97, 183, 209
Electrokinetics, 39
Electromyography (EMG) 6, 7, 11, 84, 86, 87, 97, 106, 110, 111, 112, 157, 159, 160, 173, 195, 197, 258
  and hamstrings, 86, 87, 195
  and muscle soreness, 7, 106
  trapezius, 6, 106
  trunk flexion-reextention, 195, 196, 198
Electrostatic repulsive force, 40, 63
Ellipsoid joint. *See* Condyloid joint
Endomysium, 27, 29, 48, 63, 75, 110
Endoneurium, 67
Endorphin, 101, 102, 104
Enzymes, 51, 93, 109, 112, 155
Epicondylitis, 253, 275
Epimysium, 27, 48, 49, 63, 110
Epineurium, 67, 69
Equilibrium length, 63
Estrogen, 10, 120, 121, 210
Ethnicity, 90, 148
Exhale. *See* Expiration
Expiration, 98, 99, 100, 101, 151, 152, 167, 279
Extensibility, 3, 22, 23, 24, 53, 54, 61, 127
  defined, 23
  of collagen, 127
  effects of temperature on, 61, 127
  effects of warm-up on, 127
  GAGs, 117
Extracellular matrix (ECM), 33, 34, 67, 90
Eye coordination/positioning, 99, 100, 172, 196

F

Facets. *See* Vertebral disk
Facilitation, 30, 165
Faithfulness, 139
Fall(s), 207, 208, 209, 227
Fascia, 8, 10, 17, 36, 41, 47, 48, 49, 50, 65, 89, 132, 177, 195, 196, 215, 216, 217, 218, 219, 237, 243, 244, 271
  function, 48, 49
  limits of flexibility (ROM), 47, 48, 52, 177
  lumbodorsal, 237, 238
  treatment strategies, 49, 50
  types, 48
Fascicles, 36, 37, 70
Fasciculi, 19, 48, 69, 70
Fast twitch muscles (type II), 23, 27, 29, 30, 115, 221, 224
Fat. *See* Adipose tissue

Fatigue, 7, 97, 101, 106, 148, 150, 163, 168, 178, 187, 201, 218, 219, 222, 223, 224, 226, 241, 260
Feldenkrais, 98, 170
Intrafusal. *See* Muscle spindles
Fibrils, 36, 37
Figure skating, 95, 257
Flexibility
    compensatory relative flexibility, 5
    continuum, 182, 204
    defined, 3, 4, 14
    dynamic, 3, 4, 14, 157
    functional, 4, 14, 34
    retention, 145, 146, 147
Flexibility training program 3, 5, 6, 7, 14, 23, 148, 149, 162, 185
    benefits of, 6, 7, 14, 149
    compared to strength training, 5
    defined, 5
    retention, 145, 146, 147
    specificity, 4, 5
    therapeutic muscle stretching (TMS), 5
Flexibility warm-up/cool-down program, 5
Flexion-relaxation (flexion-relaxation response), 194, 195
Foot, 215, 216
Football, 153, 184, 185, 186, 221, 222, 223, 266
Force, 53
Force deficit, 112
Fractures, 177, 178, 207
Functional techniques, 173, 174, 181
Fusimotor bias, 87

G
Gait, 85, 207
Gamma system (fibers/motor neurons), 76, 77, 78, 87, 172, 174
Gap filament. *See* Titin
Gender, 44, 89, 90, 118, 119, 120, 133, 147, 150, 227, 253, 270
Gene expression, 19, 33, 34, 35, 40
Genetics, 4, 36, 51, 89, 90, 92, 93
Genu recurvatum (swayback knee)
Geriatric population (aged/elderly/old/senior), 119, 130, 153, 193, 194, 195, 198, 202, 204, 205, 206, 207, 208, 209, 211
Glaucoma, 200, 208
Glutamate, 20
Glycine, 39, 43
Glycosaminoglycans (GAGs), 33, 39, 40, 47, 50, 117
Golf, 98, 158, 198, 273, 274, 275, 276, 277
Golgi tendon organs (GTOs)
    autogenic inhibition, 80, 82, 83, 101, 172, 173, 259
    function, 44, 77, 78, 79, 81, 87, 101, 162, 168, 172, 177
    influence of sleep on, 131
    location and structure, 78, 79
    misconceptions, 80, 83
    momentarily depressed, 168
    relationship to weight training, 271
    sensory receptor, 44, 77, 78, 79, 81, 162, 165, 173
Goniometer/Goniometry, 4, 89, 150, 228, 239
Grades of movement
    Kaltenborn, 175
    Maitland, 175
Gravity, 178
Gravity inversion. *See* Inversion
Groin, 114, 181, 190, 225
Growing pains and growth, 17, 18
Ground substances, 38, 39, 47

GTOs. *See* Golgi tendon organs
Gymnast(s), 13, 47, 77, 106, 134, 152, 164, 198, 259
Gymnastics, 95, 98, 181, 187, 190, 197, 198, 243, 257

H
Handball, 190, 258, 267
Handedness. *See* Laterality
Heart, 29, 65, 98, 102, 148, 178, 202
Heart rate, 97, 99, 127, 130, 167, 184
Hernia, 167, 178, 200, 202
Hip, 4, 15
    acetabulum, 227
    abduction, 153, 226, 228, 229, 230, 231
    adduction, 137, 229, 230, 231
    congenital dislocation, 120
    extension, 18, 31, 126, 137, 221, 224, 262, 268
    flexion, 103, 118, 137, 221, 223, 225, 226, 228, 229, 230, 231, 275
    hyperextension, 206
    lateral (external) rotation, 137, 225, 227, 230, 231, 278
    medial (internal) rotation, 18, 206, 226, 227, 230, 231, 268
Histamine, 81
Hold-Relax (HR), 101, 147, 164, 173, 183
Homeostasis, 145, 156
Hooke's law, 55
Hormone(s), 89, 120, 121, 130, 131, 136, 147, 210, 271
Hurdler's stretch (modified), 41, 99, 187, 188, 203, 239, 243
    inverted (single and double leg), 41, 187, 189, 203
Hurt-pain-agony strategy, 135
Hyaluronic acid, 39, 50
Hydration, 38, 71
Hydrogen bonds, 38
Hydroxylysine, 43
Hydroxyproline (OHP), 39, 43, 110
Hyperbaric oxygen therapy, 116
Hyperextension, 89
Hypermobility, 3, 4, 17, 88, 89, 90, 182, 183, 184, 185, 253, 280
Hypermobility syndrome, 88, 90, 93, 220, 252, 280
Hyperplasia, 86
Hypertonic, 30
Hypertrophy, 33, 86, 269, 271, 272
Hypoactive SSRs, 84
Hypomobility, 182
Hysteresis, 46, 47, 57, 58
H-zone, 20, 25, 27

I
I-band, 20, 21, 22, 25, 28
I-bridge, 20, 22, 24, 25
Ice, 61, 104, 116, 148, 156, 218, 219
Ice hockey, 5, 225
Ideokinetic imagery, 136, 137
Imagery, 135, 136, 137, 172
Immobilization, 23, 29, 32, 33, 50, 148, 156, 187, 218
Impingement, 254, 265
Inflammation, 81, 91, 104, 108, 109, 110, 112, 114, 115, 116, 117, 132, 142, 147, 148, 149, 178, 179, 207, 208, 216, 218, 253, 265
Inhale. *See* Inspiration
Inhibition/Inhibitory, 30, 79, 165
Injury
    Causes, 8, 11, 12, 31, 121, 127, 128, 131,

132, 142, 151, 158, 162, 163, 167, 179, 180, 182, 183, 184, 185, 186, 187, 188, 189, 190, 191, 192, 193, 194, 195, 196, 197, 198, 201, 202, 207, 208, 209, 210, 211, 216, 217, 218, 219, 220, 221, 222, 223, 224, 225, 226, 236, 240, 241, 242, 252, 253, 260, 261, 265, 266, 267, 268, 269, 273, 274, 275, 276, 278, 280
    eccentric contraction, 11, 29, 221
    prevention, 11, 12, 13, 14
    reduction, 97
Inspiration, 98, 99, 100, 151, 152, 279
Integrins, 33, 67
Intraabdominal pressure, 196
Intrafusal fibers. *See* Muscle spindles
Inversion, 178, 187, 200, 201, 203
Ischemia, 7, 69, 81, 111, 115
Isodesmosine, 43
Isoform, 23, 29, 32, 34, 40, 77, 86, 146
Isolation, 152

J
Javelin, 198, 266
Jogging. *See* Running
Joint(s)
    capsule, 18, 47, 49, 81, 92, 129, 149, 187, 220, 226, 228, 237, 248, 251, 265, 267
    defined, 15
    hypermobility, 4, 88, 89, 90, 96, 183, 184, 185, 280
    immobilized, 32
    instability, 3, 4, 178, 182
    laxity, 3, 4, 17, 88, 89, 90, 91, 92, 93, 95, 96, 120, 121, 182, 183, 184, 185, 210, 268
    resistance to movement, 47, 49
    risk of injury, 13, 49, 93, 185, 280
Joint classifications
    amphiarthroses, 15
    ball-and-socket, 15, 227, 239, 247
    condyloid (ellipsoid), 15
    diarthroses, 15
    hinge, 15, 220
    pivot, 15
    plane (gliding), 15
    saddle, 16
    synarthroses, 15
Joint play, 18, 161
Judo, 198, 202, 243
Jumping, 58, 258, 259

K
Kaltenborn's three grades of movement, 174
Karate, 158
Kinetic chain, 13
Knee(s)
    extension, 18, 220, 221, 224, 258
    flexion, 31, 118, 126, 220, 221, 224, 225, 258, 263, 274
    hyperextension (genu recurvatum, sway-back), 89, 193, 220
    hyperflexion, 188, 189, 190, 191, 219
    risk of injury, 184, 187, 188, 189, 190, 191, 192, 261, 278
Kyphosis, 7, 147, 232

L
Lactic acid, 81, 117
    theory of, 110
Laser, 7, 105, 225
Laterality, 8, 118, 125, 133, 266, 267, 268
Laxity. *See* Joint(s), laxity
Ligament, 9, 36, 41, 65, 81, 89, 116, 121, 132, 133, 147, 177, 187, 188, 189, 190, 191, 193, 198, 207, 215, 216, 228, 229, 230,

231, 232, 236, 237, 238, 239, 240, 241, 243, 244, 246
composition, 47
defined, 47
hypermobility/laxity, 121
injury, 8, 9, 116, 184, 198, 241
mechanoreceptors, 47, 81
restricted range of motion, 147
names of
  anterior cruciate, 121
  anterior ligament, 253
  anterior longitudinal, 237, 238, 243
  anterior talofibular, 216, 217
  anterior tibiotalar, 216, 217
  calcaneofibular, 216, 217, 218
  coracoacromial, 248
  coracohumeral, 247, 249, 250, 251
  costoclavicular, 251
  cruciate, 220
  deltoid, 216, 217, 218
  dorsal radiocarpal, 253, 253, 254
  dorsal radioulnar, 253, 253
  fibular collateral, 220
  glenohumeral, 129, 247, 249
  iliofemoral, 228, 229, 230, 231
  interclavicular, 251
  interosseous talocalcaneal, 217
  interphalangeal, 121
  interpubic, 120
  interspinous, 237, 238, 243
  intertransverse, 237, 238, 239, 243, 244
  ishiofemoral, 228, 231
  lateral collateral, 216
  ligamentum flava/flavum, 47, 195, 237, 238, 239, 243
  ligamentum nuchae, 47
  liagamentum teres, 228
  medial collateral, 187, 216
  palmar radiocarpal, 253, 254
  palmar ulnocarpal, 253
  plantar collateral, 253
  posterior capsular, 252
  posterior cruciate, 190, 220
  posterior longitudinal, 237, 238, 243
  posterior sternoclavicular, 251
  posterior talofibular, 216
  posterior tibiotalar, 216
  pubofemoral, 228, 229, 230, 231
  radial, 253
  radial collateral, 253
  sternoclavicular, 251
  supraspinal, 193, 237, 238, 241, 242, 243
  talocalcaneal, 216
  tibial collateral, 220, 276
  tibionavicular, 216
  transverse humerus, 247
  ulnar, 253
  ulnar collateral, 253, 254
  volar radioulnar, 253
Lingering after-discharge (postcontractile), 129, 166, 167, 170, 172
Localized spasm of motor units, 111, 117
Loose-packed position, 18
Lordosis, 193, 195, 196, 197, 232, 239, 241, 242, 249
  back bowed in (BBI), 197, 198
  faulty reextension, 193, 198, 240, 241, 242, 243
Low back pain (LBP), 8, 9, 10, 14, 101, 131, 175, 196, 198, 207, 268
Lumbar pelvic rhythm, 196, 224, 240, 241, 242
Lumbar region, 5, 8, 9, 130, 151, 186, 187, 195, 226, 232, 238, 239

flexion, 119, 130, 131, 132, 174, 198, 238, 239, 240, 241, 242
extension, 130, 131, 238, 239, 276
lateral flexion, 119, 130, 238, 239
rotation, 276
Lungs, 98, 99, 202, 272, 279
Lysine, 20

M
Maitland's five grades of movement, 174
Manipulation, 50, 67, 91, 98, 100, 102, 121, 161, 174, 175, 176, 177, 178, 181
  benefits, 47, 102, 121, 175, 177
  defined and described, 175
  as different from chiropractic adjustments, 175
  osteopathic, 85
  risks, 67, 91
Marfan's syndrome, 88, 91, 92, 280
Martial arts, 95, 106, 157, 179, 181, 187, 202
Massage, 7, 11, 50, 91, 98, 101, 102, 103, 148, 177, 219, 225, 280
Massage therapy/therapist, 142
M-bridge, 24, 25
Mechano-growth factors (MGF), 34
Mechanoreceptors (articular), 44, 79, 80, 81, 87
Medical (physical) examination, 149, 178, 208
Medication (drug, medicine), 91, 106, 148, 149, 167, 192, 208, 209, 210, 218, 219
Meditation, 23
Memory trace, 83, 85
Menisci (meniscus), 81, 176, 187, 188, 189, 190, 191, 192, 220, 226
Menstruation, 121
Meridian trigger points, 104, 105
Microfibrils, 36, 37
Microwave, 103
Middle aged, 198
M-line, 20, 28
Military (army), 147, 186, 201, 219
Mobilization, 18, 50, 85, 91, 100, 103, 104, 161, 174, 175, 177, 178, 181
  benefits of, 29, 39
  effects of breathing on, 100
  effects on cross-links, 39
  hypermobility, 91
  neural plasticity implications, 85
  traction, 29
Modulus of elasticity, 55
Monoarticular muscles, 31
Morning exercises, 195, 196
Morning stiffness, 55, 132, 133
Motion, types of
  abduction, 16
  adduction, 16
  circumduction, 17
  dorsiflexion, 17
  eversion, 17
  extension, 16
  flexion, 16
  inversion, 17
  pronation, 17
  protraction, 17
  retraction, 17
  rotation, 16
  supination, 17
mRNA, 32, 33, 50
Muscle
  agonist, 162, 163, 164, 165, 167, 168, 170, 171, 173
  antagonist, 162, 163, 164, 165, 167, 168, 169, 170, 171, 173
  architecture, 29, 32

control, 31
imbalance, 30, 162
names of
  adductor brevis, 225, 229, 231
  abductor carpi radialis longus, 254
  adductor longus, 225, 229, 231
  adductor magnus, 225, 229, 231
  anconeus, 252
  biceps brachii, 82, 106, 129, 152, 252, 253
  biceps femoris, 87, 221, 223, 229
  brachialis, 252
  brachioradialis, 252, 253
  calf, 164, 187, 189, 191, 258, 259, 261, 271
  cervicis, 243, 246
  coraco-brachialis, 249
  deltoid, 129, 248, 249, 250, 251, 267
  diaphragm, 99, 100
  erector spinae, 9, 98, 191, 192, 193, 194, 195, 196, 197, 232, 237, 239, 240, 241, 242, 243
  extensor carpi radialis brevis, 254
  extensor carpi radialis longus, 254
  extensor carpi ulnaris, 254
  extensor digitorum longus, 31, 45, 62, 65, 161, 218, 219
  extensor hallucis longus, 218, 219
  extensor pollicis brevis, 254
  extensor oblique. *See* Obliquus externus abdominus
  flexor carpi radialis, 254
  flexor carpi ulnaris, 254
  flexor digitorum longus, 154, 217, 218
  flexor hallucis longus, 217, 218
  gastrocnemius, 10, 29, 30, 66, 82, 153, 217, 218, 220, 223, 275
  gemellus inferior, 227, 231
  gemellus superior, 227, 231
  gluteals, 9, 227, 229, 231, 261, 262
  gluteus maximus, 30, 194, 195, 227, 229, 231
  gluteus medius, 30, 194, 227, 228, 229, 231
  gluteus minimus, 30, 227, 228, 229, 231
  gracilis, 225, 231
  hamstrings, 8, 12, 29, 30, 32, 86, 87, 90, 102, 103, 114, 119, 122, 124, 136, 137, 142, 146, 147, 152, 153, 155, 160, 164, 173, 175, 181, 182, 186, 187, 188, 190, 191, 192, 193, 194, 195, 196, 206, 217, 220, 221, 222, 223, 224, 225, 226, 228, 229, 232, 239, 240, 241, 258, 263, 273
    anterior tilt, 152, 153, 224
    injury, 31, 186, 222, 223, 224
    sit-and-reach test, 122, 123, 124, 223
    straight-leg-raising-test, 223, 239
    and x-rated stretches
  iliacus, 226, 229, 262
  iliopsoas, 30, 226
  iliotibial, 278
  infraspinatus, 129, 249, 251
  intercostals, 99, 272, 279
  internal oblique. *See* Obliquus abdominus
  intertransversarii, 244
  latissimus dorsi, 129, 249, 250, 251, 252
  levator scapulae, 30, 251, 252
  longus (longissimus) capitis, 243, 244
  obliquus capitis inferior, 243, 244, 246

Muscle *(continued)*
  obliquus capitis superior, 243, 244, 246
  obliquus externus abdominus, 237, 238, 239
  obliquus internus abdominus, 196, 237, 238, 239
  obturator externus, 227, 228, 231
  obturator internus, 227, 231
  palmaris longus, 254
  pectineus, 225, 229, 231
  pectoral, 8, 272
  pectoralis major, 30, 129, 249, 250, 251, 252
  pectoralis minor, 251, 252
  peroneus brevis, 217, 218, 219
  peroneus longus, 217, 218, 219
  peroneus tertius, 218, 219
  piriformis, 30, 227, 228, 231
  plantaris, 66, 217, 218
  popliteus, 218
  pronator quadratus, 253
  pronator teres, 252, 253
  psoas major, 226, 262
  psoas minor, 226
  quadratus lumborum, 30, 237
  quadriceps (femoris), 106, 137, 173, 189, 190, 221, 222, 225, 226, 227, 229, 231, 258, 261, 262, 263
  rectus abdominis, 30, 238
  rectus capitis anterior, 243
  rectus capitis lateralis, 243, 244, 246
  rectus capitis posterior major, 243, 244, 246
  rectus capitis posterior minor, 243, 244
  rectus femoris, 29, 30, 220
  rhomboids, 8, 30, 129, 251, 252
  sacrospinalis, 98
  sartorius, 225, 229, 231
  scalenes, 30, 243
  scapularis, 250
  semimembranosus, 221, 229
  semispinalis capitis, 243, 246
  semispinalis cervicis, 243
  semitendinosus, 221, 229
  serratus anterior, 30, 249, 251
  soleus, 31, 101, 217, 218, 219, 271, 275
  splenius capitus, 243, 246
  splenius cervicis, 243
  sternocleidomastodeus (SCM), 30, 243, 246
  subclavius, 251
  subscapularis, 129, 251
  supinator, 253
  supraspinatus, 129, 248, 251
  tensor fascia lata, 30, 225, 226, 229, 231
  teres major, 129, 249, 250, 251
  teres minor, 129, 249, 250, 251
  tibialis anterior, 30, 45, 154, 217, 218, 219
  tibialis posterior, 30, 217, 218
  trapezius, 7, 8, 30, 106, 175, 243, 249, 251, 252
  transverse abdominis, 196
  triceps brachii, 82, 129, 168, 250, 252
  triceps surae, 29, 101, 103, 106, 124, 218
  vastus intermedialius, 220, 225
  vastus lateralis, 30, 220, 225
  vastus medialis, 30, 220, 225
Muscle bound, 128
Muscle energy techniques (MET), 85, 173, 174, 181

Muscle injury, pain and soreness, 7, 10, 11, 14, 27, 29, 45, 49, 108, 109, 110, 111, 112, 113, 114, 115, 116, 117, 162
Muscle spindles, 23, 27, 75, 76, 77, 78, 79, 81, 82, 83, 86, 87, 86, 101, 103, 162, 164, 165, 166, 167, 174, 195, 259
  cybernetic stretch, 136
  effects of breathing on, 99
  effects of sleep on, 131
  lingering-after-discharge, 166, 168, 173
  myosin, 77, 86
  nuclear bag intrafusal fiber, 75
  nuclear chain intrafusal fiber, 75
  primary endings, 75, 76, 81, 82, 172, 174
  secondary endings, 75, 76, 81, 82, 172
  sensitivity, 23, 75, 76, 77, 78, 82, 86, 87, 103, 164, 166, 172
  strain-counterstrain, 174
Muscle-tendon unit (junction), 3, 4, 11, 12, 13, 33, 46, 55, 62, 64, 78, 79, 114, 128, 154, 155, 159, 161, 184, 186, 259
Muscle tuning, 54
Muscular imbalance (strength), 8, 162, 219, 265
Musicians/Music, 44, 90, 106, 278, 279, 280, 281
Myofascial release technique (MRT), 50
Myofibril, 19, 20, 32, 37
Myofibrillogenesis, 33, 34
Myofilament, 19, 20, 21, 25, 26, 27, 28, 32, 37, 109, 112, 113
Myogenic, 32
Myosin, 19, 20, 21, 22, 24, 25, 26, 27, 28, 31, 32, 35, 37, 56, 62, 63, 64, 73, 97, 109, 112
Myotendon junction, 45, 166

N
Nebulin, 63
Nerve(s), 67, 68, 69, 70, 71
Neuron, 81
Nocieptive substances, 7
Nociceptors, 80, 81
Nonsteroidal anti-inflammatory drugs (NSAIDs), 11, 91, 116, 219
Nontraditional stretching devices, 180, 181
Nucleus pulposus. *See* Vertebral disk
Nutrition, 51, 52

O
Osgood-Schlatter disease, 189
Osteoarthritis, 90, 92, 184
Osteogenesis imperfecta (OI), 88, 92
Osteokinematics, 15, 182
Osteology, 15
Osteopath/Osteopathy, 47, 49, 81, 121, 142, 192
Osteophytes, 18, 217
Osteoporosis, 178, 202, 207
Os trigonum, 217
Overcompliance, 140, 142
Overload, 145, 153
Overstretching principle, 145, 153, 156
Oxygen, 6, 65, 66, 67, 81, 97, 110, 116, 127, 163, 271

P
Pain (discomfort), 3, 5, 7, 9, 14, 27, 49, 57, 58, 59, 81, 91, 102, 111, 115, 130, 135, 139, 147, 150, 155, 173, 265
  contraindications for stretching, 59, 135
  limits of flexibility (ROM), 5, 49
  muscle soreness, 7, 27, 128, 130
  pregnancy, 120
  threshold/tolerance level, 5, 58
Parallel elastic component (PEC), 62, 63, 64
Passive
  Accessory component/motion, 161

  adequacy zone, 161, 164
  flexibility/ROM, 4, 5
  inadequacy, 161, 164
  physiologic component/motion, 161
  stretch, 3, 45, 58, 161, 162, 163, 181, 271
    defined and described, 161
    goals, 161
    measured, 5
    partner communication, 162
    tension (applied), 4, 79, 87, 110
      effects on GTOs, 162
      limits flexibility (ROM), 5
    tension (resistance, resting), 20, 24, 29, 3, 32, 59, 63
Passive-active flexibility/stretching, 162
Pelvic rotation/tilt, 8, 10, 99, 119, 152, 153, 193, 223, 226, 229, 230, 231, 232, 239, 240, 241, 242
Pelvis, classifications of, 120
Performance, 23, 127
Perimysium, 27, 48, 49, 63, 110
Perineurium, 67, 68, 69
Periorbital petechiae, 201
Permanent set, 56, 58
Pes cavus, 215, 277
Pes planus, 215, 277
PEVK, 20, 22, 27
Physical
  fitness, 4
  therapist 3, 5, 13, 29, 33, 49, 50, 67, 81, 100, 103, 121, 139, 142, 150, 187, 192, 202, 265
  therapy, 70, 85, 147, 174
Physically challenged, 204
  disability, 210, 211
  impairment, 210, 211
Physician, 3, 13, 103, 139, 142, 188, 193, 265
  medical doctor, 49, 81, 121, 192
  medical practitioner, 49, 67
  orthopedic, 187, 190, 193
  surgeon, 193, 203
Piezoelectric effect, 39
Plantar aponeurosis, 215
Plantar fascia, 216, 217
Plantar fasciitis, 216, 217
Plantar flexion. *See* Ankle(s)
Plastic changes/deformations, 45, 60, 61, 71
Plasticity, mechanical, 56, 57
Plasticity, neurophysiological, 77, 83, 84, 85, 86, 87
Plastic stretch, 56
Pliés, 217, 277
Plow, the, 187, 202, 203, 243
Plyometrics, 158
Pointe (en), 215, 216, 277
Popping hypothesis, 27, 62, 112, 113
Posture, 7, 8, 10, 14, 23, 25, 57, 131, 177, 224, 272
  forward head, 202
  relationship to flexibility, 7, 8
  relationship to LBP, 8, 57
Power lifting/training, 5, 125, 193, 196, 269
Pregnancy, 7, 107, 120, 121, 133, 147, 178, 179, 189, 201, 204, 209, 210, 211, 212, 227
Pretibial periostitis (shinsplints), 12, 219
Principle of No Absolute No-Nos, 204
Progressive deep muscle relaxation (PDMR), 105
Progressive velocity flexibility program (PVFP), 158, 159
Progesterone, 10, 210
Proline, 20, 22, 39, 43

Proprioceptive neuromuscular facilitation (PNF), 56, 86, 97, 101, 103, 148, 152, 153, 154, 156, 157, 164, 165, 166, 167, 168, 169, 170, 171, 172, 173, 181, 206, 259
    cramps, 181
    diagonal plane, 167, 168, 169
    neural plasticity, 85
    one plane, 168
    relaxation, 167
    risk, 167, 170
    spiral plane, 167, 168, 169
Proteoglycans, 33, 40, 45
Psycho-Cybernetics, 135, 136
Psychosomatic disorder, 138
Psychosomatic medicine, 138
Puberty, 17, 18, 118

R
Race, elasticity differences in, 47, 124
Race, flexibility differences in, 124, 133
Rack system, 181
Racquetball, 251, 253
Range of motion (ROM) 3, 4, 5, 9, 10, 12, 33
    limitations to, 4, 5
    measured, 8, 9, 10, 150
    relationship to performance, 4
Receptor tonus, 105
Record keeping, 150
Reflex
    autogenic inhibition, 79, 82, 83, 259
    clasped knife, 83, 177
    H (Hoffman), 83
    inverse myotatic, 62, 82, 83, 87, 148
    knee jerk (patella reflex), 82, 131
    positive support reaction, 156, 196
    reciprocal innervation, 82, 86, 87, 101, 127, 137, 148, 156, 172
    stretch (myotatic), 81, 82
Relaxation
    advantages of, 6, 7, 97, 136, 137, 151
    defined, 97
    measuring, 97
    methods of facilitating, 98, 99, 100, 101, 102, 103, 104, 105, 106, 107, 128, 136, 137
    muscular, 6, 25, 27, 97, 136, 137, 172, 173
        molecular (chemical) basis, 27
        ultrastructural (physical) basis, 25
    psychological, 98, 105, 128
    timing, 151
Relaxation response, 105
Relaxin, 120, 147, 210
Renshaw cell, 172
Repeated contractions (RC), 168, 169, 170, 171
Resistance training. *See* Strength training
Respiration, 172
Respiratory synkinesis, 98
Resting length, 63
Resting tension, 23, 24, 28, 63
Retrotorsion, 267
Retroversion, 227, 228
Rheumatoid arthritis, 55, 92, 104, 132, 178, 207
Rhythmic gymnastics, gymnasts, 29, 198
Rhythmic initiation (RI), 170, 171
Rhythmic stabilization, 170, 171
Ribs (rib cage), 233, 238, 239, 247, 272-273
R.I.C.E., 116
Rowing, 5, 98
Runner(s), 13, 23, 29, 110
Running (jogging), 27, 29, 54, 58, 91, 98, 127, 128, 135, 161, 185, 187, 207, 217, 219, 222, 223, 231, 259, 260, 265
    analysis of, 260, 261, 262, 263

economy, 161, 207, 222, 223, 259, 260
    hurt-pain-agony strategy, 135
    injury, 29, 91, 186, 217, 219, 222, 223, 231, 260, 261
    respiratory patterns, 98
    relationship of warm-up and injury, 127, 128, 186
    stride, 207, 223, 260, 261
Rhythmic gymnastics, 23, 95

S
Safety, 148, 149, 156, 241
SAID principle (specific adaptation to imposed demands), 153
Sarcolemma, 25, 33, 34, 41, 48, 59, 63
Sarcomere(s) 7, 17, 23, 24, 25, 26, 27, 31, 32, 33, 34, 35, 37, 38, 45, 48, 59, 62, 63, 64, 65, 67, 86, 89, 110, 112, 113, 115, 146
    composition and structure, 19, 20, 21, 22, 23, 37, 38
    decreased number, 32, 115
    effects of immobilization, 31, 32, 33
    effects of stretch, 22, 23, 33, 34
    increased number, 31, 32, 33
    theoretical limit of elongation, 27, 28, 35
Sarcoplasm, 59, 63, 75
Sarcoplasmic reticulum, 25, 27, 108
Scapulohumeral rhythm, 248, 249, 250
Scar, 39, 70, 92, 115, 116, 117, 129, 142, 149, 195
Schwartz-Jampel syndrome, 23
Sciatic nerve, 192, 228, 240
Sciatica, 70
Scoliosis, 147, 177, 232
Screwing the knee, 278
Series elastic component (SEC), 62, 63, 64, 110, 158
Servo-mechanism, 134, 136
Sex, 14
S-filament, 63
Shear, 53, 54
Shinsplints. *See* Pretibial periostitis, 189
Shortwave, 103
Shot-putters, 23
Shoulder joints (glenohumeral), 4, 55, 61, 63, 118, 128, 129, 130, 204, 247, 248, 249, 250, 251, 252, 265, 266, 267
    abduction, 248, 249
    adduction, 249, 250
    depression, 247
    extension, 126, 250
    external (lateral or outward) rotation, 125, 128, 266, 267, 268
    flexion (elevation), 118, 126, 206, 247, 249, 250, 252
    horizontal extension (transverse abduction), 251
    horizontal flexion (transverse adduction), 251
    hyperextension, 250
    internal (medial) rotation, 125, 128, 129, 250, 251, 266, 267, 268
    lateral rotation, 130, 251
Shoulderstand, 187, 201, 202, 203
Singing, 98
Sit-and-reach test (toe-touch), 8, 118, 121, 122, 123, 124, 147, 206, 223, 224, 259
Sitting (in a chair), 119, 148, 198
Skiers, 126
Skin 47, 50, 79, 89, 92, 93, 97, 116, 147, 179, 195, 212
    EDS, 92
    measuring relaxation, 97

Skinfold, 121, 122, 124
Sleep, 13, 14, 130, 183, 252
Sliding-filament theory, 25, 27, 35, 63
Slow reversal (SR), 165, 170, 171
Slow reversal-hold (SRH), 170, 171
Slow reversal-hold relax (SRHR), 170, 171
Slow twitch muscles (type I), 23, 27, 29, 30, 115
Soccer (European football), 12, 125, 222, 223
Social facilitation, 134
Social psychology, 134
Spasm
    contracture, 30
    hypothesis of localized spasm of motor units, 111
    muscle action potentials, 11
    treatment of, 10, 11, 102, 104, 106, 115, 116, 117, 174, 178
Spastic muscles, spasticity, 29, 30, 32, 84, 104, 147
Specificity, 4, 5, 12, 14
Spectators. *See* Audience
Spherule, 37, 38
Spinal cord, 14, 75, 77, 81, 82, 83, 84, 85, 104, 164, 202
Spinal stretch reflex, 83, 84, 85, 131
Split, 4, 134, 136, 137, 181, 225, 227, 229, 263
Split leap, 7, 226
Spondylolysis, 198
Sprain
    ankle, 12, 85, 142, 184, 186, 216, 217
    joint, 13
    ligamentous tissues, 58, 142, 202
    mechanical, 56
    neural plasticity, 85
    terminology, 56, 114
Sprinting. *See* Running
Squat training, 184
Standing straight-leg toe touch, 187, 191, 192, 193, 194, 195, 196, 197, 198, 203, 241
Standing torso twist, 187, 198, 200, 203
Static
    flexibility, 3, 4, 14, 54, 55, 159
    stretching, 11, 47, 58, 60, 61, 85, 87, 101, 103, 106, 110, 111, 146, 151, 153, 154, 157, 163, 182, 187, 206, 225, 258, 259
        active, 153, 154
        advantages, 60, 61, 111, 159, 172
        arguments against, 11, 160, 258, 259
        combined with heat, 102, 103
        compared to PNF, 225
        decreased electrical activity, 11, 111, 159, 160
        functional stretching flexibility components, 4
Stature, recovery of, 131, 132, 133
Stiffness, 4, 12, 54, 54, 55, 59, 61, 62, 63, 66, 82, 102, 103, 131, 132, 146, 258, 259, 260
    factors, 29, 31, 32, 39, 48, 49, 59, 60, 61, 62, 63, 66, 82, 110, 131, 132, 258
    maximal performance, 54, 146, 258, 259, 260, 259
    meaning or significance to different disciplines, 55, 150
    muscle injury and soreness, 12, 29, 49, 54, 55, 110, 259, 260
    relationship to aging, 48
    relationship to collagen, 32
    relationship to sleep, 132
    relationship to temperature, 61, 102, 103, 132
    relationship to titin, 32, 63

Straight-leg-raising test (SLR), 32, 63, 130, 153, 161, 175, 223, 224, 228, 229
Strain, 29, 54, 55, 62, 114, 115, 142, 186, 253
  injury, 29, 62, 128, 142, 185, 186, 194, 195, 253
  muscle, 13, 29, 55, 58, 62, 115, 128, 142, 186, 187, 193
  lower back, 194
Strain-counterstrain, 173, 174, 181
Streaming potentials, 33, 34, 39, 40, 41, 59
Strength and aging, 129, 130
Strengthening, 9, 13, 184, 185, 265
Strength imbalance/ratios, 129, 221, 222, 223
Strength training (resistance), 5, 56, 86, 128, 129, 130, 133, 184, 203, 225
Stress, 54
  classifications of, 54
  direction of, 54
  injury, 136
  psychological, 6, 136
Stress-relaxation, 14, 56, 59, 61, 101, 154, 158, 160, 166
Stress-strain curve, 23, 45, 55, 57, 58, 59, 70, 154
Stretch reflex, 64, 65, 81, 82, 84, 87, 97, 101, 158, 160, 162, 164, 192
Stretch response, 64
Stretch tolerance, 5, 12, 13, 87, 147, 166
Stretching, 5
  benefits of, 33
  cheating, 225
  controversy, 183, 184, 185, 186
  defined, 53
  duration, 147, 153, 154, 157
  frequency, 154, 155, 157
  intensity, 155, 157
  effects on blood flow, 65, 66
  effects on oxygen consumption, 66
  isolation of muscle or muscle group, 152
  modulating gene expression, 33, 34
  multi-directional, 152
  negative effects, 258
  placement and timing of the stretching program, 155
  self-stretching, 5
  stabilization, 152, 153
  therapeutic, 5, 149
Stretching machines, 180, 181, 182
Stroke, 30, 32, 106, 159, 198
Subluxation, 47, 121, 174, 175, 182, 193
Sumo wrestling, 124, 269
Surgery, 12, 92, 126, 167, 177, 182, 201, 218
Swimmers and Swimming, 5, 10, 91, 98, 125, 130, 134, 135, 151, 180, 259, 263, 264, 265
Symmetry, 14

T
Table tennis, 251
Tai chi, 98, 170, 206
Talocrural joint. *See* Ankle
Tandem Ig (Ig domains), 22, 27
Tanner staging assessment (TS), 17, 119
T-bar, 105
Temperature 47, 59, 71, 89, 102, 103, 104, 126, 127, 128, 130, 131, 148, 152, 155, 165
  cold, 61, 103, 104
  connective tissue, 61, 71
  heat, 61, 102, 103
Tendon(s), 36, 41, 45, 46, 47, 58, 64, 65, 86, 87, 89, 127, 154, 177
  aging of, 41

application of tensile force, 45, 46, 47, 58
  effects of training, 47, 58, 86
  function and organization, 37, 44
  GTOs, 41
  injuries, 218
  relation to sarcomeres, 64
  stress-strain curve, 45, 46, 47
Tennis 5, 125, 218, 251, 253, 257, 266, 267, 268
Tennis, elbow. *See* Epicondylitis
Tennis leg, 218
Tennis shoulder, 267
Tensegrity models, 33, 34
Tensile force/load, 53, 59, 60, 61, 68, 116
Terminology, 3, 53
Therapeutic muscle stretching (TMS), 5
Thermal transition, 61
Thick filament. *See* Myosin
Thin filament. *See* Actin
Thixotrophy, 56, 166
Throwing, 125, 126, 265, 266, 267, 268
Thumb, 4, 16, 89, 90
Thightness, 55
Titin (connectin, gap filament), 20, 21, 22, 23, 24, 27, 28, 29, 32, 34, 35, 37, 40, 63, 64, 86
Torture, 142, 179
Tourne-hanche, 179
Traction, 85, 105, 160, 161, 177, 178, 179, 181
  benefits, 29, 57, 58, 105, 177, 178
  classifications, 177, 178
  compared to stretching, 85
  parameters, 179
Training, 5, 23, 54, 89, 111, 113, 114, 118, 119, 128, 129, 130, 148, 187
Transcutaneous electrical nerve stimulation (TENS), 91, 225
Transduction, 33, 40
Trauma, 7, 23, 114, 125, 131, 201, 227, 254
Trigger point(s), 7, 49, 105, 138, 174
Troponin, 25, 27
T-tubules, 25, 108
Turnout, 151, 228, 231
Two-joint muscle. *See* Biarticular

U
Ultimate strength, 29, 56
Ultrasonography, 41
Ultrasound, 7, 103, 116, 127
Upper body torque (UBT)
Uptrain, 83, 84

V
Valine, 20
Valsalva, 98, 100, 167
Vascular system, 65, 66, 67
Vein, 65
Vertebral disk, 8, 9, 40, 122, 131, 151, 155, 192, 193, 194, 197, 199, 232, 233, 234, 235, 236, 237, 238, 240
  annulus fibrosus, 132, 176, 202, 234-236, 237, 238, 239
  articular process
  facets, 15, 131, 178, 234, 238, 239, 243, 246
  hydration, 131, 234
  lamina, 233, 234
  nucleus pulposus, 176, 178, 202, 234, 235, 236
  pedicle, 233, 234
  spinous process, 233, 234, 243
  transverse process, 233, 234
  vertebral arch, 233, 234

vertebral body, 233, 235, 243
Vertebral region(s)
  cervical, 130, 175, 196, 198, 201, 202, 205, 206, 232, 243, 244, 246, 275
  coccygeal, 232
  lumbar, 5, 8, 9, 132, 119, 151, 174, 178, 187, 188, 198, 229, 232, 234, 236, 238, 239, 276
  sacral, 232
  thoracic, 5, 7, 8, 202, 232, 234, 238, 239, 272
Vertebral (spinal) trunk
  extension, 130
  flexion, 119, 130, 239
  hyperextension, 198, 239, 264
  lateral flexion (side bending), 237. 238
Viscoelastic (deformation), 13, 57, 124
Viscosity, 47, 57, 127, 158
Vitamins, 51

W
Walking, 98
Warm-down, 5
Warm-up, 11, 13, 61, 101, 104, 111, 107, 114, 117, 126, 127, 128, 133, 146, 147, 149, 150, 155, 156, 157, 160, 163, 185, 202, 209, 218, 226, 252, 253, 254, 258, 261, 275, 276, 280
  affecting flexibility, 13, 57, 127, 133, 147, 150
  benefits, 11, 57, 114, 126, 127, 128, 254
  categories, 126
  improper, 126, 128, 219, 226
  relationship to muscle injury and soreness, 11, 114, 126, 127, 128, 135, 186
  relationship to running, 186, 187, 261
  viscosity, 57, 127
Water, 39, 40, 43, 44, 50, 52, 110, 117, 234
Water Polo, 263, 265
Water skiing, 222
Weak muscles, 30
Weightlifters/lifting, 55, 98, 128, 184, 185, 190, 194, 195, 196, 197, 269, 270
Weight training, 128, 129, 130, 223
Wolff's law, 18
Wrestling, 187, 190, 198, 202, 243, 269
Wrist, 15, 118, 204, 253, 254, 275
  extension, 18, 253, 254, 280
  flexion, 253, 254, 276, 280
  radial deviation (abduction), 253, 254, 276, 280
  ulnar deviation (adduction), 253, 254, 275, 276, 280

X
X-ray, 178, 202

Y
Yawning, 183
Yield point, 28, 56
Yoga, 6, 7, 29, 70, 77, 86, 95, 101, 105, 138, 142, 147, 148, 170, 179, 187, 188, 189, 191, 198, 201, 202, 206, 210, 231, 243
  asanas, 6, 7, 95, 187, 202
  breathing, 6, 101
  goals, 6, 7
  hatha, 23, 159
  neural plasticity, 86
  Sutras, 6

Z
Z-band/disc/line, 19, 20, 21, 22, 24, 25, 28, 33, 63, 64, 108, 109

About the Author

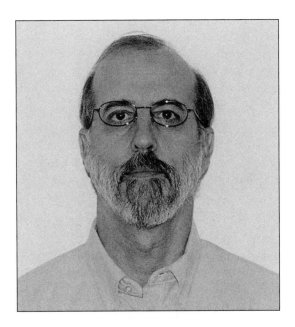

Michael J. Alter, MS, is a former gymnast, coach, and nationally certified men's gymnastics judge. Currently a high school history teacher, Alter has authored two previous editions of *Science of Flexibility*, as well as the *Sport Stretch* series.

Michael has been a guest lecturer at annual meetings across the country, including the Chiropractic Sports Science Symposium and the Scientific Meeting of the North American Society of Pediatric Exercise Medicine. He earned his master's degree in health education from Florida International University.

In his leisure time, Michael enjoys working out, writing, and listening to classical music.

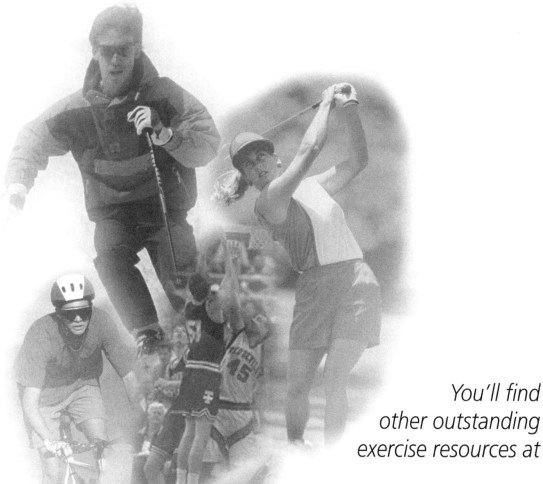